Essentials of Medical Language

Third Edition

David M. Allan, MA, MD

Karen D. Lockyer, BS, RHIT, CPC

Mc
Graw
Hill
Education

ESSENTIALS OF MEDICAL LANGUAGE, THIRD EDITION

1 2 3 4 5 6 7 8 9 0 RMN/RMN 1 0 9 8 7 6 5

ISBN   978-0-07-351379-9
MHID   0-07-351379-2

Senior Vice President, Products & Markets: *Kurt L. Strand*
Vice President, General Manager, Products & Markets: *Marty Lange*
Vice President, Content Design & Delivery: *Kimberly Meriwether David*
Managing Director: *Chad Grall*
Brand Manager: *William Mulford*
Director, Product Development: *Rose Koos*
Product Developer: *Yvonne Lloyd*
Marketing Manager: *Harper Christopher*
Digital Product Analyst: *Katie Ward*
Director, Content Design & Delivery: *Linda Avenarius*
Program Manager: *Faye M. Herrig*
Content Project Managers: *Jane Mohr, Christina Nelson, and Judi David*
Buyer: *Susan K. Culbertson*
Design: *Tara McDermott*
Cover Design: *Studio Montage, St. Louis, MO*
Content Licensing Specialist: *Carrie K. Burger*
Cover Image: *MedicalRF.com*
Compositor: *Laserwords Private Limited*
Printer: *R. R. Donnelley*

Library of Congress Cataloging-in-Publication Data

Allan, David, 1942-
    Essentials of medical language/David M. Allan, MA, MD, Karen D. Lockyer,
BS, RHIT, CPC.—Third edition.
        pages cm
    Includes index.
    ISBN 978-0-07-351379-9 (alk. paper)
    1. Medicine—Terminology—Programmed instruction. 2. Communication in
medicine—Programmed instruction.   I. Lockyer, Karen.   II. Title.
    R123.A44 2016
    610.1'4—dc23
                                                          2014046564

www.mhhe.com

Brief Contents

Contents

Chapter 3
The Integumentary System: *The Essentials of the Language of Dermatology* 31

Chapter 4
The Skeletal System: *The Essentials of the Language of Orthopedics* 57

Chapter 5
Muscles and Tendons: *The Essentials of the Languages of Orthopedics and Rehabilitation* 91

Chapter 6
The Cardiovascular and Circulatory Systems: *The Essentials of the Language of Cardiology* 109

Chapter 7

The Blood, Lymphatic, and Immune Systems: *The Essentials of the Languages of Hematology and Immunology 137*

Chapter 8

The Respiratory System: *The Essentials of the Language of Pulmonology 169*

Chapter 9
The Digestive System: *The Essentials of the Language of Gastroenterology* 191

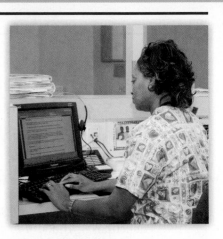

Chapter 10
The Nervous System and Mental Health: *The Essentials of the Languages of Neurology and Psychiatry* 223

Chapter 11
Special Senses of the Eye and Ear: *The Essentials of the Languages of Ophthalmology and Otology* 257

Chapter 12
The Endocrine System: *The Essentials of the Language of Endocrinology* 293

Chapter 13
The Urinary System: *The Essentials of the Language of Urology* 311

WHAT HELPS STUDENTS LEARN MEDICAL TERMINOLOGY

THIS TEXTBOOK INCORPORATES FEATURES DESIGNED TO ADDRESS THESE FOUR FACTORS:

Motivation to learn	→	In order for students to be motivated to learn, what they are learning must be meaningful and relevant. To ensure the chapters in *Essentials of Medical Language* fit these criteria, the student is asked to step into the role of an allied health professional in each chapter. Authentic patient cases are used to illustrate how medical language is used on the job.
Retention of the material	→	When students encounter new medical terms within the context of a patient case, they are able to remember it more effectively. In addition, each chapter presents medical terms from one body system or medical specialty, which further serves to "tie it all together" to help students retain the knowledge and skills.
Opportunities for application and practice	→	Practice makes perfect. This is especially true for learning medical terminology. This textbook provides many opportunities for students to apply what they are learning. Exercises are included in the lessons, and are available in Connect for practice. Chapter review questions are also included in Connect to reinforce students' mastery of the terminology in each chapter.
Readily available information	→	In this book, all the information needed for a specific topic is presented in self-contained two-page spreads. On the left-hand page, new medical terms are introduced. On the right-hand page, for each new term, the pronunciation, color-coded word elements, and definition are provided in a *Word Analysis and Definition (WAD) Table*.

Essentials of Medical Language will help you learn the terminology and language of modern health care in a way that bridges the gap between the classroom and a clinical setting.

RELEVANT MATERIALS—YOUR MOTIVATION TO LEARN!
Essentials of Medical Language 3e provides you with terminology, exercises, images and examples you can apply to other courses and within your career. You will step into the role of a health professional in every chapter and experience medical language illustrated through authentic patient cases.

BODY SYSTEMS AND MEDICAL SPECIALTIES—REMEMBER AND APPLY THE MATERIAL!
Encountering new medical terms within the context of each patient case will help you remember them more effectively. Every chapter presents medical terms from one body system or medical specialty, which helps tie it all together!

APPLICATION AND PRACTICE—YOUR KEY TO MASTERING MEDICAL TERMINOLOGY!
Practice makes perfect, especially when you are learning medical terminology. You will have plenty of opportunity to apply what you learn through exercises during the lessons and at the end of every chapter. Additional practice opportunities and exercises are available through LearnSmart and Connect (see pages xv and xiv).

TO THE INSTRUCTOR

McGraw-Hill Education knows how much effort it takes to prepare for a new course. Through focus groups, symposia, reviews, and conversations with instructors like you, we have gathered information about what materials you need in order to facilitate successful courses. We are committed to providing you with high-quality, accurate instructor support.

MEETING YOUR NEEDS

New to This Edition!

1. The third edition contains 120 fewer text pages than the previous edition. This has been achieved by focusing on essential terms, disorders, and procedures and by changing the layout of the text on each page.

2. The book's artwork has been updated with 40 new figures and labeling has been reduced to allow greater focus on the terms.

3. Each body system chapter includes new sections on diagnostic and therapeutic procedures and coverage of pharmacological terms.

4. More word construction and deconstruction exercises have been added to the Test Bank in *Connect*.

5. The learning outcomes have been revised and updated.

6. The learning outcomes have been tagged numerically and related to all questions in the Test Bank and to the exercises and activities in *Connect*.

7. The learning outcomes have been mapped to the content, with lessons and topics within the lessons in each chapter directly correlated to the outcome it satisfies.

8. The Word Analysis and Definition (WAD) tables and review exercises have been updated and expanded.

9. The contextual Case Reports have been emphasized within well-defined boxes. Each spread with a Case Report includes exercises that review the Case Report.

10. The exercises in the Test Bank move from easy to more difficult based on Bloom's taxonomy.

When you use *Essentials of Medical Language,* you will be supported at every point in the program. Each chapter in the book is broken down into lessons, and the Instructor's Manual provides lesson plans and additional materials for each lesson. Following are features of the textbook designed to address student needs.

Lesson-Based Approach

Each chapter of *Essentials of Medical Language* is divided into lessons covering different aspects of the overall chapter subject. Lessons within a chapter break down into topics. Each topic is designed so your students will not have to flip back and forth when completing exercises or looking at figures, tables, and boxes. All main concepts and ideas presented in topics begin and end within a two-page "spread." These spreads help learning flow smoothly by ensuring that valuable class and reading time is not wasted on flipping pages.

You Are . . . Your Patient Is . . . Case Scenarios

Each chapter and most lessons begin by immediately placing your students in the role of an allied health professional faced with a situation in which medical communication is necessary. Many different professional allied health and LPN-level nursing roles are utilized so your students can "experience" various specialties and positions. The patient cases introduced at the beginning of the chapters and lessons are referenced throughout the lessons to further unify the students' experience.

Chapter Outcomes and Lesson Objectives

The major learning outcomes for each chapter are presented in the beginning so you and your students can focus on what they need to know and be able to do by the end of the chapter. Each lesson has outcome-based learning objectives. Accomplishing each lesson's objectives helps ensure students will be able to achieve the chapter outcomes and, ultimately, the goal of the textbook: to help them learn the essential terminology and language of modern health care.

Word Analysis and Definition Tables (WAD)

Each lesson contains tables listing important medical terms and their pronunciation, elements, and definition. Prefixes, suffixes, and combining forms are color-coded. These tables provide your students with an at-a-glance view of the terms covered. The tables are excellent for reference as well as for studying and reviewing.

Exercises

In addition to the exercises at the end of topic areas in the book, the chapter review exercises are included in the Test Bank in *Connect* (**http://connect.mheducation.com**). All these exercises are graded in their difficulty according to Bloom's Taxonomy and are tied to Chapter Learning Outcomes.

Attention is given to developing skills in spelling, forming plurals, using accepted abbreviations, writing medical language, and pronunciation. The exercises take the learner beyond memorization and teach how to think critically about the realistic application of the medical language being learned.

A ONE-STOP SPOT TO PRESENT, DELIVER, AND ASSESS DIGITAL ASSETS AVAILABLE FROM MCGRAW-HILL: MCGRAW-HILL ESSENTIALS OF MEDICAL TERMINOLOGY

McGraw-Hill Connect® Essentials of Medical Terminology provides online presentation, assignment, and assessment solutions. It connects your students with the tools and resources they'll need to achieve success. With Connect, you can deliver assignments, quizzes, and tests online. A robust set of questions and activities, including all of the lesson and end-of-chapter exercises, case studies, animation questions, and interactives, are presented and aligned with the textbook's learning outcomes. As an instructor, you can edit existing questions and author entirely new problems. Connect enables you to track individual student performance—by question, by assignment, or in relation to the class overall—with detailed grade reports. You can integrate grade reports easily with learning management systems (LMSs), such as Blackboard, Desire2Learn, and eCollege, plus much more.

   Connect Essentials of Medical Terminology also provides students with 24/7 online access to an ebook. This media-rich version of the textbook is available through the McGraw-Hill Connect platform and allows seamless integration of text, media, and assessments. To learn more, visit **http://connect.mheducation.com. Connect Insight™** is the first and only analytics tool of its kind, which highlights a series of visual data displays—each framed by an intuitive question—to provide at-a-glance information regarding how your class is doing. As an instructor or administrator, you receive an instant, at-a-glance view of student performance matched with student activity. It puts real-time analytics in your hands so you can take action early and keep struggling students from falling behind. It also allows you to be empowered with a more valuable, transparent, and productive connection between you and your students. Available on demand wherever and whenever it's needed, Connect Insight travels from office to classroom!

A SINGLE SIGN-ON WITH CONNECT AND YOUR BLACKBOARD COURSE: MCGRAW-HILL EDUCATION AND BLACKBOARD

Blackboard, the Web-based course management system, has partnered with McGraw-Hill Education to better allow students and faculty to use online materials and activities to complement face-to-face teaching. Blackboard features exciting social learning and teaching tools that foster active learning opportunities for students. You'll transform your closed-door classroom into communities where students remain connected to their educational experience 24 hours a day. This partnership allows you and your students access to McGraw-Hill's Connect and Create right from within your Blackboard course—all with a single sign-on. Not only do you get single sign-on with Connect and Create, but you also get deep integration of McGraw-Hill Education content and content engines right in Blackboard. Whether you're choosing a book for your course or building *Connect* assignments, all the tools you need are right where you want them—inside Blackboard. Gradebooks are now seamless. When a student completes an integrated Connect assignment, the grade for that assignment automatically (and instantly) feeds into your Blackboard grade center. McGraw-Hill Education and Blackboard can now offer you easy access to industry-leading technology and content, whether your campus hosts it or we do. Be sure to ask your local McGraw-Hill Education representative for details. *Still want a single sign-on solution using another learning management system?* See how **McGraw-Hill Compus®** (**http://mhcampus.mhhe.com/**) makes the grade by offering universal sign-on, automatic registration, gradebook synchronization, and open access to a multitude of learning resources—all in one place. MH Campus supports Active Directory, Angel, Blackboard, Canvas, Desire2Learn, eCollege, IMS, LDAP, Moodle, Moodlerooms, Sakai, Shibboleth, WebCT, Brain-Honey, Campus Cruiser, and Jenzibar eRacer. Additionally, MH Campus can be easily connected with other authentication authorities and LMSs.

CREATE A TEXTBOOK ORGANIZED THE WAY YOU TEACH: MCGRAW-HILL CREATE

With **McGraw-Hill Create™,** you can easily rearrange chapters, combine material from other content sources, and quickly upload content you have written, such as your course syllabus or teaching notes. Find the content you need in Create by searching through thousands of leading McGraw-Hill Education textbooks. Arrange your book to fit your teaching style. Create even allows you to personalize your book's appearance by selecting the cover and adding your name, school, and course information. Order a Create book and you'll receive a complimentary print review copy in three to five business days or a complimentary electronic review copy (eComp) via e-mail in minutes. Go to **www.mcgrawhillcreate.com** today and register to experience how McGraw-Hill Create empowers you to teach *your* students *your* way.

RECORD AND DISTRIBUTE YOUR LECTURES FOR MULTIPLE VIEWING: MY LECTURES—TEGRITY

McGraw-Hill Tegrity® records and distributes your class lecture with just a click of a button. Students can view it anytime and anywhere via computer, iPod, or mobile device. It indexes as it records your PowerPoint presentations and anything shown on your computer, so students can use keywords to find exactly what they want to study. Tegrity is available as an integrated feature of **McGraw-Hill *Essentials of Medical Terminology*** and as a stand-alone product.

MCGRAW-HILL EDUCATION'S ADAPTIVE SUITE

New from McGraw-Hill Education, LearnSmart Advantage® is a series of adaptive learning products fueled by LearnSmart. Since 2009, it has been the most widely used and intelligent adaptive learning resource proven to improve learning. Developed to deliver demonstrable results in boosting grades, increasing course retention, and strengthening memory recall, the LearnSmart Advantage series spans the entire learning process from course preparation to providing the first adaptive reading experience, and it's found only in SmartBook. Distinguishing what students know from what they don't, and honing in on concepts they are most likely to forget, each product in the series helps students study smarter and retain more knowledge. A smarter learning experience for students coupled with valuable reporting tools for instructors, and available in hundreds of course areas, LearnSmart Advantage is advancing learning like no other products in higher education today. **Go to www.LearnSmartAdvantage.com** for more information.

LearnSmart® is one of the most effective and successful adaptive learning resources available on the market today and is again available for *Essentials of Medical Terminology*. More than 2 million students have answered more than 1.3 billion questions in LearnSmart since 2009, making it the most widely used and intelligent adaptive study tool. It has proven to strengthen memory recall, keep students in class, and boost grades. Students using LearnSmart are 13% more likely to pass their classes and 35% less likely to drop out. This revolutionary learning resource is available only from McGraw-Hill Education, so join the learning revolution, and start using LearnSmart today!

SmartBook® is the first and only adaptive reading experience currently available. SmartBook personalizes content for each student in a continuously adapting reading experience. Reading is no longer a passive and linear experience, but an engaging and dynamic one where students are more likely to master and retain important concepts, thus coming to class better prepared. Valuable reports provide instructors with insight into how students are progressing through textbook content, and are useful for shaping in-class time and assessments. As a result of the adaptive reading experience found in SmartBook, students are more likely to retain knowledge, stay in class, and get better grades. This revolutionary technology is available only from McGraw-Hill Education for hundreds of course areas as part of the LearnSmart Advantage series.

Instructors' Resources

The Instructor Online Learning Center is available through your Connect course. Your McGraw-Hill sales representative can provide you with the access you need to easily prepare for using *Essentials of Medical Language,* 3e. Our Online Learning Centers include:

- The Instructors' Manual, which contains valuable information that makes course prep a snap!
  - This manual includes information about student learning styles and instructor strategies; innovative learning activities; assessment techniques and strategies; classroom management tips; and answer keys.
  - **Lesson Planning Guide.** Our Lesson Planning Guide comes complete with a customizable lesson plan for each of the lessons in this text. Each plan contains a step-by-step 50-minute teaching plan

and master copies of handouts. Use these lessons alone or combined to accommodate different class schedules—you can even revise them to reflect your preferred topic or sequence. Each lesson plan is designed to be used with a corresponding PowerPoint® presentation that is also available on the OLC.

- **PowerPoint® Lecture Outlines.** The PowerPoint lectures with speaking notes correlate to the Lesson Plans mentioned above and include the art and photos from the text. Covering the most important parts of every lesson, the slides are customizable to fit your course needs.
- **McGraw-Hill's EZ-Test Generator,** which makes creating tests easy!
  - This flexible electronic testing program allows instructors to create tests correlated to every chapter and learning outcome. Accommodating a variety of question types tied to Bloom's taxonomy, EZ-Test allows instructors to create multiple versions of the tests and then export to a course management system, such as Blackboard. EZ-Test Online gives you a place online to quickly and easily administer the exams you create.

Contextual Approach Promotes Active Learning

Chapters in the textbook are organized by body system in accordance with an overall anatomy and physiology (A & P) approach. Lessons introduce and define terminology through the context of A & P, pathology, and clinical and diagnostic procedures/tests. The organization of the body systems into chapters is based on an "outside to inside" sequence that reflects a physician's differential diagnosis method used during an examination.

To provide students with an authentic context, the medical specialty associated with each body area or system is introduced along with relevant anatomy and physiology. Students actually step into the role of an allied health professional associated with each specialty. Patient cases and documentation are used to illustrate the real-life application of medical terminology in modern health care: to care for and communicate with patients and to interact with other members of the health care team.

The A & P organizational approach, used in conjunction with an authentic medical setting and patient cases, encourages student motivation and facilitates active, engaged learning.

Innovative Pedagogical Aids Provide a Coherent Learning Program

Each chapter is structured around a consistent and unique framework of pedagogic devices. No matter what the subject matter of a chapter, the structure enables students to develop a consistent learning strategy, making *Essentials of Medical Language* a superior learning tool.

YOU ARE COMMUNICATING WITH . . .

Each chapter opens by placing the student in the role of an allied health professional related to the specialty and associated body systems/areas covered by the chapter. The student is also introduced to a patient and given information about the patient's case.

Muscles and Tendons
The Essentials of the Languages of Orthopedics and Rehabilitation

CHAPTER 5

Learning Outcomes

The **appendicular skeleton**, which includes the bones of the upper and lower limbs, is attached to the **axial skeleton** through joints and muscles. Understanding the terminology that identifies and describes the muscles and tendons of the limbs and trunk is vital to your knowledge of the human body. Information in this chapter provides correct medical terminology to:

LO 5.1 Use roots, combining forms, suffixes, and prefixes to construct and analyze (deconstruct) medical terms related to muscles and tendons and rehabilitation medicine.

LO 5.2 Spell and pronounce correctly medical terms related to muscles and tendons and rehabilitation medicine in order to communicate them with accuracy and precision in any health care setting.

LO 5.3 Define accepted abbreviations related to muscles and tendons and rehabilitation medicine.

LO 5.4 Relate the three different types of muscle to their structures, functions, and disorders.

LO 5.5 Identify diagnostic and therapeutic methods for disorders of the muscles and tendons.

LO 5.6 Describe the muscles and tendons of the trunk, shoulder girdle, and upper limbs and their disorders.

LO 5.7 Describe the muscles and tendons of the pelvic girdle and lower limbs and their disorders.

LO 5.8 Identify the goals of rehabilitation medicine and the health professionals involved in a rehabilitation program.

LO 5.9 Apply your knowledge of the medical terms of the muscles and tendons, their disorders and rehabilitation medicine to documentation, medical records, and medical reports.

LO 5.10 Translate the medical terms of the muscles and tendons and their disorders and rehabilitation medicine into everyday language in order to communicate clearly with patients and their families.

Case Report 5.1

You are . . .
. . . an orthopedic technologist working with orthopedist Kenneth Stannard, MD, in Fulwood Medical Center.

You are Communicating with . . .
Mr. Bruce Adams, a 55-year-old construction worker who presents with severe pain in his right shoulder.

Mr. Adams' pain began 3 or 4 months ago; it is worse at the end of the workday and when he lifts his arm above his head. During the past week, the pain has woken him from sleep. Mr. Adams' primary care physician has given him pain medication, advised him to stop working, and referred him to Dr. Stannard for diagnosis and treatment. A physical examination shows that Mr. Adams' pain is noticeably limiting all the **passive** and **active** movements of his right shoulder, including his ability to lift weight.

LEARNING OUTCOMES

At the same time, **Learning Outcomes** are presented to let students know what they will learn in the chapter. This technique immediately engages students, motivating them to read on to learn how this patient's case (and their role in the patient's care) relates to the medical terminology being introduced in the chapter.

LESSON-BASED ORGANIZATION

The chapter content is broken down into chunks, or lessons, to help students digest new information and relate it to previously learned information. Rather than containing many various topics within a chapter, these lessons group the chapter material into logical, streamlined learning units designed to help students achieve the chapter outcomes. Lessons within a chapter build on one another to form a cohesive, coherent experience for the learner.

Each lesson is based on specific **Lesson Objectives** designed to support the students' achievement of the overall chapter outcomes.

Each lesson in a chapter contains an Introduction, Lesson Objectives, Lesson Topics, Word Analysis and Definition Tables, and Lesson Exercises. Within each lesson, all topics and information are presented in **self-contained two-page spreads.** This means students will no longer have to flip back and forth to see figures on one page that are described on another.

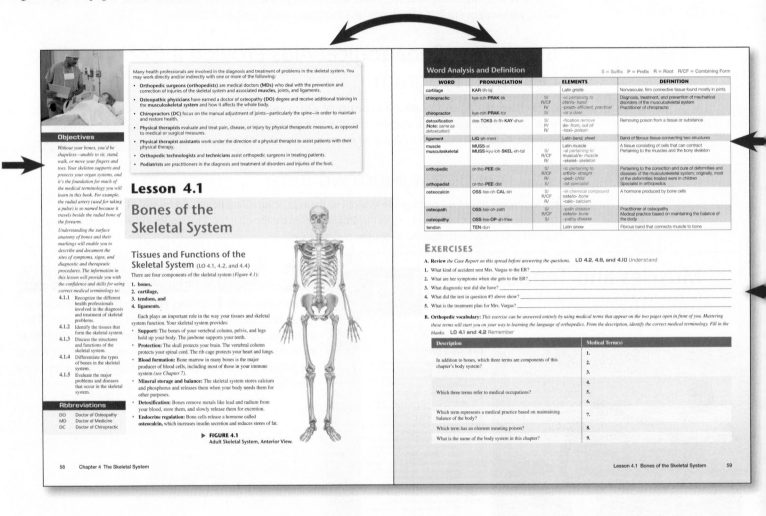

WORD ANALYSIS AND DEFINITION TABLES

The medical terms covered in each lesson are introduced in context, either within a patient case or in the lesson topics. To facilitate easy reference and review, the terms are also listed in tables as a group. The **Word Analysis and Definition (WAD) Tables** list each term and its pronunciation, elements, and definition in a concise, color-coded, at-a-glance format.

LESSON AND CHAPTER EXERCISES

Topics within a chapter end with exercises designed to allow students to check their basic understanding of the terms they just learned. These "checkpoints" can be used by instructors as assignments or for self-evaluation by students.

In *Connect* you will find additional review exercises that ask students to apply what they learned in all lessons of a chapter. These exercises reinforce learning and help students go beyond mere memorization to think critically about the medical language they use. In addition to reviewing and recalling the definitions of terms learned in the chapter, students are asked to use medical terms in new and different ways to ensure a thorough understanding.

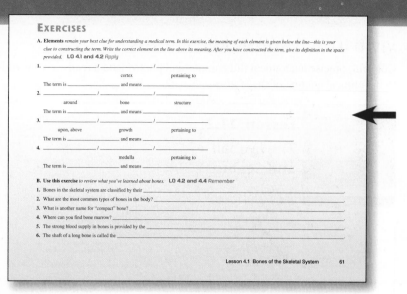

CHAPTER REVIEW IN CONNECT

Vivid Illustrations and Photos

Colorful, precise anatomical illustrations and photos lend a realistic view of body structures and correlate to the clinical context of the lessons.

Lesson 11.2
The Eyeball and Seeing

Objectives

Although your eyeball may appear to be solid, it's actually a hollow sphere that measures around 1 inch in diameter. Knowledge of its terminology, structure, and function allows you to understand how we see and what major problems and disorders can arise with the eye. In this lesson, the information will enable you to use correct medical terminology to:

11.2.1 Identify the principal structures of the eyeball and their functions.

11.2.2 Explain the role of the cornea and the problems that can occur in that structure.

11.2.3 Describe the structures and functions of the lens and its associated structures.

11.2.4 Link the different components of the retina to their functions.

11.2.5 Discuss disorders of the eyeball.

Keynotes

- The cornea protects the eye and, by changing shape, provides about 60% of the eye's focusing power.
- The iris controls the amount of light entering the eye.
- The lens changes its shape to focus rays of light on the retina.
- Medical shorthand for a quick, normal eye examination can be PERRLA: Pupils Equal, Round, Reactive to Light and Accommodation.

The Eyeball (Globe)
(LO 11.5)

The functions of the eyeball are to continuously:

1. **Adjust** the amount of light it lets in to reach the retina;

2. **Focus** on near and distant objects; and

3. **Produce** images of those objects and instantly transmit them to the brain.

As shown earlier in this chapter, the front of the eyeball is covered by the conjunctiva. This thin layer of tissue lines the inside of the eyelids and curves over the eyeball to meet the **sclera** (*Figure 11.9*), the tough, white outer layer of the eye.

At the center of the front of the eye is the **cornea**, a transparent, dome-shaped membrane. The cornea has no blood supply and obtains its nutrients from tears and from fluid in the anterior chamber behind it.

When light rays strike the eye, they pass through the cornea. Because of its dome curvature, those rays striking the edge of the cornea are bent toward its center. The light rays then go through the **pupil**, the black opening in the center of the colored area (the **iris**) in the front of the eye.

The iris controls the amount of light entering the eye. For example, when you're in the dark outside at night the iris opens (**dilates**) to allow more light into the eye. When you're in bright sunlight or in a well-lit room, the iris closes (**constricts**) to allow less light into the eye.

After traveling through the pupil, the light rays pass through the transparent **lens**. This lens can become thicker and thinner, enabling it to bend light rays and focus them on the **retina** at the back of the eye. Accommodation is the process of changing focus, and **refraction** is the process of bending light rays.

The lens does not contain blood vessels (**avascular**) or nerves, and with increasing age, it loses its elasticity. Because of this reduced elasticity, when you reach your forties, your eyes may have difficulty focusing on near objects, a condition called **presbyopia**.

▲ FIGURE 11.9
Anatomy of the Eyeball.

Labels: Cranial nerve II (optic); Optic disc (blind spot); Fovea centralis; Retina; Sclera; Lens; Iris; Cornea; Pupil

---

tory tests for it. The only treatment options are pain management, physiotherapy, and stress reduction.

▲ FIGURE 5.3
RICE Treatment.

Lesson 4.2 (cont'd)

Skull and Face (LO 4.2 and 4.6)

The Skull (LO 4.2 and 4.6)

When you glance at your face in the mirror, chances are you're not thinking about what's behind your brown eyes or your slightly crooked smile. You see one image—not its layers, pieces, or parts. However, the human skull (*Figure 4.9*) is made up of 22 separate bones. Your **cranium**, the upper part of the skull that encloses the **cranial** cavity and protects the brain, contains 8 of these 22 bones; your facial skeleton contains the rest.

The bones of the cranium are joined together by sutures (joints that appear as seams), which are covered on the inside and outside by a thin layer of connective tissue. These bones have the following functions:

1. The **frontal** bone forms the forehead, roofs of the (eye) orbits, and part of the floor of the cranium and contains a pair of right and left frontal sinuses above the orbits.

2. **Parietal** bones form the bulging sides and roof of the cranium.

3. The **occipital** bone forms the back of and part of the base of the cranium.

4. **Temporal** bones form the sides of and part of the base of the cranium.

5. The **sphenoid** bone forms part of the base of the cranium and the orbits.

6. The **ethmoid** bone is hollow and forms part of the nose, the orbits, and the ethmoid sinuses.

These bones of the skull provide protection for the brain and the organs of vision, taste, hearing, equilibrium, and smell.

The lower part of the skull houses the bones of the facial skeleton (*Figure 4.10*). These bones do the following:

1. **Maxillary** bones form the upper jaw (**maxilla**), hold the upper teeth, and are hollow, forming the maxillary sinuses.

2. **Palatine** bones are located behind the maxilla and cannot be seen on a lateral view of the skull.

3. **Zygomatic** bones are the prominences of the cheeks (cheekbones) below the eyes.

4. **Lacrimal** bones form the medial wall of each orbit.

5. **Nasal** bones form the sides and bridge of the nose.

6. The **mandible** is the lower jawbone, which holds the lower teeth. The mandible articulates (joins) with the temporal bone to form the **temporomandibular joint (TMJ).**

The bones of the facial skeleton provide a frame on which the muscles and other tissues of the face facilitate eating, facial expressions, breathing, and speech.

The third component of the axial skeleton, the rib cage, is discussed in Chapter 8, "Respiratory System."

▲ FIGURE 4.9
Skull, Right Lateral View.

Labels: Parietal bone; Sphenoid bone; Occipital bone; Temporal bone; Frontal bone; Ethmoid bone; Nasal bone; Lacrimal bone; Maxilla; Zygomatic bone; Mandible

▲ FIGURE 4.10
Facial Bones.

Labels: Nasal bone; Palatine bone; Maxilla; Mandible

Abbreviation

TMJ	temporomandibular joint

TABLES

Meaningful tables aid in summarizing concepts and lesson topics.

KEYNOTES AND ABBREVIATIONS

Keynotes and Abbreviations offer students additional information correlating to the lesson.

Lesson 4.1 (cont'd) Bone Fractures (FXs) (LO 4.2 and 4.5)

▼ **TABLE 4.1**
CLASSIFICATION AND DEFINITION OF BONE FRACTURES

Name	Description	Reference
Closed (also called **simple** fracture)	A bone is broken, but the skin is not broken.	Figure 4.6g
Open (also called **compound** fracture)	A fragment of the fractured bone breaks the skin, or a wound extends to the site of the fracture.	Figure 4.6e
Displaced	The fractured bone parts are out of line.	Figure 4.6e
Complete	A bone is broken into at least two fragments.	Figure 4.6a
Incomplete	The fracture does not extend completely across the bone. It can be hairline, as in a stress fracture in the foot, when there is no separation of the two fragments.	Figure 4.6a
Comminuted	The bone breaks into several pieces, usually two major pieces and several smaller fragments.	Figure 4.6b
Transverse	The fracture is at right angles to the long axis of the bone.	Figure 4.6b
Impacted	The fracture consists of one bone fragment driven into another, resulting in shortening of a limb.	Figure 4.6c
Spiral	The fracture spirals around the long axis of the bone.	Figure 4.6d
Oblique	The fracture runs diagonally across the long axis of the bone.	Figure 4.6d
Linear	The fracture runs parallel to the long axis of the bone.	Figure 4.6f
Greenstick	This is a partial fracture. One side breaks, and the other bends.	Figure 4.6g
Pathologic	The fracture occurs in an area of bone weakened by disease, such as cancer.	—
Compression	The fracture occurs in a vertebra from trauma or pathology, leading to the vertebra being crushed.	—
Stress	This is a fatigue fracture caused by repetitive, local stress on a bone, as occurs in marching or running.	—

▲ **FIGURE 4.6**
Bone Fractures.

Healing of Fractures (LO 4.2 and 4.5)

When a bone is fractured, blood vessels bleed into the fracture site, forming a hematoma (*Figure 4.7a*). After a few days, bone-forming cells called **osteoblasts** move in and start to produce new bone cells (osteocytes), which form a **callus** (*Figure 4.7b*). Osteoblasts continue to produce bone cells, which form **cancellous** (spongy) bone to replace the callus (*Figure 4.7c*). As more bone cells form, the spongy bone structure is replaced by compact bone, which fuses together the bone segments (*Figure 4.7d*). Uncomplicated fractures take 8 to 12 weeks to heal. (Surgical procedures to help fractures heal are shown in Lesson 4.4.)

▶ **FIGURE 4.7**
Healing of Bone Fracture.

Abbreviation

Fx	fracture

Lesson 4.1 (cont'd) Diseases of Bone
(LO 4.2 and 4.5)

Keynote

- Osteomalacia occurs in some developing nations and occasionally in this country when children drink soft drinks instead of milk fortified with vitamin D.

Abbreviations

BMD	bone mineral density
DEXA	dual energy x-ray absorptiometry
FDA	Food and Drug Administration
IU	international unit(s)
mg	milligram

One of the major bone diseases is **osteoporosis**, which results from a loss of bone density (*Figure 4.4*). More common in women than in men, the incidence of osteoporosis increases with age. In the United States alone, 10 million people are living with osteoporosis and 18 million more have low bone density (**osteopenia**).

Osteopenia puts people at risk for developing osteoporosis.

In women, production of the hormone estrogen decreases after menopause, weakening the body's protection against bone loss and potentially resulting in fragile, brittle bones. In men, lower levels of testosterone have a similar but less noticeable effect.

Women at risk for osteoporosis should have a bone mineral density (**BMD**) screening using a **DEXA** scan, which is a measuring device that uses low-energy radiation beams. Men and women over 50 are often advised to follow a daily regimen of 1,200 milligrams (**mg**) of calcium, 400 to 600 international units (**IU**) of vitamin D, and 15 minutes of real sun exposure. In addition, there are several **FDA**-approved medications available for treating osteoporosis.

Other bone diseases that may not be as prevalent or publicized as osteoporosis are the following:

Osteomyelitis: an inflammation in a bone area caused by a bacterial infection, such as staphylococcus.

Osteomalacia: a disease (known as **rickets** in children) caused by vitamin D deficiency where the calcium-lacking bones become soft and flexible, lose their ability to bear weight, and become bowed.

Achondroplasia: a very rare condition where the long bones stop growing in childhood, but the axial skeleton bones are not affected (*Figure 4.5*). People with this condition are short in stature, with the average adult measuring about 4 feet tall. Although intelligence and life span are normal, the disease is caused by a spontaneous gene mutation that then becomes a dominant gene for succeeding generations.

Osteogenesis imperfecta: a rare genetic disorder producing very brittle bones that are easily fractured or broken, often **in utero** (while inside the uterus).

Primary bone cancer is found in three forms:

1. **Osteogenic sarcoma** occurs most often in bone cells around the knee in adolescents.
2. **Ewing sarcoma** occurs most often in children and adolescents.
3. **Chondrosarcoma** arises in cartilage cells, often in the pelvises of older people.

Case Report 4.1 (continued)

On questioning, Amy Vargas demonstrated many of the risk factors for osteoporosis, including family history, lack of exercise, cigarette smoking, inadequate diet, postmenopause, and increasing age.

Normal bone   Osteoporotic bone

ACKNOWLEDGMENTS

I wish to thank the talented efforts of a group of dedicated individuals at McGraw-Hill Education who have made this book and its digital ancillary products come together: Chad Grall, Managing Director, Health Professions, for championing this book through the approval process; William Mulford, Executive Brand Manager, for his skillful leadership; Yvonne Lloyd, Product Developer, for her ability to get things done so smoothly; Jane Mohr, Lead Full-Service Content Manager, for keeping the project on track; Katherine Ward, Digital Product Analyst, for skillfully managing the integration of the digital products; Harper Christopher, Executive Marketing Manager, for organizing the positioning of the book; and Kimberly Bauer, Market Development Manager, who will conduct live reviews of the content and digital exercises.

I also wish to thank Ramya T. of SPi Global for managing the copyediting and proofreading and Verabaghu Nagarajan of Lumina Datamatics for obtaining the necessary photographs and diagrams.

David Allan, MD
Author

3e Reviewers

Theresa Allyn, BS, MEd
Edmonds Community College

Rachel Basco, BS, MHS
Bossier Parish Community College

Michael Battaglia, MS
Greenville Technical College

Carole Berube, MA, BSN, MSN
Bristol Community College

Carlos Cuervo, MD
Florida National University

Robert E. Fanger, BS HCM, MSEd
Del Mar College

Kenneth D. Franks
Bossier Parish Community College

Mary W. Hood MS ARR(R)(CT)
William Rainey Harper College

Harold N. Horn MA
Lincoln Land Community College

William J. Horton, RHIA
Hutchinson Community College

Heather Kies, MHA, CMA (AAMA)
Goodwin College

Amy Kuehnl, BS
Central Ohio Technical College

James Lynch, MD
Florida Southern College

David McBride, MA, RT(R) (CT) (MR)
Westmoreland County Community College

Steve Moon, MS CMI, FAMI
The Ohio State University

Charlotte Susie Myers, MA
Kansas City Kansas Community College

Professor Eva Oltman, MEd, CPC, CPC-I
Jefferson Community and Technical College

Mirella G Pardee, MSN, MA, RN
The University of Toledo

Irma Rodriguez
South Texas College

Dr. Beth Roraback
Greenville Technical College, Spartanburg Community College

Amy Bolinger Snow, MS
Greenville Technical College

Brian S. Spence
Tarrant County College

Alice L. Spencer, BS, MT, MS, CQA (ASQ)
National College-Florence, Kentucky

Leesa Whicker, CMA (AAMA), BA
Central Piedmont Community College

Reviewers of Previous Editions

Kathryn G. Aguirre, MA
UEI College–El Monte Campus

Vanessa Austin, RMA, CAHI
Clarian Health Ed Sciences

Dr. Joseph H. Balabat, MD, RMA, RPT
Sanford-Brown Institute, New York

Dr. Seth Balogh, BS, MS, PhD
Brookline College

Sue Biedermann, MSHP, RHIA, FAHIMA
Texas State University–San Marcos

Bonnie Bonner, RDA, LVN
Franklin Career College

Quiana Bost, RMA
Bohecker College–Cincinnati

Dorisann Brandt, MSPT
Greenville Technical College

Bill Burke, BA
Madison Area Technical College; Blackhawk Technical College

Jennifer Campbell, BS, M.Ed
Tulsa Community College

Kim Carlson, M.Ed
Delta College of Arts and Technology

Marie Cissell, MN, RN, C
South Dakota State University

Ursula Cole, M.Ed, CMA, AAMA
Harrison College

Rosalind Collazo, CMA
ASA Institute of Business and Technology

Christina Rauberts Conklin, AA, RMA
Keiser University

Dr. Brian Conroy, MD
Lehigh Valley College

Kimberly Corsi, LRCP, CCS
Davenport University

Debra Mishoe Downs, LPN, AAS, RAM (AMT)
Okefenokee Technical College

Pat Dudek, RNM CHI, RMA
McCann School of Business and Technology

Tim Feltmeyer, MS

Erie Business Center

Jean Fennema, BA
Pima Medical Institute

Lance Followell, BS
Fremont College

Joanne Habenicht, MPA, RT, BS, ARRT
Manhattan College

Gregory Hartnett, BS, CPC
Sanford-Brown, Iselin, New Jersey

Diana Hollwedel, LPN
Career Institute of Florida

Susan Horn, AAS, CMA
Indiana Business College–Lafayette

Janet Hunter, MS, MBA
Northland Pioneer College

Judy Johnson, RN
Nashville State Community College

Tim Jones, BA, MA
Oklahoma City Community College; University of Oklahoma

Angela C. Jording, CMA
Fortis College

Judith Karls, RN, BSN, M.Ed
Madison Area Technical College

Shelli Lampi, PhD, RDH, NREMT
Dunwoody College of Technology

Sandra Lehrke, RN, LNC, RMA
Anoka Technical College

Nelly Mangarova, MD
Heald College

Pam McConnell, MA, AS
High Tech Institute

Jacqueline McNair, MA, RHIT
Baltimore City Community College

Cari McPherson, LP, N.II, AHI
Ross Medical Education Center

Susan Meeks, CPC-A
Milan Institute

Roxanna Montoya, M.Ed
Pima Medical Institute

Steve Moon, MS, CMI, FAMI
Ohio State University, College of Medicine

Cathleen Murphy, DC
Katherine Gibbs School

Sheila Newberry, M.Ed, RHIT
Remington College

Evie O'Nan, RMA
National College

Jennifer S. Painter,
Ohio Business College

Fred Pearson, PhD
Brigham Young University–Idaho

Adrienne Reeves, BS, M.Ed
Westwood College

Becky Rodenbaugh, MBA, CMA
Baker College of Cadillac

Janette Rodriguez, RN, LNC RMA
Woot Tobe Coburn School, Manhattan, New York

Shawn Marie Russell, BA, CPC
University of Alaska–Fairbanks

Rebecca Schultz, PhD
University of Sioux Falls

Gene Simon, RHIA, RMD
Florida Career College

Donna Slovensky, PhD, RHIA, FAHIMA
University of Alabama–Birmingham

Susan Stockmaster, CMA (AAMA), MHS
Trident Technical College

Catherine A. Teel, AST, Health Care
    Technology, RMA
McCann School of Business and Technology

Lenette Thompson, CST
Piedmont Technical College

Jonathan Thorsen, BS, RRT
Long Beach Community College

Margaret A. Tiemann, RN, BS
St. Charles Community College

Lori A. Warren, MA, RN, CPC, CPC-I,
    CCP, CLNC
Spencerian College–Louisville, KY

Kathryn Whitley, MSN, FNP
Patrick Henry Community College

Stacy Wilson, MT/PBT, CMA, MHA
    Program Chair
Cabarrus College of Health Sciences

Kathy Wishon, RN
North Metro Tech

Dr. Barbara Worley, DPM, BS, RMA, Program
    Manager, Medical Assisting
King's College

Carole A. Zeglin, MS, BS, RMA
Westmoreland County Community College

Daphne Zito, M.Ed, LPN
Katharine Gibbs School

Susan Zolvinski, BS, MBA
Brown Mackie College

**Digital and Instructor Resource Content
  Development**
Special thanks to the instructors who assisted with
    the development of Connect and SmartBook.

Rachel Basco, BS, MHS
Bossier Parish Community College

Lorna Cassano
Bucks County Community College

Kenneth D. Franks
Bossier Parish Community College

Judy Hurtt, MEd
East Central Community College

Judith Karls, RN, BSN, MSE
Madison Area Technical College

Vicky Navaroli, PhD
Goodwin University

Mirella G Pardee, MSN, MA, RN
The University of Toledo

Brian S. Spence
Tarrant County College

David M. Allan

David Allan received his medical training at Cambridge University and Guy's Hospital in England. He was Chief Resident in Pediatrics at Bellevue Hospital in New York City before moving to San Diego, California.

Dr. Allan has worked as a family physician in England, a pediatrician in San Diego, and Associate Dean at the University of California, San Diego School of Medicine. He has designed, written, and produced more than 100 award-winning multimedia programs with virtual reality as their conceptual base. Dr. Allan resides happily in San Diego.

Karen D. Lockyer

Karen Lockyer holds a degree in Health Information (RHIT), a national coding certification (CPC), and a BS from Rutgers University. She is also a credentialed member of AHIMA (American Health Information Management Association) and AAPC (American Academy of Professional Coders).

Mrs. Lockyer has worked in medical practice administration and the Health Information Management fields for many years. She has taught medical terminology for high school, community college, and workforce development areas at the National Institutes of Health and the federal government's Office of Personnel Management. She has also taught coding and billing for undergraduate and certificate programs at the community college level.

Learning the Essentials of Medical Language

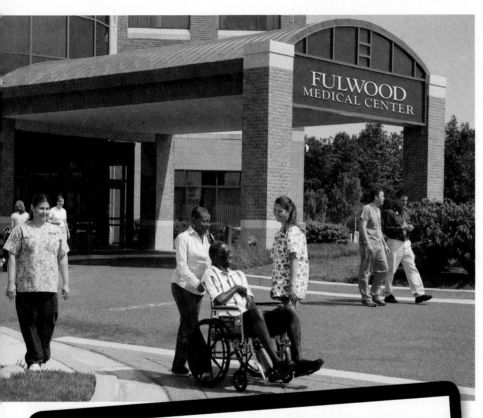

Learning Outcomes

In order to get the most out of your learning experiences and this textbook, you need to:

LO W.1 Establish a commitment to learn medical terminology.

LO W.2 Recognize the knowledge and skills you will need to be an active learner.

LO W.3 Understand how the contextual approach of this book promotes active learning.

LO W.4 Utilize the pedagogical devices used in each chapter and lesson.

LO W.5 Use the vivid illustrations, photos, and tables in the book to enhance understanding of the concepts being taught.

LO W.6 Solve the exercises in each lesson and at the end of each chapter to demonstrate understanding of the material.

LO W.7 Implement the effective organizational strategies and study habits described in this chapter of the book.

LO W.8 Understand how a commitment to lifelong learning will enhance your professionalism.

LO W.9 Differentiate the roles of the various members of a health care team in different medical specialties and settings.

Case Report W.1

You are . . .

. . . a student preparing for a career as a health professional and allied health care worker.

You are communicating with . . .

. . . many different health professionals in health care teams as you go through an externship at Fulwood Medical Center. The center comprises a medical office building with physicians in a wide range of primary care, medical specialties, and complementary medicine therapies; a 300-bed hospital with a busy Emergency Room and operating rooms; a laboratory, pharmacy, X-Ray Department, Physiotherapy Department, and Patient Education Unit that serve both the hospital and the medical offices.

Between attending classes, doing your externship, working part-time, and bringing up two children, you have a full schedule. The knowledge and skills you are learning in the classroom and at Fulwood Medical Center will prepare you for a successful future.

▲ FIGURE W.1
Direct Communication
with Doctor and Patient.

Case Report W.2

You are . . .

. . . Luis Guitterez, a certified medical assistant (CMA) working with Susan Lee, MD, a primary care physician at Fulwood Medical Center.

You are communicating with . . .

. . . Dr. Lee and Mrs. Martha Jones, a patient.

Luiz Guitterez, CMA: Dr. Lee, this is Mrs. Martha Jones, who is a type **2 diabetic** with **retinopathy** and **neuropathy.** She had a routine appointment with us today. Her temperature is 97.8, pulse 120, respirations 24, blood pressure 100/50.

Mrs. Martha Jones: Dr. Lee, I've had a cough and cold for the past few days, and today I'm feeling drowsy and nauseous and my chest hurts.

Dr. Lee: Did you give yourself your morning insulin?

Mrs. Jones: I can't remember.

Dr. Lee: Luis, she's confused, has **tachycardia** and **tachypnea,** and is **hypotensive.** I'm concerned she is going into diabetic **ketoacidosis.** Get the glucometer and test her blood glucose while I examine her. She may have **pneumonia.**

(Note: The pronunciations and meanings of the medical terms used in this Case Report are on page W-9.)

Keynote

As a health professional, you are part of a team of medical and other professionals who provide health care services designed to improve the health and well-being of their patients.

The Health Care Team (LO W.9)

Fulwood Medical Center is a realistic health care setting that allows you to experience the use of medical language. Each chapter in this book focuses on the medical terminology used in a specific medical specialty and the body systems related to that specialty. A variety of health professionals make up the teams caring for patients in each medical specialty.

The team leader is a medical doctor, or physician, who can be an **MD** (doctor of medicine) or a **DO** (doctor of osteopathy). Most **managed care systems** require the patient to have a **primary care physician.** This physician can be a **family practitioner, internist,** or **pediatrician** (for children) and is responsible for the continuing overall care of the patient. In managed care, the primary care physician acts as the "gatekeeper" for the patient to enter the system, supervising all care the patient receives.

If needed medical care is beyond the expertise of the primary care physician, the patient is referred to a medical specialist whose expertise is based on a specific body system or even a part of a body system. For example, a **cardiologist** has expertise in diseases of the heart and vascular system, whereas a **dermatologist** specializes in diseases of the skin and an **orthopedist** in problems with the musculoskeletal system. A **gastroenterologist** is an expert in diseases of the whole digestive system, whereas a **colorectal surgeon** specializes only in diseases of the lower gastrointestinal tract.

Other health professionals work under the supervision of the physician and provide direct care *(Figure W.1)* to the patient. These can include a **physician assistant, nurse practitioner, medical assistant,** and, in specialty areas, different therapists, technologists, and technicians with expertise in the use of specific therapeutic and diagnostic tools.

Still other health professionals on the team provide indirect patient care *(Figure W.2)*. These include **administrative medical assistants,**

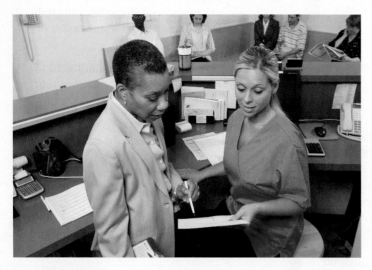

▲ FIGURE W.2
Administrative medical assistants are among the health professionals who provide indirect care to patients.

transcriptionists, **health information technicians, medical insurance billers,** and **coders,** all of whom are essential to providing high-quality patient care.

As you study the language of each medical specialty at Fulwood Medical Center, you will also meet the members of each specialty's health care team and learn more about their roles in caring for the patient.

"Why Do I Need to Learn Medical Terminology?"
Communication Needs

Throughout your career as a health professional, you will need to communicate with other health professionals. This need is present whether you are providing direct patient care—for example, as a CMA like Luis Guitterez—or whether you are providing indirect patient care—for example, as a medical transcriptionist, biller, or coder. In this book, you will find all the medical terms necessary to equip yourself with the essential medical vocabulary needed for work and further study in any of the allied health professional careers.

As you can see in Case Report W.2, health professionals use specific terms and a different language to describe to each other situations they encounter each day. You need to be able to understand, spell, and pronounce the terms they use.

Modern medical terminology is an artificial language constructed over centuries using words and elements from Greek and Latin origins (where healing professions began). Some 15,000 or more words are formed from 1,200 Greek and Latin roots. New words are being added continually as new medical discoveries are made. Medical terminology enables health professionals from different fields, different specialties, and different countries to communicate clearly and precisely with each other. Every profession has its own language *(Figure W.3)*.

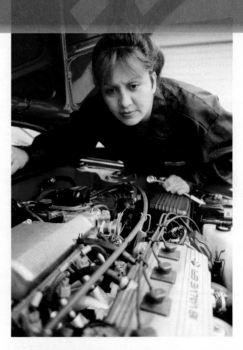

▲ **FIGURE W.3**
Every Profession Has Its Own Language
You may have difficulty understanding your auto mechanic when she tells you that the expansion valve, evaporator core, and orifice tubes in your air-conditioning system need to be replaced.

Listening, Speaking, Reading, Writing, and Critical Thinking

Daily in your practice as a health professional you will:

Listen to information from physicians about patient care, and carry out their instructions.

Listen to patients describing their symptoms, and translate their descriptions into medical terms.

Speak to physicians and other health professionals to report information and ask questions.

Speak to patients to translate and clarify information given to them by physicians and other health professionals.

Read physicians' comments and treatment plans in patient medical records and insurance reports.

Read the results of physical examinations, procedures, and laboratory and diagnostic tests.

Write to document actions taken by yourself and other members of the health care team *(Figure W.4)*.

Write to precisely record verbal orders, test results given over the phone, and other phone messages.

Think critically to evaluate medical documentation for accuracy.

Think critically to analyze and discover the meaning of unfamiliar medical terms using the strategies outlined in *Chapter 1* of this book.

▲ **FIGURE W.4**
Accurate Documentation of Care Is Critical.

IF YOU CANNOT SPEAK AND UNDERSTAND THE LANGUAGE, YOU CANNOT JOIN THE CLUB.

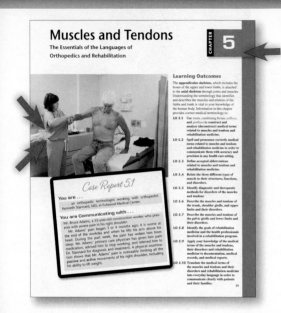

"What's Unique About This Book?"

Although the chapters in this book are organized by body system, as in many other textbooks on medical terminology, this book has many unique features that enhance learning, create interest, and provide a consistent learning strategy for you.

Each chapter is broken down into lessons; each lesson is broken down into self-contained topic areas so that there are smaller "chunks" of information to master.

You Are . . . You Are Communicating With . . .

At the beginning of each chapter and lesson, you are placed in the role of a health professional in a field related to the body system and medical specialty covered in the material. At the same time, learning objectives (**LOs**) are presented for each chapter and lesson. These techniques immediately engage your attention, motivate you to read on to discover how this patient's diagnosis and care progress, and illustrate the medical terminology being introduced in the lessons.

Word Analysis And Definition

All the information needed for a topic area is presented in self-contained two-page spreads. On the left-hand page, the new medical terms are introduced. On the right-hand page, for each new medical term the pronunciation, color-coded word elements, and definition are provided in a **Word Analysis and Definition (WAD)** box. For example, in Case Report W.2 earlier in this chapter, the medical terms diabetic, retinopathy, neuropathy, tachycardia, tachypnea, hypotensive, ketoacidosis, glucometer, and pneumonia were used. On the right-hand page here, you can see an example of how these terms are analyzed. All these terms will appear again in the appropriate body-system chapter.

Also, below each WAD are exercises that test your understanding of key components of the terminology analyzed in the WAD.

Exercises

In addition to the exercises at the end of each topic area, there are chapter review questions exercises included in Connect (see below).

Attention is given to developing skills in pronunciation, spelling, forming plurals, using abbreviations, and writing medical language. The exercises take you beyond memorization and teach you to think critically about the realistic application of the medical language you are learning.

Keynotes

- Study Hints provide ways to help retain knowledge.
- Abbreviation Boxes show commonly accepted abbreviations.
- Illustrations and photos are vivid and clear and correlate precisely to the appropriate terms in the text.

≣ connect

A ONE-STOP SPOT TO PRESENT, DELIVER, AND ASSESS DIGITAL ASSETS AVAILABLE WITH ESSENTIALS OF MEDICAL LANGUAGE:

McGraw-Hill Connect® Essentials of Medical Language provides online presentation, assignment, and assessment solutions. It connects students with the tools and resources they'll need to achieve success. With *Connect,* students can complete assignments, quizzes, and tests online. A robust set of questions and activities, including all of the lesson exercises and end-of-chapter questions, additional case studies, and interactives, are presented and aligned with the textbook's learning outcomes.

Connect Essentials of Medical Language also provides students with 24/7 online access to an ebook. This media-rich version of the textbook is available through the McGraw-Hill Education Connect platform and allows seamless integration of text, media, and assessments. To learn more, visit **http://connect.mheducation.com**.

≣LEARNSMART ADVANTAGE

MCGRAW-HILL EDUCATION'S ADAPTIVE SUITE

New from McGraw-Hill Education, LearnSmart Advantage is a series of adaptive learning products, which include LearnSmart, Smartbook, LearnSmart Prep, LearnSmart Achieve, and Learnsmart Labs. Since 2009, LearnSmart has been the most widely used and intelligent adaptive learning resource proven to improve learning. Developed to deliver demonstrable results in boosting grades, increasing course retention, and strengthening memory recall, the LearnSmart Advantage series spans the entire learning process from course preparation to providing the first adaptive reading experience, and it's found only in SmartBook. Distinguishing what students know from what they don't, and honing in on concepts they are most likely to forget, each product in the series helps students study smarter and retain more knowledge. A smarter learning experience for students coupled with valuable reporting tools for instructors, and available in hundreds of course areas, LearnSmart Advantage is advancing learning like no other products in higher education today. **Go to www.LearnSmartAdvantage.com** for more information.

Word Analysis and Definition

S = Suffix   P = Prefix   R = Root   R/CF = Combining Form

WORD	PRONUNCIATION	ELEMENTS		DEFINITION
diabetes mellitus	dye-ah-**BEE**-teez **MEL**-ih-tus		diabetes, Greek *a siphon* mellitus, Latin *sweetened with honey*	Metabolic syndrome caused by absolute or relative insulin deficiency and/or insulin ineffectiveness
diabetic (adj)	dye-ah-**BET**-ik	S/ R/	-ic *pertaining to* diabet- *diabetes*	Pertaining to or suffering from diabetes
hypotension	HIGH-poh-**TEN**-shun	S/ P/ R/	-ion *action, condition* hypo- *below* -tens- *pressure*	Persistent low arterial blood pressure
hypotensive (adj)	HIGH-poh-**TEN**-siv	S/	-ive *pertaining to, quality of*	Pertaining to or suffering from hypotension
ketoacidosis	KEY-toe-ass-ih-**DOE**-sis	S/ R/CF R/CF	-sis *abnormal condition* ket/o- *ketone* -acid/o- *acid*	Excessive production of ketones, making the blood acidic
neuropathy	nyu-**ROP**-ah-thee	S/ R/CF	-pathy *disease* neur/o- *nerve*	Any disorder affecting the nervous system
pneumonia (**Note:** *The initial "p" is silent.*)	new-**MOH**-nee-ah	S/ R/	-ia *condition* pneumon- *air, lung*	Inflammation of the lung parenchyma
retinopathy	ret-ih-**NOP**-ah-thee	S/ R/CF	-pathy *disease* retin/o- *retina*	Any disease of the retina
tachycardia	tack-ih-**KAR**-dee-ah	S/ P/ R/	-ia *condition* tachy- *rapid* -card- *heart*	Rapid heart rate, above 100 beats per minute
tachypnea	tack-ip-**NEE**-ah	P/ R/	tachy- *rapid* -pnea *breathe*	Rapid breathing

The elements of a term are discussed in Chapter 1.

SmartBook is the first and only adaptive reading experience currently available. SmartBook personalizes content for each student in a continuously adapting reading experience. Reading is no longer a passive and linear experience, but an engaging and dynamic one where students are more likely to master and retain important concepts, thus coming to class better prepared. Valuable reports provide instructors with insight into how students are progressing through textbook content, and are useful for shaping in-class time and assessments. As a result of the adaptive reading experience found in SmartBook, students are more likely to retain knowledge, stay in class, and get better grades. This revolutionary technology is available only from McGraw-Hill Education for hundreds of course areas as part of the LearnSmart Advantage series.

EXERCISES

Elements *are your best tool for understanding medical terms. In the chart below, the elements are listed in column 1. Identify the meaning of each element in column 2, and give an example of a term containing that element in column 3. Some terms will apply to more than one element. The first one is done for you.*

Element	Meaning of Element	Medical Term Containing This Element
hypo	below	hypotension
tens		
ion		
neuro		
retino		
pathy		
ia		
pneumon		
pnea		
tachy		

1. Choose any term from column 3, and use it in a sentence of your choice:

_____

_____

_____

"What Is Lifelong, Active Learning?"

Lifelong Learning

Your current training in medical terminology is necessary for you to be able to continue your education in your health care profession. But it is important to recognize that school is only one of the many places where you acquire knowledge.

You also acquire knowledge:

- Each time you ask a question about a patient or a report and receive an answer.

- Each time you analyze an unfamiliar medical term and discover its meaning.

- Each time you interact with a patient and see how that patient is coping with his or her problems *(Figure W.5)*.

All these are opportunities for learning to discover **your own** answers to **your own** problems or lack of knowledge.

This type of knowledge—discovered through your own experience and driven by your own needs and goals—is genuine, real, and trustworthy for you. It is not like what you learn in school, which is determined by some distant authority.

The authentic knowledge you gain from solving your own problems, whether by yourself or with the help of other people or resources, motivates you to acquire still more knowledge and helps you grow as a person and as a professional.

Throughout your working life, additional classroom training will be needed to keep your skills and professional knowledge up to date with new developments in medicine. You will also continue to learn through your own experience. Everything you do in life can result in learning.

Your own experience and judgment become your most valuable resources for making your life vibrant, strong, creative, and what *you* want *it* to be.

Your own experience and judgment maximize your professional and personal success.

Your own learning never ends.

▲ **FIGURE W.5**
Every Patient Interaction Is an Opportunity for Learning.

Keynote

Novelist Lillian Smith said, "When you stop learning, stop listening, stop looking, and stop asking new questions, then it is time to die."

Actively Experiencing Medical Language

Medical terms were created to provide health care professionals a way to communicate with each other and document the care they provide. To provide effective patient care, all health care professionals must be fluent in medical language. One misused or misspelled medical term on a patient record can cause errors that can result in injury or death to patients, incorrect coding or billing of medical claims, and possible fraud charges.

When medical terms are separated from their intended context, as they are in other medical terminology textbooks, it is easy to lose sight of how important it is to use them accurately and precisely. Learning medical terminology in the context of the medical setting reinforces the importance of correct usage and precision in communication.

During your externship at Fulwood Medical Center, you will *experience* medical language. Just as in a real medical center, you will encounter and apply medical terminology in a variety of ways. Actively experiencing medical language will help ensure that you are truly learning, and not simply memorizing, the medical terms in each chapter. Memorizing a term allows you to use it in the same situation (e.g., repeating a definition) but doesn't help you apply it in new situations. Whether you are reading chart notes in a patient's medical record *(Figure W.6)* or a description of the treatment prescribed by a physician, you will see medical terms being used for the purpose they were intended.

▲ **FIGURE W.6**
Medical assistant interacts with a physician.

Active Learning

It's no good sitting back and expecting someone else to pour knowledge into your head. You have to **actively work at learning** *(Figure W.7)*.

Get the Most Out of Lectures

- *Prepare* for your classroom experiences. Preview the book chapter before class *(Figure W.7)*, and the material will be much easier to understand.
- *Listen actively.* You cannot do this if you are looking at your cell phone, daydreaming, or worrying about what you have to get for dinner.
- *Ask* a question if you do not comprehend something the instructor is saying.
- *Write* good notes. Focus on the main points, and capture key ideas; review and edit your notes within 24 hours of the class.

Get the Most Out of Reading

- *Concentrate* on what you are reading. Review the titles, objectives, headings, and visuals for each lesson to identify what the lesson is all about.
- *Read* actively using the SQ3R method (see the Study Hint) to help you.
- *Write* down any questions you have.

Study with a Partner or Group

- *Find* a study partner. Schedule study dates, compare notes, talk through concepts and questions, and quiz each other.
- *Establish* a small study group, including your study partner. Again, compare notes and quiz each other.

Perform Well on Tests

- *Read* the directions carefully, and scan the entire test so that you know how long it is and what types of activities it contains.
- *Answer* the easy questions or sections first so that you finish as much as possible before doing the difficult questions, which might slow you down.
- *Use* any extra time, after you have finished the test, to check that you have answered all the questions and then to confirm your answers.

Know and Motivate Yourself

- What type of learner are you? **Visual**—who responds best by **seeing** information. **Auditory**—who works best by listening. **Tactile**—who prefers hands-on applications. Recognize your type and motivate yourself by emphasizing your best method of learning to help achieve your goals.

A few months of committed study now is a small price to pay for a lifetime of professionalism.

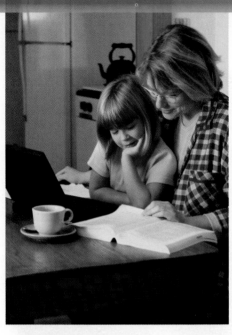

▲ **FIGURE W.7**
Identify your own personal preferences for learning, and seek out the resources that will best help you with your studies. Recognize your weaknesses, and try to compensate for or work to improve them.

Study Hint

The SQ3R model for reading is a successful equation for studying:

Survey what you are going to read.

Question what you are going to learn after the preview.

Read the assignment.

Recite. Stop every once in a while, look up from the book, and put what you've just read into your own words.

Review. After you've finished, review the main points.

▲ FIGURE W.8
An Evening at Home.

Case Report W.3

Your first day of externship at Fulwood Medical Center went well. You enjoyed being in the Primary Care Clinic with Dr. Lee and Luis Guitterez, CMA. You wonder if this could be a career choice for you. Now it's 6:15 p.m. at home, and you have yet to feed the kids, get them to bed, pay some bills, pick up around the house, and review a whole chapter in your medical terminology text to prepare for a test in class tomorrow. How are you going to do all this?

"How Can I Help Myself Learn Better?"

You have a lot of time and money invested in your education. To succeed, you need to be able to focus and manage your time and your studies. To manage the difficulties described in Case Report W.3 *(Figure W.8),* you need to:

- *Recognize* the stresses in your life at different times.

- *Prioritize* mentally, and handle each task in the order of importance. In this case, eat a healthy meal with your kids, enjoy putting them to bed, pay the bills, and then relax (or meditate) for 10 minutes. When you are relaxed, settle down to review the text, and go to bed at a reasonable hour. Picking up around the house will have to wait because study and sleep are a higher priority. Sounds too easy? What other choices do you have to be able to study in an effective way?

- *Actively develop a support group.* Enlist the support of your spouse, parents, siblings, friends—any people you can trust and rely on. If you have a test every Thursday, get one of them to come over Wednesday night and put the kids to bed while you go over to his or her house or the library to study.

- *Find your own space.* Create a place where you keep everything for your courses at your fingertips, clutter-free.

- *Study when you are most productive.* Are you a night owl or an early bird? Set a daily study time for yourself.

- *Balance your life.* While studying should be a main focus, plan time for family, friends, leisure, exercise, and sleep.

- *Resist distractions.* Avoid the temptation to surf the Web, send instant messages, and make phone calls. Stick to your schedule.

- *Be realistic* when planning—know your limits and priorities.

- *Be prepared* for the unexpected (child's illness, your illness, inclement weather) that can turn your schedule into shambles.

- *Reprioritize* daily on the basis of schedule disruptions and other conflicts.

- *Identify* clear goals for what you need to get done today, this week, this month, before the end of the semester, and so on.

EXERCISES

Write out *all of your activities for a typical week. On average, how many hours each week do you spend sleeping, grooming, eating, working, running errands, studying, attending your children's activities, and watching TV? Add all the hours up. There are 168 hours in the week. How many hours do you have left for studying? A sample time budget is shown below.*

Activity	Number of Hours per Day	Number of Days per Week	Number of Hours per Week
Sleeping	8	7	56
Grooming	1	7	7
Meals: preparation, eating, cleanup	1	7	7
Cleaning, laundry	1	3	3
Commuting to and from school	1	5	5
In class	4	5	20
Doing errands	1	3	3
Family time	3	7	21
Church, workout, hobbies			5
Job			30
Friends, going out, TV, entertainment			6
TOTAL			163
TOTAL HOURS IN A WEEK			168
Hours remaining for study			5

- Are 5 hours enough for study?
- When are they available?
- What can you do to increase them?

Study hours should be spent in a setting that allows you to concentrate on your work and not be distracted. Turn off your cell phone and TV. The biggest question to ask yourself is, "Am I investing my time wisely?" If not, how can you budget your time differently so that more time is spent on higher-priority activities?

The Anatomy of Medical Terms

The Essential Elements of the Language of Medicine

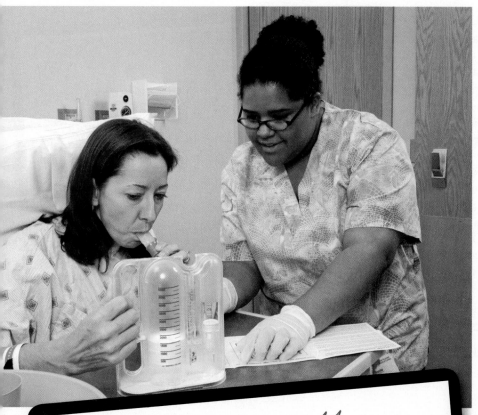

CHAPTER 1

Learning Outcomes

The technical language of medicine has been developed logically from Latin and Greek roots. In fact, it was in Latin and Greek cultures that the concept of treating patients began. Medical terms are built from their individual parts, or **elements,** which form the **anatomy** of the word. The information in this chapter will enable you to:

LO 1.1 Select the roots, combining vowels and combining forms of medical terms.

LO 1.2 Demonstrate the importance of suffixes and prefixes in forming medical terms.

LO 1.3 Construct (build) medical terms from separate elements.

LO 1.4 Deconstruct (break down) medical terms into their elements.

LO 1.5 Use correctly the plurals of medical terms.

LO 1.6 Articulate the correct pronunciations of medical terms.

LO 1.7 Demonstrate precision and accuracy in documentation and other written and verbal communication of medical terms.

Case Report 1.1

You are . . .

. . . a **respiratory therapist** working with Tavis Senko, MD, a pulmonologist at Fulwood Medical Center.

You are communicating with . . .

. . . Mrs. Sandra Schwartz, a 43-year-old woman referred to Dr. Senko by her primary care physician, Dr. Andrew McDonald, an **internist.** Mrs. Schwartz has a persistent abnormality on her chest X-ray. You have been asked to determine her **pulmonary** function prior to a scheduled **bronchoscopy.**

This summary of a Case Report illustrates for you the use of some simple medical terms. Modern health care and medicine have their own language. The medical terms all have precise meanings, which enable you, as a health professional, to communicate clearly and accurately with other health professionals involved in the care of a patient. This communication is critical for patient safety and the delivery of high-quality patient care.

Lesson 1.1

The Construction of Medical Words

Objectives

Your confidence in using and understanding the medical terms in this book will increase as you become familiar with the logic of how these terms are constructed. The information in this lesson will enable you to:

1.1.1 Build and construct medical terms using their elements.

1.1.2 Select and identify the meaning of essential medical term **roots**.

1.1.3 Define the elements **combining vowel** and **combining form**.

1.1.4 Identify the **combining vowel** and **combining form** of essential medical terms.

1.1.5 Define the elements **suffix** and **prefix**.

1.1.6 Select and identify the meaning of the **suffixes** and **prefixes** of essential medical terms.

Roots

- A **root** is the constant foundation and core of a medical term.
- **Roots** are usually of Greek or Latin origin.
- All medical terms have *one* or *more* **roots**.
- A **root** can appear anywhere in the term.
- More than one **root** can have the same meaning.
- A **root** plus a **combining vowel** creates a **combining form**.

Roots (LO 1.1)

Every medical term has a **root**—the element that provides the core meaning of the word. For example, in Case Report 1.1:

- The word *pneumonia* has the **root** *pneumon-*, taken from the Greek word meaning *lung* or *air*. The Greek root *pneum-* also means *lung* or *air*. *Pneumonia* is an infection of the lung tissue.

- Dr. Tavis Senko is a *pulmonologist*. The root *pulmon-* is taken from the Latin word meaning *lung*. A *pulmonologist* is a specialist who treats lung diseases.

> *Case Report 1.1 (continued)*
>
> From her medical records, you can see that 2 months ago Mrs. Schwartz developed a right upper lobe (RUL) **pneumonia**. After treatment with an **antibiotic**, a follow-up chest X-ray (CXR) showed some residual collapse in the right upper lobe and a small right **pneumothorax**. Mrs. Schwartz has smoked a pack a day since she was a teenager. Dr. Senko is concerned that she has lung cancer and has scheduled her for a **bronchoscopy**.

Combining Forms (LO 1.1)

Roots are often joined to other elements in a medical term by adding a **combining vowel**, such as the letter "o," to the end of the **root**, like *pneum-*, to form **pneum/o-**.

| pneum-
root
lung or air | + | -o-
combining vowel | = | pneum/o-
combining form |

Throughout this book, whenever a term is presented, a **slash** (/) will be used to separate the combining vowel from the **root**. Other examples of this approach are as follows:

- Adding the **combining vowel** "o" to the Latin **root** *pulmon-* makes the **combining form** *pulmon/o-*.

| pulmon-
root
lung | + | -o-
combining vowel | = | pulmon/o-
combining form |

Any vowel, "a," "e," "i," "o," or "u," can be used as a **combining vowel**.

- The root *respir-* means *to breathe*. Adding the **combining vowel** "a" makes the **combining form** *respir/a-*.

| respir-
root
to breathe | + | -a-
combining vowel | = | respir/a-
combining form |

- The **root** *bronch-* is derived from the Greek word for *windpipe* and is one of the two subdivisions of the trachea that carry air to and from the lungs. Adding the **combining vowel** "o" to the **root** *bronch-* makes the **combining form** *bronch/o-*.

bronch-
root
bronchus

+

-o-
combining vowel

=

bronch/o
combining form

Combining Forms

- Combine a **root** and a combining vowel.
- Can be attached to another **root** or **combining form**.
- Can precede another word element called a **suffix**.
- Can follow a **prefix**.

Many medical terms contain more than one **root**; when two roots occur together, they are always joined by a **combining vowel**, as in the following example:

- The word **hemopneumothorax** has the **root** *hem-*, from the Greek word meaning *blood*, and the **root** *pneum-*, from the Greek word meaning *air* or *lung*, and the **suffix** *-thorax*, from the Greek word meaning *chest*. The **combining vowel** "o" joins these two roots together to make the **combining form**, *pneum/o-*. A **hemopneumothorax** is the presence of air and blood in the space that surrounds the lungs in the chest. As blood and air fill the pleural cavity, the lungs cannot expand and respiration is not possible, thus forceing the affected lung to collapse.

hem-
root
blood

+

-o-
combining vowel

+

pneum-
root
lung or air

+

-o-
combining vowel

+

-thorax
suffix
chest

=

hemopneumothorax
blood or air in the chest

Keynotes

- Throughout this book, look for the following patterns:

    Roots, combining forms, and combining vowels will be colored red.

    Prefixes will be colored green.

    Suffixes will be colored blue.

- Different roots can have the same meaning. *Pulmon-* and *pneumon-* both mean *lung, air*.

EXERCISES

A. Review *what you have just learned about the roots and combining forms on the two pages spread open in front of you. Fill in the blanks.* **LO 1.1** *Remember*

1. Which element is the core or foundation of every medical term? _____

2. Give two examples of the element named in question #1 above: _____

3. If a **combining vowel** is added to the element in question #1, what is the name of the new element? _____

4. Give an example of a **root** that has become a **combining form**:

    _____ + _____ = _____

    Root   Combining vowel   Combining form (Don't forget the slash!)

5. More than one element can have the same meaning in medical terminology.

    Give an example from the elements on these two pages:

    _____ and _____

    both mean _____

6. Give an example of a term using each element in the above question:

    _____ means _____

    _____ means _____

Study Hint

Even though both these elements mean the same thing, they are not interchangeable. Only certain elements belong with certain terms, and you must know them.

7. The following terms have not been introduced yet, but the principle remains the same. The root/combining form will always carry the same meaning. Circle the roots/combining forms that you recognize, and provide the meaning of the root or combining form on the blank line.

7a. *Pneumonectomy, pneumonitis,* and *pneumococcal* all pertain to the _____.

7b. *Respirator* and *respiratory* both pertain to _____.

Lesson 1.1 (cont'd)

Suffixes

- A suffix is a group of letters attached to the end of a root or combining form.
- A suffix changes the meaning of the word.
- If the suffix begins with a consonant, it must follow a combining vowel.
- If the suffix begins with a vowel, no combining vowel is needed.
- A few medical terms can have two suffixes.
- A suffix always appears at the end of a term.
- Suffixes that are different can have the same meaning.

Keynote

Adjectival suffixes meaning *pertaining to:*

-ac, -al, -ale, -alis, -ar, -aris, -ary, atic, -ative, -eal, -ent, -etic, -ial, -ic, -ica, -ical, -ine, -ior, -iosum, -ious, -istic, -ius, -nic, -ous, -tic, -tiz, -tous, -us.

Suffixes (LO 1.2)

A suffix is an element added to the end of a root or combining form to give it a new meaning. You can add different suffixes to the same root to build new words, all with different meanings. For example:

- Add the suffix *-ary* to the root *pulmon-* to create the term **pulmonary.** The suffix *-ary* means *pertaining to* or *relating to.* The adjective **pulmonary** means *pertaining to the lung.* **Pulmonary circulation** means the *passage of blood through the lungs.*

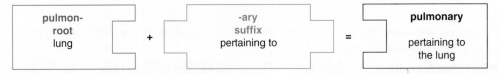

- Add the suffix *-logy* to the combining form *pulmon/o-* to make the term **pulmonology.** The suffix *-logy* means *study of.* **Pulmonology** is the study of the structure, functions, and diseases of the lungs.

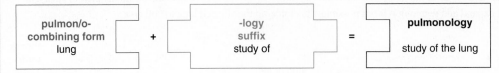

- Add the suffix *-ia* to the root *pneumon-* to make the term **pneumonia.** The suffix *-ia* means *a condition of.* **Pneumonia** is a condition of the lungs that involves an infection of the lung tissue.

- Add the suffix *-ation* to the root *respir-* to make the term **respiration.** The suffix *-ation* means *a process.* **Respiration** is the process of breathing in and out.

- Add the suffix *-itis* to the root *bronch-* to make the term **bronchitis.** The suffix *-itis* means *inflammation.* **Bronchitis** is an inflammation of the bronchial tubes.

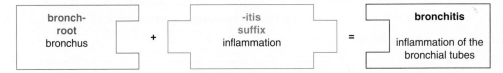

Although most roots are specific to body systems and medical specialties, suffixes are universal and can be applied to all body systems and specialties.

One user-friendly design concept of this book is that all the information you will need for any given topic is presented on the left-hand page of the two-page spread open in front of you. As part of this, you will find a Word Analysis and Definition (WAD) box on the right-hand side of each two-page spread. This section provides the elements, definition, and pronunciation of every new and repeated significant medical term that appears in the two-page spread.

Review all the terms in the WAD before you start any exercise.

Word Analysis and Definition

S = Suffix   P = Prefix   R = Root   R/CF = Combining Form

WORD	PRONUNCIATION	ELEMENTS		DEFINITION
bronchitis	brong-**KI**-tis	S/ R/	-itis *inflammation* *bronch- bronchus*	Inflammation of the bronchi
pneumonia	new-**MOH**-nee-ah	S/ R/	-ia *condition* *pneumon- lung, air*	Inflammation of the lung parenchyma (tissue)
pneumonitis (**same as** *pneumonia*)	new-moh-**NI**-tis	S/	-itis *inflammation*	
pulmonary	**PULL**-moh-**NAR**-ee	S/ R/	-ary *pertaining to* *pulmon- lung*	Pertaining to the lungs
pulmonology	**PULL**-moh-**NOL**-oh-jee	S/ R/CF	-logy *study of* *pulmon/o- lung*	Study of the lungs, or the medical specialty of disorders of the lungs
pulmonologist	**PULL**-moh-**NOL**-oh-jist	S/	-logist *one who studies, specialist*	Specialist in treating disorders of the lungs
respiration	**RES**-pih-**RAY**-shun	S/ R/	-ation *process* *respir- to breathe*	Process of breathing; fundamental process of life used to exchange oxygen and carbon dioxide
respiratory (adj)	**RES**-pih-rah-tor-ee	S/	-atory *pertaining to*	Pertaining to respiration

EXERCISES

Elements: *It is important for you to recognize the identity of an element. Is it a root, combining form, or suffix? This will help you to determine its place in the term when you are building terms.*

A. Build the appropriate medical term *to match the definitions given. The placement of the elements is noted for you under the line; each different element is separated on the line. Write the correct elements on the line. The first one is done for you.*   **LO 1.1 and 1.2** *Apply*

1. Study of the lungs: _____pulmon/o_____/_____logy_____
                           R/CF   S

2. Pertaining to the lung: _____/_____
               R/CF   S

3. The process of breathing: _____/_____
               R/CF   S

4. Condition of the lung: _____/_____
               R/CF   S

5. Use any one of the preceding terms in a sentence of your choice—one that is *not* a definition from above.

   _____
   _____

6. Choose another term from above and use it in patient documentation that you write below.

   _____
   _____

B. Deconstruct (break down) each of the following medical terms into its elements and give its meaning.   **LO 1.1, 1.2, and 1.4** *Analyze*

1. Bronchitis: _____/_____
                 R/CF   S
       Meaning:_____

2. Pulmonologist: _____/_____
                 R/CF   S
       Meaning:_____

C. Answers *to all questions in this exercise can be found on the two-page spread open in front of you.*   **LO 1.1, 1.2, and 1.7** *Remember*

1. What is another term for inflammation of the lung? _____

2. Which term is a body process? _____

3. Which suffix can be applied to a specialist? _____

Prefixes (LO 1.2)

Prefixes

- A **prefix** always appears at the beginning of a term.
- A **prefix** precedes a **root** to change its meaning.
- **Prefixes** can have more than one meaning.
- **Prefixes** never require a **combining vowel**.
- An occasional medical term can have two **prefixes**.
- Not every term has a **prefix**.

Practical Points

- A **root** can start a term and does not become a **prefix**.
- A **root** can end a term and does not become a **suffix**.

A **prefix** is an element added to the beginning of a **root** or **combining form** to further expand the meaning of a medical term. **Prefixes** usually indicate time, number, color, or location. Examples of **prefixes** defining time are as follows:

- The term **mature** can refer to an infant born after a normal length of pregnancy, between 37 and 42 weeks.
- An infant born before 37 weeks is called **premature**. The **prefix** *pre-* means *before.* **Premature** means that the infant was born *before 37 weeks.*
- An infant born after 42 weeks is called **postmature**. The **prefix** *post-* means *after.* **Postmature** means that the infant was born *after 42 weeks.*

- The term **natal** contains the **root** *nat-* (*birth* or *born*) and the **suffix** *–al* (*pertaining to*); it means *pertaining to birth.*
- Add the **prefix** *pre-* (*before*) to form **prenatal,** which means *the time before birth.*
- Add the **prefix** *post-* (*after*) to form **postnatal,** which means *the time after birth.*
- Add the **prefix** *peri-* (*around*) to form **perinatal,** which means *around the time of birth.* This includes the time immediately *before, during,* and *directly after birth.*

Examples of **prefixes** indicating number are as follows:

- The term **lateral** contains the **root** *later-* (*side*) and the **suffix** *–al* (*pertaining to*). **Lateral** means *pertaining to a side of the body.*
- Add the **prefix** *uni-* (*one*) to form **unilateral,** which means *pertaining to one side of the body only.*
- Add the **prefix** *bi-* (*two*) to form **bilateral,** which means *pertaining to both sides of the body.*

Examples of prefixes indicating location are as follows:

- The term **gastric** contains the **root** *gastr-* (*stomach*) and the **suffix** *–ic* (*pertaining to*). **Gastric** means *pertaining to the stomach.*
- Add the **prefix** *epi-* (*above*) to form **epigastric,** which means *pertaining to above the stomach.*
- Add the **prefix** *hypo-* (*below*) to form **hypogastric,** which means *pertaining to below the stomach.*

Examples of **prefixes** indicating size are as follows:

- The **root** *-cyte* means *cell.*
- Add the **prefix** *macro-* (*large*) to form **macrocyte,** which means *a large cell.*
- Add the **prefix** *micro-* (*small*) to form **microcyte,** which means *a small cell.*

WORD	PRONUNCIATION	ELEMENTS		DEFINITION
gastric	GAS-trik	S/	-ic *pertaining to*	Pertaining to the stomach
		R/	gastr- *stomach*	
epigastric	ep-ih-GAS-trik	P/	epi- *above*	Abdominal region above the stomach
hypogastric	high-poh-GAS-trik	P/	hypo- *below*	Abdominal region below the stomach
lateral	LAT-er-al	S/	-al *pertaining to*	Pertaining to one side of the body
		R/	later- *side*	
bilateral	by-LAT-er-al	P/	bi- *two*	Pertaining to both sides of the body
unilateral	you-nih-LAT-er-al	P/	uni- *one*	Pertaining to one side of the body only
macrocyte	MACK-roh-site	P/	macro- *large*	Large cell
		R/	-cyte *cell*	
macrocytic (adj)	mack-roh-SIT-ik	S/	-ic *pertaining to*	Pertaining to a macrocyte
(Note: *The "e" in* cyte *is deleted to allow the word to flow.*)				
mature	mah-TYUR		Latin *ready*	Fully developed
postmature	post-mah-TYUR	P/	post- *after*	Infant born after 42 weeks of gestation
		R/	-mature *fully developed*	
premature	pree-mah-TYUR	P/	pre- *before*	Occurring before the expected time; e.g., an infant born before 37 weeks of gestation.
microcyte	MY-kroh-site	P/	micro- *small*	Small cell
		R/	-cyte *cell*	
microcytic (adj)	my-kroh-SIT-ik	S/	-ic *pertaining to*	Pertaining to a small cell
(Note: *The "e" in* cyte *is deleted to allow the word to flow.*)				
natal	NAY-tal	S/	-al *pertaining to*	Pertaining to birth
		R/	nat- *birth, born*	
perinatal	per-ih-NAY-tal	P/	peri- *around*	Around the time of birth
postnatal	post-NAY-tal	P/	post- *after*	After the birth
prenatal	pree-NAY-tal	P/	pre- *before*	Before the birth
pneumothorax	new-moh-THOR-ax	R/CF	pneum/o- *air, lung*	Air in the pleural cavity
		S/	-thorax *chest*	

EXERCISES

Prefixes: *Solid knowledge of prefixes will quickly help increase your medical vocabulary. A good example is the Word Analysis and Definition (WAD) entry for* natal. *The addition of three different prefixes builds three new medical terms.*

A. *To begin this exercise, underline every prefix in the bolded terms below. Answer the first question, and then build the correct term on the line next to the definitions in 2 through 4. Follow the instructions for question 5.*   **LO 1.1, 1.2, and 1.4** *Apply*

natal   prenatal   postnatal   perinatal

1. The term *natal* means _____

2. Pertaining to around the time of birth: _____ / _____ / _____
                                                P   R/CF   S

3. Pertaining to after the birth: _____ / _____ / _____
                                        P   R/CF   S

4. Pertaining to before the birth: _____ / _____ / _____
                                        P   R/CF   S

5. In 2 through 4 above, circle the word in the definition that is the clue to the correct prefix to use in the term.

B. Review *the prefixes for number, location, and size. Check (✔) the correct box for the category, and write the meaning for every prefix in the chart.*
LO 1.2 *Remember*

Prefix	Number	Location	Size	Prefix Means
1. hypo				
2. uni				

Lesson 1.2

Word Deconstruction, Plurals, Pronunciation, and Precision

Objectives

*When you see an unfamiliar medical term, you can learn its meaning by **deconstructing** it—reducing it to its basic elements. In this lesson you will learn to:*

1.2.1 Break down or deconstruct a medical term into its elements.

1.2.2 Use word analysis to help ensure the precise use of medical terms.

1.2.3 Use the word elements to analyze and determine the meaning of the term.

1.2.4 Apply the correct pronunciation to medical terms.

Case Report 1.2

You are . . .

. . . a medical assistant working in the office of Lokesh Bannerjee, MD, a cardiologist in Fulwood Medical Center.

You are communicating with . . .

. . . the 70-year-old wife and the 45-year-old son of James Donovan, a 75-year-old man who will be admitted to the hospital's acute care **cardiology** unit.

Dr. Bannerjee has **diagnosed** Mr. Donovan with an acute myocardial infarction **(AMI)**, confirmed by changes in his **electrocardiogram (ECG/EKG).** One of your tasks is to explain Mr. Donovan's **diagnosis** and reasons for admission to the hospital to Mrs. Donovan and her son. While Mr. Donovan is waiting to be admitted, he is receiving oxygen through nasal prongs. He is **hypotensive,** and an intravenous **(IV)** infusion of normal saline has been started. His medical record indicates that he is being seen in the neurology clinic for early dementia.

The bold terms in the Case Report are used as examples in the text and/or are deconstructed in the Word Analysis and Definition box (opposite page).

Keynotes

- Always begin deconstructing a medical term by identifying its suffix.
- Abbreviations are listed in Abbreviations Boxes throughout the book.

Abbreviations

AMI	acute myocardial infarction
CXR	chest x-ray
ECG/ EKG	electrocardiogram
IV	intravenous

Word Deconstruction (LO 1.1, 1.2, and 1.4)

When you see an unfamiliar medical term, first identify the **suffix.** Take the term **cardiologist.** Here, the **suffix** at the end of the word is *-logist,* which means *one who studies and is a specialist in.* This leaves the element *cardi/o-,* which is the **combining form** for *heart.* The term **cardiologist** means *a specialist in the heart and its diseases.* It has a **combining form** and a **suffix.**

In the term **myocardial,** the **suffix** at the end of the word is **-al,** which means *pertaining to,* as you learned earlier in this chapter. The **combining form** *my/o-,* which means *muscle,* is at the beginning of the word. The **root** *-cardi-,* which means *heart,* is in the middle of the word. So, the term **myocardial** means *pertaining to the heart muscle.* It has a **combining form,** a **root,** and a **suffix.**

Changing the **suffix** to *-um,* meaning *a structure,* results in the term **myocardium,** *the structure called the heart muscle.*

The term **cardiomyopathy** contains the **suffix -pathy,** meaning *a disease,* the **combining form** *cardi/o-,* meaning the *heart,* and the **combining form** *my/o-,* meaning *muscle.* When you put this all together, the term **cardiomyopathy** means *a disease of the heart muscle.*

The term **ischemia** has the **suffix** *-emia,* which means *a blood condition.* The **root** *isch-* means *to block.* **Ischemia** means *a blockage of blood flow.* The term **myocardial ischemia** means *a blockage of blood flow to the heart muscle*—better known as a heart attack.

WORD	PRONUNCIATION	ELEMENTS		DEFINITION
cardiologist	kar-dee-**OL**-oh-jist	S/	-logist *one who studies and is a specialist in*	A medical specialist in the diagnosis and treatment of disorders of the heart
		R/CF	cardi/o- *heart*	
cardiology	kar-dee-**OL**-oh-jee	S/	-logy *study of*	Medical specialty of diseases of the heart
cardiomyopathy	KAR-dee-oh-my-**OP**-ah-thee	S/	-pathy *disease*	Disease of the heart muscle, the myocardium
		R/CF	cardi/o- *heart*	
		R/CF	-my/o- *muscle*	
diagnosis (noun)	die-ag-**NO**-sis	P/	dia- *complete*	The determination of the cause of a disease
		R/	-gnosis *knowledge of an abnormal condition*	
diagnoses (pl)	die-ag-**NO**-seez			
diagnostic (adj)	die-ag-**NOS**-tik	S/	-tic *pertaining to*	Pertaining to or establishing a diagnosis
(Note: *The "is" in -gnosis is deleted to allow the word to flow.*)				
diagnose (verb)	die-ag-**NOSE**	R/	-gnose *recognize an abnormal condition*	To make a diagnosis
electrocardiogram	ee-lek-troh-**KAR**-dee-oh-gram	S/	-gram *record*	Record of the heart's electrical signals
		R/CF	electr/o- *electricity*	
		R/CF	-cardi/o- *heart*	
hypertensive (adj)	**HIGH**-per-**TEN**-siv	S/	-ive *pertaining to*	Pertaining to or suffering from high blood pressure
		P/	hyper- *excessive*	
		R/	-tens- *pressure*	
infarct	in-**FARKT**	P/	in- *in*	An area of cell death resulting from blockage of its blood supply
		R/	-farct *area of dead tissue*	
infarction	in-**FARK**-shun	S/	-ion *action, condition*	Sudden blockage of an artery
ischemia	is-**KEY**-me-ah	S/	-emia *a blood condition*	Lack of blood supply to tissue
		R/	isch- *to block*	
ischemic (adj)	is-**KEY**-mik	S/	-emic *pertaining to a condition of the blood*	Pertaining to the lack of blood supply to tissue
myocardial (adj)	MY-oh-**KAR**-dee-al	S/	-al *pertaining to*	Pertaining to heart muscle
		R/CF	my/o- *muscle*	
		R/	-cardi- *heart*	
myocardium	MY-oh-**KAR**-dee-um	S/	-um *structure*	All the heart muscle
prognosis (noun)	prog-**NO**-sis	P/	pro- *before, project forward*	A forecast of the probable course and outcome of a disease
		R/	-gnosis *knowledge of an abnormal condition*	

Changing the suffix *-emia* to *-emic,* which means *pertaining to a condition of the blood,* creates a new term, **ischemic,** that is an adjective. It means *pertaining to a blockage of blood flow.* It has a **root** and a **suffix.**

EXERCISES

Precision in communication: *In addition to using the precise medical terms and speaking and spelling them correctly, you must use the appropriate form of the term as well.*

A. Reread the WAD entry for diagnosis. *Note that there are singular and plural forms of the term, as well as the noun, adjective, and verb forms. Insert the correct form of the term in the documentation below.*   **LO 1.1, 1.2, and 1.7** *Apply*

Note:	A noun is a person, place, or thing.	Singular: One
	A verb denotes action.	Plural: More than one
	An adjective usually describes something.	

1. The primary _____ for this patient is myocardial ischemia.

2. Dr. Bannerjee is unable to _____ this patient until he receives the lab results.

3. The _____ tests have been ordered for this patient first thing in the morning.

4. It is possible for this patient to have multiple _____ if there is more than one condition present.

B. Challenge your new knowledge *used in questions 1–4 above.*   **LO 1.4 and 1.7** *Apply*

1. Which sentence contains the verb form of the term?   _____

2. Which sentence contains the plural form of the term?   _____

3. Which sentence contains the singular noun?   _____

4. Which sentence contains an adjective form?   _____

Lesson 1.2

Communication

Some medical terms are pronounced the same but spelled differently. For example:

- Both *ilium* and *ileum* are pronounced **ILL**-ee-um. *Ilium* is a bone in the pelvis; *ileum* is a segment of the small intestine.

- Both *mucus* and *mucous* are pronounced **MYU**-kus. *Mucus* is a noun and is the name of a fluid secreted by *mucous* (adjective) membranes that line body cavities.

A medical term may relate to more than one anatomical structure.

- The term *cervical* means relating to a neck in any sense.

- It can pertain to the neck that joins the head to the trunk with the cervical vertebrae.

- It can also pertain to the cervix of the uterus, with its cervical canal.

Some words, when incorrectly pronounced, sound the same. For example:

- The term *prostate,* pronounced **PROS**-tate, refers to the gland at the base of the male bladder. The term *prostrate* means to be physically weak or exhausted, or to lie flat on the ground.

- Train your ear to hear the differences—*reflex* is not *reflux.*

Many medical terms form a verb, a noun, a plural, and an adjective, and you have to know them all, as in diagnose, diagnosis, diagnoses, and diagnostic (see the WAD on the previous spread).

Plurals (LO 1.5)

Many words in the English language allow you to change them from singular to plural by adding an "s." For medical terms, this rarely happens, as these plurals are formed in ways that were once logical to Greeks and Romans but now have to be learned by memory in English. Examples of medical terms with Greek and Latin plurals are shown in *Table 1.1.*

Throughout this book, the Greek and Latin plurals of medical terms appear in the Word Analysis and Definition box with the singular medical term, as with the term **diagnosis** in the previous spread.

▼ **TABLE 1.1**

SINGULAR AND PLURAL FORMS

Singular Ending	Plural Ending	Examples
-a		axilla
	-ae	axillae
-ax		thorax
	-aces	thoraces
-en		lumen
	-ina	lumina
-ex		cortex
	-ices	cortices
-is		diagnosis
	-es	diagnoses
-is		epididymis
	-ides	epididymides
-ix		appendix
	-ices	appendices
-ma		carcinoma
	-mata	carcinomata
-on		ganglion
	-a	ganglia
-um		septum
	-a	septa
-us		viscus
	-era	viscera
-us		villus
	-i	villi
-us		corpus
	-ora	corpora
-x		phalanx
	-ges	phalanges
-y		ovary
	-ies	ovaries
-yx		calyx
	-ices	calices

Pronunciation (LO 1.6)

Being able to pronounce words correctly is essential to effective communication. In the medical world, this concept is especially important. As a health professional, you will routinely use medical terms and your colleagues must be able to understand what you are saying. Correct pronunciation is crucial to patient safety and your ability to provide high-quality patient care.

Throughout this book, the pronunciation of medical terms is spelled out phonetically using modern English forms to show you exactly how the terms are pronounced. The word part to be emphasized is shown in bold, uppercase letters.

For example, **pulmonary** is phonetically written **PUL**-moh-nar-ee, and **pulmonology** is written **PUL**-moh-**NOL**-oh-jee. This illustrates that words derived from the same **root** can have their emphasis placed on different parts of the word and that the emphasized part can be from different elements. The emphasized syllable **NOL** comes partly from the **combining form** *pulmon/o-* and partly from the **suffix** *-logy.* You can hear glossary terms pronounced correctly by visiting the audio glossary in Connect® (connect.mheducation.com).

Word Analysis and Definition

WORD	PRONUNCIATION	ELEMENTS		DEFINITION
axilla axillae (pl) axillary (adj)	AK-sill-ah AK-sill-ee AK-sill-air-ee	 S/ R/	Latin *armpit* -ary *pertaining to* axill- *armpit*	Medical term for the armpit Pertaining to the armpit
dementia	dee-**MEN**-she-ah	S/ P/ R/	-ia *condition* de- *without* -ment- *mind*	Chronic, progressive, irreversible loss of intellectual and mental functions
ganglion ganglia (pl)	GANG-lee-on GANG-lee-ah		Greek *a swelling* or *knot*	A fluid-filled cyst or a collection of nerve cells outside the brain and spinal cord
ileum ilium ilia (pl)	ILL-ee-um ILL-ee-um ILL-ee-ah		Latin *to twist* or *roll up* Latin *groin*	Third portion of the small intestine. Large wing-shaped bone at the upper and posterior part of the pelvis
mucus (noun) mucous (adj) mucosa	MYU-kus MYU-kus myu-**KOH**-sah	 S/ R/ S/	Greek *slime* -ous *pertaining to* muc- *mucus* -osa *full of; like*	Sticky secretion of cells in mucous membranes Pertaining to mucus or the mucosa Lining of a tubular structure that secretes mucus
prostate prostrate prostration (noun)	**PROS**-tate pros-**TRAYT** pros-**TRAY**-shun		Greek *one who stands before* Latin *to stretch out*	Organ surrounding the urethra at the base of the male urinary bladder To lay flat or to be overcome by physical weakness and exhaustion
reflex reflux	**REE**-fleks **REE**-fluks		Latin *bend back* Latin *backward flow*	An involuntary response to a stimulus Backward flow
septum septa (pl)	**SEP**-tum **SEP**-tah		Latin *a partition*	A thin wall separating two cavities or two tissue masses

EXERCISES

A. Medical language: *Many terms in medicine sound and/or look very similar. The difference of only one letter can make a new term. Train your eye and ear to know the difference. Circle the correct choice of terms in the following documentation.* **LO 1.6 and 1.7** *Remember*

1. The patient's nasal (mucus/mucous) membrane is severely infected.

2. Schedule this patient for a (prostrate/prostate) exam at his next annual physical.

3. The doctor checked the (reflex/reflux) in the patient's knee.

4. The patient's (ilium/ileum) was severely fractured in the motor vehicle accident.

B. Plurals: *Circle the correct form of the plural in the following sentences.* **LO 1.5** *Remember*

1. Because of additional medical problems needing treatment, this patient's insurance claim form will have multiple (diagnoses/diagnosis).

2. Check both (axilla/axillae) for any evidence of enlarged lymph nodes.

3. Several (septa/septum) exist in the body—e.g., in the heart and in the nose.

4. A cluster of (ganglia/ganglion) has formed on her left wrist.

C. Terminology challenge: *Use your knowledge of the new medical terms you have learned in this chapter and answer the following questions.*
LO 1.7 *Apply*

1. The term *cervical* can apply to two different places in the body. Where are they?

_____

_____

2. The terms *ileum* and *ilium* are pronounced the same but are in two different body systems. Where are they?

_____

_____

Lesson 1.2 (cont'd)   Precision in Communication (LO 1.7)

Keynotes

- Many words, when they are written or pronounced, have an element that if misspelled or mispronounced gives the intended word an entirely different meaning. A treatment response to the different meaning could cause a medical error or even the death of a patient.

- Precision in written and verbal communication is essential to prevent errors in patient care.

- The medical record in which you document a patient's care and your actions is a legal document. It can be used in court as evidence in professional medical liability cases.

Abbreviation

IV   intravenous

Keynotes

- Communicate verbally and in writing with attention to detail, accuracy, and precision.

- When you understand the individual word elements that make up a medical term, you are better able to understand clearly the medical terms you are using.

It's important for you to note that being accurate and precise in both your written and verbal communication with your health care team can save someone's life. Each year in the United States, more than 400,000 people die because of drug reactions and medical errors, many of which are the result of poor communication. On the next page, you will find some specific examples of how certain medical terms could be seriously miscommunicated and misinterpreted.

In the above Case Report involving Mr. Donovan, if **hypotensive** (suffering from **low** blood pressure) were confused with **hypertensive** (suffering from **high** blood pressure), incorrect and dangerous treatments could be prescribed.

Case Report 1.2 (continued)

Mr. Donovan is waiting to be admitted to the hospital and is receiving oxygen through nasal prongs. He is **hypotensive**, and an **intravenous (IV) infusion** of normal saline has been started. According to his medical record, he is being seen in the **neurology** clinic for early dementia.

- In the word **hypotensive,** the suffix *-ive* means *pertaining to.* The prefix *hypo-* means *below or less than normal.* The root *-tens-* means *pressure.* The term **hypotensive** means *pertaining to or suffering from a below normal or low blood pressure.*

- In the word **hypertensive,** the prefix *hyper-* means *above or higher than normal.* The term **hypertensive** means *pertaining to or suffering from an above normal or high blood pressure.*

To deconstruct the term **hypotensive,** start with the suffix *-ive,* which means *pertaining to* or *suffering from.* Next, the prefix *hypo-* means *below or less than normal.* Then the root *-tens-* means *pressure.* Now, place the pieces together to form a word meaning *suffering from a below-normal pressure* or *low blood pressure.*

| HYPO-
prefix
below normal | + | -TENS-
root
pressure | + | -IVE
suffix
suffering from | = | **HYPOTENSIVE**
suffering from low blood pressure |

Also in the above Case Report, the term **neurology,** the specialty of the nervous system *(see Chapter 10),* can sound very similar to **urology,** the study of the urinary system *(see Chapter 13).* In the urinary system, if a patient's **ureter** (the tube from the kidney to the bladder) were confused with the **urethra** (the tube from the bladder to the outside), the consequences could be serious.

As you can see from the above examples, your ability to correctly identify, spell, and pronounce different medical terms is essential. Being a health professional requires the utmost attention to detail, as a patient's life could be in your hands. Incorrect spelling and poor pronunciation not only reflect badly on you and your health team—it could also be a matter of life and death.

WORD	PRONUNCIATION	ELEMENTS		DEFINITION
cervical (adj)	SER-vih-kal	S/ R/	-al *pertaining to* cervic- *neck*	Pertaining to the cervix or to the neck region
cervix	SER-viks		Latin *neck*	Lower part of the uterus
hypertension	HIGH-per-TEN-shun	S/ P/ R/	-ion *condition, action* hyper- *above normal* -tens- *pressure*	Persistent high arterial blood pressure
hypertensive (adj)	HIGH-per-TEN-siv	S/	-ive *pertaining to*	Pertaining to or suffering from high blood pressure
hypotension hypotensive (adj)	HIGH-poh-TEN-shun HIGH-poh-TEN-siv	P/	hypo- *below normal*	Persistent low arterial blood pressure Pertaining to or suffering from low blood pressure
infusion	in-FYU-zhun	P/ R/	in- *in* -fusion *to pour*	Introduction of a substance other than blood intravenously
transfusion	trans-FYU-zhun	P/	trans- *across, through*	Transfer of blood or a blood component from a donor to a recipient
intravenous	IN-trah-VEE-nus	S/ P/ R/	-ous *pertaining to* intra- *within, inside* -ven- *vein*	Inside a vein
neurology	nyu-ROL-oh-jee	S/ R/CF	-logy *study of* neur/o- *nerve*	Medical specialty of disorders of the nervous system
neurologist	nyu-ROL-oh-jist	S/	-logist *one who studies and is a specialist in*	Medical specialist in disorders of the nervous system
protocol	PRO-toe-kol		Latin *contents page of a book*	Detailed plan; in this case, for a regimen of therapy
ureter	you-REE-ter		Greek *urinary canal* Greek *passage for urine*	Tube that connects a kidney to the urinary bladder
urethra urology	you-REE-thrah you-ROL-oh-jee	S/ R/CF	-logy *study of* ur/o- *urine*	Canal leading from the bladder to the outside Medical specialty of disorders of the urinary system
uterus	YOU-ter-us		Latin *womb*	Organ in which an egg develops into a fetus
vertebra vertebrae (pl)	VER-teh-brah VER-teh-brae		Latin *bone in the spine*	One of the bones of the spinal column

EXERCISES

A. Patient documentation: *Read the following excerpts from patient charts and insert the correct medical term from the above Word Analysis and Definition (WAD) box. Always review the WAD before you start the exercise.*   **LO 1.7** *Apply*

1. This patient has several badly fractured _____ in his spinal column.

2. This patient has nerve damage. Refer him to the department of _____.

3. Schedule this patient for an _____ of chemotherapy drugs today.

4. This patient has low blood pressure—he is _____ and anemic.

5. I am ordering an immediate _____ of 2 units of whole blood for this patient.

6. Send this patient for _____ x-rays of his neck immediately.

B. Brain teaser: *Challenge yourself to analyze the question and insert the correct answers.*   **LO 1.1, 1.2, and 1.7** *Analyze*

1. If a medical specialist in the study of disorders of the nervous system is a neurologist, what is a medical specialist in the study of disorders of the urinary system called?

   (Hint: Use your knowledge of suffixes and roots to help you.)

2. What element is the difference between high blood pressure and low blood pressure? _____

3. What substances go through an infusion? _____

4. What substances go through a transfusion that do not go through an infusion? _____

Chapter Review exercises, along with additional practice items, are available in Connect!

The Body as a Whole

The Essentials of the Language of Anatomy

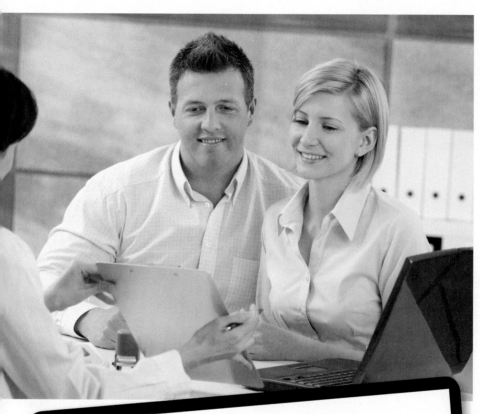

CHAPTER 2

Case Report 2.1

You are . . .

. . . a certified medical assistant (CMA) employed as an in vitro fertilization coordinator in the Assisted Reproduction Clinic at Fulwood Medical Center.

You are communicating with . . .

. . . Mrs. Mary Arnold, a 35-year-old woman who has been unable to **conceive. In vitro fertilization (IVF)** was recommended. After **hormone** therapy, several healthy and mature eggs were recovered from her **ovary**. The eggs were combined with her husband's **sperm** in a laboratory dish where **fertilization** occurred to form a single cell, called a **zygote**. The cells were allowed to divide for five days to become **blastocysts**, and then four blastocysts were implanted in her uterus.

Your role is to guide, counsel, and support Mrs. Arnold and her husband through the implementation and follow-up for the IVF process.

Learning Outcomes

Effective medical treatment recognizes that each organ, tissue, and cell in your body, no matter where it's located, is connected to and functions in harmony with every other organ, tissue, and cell. To understand these concepts, you need to be able to:

LO 2.1 Use roots, combining forms, suffixes, and prefixes to construct and analyze (deconstruct) medical terms related to the anatomy and physiology of the body as a whole.

LO 2.2 Spell and pronounce correctly medical terms related to the body as a whole in order to communicate with accuracy and precision in any health care setting.

LO 2.3 Discuss the medical terms associated with cells and tissues.

LO 2.4 Describe the primary tissue groups and their functions.

LO 2.5 Relate individual organs and organ systems to the organization and function of the body as a whole.

LO 2.6 Integrate the medical terms of the different anatomic positions, planes, and directions of the body into everyday medical language.

LO 2.7 Describe the nine regions of the abdomen.

LO 2.8 Map the body cavities.

LO 2.9 Apply your knowledge of the medical terms of the body as a whole to documentation, medical records, and medical reports.

LO 2.10 Translate the medical terms of the body as a whole into everyday language in order to communicate clearly with patients and their families.

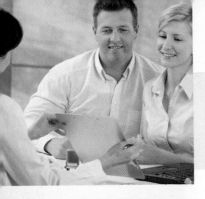

Lesson 2.1

Composition of Body and Cells

Objectives

All the different elements of your body interact with each other to support constant change as your body reacts to your environment and to the nourishment you give it. To understand the structure and function of the elements of your body, you need to be able to:

2.1.1 Name the medical terms associated with cells, tissues, and organs.

2.1.2 Discuss the medical terminology for the major structures and functions of a cell.

Composition of the Body (LO 2.1 and 2.2)

- The whole body or organism is composed of **organ systems** *(Figure 2.1)*.
  - Organ systems are composed of **organs.**
    - Organs are composed of **tissues.**
      - Tissues are composed of **cells.**
        - Cells are composed in part of **organelles.**
          - Organelles are composed of **molecules.**
            - Molecules are composed of **atoms.**

Organism   Body system   Organ   Tissue   Cell   Organelle   Molecule   Atom

▲ **FIGURE 2.1**
Composition of the Body.

The Cell (LO 2.3)

The result of the **fertilization** of an egg by a sperm is a single fertilized cell called a **zygote** *(Figure 2.2)*. This process is also called **conception.** This zygote is the origin of every cell in your body. It divides and multiplies into trillions of cells, which become the basic unit of every tissue and organ. These cells are responsible for the structure and all the functions of your tissues and organs.

Cytology is the study of cell structure and function, and this forms the basis of the knowledge of the anatomy and physiology of every tissue and organ.

▲ **FIGURE 2.2**
Fertilization of Egg by Single Sperm.

Case Report 2.1 (continued)

Mrs. Arnold achieved pregnancy and delivered a healthy girl at term.

Word Analysis and Definition

S = Suffix   P = Prefix   R = Root   R/CF = Combining Form

WORD	PRONUNCIATION		ELEMENTS	DEFINITION
cell	SELL		Latin *a storeroom*	The smallest unit of the body capable of independent existence
conception	kon-**SEP**-shun		Latin *something received*	Fertilization of the egg by sperm to form a zygote
cytology	**SIGH**-tol-oh-jee	S/ R/CF	-logy *study of* cyt/o- *cell*	Study of the cell
cytologist	**SIGH**-tol-oh-jist	S/	-logist *one who studies, a specialist*	Specialist in the structure, chemistry, and pathology of the cell
fertilization (noun)	FER-til-eye-**ZAY**-shun	S/ R/	-ation *process* fertiliz- *to make fruitful*	Union of a male sperm and a female egg
fertilize (verb) in vitro	FER-til-ize en-**VEE**-troh		Greek *to bear* Latin *glass*	Penetration of the egg by sperm In vitro fertilization is the process of combining sperm and eggs in a laboratory dish and placing resulting embryos inside a uterus
organ	OR-gan		Latin *instrument, tool*	Structure with specific functions in a body system
organelle	OR-gah-nell	S/ R/	-elle *small* organ- *organ*	Part of a cell having specialized function(s)
organism	OR-gan-izm	S/	-ism *condition, process*	Any whole living, individual plant or animal
tissue	TISH-you		Latin *to weave*	Collection of similar cells
zygote	ZYE-goat		Greek *yolk*	Cell resulting from the union of sperm and egg

EXERCISES

A. Review *the terms in the WAD box above and the text on the opposite page before answering the questions. Pay careful attention to word elements and meanings. Fill in the blanks.*   **LO 2.1 and 2.3** *Remember*

1. Put the following terms in ascending order of their size:

organism	cells	molecules	organs
organ systems	organelles	atoms	tissues

    a. _____

    b. _____

    c. _____

    d. _____

    e. _____

    f. _____

    g. _____

    h. _____

B. Review the WAD *before answering the questions.*   **LO 2.1 and 2.2** *Apply*

1. The suffix _____ means *study of.* The suffix that means *specialist (in the study of)* is _____.

2. What part of *cyt/o* makes it a combining form rather than a root? _____

3. What is the medical term for *union of a male sperm and a female egg?* _____

4. What suffix in the WAD describes the size of something? _____

5. What does a cytologist study? _____

Structure and Function of Cells (LO 2.3)

As the zygote divides, every cell it creates becomes a complex little factory that carries out these basic life functions:

• **Manufacture** of **proteins** and **lipids;**

• **Production** and use of energy;

• **Communication** with other cells;

• **Replication** of **deoxyribonucleic acid (DNA);** and

• **Reproduction** of itself.

All cells contain a fluid called **cytoplasm** (intracellular fluid) surrounded by a cell **membrane** *(Figure 2.3)*. Your cell membrane—made of **proteins** and **lipids**—allows water, oxygen, glucose, **electrolytes, steroids,** and alcohol to pass through it. On the outside of the cell membrane, you have receptors that bind to chemical messengers like **hormones** sent by other cells. These are the chemical signals by which your cells communicate with each other.

Organelles (LO 2.2)

Organelles are small structures in the cytoplasm of the cell that carry out special **metabolic** tasks (the chemical processes that occur in the cell).

The **nucleus** is the largest organelle *(Figure 2.3)*. It is surrounded by its own membrane and directs all the cell's activities. The 46 molecules of DNA in the nucleus form 46 **chromosomes.**

A **nucleolus** is a small, dense body composed of **ribonucleic acid** (**RNA**) and protein found in the nucleus. It is involved in the manufacture of proteins from simple materials—a process called **anabolism.**

Mitochondria are the cell's powerhouses. They produce energy by breaking down compounds like glucose and fat in a process called **catabolism.**

• **Metabolism** is the sum of the constructive processes of anabolism and the destructive processes of catabolism within a cell (**intracellular).**

The **endoplasmic reticulum** manufactures steroids, cholesterol and other lipids, and proteins. It also detoxifies alcohol and other drugs.

Apical surface of cell · Receptors · Cytoplasm · Cell membrane · Endoplasmic reticulum · Nucleus · Nucleolus · Mitochondrion

▲ **FIGURE 2.3**
Structure of a Representative Cell.

Word Analysis and Definition

WORD	PRONUNCIATION	ELEMENTS		DEFINITION
anabolism	an-**AB**-oh-lizm	S/ R/	-ism *process, condition* anabol- *build up*	The buildup of complex substances in the cell from simpler ones as a part of metabolism
catabolism	kah-**TAB**-oh-lizm	S/ R/	-ism *process, condition* catabol- *break down*	The breakdown of complex substances into simpler ones as a part of metabolism
chromosome	**KROH**-moh-sohm	S/ R/CF	-some *body* chrom/o- *color*	Body in the nucleus that contains DNA and genes
cytoplasm	**SIGH**-toh-plazm	S/ R/CF	-plasm *something formed* cyt/o- *cell*	Clear, gelatinous substance that forms the substance of a cell, except for the nucleus
deoxyribonucleic acid (DNA)	dee-**OCK**-see-rye-boh-nyu-**KLEE**-ik **ASS**-id		deoxyribose *a sugar* nucleic acid *a protein*	Source of hereditary characteristics found in chromosomes
electrolyte	ee-**LEK**-troh-lite	S/ R/CF	-lyte *soluble* electr/o- *electricity*	Substance that, when dissolved in a suitable medium, forms electrically charged particles
hormone	**HOR**-mohn		Greek *set in motion*	Chemical formed in one tissue or organ and carried by the blood to stimulate or inhibit a function of another tissue or organ
hormonal (adj)	hor-**MOHN**-al	S/ R/	-al *pertaining to* hormon- *hormone*	Pertaining to a hormone
intracellular	in-trah-**SELL**-you-lar	S/ P/ R/	-ar *pertaining to* intra- *within* -cellul- *small cell*	Within the cell
lipid	**LIP**-id		Greek *fat*	General term for all types of fatty compounds; for example, cholesterol, triglycerides, and fatty acids
membrane membranous (adj)	**MEM**-brain **MEM**-brah-nus	S/ R/	Latin *parchment* -ous *pertaining to* membran- *cover, skin*	Thin layer of tissue covering a structure or cavity Pertaining to a membrane
metabolism	meh-**TAB**-oh-lizm	S/ R/	-ism *condition, process* metabol- *change*	The constantly changing physical and chemical processes occurring in the cell that are the sum of anabolism and catabolism
metabolic (adj)	met-ah-**BOL**-ik	S/	-ic *pertaining to*	Pertaining to metabolism
mitochondria (pl)	my-toe-**KON**-dree-ah	S/ R/CF R/	-ia *condition* mit/o- *thread* -chondr- *granule*	Organelles that generate, store, and release energy for cell activities
mitochondrion (singular)	my-toe-**KON**-dree-on	S/	-ion *condition*	
nucleolus	nyu-**KLEE**-oh-lus	S/ R/CF	-lus *small* nucle/o- *nucleus*	Small mass within the nucleus
nucleus nuclear (adj)	**NYU**-klee-us **NYU**-klee-ar	S/ R/	Latin *command center* -ar *pertaining to* nucle- *nucleus*	Functional center of a cell or structure Pertaining to a nucleus
protein	**PRO**-teen		Greek *protein*	Class of food substances based on amino acids
ribonucleic acid (RNA)	RYE-boh-nyu-**KLEE**-ik **ASS**-id	S/ P/ R/	-ic *pertaining to* ribo- *from ribose, a sugar* -nucle- *nucleus*	The information carrier from DNA in the nucleus to an organelle to produce protein molecules
steroid	**STAIR**-oyd	S/ R/	-oid *resembling* ster- *solid*	Large family of chemical substances found in many drugs, hormones, and body components

Exercise

A. *Knowledge of elements is your best clue to determining the meaning of medical terminology. Deconstruct the elements in these questions to find your answers. Review the WAD before attempting to answer the questions. Circle the BEST ANSWER to the question.* **LO 2.3** *Analyze*

1. Which term relates to electrically charged particles?

   protein   hormonal   electrolyte

2. Which term relates to change?

   steroid   metabolic   lipid

3. Which term has an element meaning "condition"?

   metabolism   cytoplasm   hormone

4. What is a thin layer of tissue that covers a structure or cavity?

   lipid   membrane   hormone

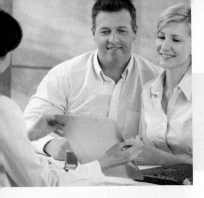

Lesson 2.2

Tissues, Organs, and Organ Systems

Objectives

Your tissues, organs, and organ systems must continually adapt and adjust in order to work in sync with each other. The information in this lesson will enable you to:

2.2.1 Define the four primary tissue groups.

2.2.2 Discuss the medical terminology for the structure and functions of each tissue group.

2.2.3 Name the organ systems.

2.2.4 Describe the medical terminology for the strucure and functions of each organ system.

Tissues (LO 2.3)

Tissues hold your body together. Each tissue is different but made of similar cells with unique materials around them manufactured by the cells. The many tissues of your body have different structures that enable them to perform specialized functions. **Histology** is the study of the structure and function of tissues. The four primary tissue groups are outlined in *Table 2.1*.

Case Report 2.2

You are . . .

. . . a physical therapy assistant employed in the Rehabilitation Unit in Fulwood Medical Center.

You are communicating with . . .

. . . Mr. Richard Josen, a 22-year-old man who injured tissues in his left knee while playing football (*Figure 2.4*). Using **arthroscopy**, the orthopedic surgeon removed his torn **anterior cruciate ligament (ACL)** and replaced it with a **graft** from his **patellar tendon.** The torn medial collateral ligament was **sutured** together. The tear in his medial **meniscus** was repaired. Rehabilitation is focused on strengthening the **muscles** around his knee joint and regaining joint mobility and stability.

▼ **TABLE 2.1**

THE FOUR PRIMARY TISSUE GROUPS (LO 2.4)

Type	Function	Location
Connective	Bind, support, protect, fill spaces, store fat	Widely distributed throughout the body, e.g., in blood, bone, cartilage, and fat
Epithelial	Protect, secrete, absorb, excrete	Cover body surface, cover and line internal organs, compose glands
Muscle	Movement	Attached to bones; found in the walls of hollow tubes, organs, and the heart
Nervous	Transmit impulses for coordination, sensory reception, motor actions	Brain, spinal cord, nerves

Adapted from David Shier, Jackie L. Butler, and Ricki Lewis, *Hole's Human Anatomy and Physiology*, 10th ed. Copyright © 2004 The McGraw-Hill Companies, Inc. Adapted with permission.

▶ **FIGURE 2.4**
Knee Anatomy.
(a) Injury to left knee.
(b) Normal knee.

Abbreviation

ACL   anterior cruciate ligament

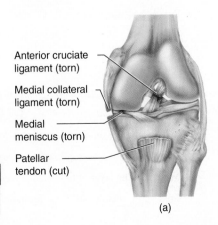

Anterior cruciate ligament (torn)

Medial collateral ligament (torn)

Medial meniscus (torn)

Patellar tendon (cut)

(a)

Femur

Cartilage

Tibia

Quadriceps muscle

Patella

Synovial fluid

Synovial membrane

Patellar tendon

(b)

Word Analysis and Definition

WORD	PRONUNCIATION	ELEMENTS		DEFINITION
arthroscopy	ar-**THROS**-koh-pee	S/	-scopy *to examine, to view*	Visual examination of the interior of a joint
		R/CF	arthr/o- *joint*	
connective tissue	koh-**NECK**-tiv **TISH**-you	S/ R/	-ive *pertaining to* connect- *join together* tissue Latin *to weave*	The supporting tissue of the body
cruciate	**KRU**-she-ate		Latin *cross*	Shaped like a cross
graft	**GRAFT**		French *transplant*	Transplantation of living tissue
histology	his-**TOL**-oh-jee	S/ R/CF	-logy *study of* hist/o- *tissue*	Study of the structure and function of cells, tissues, and organs
histologist	his-**TOL**-oh-jist	S/	-logist *one who studies, specialist*	Specialist in histology
ligament	**LIG**-ah-ment		Latin *band*	Band of fibrous tissue connecting two structures
meniscus	meh-**NISS**-kuss		Greek *crescent*	Disc of cartilage between the bones of a joint
muscle	**MUSS**-el		Latin *muscle*	A tissue consisting of contractile cells
patella (singular) patellae (pl)	pah-**TELL**-ah pah-**TELL**-ee		Latin *small plate*	Thin, circular bone embedded in the patellar tendon in front of the knee joint; also called the kneecap
patellar (adj)	pah-**TELL**-ar	S/ R/	-ar *pertaining to* patell- *patella*	Pertaining to the patella
therapy	**THAIR**-ah-pee		Greek *medical treatment*	Systematic treatment of a disease, dysfunction, or disorder
therapeutic	**THAIR**-ah-**PYU**-tik	S/ R/	-ic *pertaining to* therapeut- *treatment*	Relating to the treatment of a disease or disorder
therapist	**THAIR**-ah-pist	S/ R/	-ist *specialist* therap- *treatment*	Professional trained in the practice of a particular therapy

EXERCISES

A. Review *the Case Report on this two-page spread before answering the questions.*   **LO 2.2 and 2.4** *Analyze*

1. How was Mr. Josen injured? _____

2. What type of procedure is an arthroscopy? _____

3. Where is the patellar tendon located? _____

4. What two specific knee components were repaired? _____

5. What other component could not be repaired and required replacement? _____

B. Dictionary exercise: *When you are working in the medical field, you will be exposed to medical terms you may not recognize. Learn to use the glossary or a good medical dictionary, or practice going online to find the definitions you need. The Case Report on the opposite page contains some terms that are not defined in the WAD above.*   **LO 2.2 and 2.9** *Apply*

Use the glossary or a dictionary (or go online) to define each of the following terms and identify it as noun, verb, or adjective.

1. orthopedic   (noun, verb, adjective) _____

Definition: _____

2. collateral   (noun, verb, adjective) _____

Definition: _____

3. sutured   (noun, verb, adjective) _____

Definition: _____

Lesson 2.2 (cont'd)

Keynotes

- Different tissues are made of specialized cells that manufacture unique fluids. The epithelial layer of the connective tissue synovial membrane is an example, as it produces the lubricant synovial fluid.

- Each connective tissue has distinct functions that enable a structure or organ to function correctly.

- There are four major ligaments of the knee joint:
  1. anterior cruciate ligament (ACL)
  2. posterior cruciate ligament (PCL)
  3. medial collateral ligament (MCL)
  4. lateral collateral ligament (LCL)

Connective Tissues (LO 2.4)

The relation of structure to function in your body tissues is key. To help you understand this important connection, this lesson uses the knee joint to illustrate the structures and functions of the different tissues found in this joint.

Connective Tissues in the Knee Joint (LO 2.4)

The connective tissues in your knee joint make it possible for you to enjoy your daily life—from standing, sitting, walking, bending, and running. These tissues and their roles are listed below:

- The **bones** of the knee joint are the **femur, tibia,** and **patella** *(see Chapter 4)*. Bone is the hardest connective tissue in your body because it contains calcium mineral salts (mainly calcium phosphate). Bones have a good blood supply so they can heal well after a fracture. Bones in general are covered with a thick fibrous tissue called the **periosteum.**

- **Cartilage** has a flexible, rubbery **matrix** (in the knee as a **meniscus**) that allows it to function as a shock absorber and a gliding surface where two bones meet to form a joint. Cartilage has very few blood vessels and heals poorly—sometimes not at all. When it is injured or torn, surgery is often needed. Cartilage also forms the shape of your ear, the tip of your nose, and your larynx.

- **Ligaments** are strips or bands of fibrous connective tissue

made of **collagen** fibers. The knee joint has four major ligaments that hold it together. The blood supply to these ligaments is poor, so they do not heal well without surgery *(Figure 2.5).*

- **Tendons** are thick, strong ligaments that attach muscles to bone.

- The **joint capsule** of the knee joint encloses the joint cavity. It's made of thin, fibrous connective tissue and strengthened by fibers that extend over it from the surrounding ligaments and muscles. These features are common to most joints.

- The **synovial membrane** lines many joint capsules and secretes **synovial fluid**—a slippery lubricant stored in the joint cavity. This fluid makes joint movement almost friction-free. It distributes **nutrients** to the cartilage on the joint surfaces of bone.

- **Muscle tissue** stabilizes the joint. Extensions of the large muscle tendons in the front and the rear of the thigh are major stabilizers of the knee joint. The muscles alone extend and flex the knee joint *(see Chapter 4).*

- **Nervous tissue** carries messages between the brain and the knee structures. All the knee structures are packed with nerves, which is why a knee injury is excruciatingly painful.

Femur

Lateral collateral ligament

Lateral meniscus

Fibula

Posterior cruciate ligament

Anterior cruciate ligament

Medial meniscus

Medial collateral ligament

Tibia

▶ **FIGURE 2.5**
Ligaments of Knee Joint, with the Patellar Tendon Removed.

Anterior view

WORD	PRONUNCIATION		ELEMENTS	DEFINITION
capsule	**KAP**-syul		Latin *little box*	Fibrous tissue layer surrounding a joint or other structure
capsular (adj)	**KAP**-syu-lar	S/ R/	-ar *pertaining to* capsul- *box*	Pertaining to a capsule
cartilage	**KAR**-tih-lage		Latin *gristle*	Nonvascular, firm connective tissue found mostly in joints
collagen	**KOLL**-ah-jen	S/ R/CF	-gen *produce, form* coll/a- *glue*	Major protein of connective tissue, cartilage, and bone
matrix	**MAY**-triks		Latin mater *mother*	Substance that surrounds and protects cells, is manufactured by the cells, and holds them together
nutrient	**NYU**-tree-ent	S/ R/	-ent *end result* nutri- *nourish*	A substance in food required for normal physiologic function
periosteum	**PER**-ee-**OSS**-tee-um	S/ P/ R/	-um *tissue* peri- *around* -oste- *bone*	Fibrous membrane covering a bone
synovial	si-**NOH**-vee-al	S/ P/ R/CF	-ial *pertaining to* syn- *together* -ov- *egg*	Pertaining to the synovial membrane or fluid
tendon	**TEN**-dun		Latin *sinew*	Fibrous band that connects muscle to bone

EXERCISES

A. Construct *the medical term given by the definition.*   **LO 2.4** *Apply*

1. Fibrous membrane covering a bone: _____ / _____ / _____

                                        P   R/CF   S

2. Major protein of connective tissue: _____ / _____ / _____

                                          P   R/CF   S

3. Pertaining to the synovial membrane _____ / _____ / _____

                                          P   R/CF   S

4. Substance in food _____ / _____ / _____

                                P   R/CF   S

B. Construct *the medical term that correctly answers the question.*   **LO 2.4** *Apply*

1. What is the only term in the WAD that contains a prefix, root, and suffix? _____ / _____ / _____

                                        P   R/CF   S

2. Which term contains an element that means *glue?* _____ / _____ / _____

                                      P   R/CF   S

3. What is the only term in the WAD that contains a prefix, combining form, and suffix? _____ / _____ / _____

                                          P   R/CF   S

4. What is the term for nonvascular, firm connective tissue found mostly in joints? _____

5. What terms in this WAD do not deconstruct into elements? _____

- Homeostasis is the coordinated response of all the organs to maintain the internal physiologic stability of an organism.

Organs and Organ Systems (LO 2.5)

An **organ** is a structure composed of several tissues that work together to carry out specific functions. For example, your skin is an organ that has different tissues in it, such as epithelial cells, hair, nails, and glands *(see Chapter 3)*.

An **organ system** is a group of organs with a specific collective function, like digestion, circulation, or respiration. For example, your nose, pharynx, larynx, trachea, bronchi, and lungs all work together to achieve the total function of respiration *(see Chapter 8)*.

The different organs in an organ system are usually interconnected. For example, in the **urinary** organ system *(Figure 2.6)*, the organs are the kidneys, ureters, bladder, and urethra, and they are all connected *(see Chapter 13)*.

All your organ systems work together to ensure that your body's internal environment remains relatively constant. This process is called **homeostasis.** It ensures that cells receive adequate nutrients and oxygen. It also ensures that cell waste products are removed so your cells can function normally. Disease affecting an organ or organ system disrupts the homeostasis game plan.

Your body has 11 organ systems, as shown in *Table 2.2*. Muscular and **skeletal** are considered one organ system called the musculoskeletal system *(see Chapters 4 and 5)*. Each body system has a chapter in this book where the terms associated with it are defined.

▼ **TABLE 2.2**
ORGAN SYSTEMS LO 2.5

Organ System	Major Organs	Major Functions
Integumentary	Skin, hair, nails, sweat glands, sebaceous glands	Protect tissues, regulate body temperature, support sensory receptors
Skeletal	Bones, ligaments, cartilage	Provide framework, protect soft tissues, provide attachments for muscles, produce blood cells, store inorganic salts
Muscular	Muscles	Cause movements, maintain posture, produce body heat
Nervous	Brain, spinal cord, nerves, sense organs	Receive and interpret sensory information and, in response, stimulate muscles, glands, and other organ systems
Endocrine	Glands that secrete hormones: pituitary, thyroid, parathyroid, adrenal, pancreas, ovaries, testes, pineal, thymus	Control metabolic activities of organs
Cardiovascular	Heart, blood vessels	Move blood and transport substances throughout body
Lymphatic	Lymph vessels and nodes, thymus, spleen	Defend body against infection, return tissue fluid to blood, carry certain absorbed food molecules
Digestive	Mouth, tongue, teeth, salivary glands, pharynx, esophagus, stomach, liver, gallbladder, pancreas, small and large intestines	Receive, break down, and absorb food; eliminate unabsorbed material
Respiratory	Nasal cavity, pharynx, larynx, trachea, bronchi, lungs	Intake and output air, exchange gases between air and blood
Urinary	Kidneys, ureters, urinary bladder, urethra	Remove wastes from blood, maintain water and electrolyte balance, store and transport urine
Reproductive	Male: scrotum, testes, epididymides, vasa deferentia, seminal vesicles, prostate, bulbourethral glands, urethra, penis	Produce and maintain sperm cells, transfer sperm cells into female reproductive tract
	Female: ovaries, fallopian tubes, uterus, vagina, vulva	Produce and maintain egg cells, receive sperm cells, support development of an embryo, function in birth process

Adapted from David Shier, Jackie L. Butler, and Ricki Lewis, *Hole's Human Anatomy and Physiology, 10th ed.* Copyright © 2004 The McGraw-Hill Companies, Inc. Adapted with permission.

▲ **FIGURE 2.6**
The Urinary System.

Word Analysis and Definition

S = Suffix   P = Prefix   R = Root   R/CF = Combining Form

WORD	PRONUNCIATION		ELEMENTS	DEFINITION
abdomen	AB-doh-men		Latin *abdomen*	Part of the trunk between the thorax and the pelvis
abdominal (adj)	ab-DOM-in-al	S/ R/	-al *pertaining to* abdomin- *abdomen*	Pertaining to the abdomen
abdominopelvic	ab-DOM-ih-no-PEL-vik	S/ R/CF R/	-ic *pertaining to* abdomin/o- *abdomen* -pelv- *pelvis*	Pertaining to the abdomen and pelvis
cavity	KAV-ih-tee	S/	-ity *state, condition*	A hollow space or body compartment
cavities (pl)	KAV-ih-teez	R/	cav- *hollow space*	
cranial (adj)	KRAY-nee-al	S/ R/	-al *pertaining to* crani- *skull*	Pertaining to the cranium
cranium	KRAY-nee-um	S/	-um *structure*	The skull
diaphragm	DIE-ah-fram		Greek *diaphragm, fence*	Muscular sheet separating the abdominal and thoracic cavities
diaphragmatic (adj)	DIE-ah-frag-MAT-ik	S/ R/	-ic *pertaining to* diaphragmat- *diaphragm*	Pertaining to the diaphragm
quadrant	KWAD-rant		Latin *one quarter*	One quarter of a circle; one of four regions of the surface of the abdomen
spine	SPYN		Latin *spine*	The vertebral column or a short bony projection
spinal (adj)	SPY-nal	S/ R/	-al *pertaining to* spin- *spine*	Pertaining to the spine
thoracic (adj)	THOR-ass-ik	S/ R/	-ic *pertaining to* thorac- *chest*	Pertaining to the chest (thorax)
thorax	THOR-acks		Greek *chest*	The part of the trunk between the abdomen and the neck
umbilical (adj)	um-BILL-ih-kal	S/ R/	-al *pertaining to* umbilic- *navel (belly button)*	Pertaining to the umbilicus or the center of the abdomen
umbilicus	um-BILL-ih-kuss		Latin *navel (belly button)*	Pit in the abdomen where the umbilical cord entered the fetus

EXERCISES

A. Deconstruct the following terms *into their basic elements. Note that not every type of element will appear in every term. The only element every term needs is a root or a combining form. Fill in the blanks.* **LO 2.1 and 2.8** *Analyze*

1. diaphragmatic _____ / _____ / _____

    P   R/CF   S

2. abdominopelvic _____ / _____ / _____

    P   R/CF   S

3. umbilical _____ / _____ / _____

    P   R/CF   S

4. cranial _____ / _____ / _____

    P   R/CF   S

5. thoracic _____ / _____ / _____

    P   R/CF   S

6. cavity _____ / _____ / _____

    P   R/CF   S

B. Analyze the elements *in the terms in Exercise A to get the correct answers.* **LO 2.7 and 2.8** *Analyze*

1. Which term contains a root and a combining vowel? _____

2. Which term is a muscle that separates body cavities? _____

3. The term "quadrant" represents what number? _____

4. The term "spine" also means _____

5. What term in the WAD is a dentist likely to use? _____

Chapter Review exercises, along with additional practice items, are available in Connect!

The Integumentary System

The Essentials of the Language of Dermatology

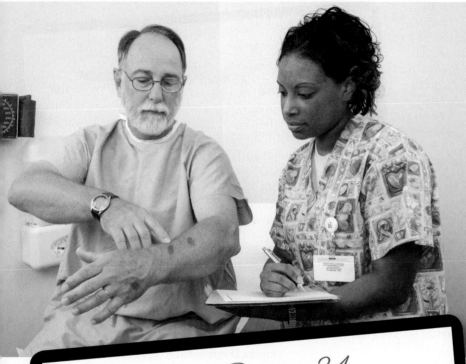

Learning Outcomes

In addition to anticipating Dr. Echols' needs for equipment to **biopsy,** diagnose, and treat the lesions, you also have to be able to communicate clearly with her in medical terms and understand her language as she communicates with you and the patient about the **etiology** (cause) and structure of the lesions. You will then need to document the medical history and treatment and communicate clearly with Mr. Andrews about the treatment of his lesions and their **prognosis.**

To perform these tasks, you must be able to:

LO 3.1 Use roots, combining forms, suffixes, and prefixes to construct and analyze medical terms related to the integumentary system.

LO 3.2 Spell and pronounce correctly medical terms and their plurals related to the integumentary system to communicate them with accuracy and precision in any health care setting.

LO 3.3 Define accepted abbreviations related to the integumentary system.

LO 3.4 Relate the anatomical structures of the integumentary system and their locations to their functions.

LO 3.5 Describe common disorders of and injuries to the skin and its accessory glands.

LO 3.6 Identify pharmacologic agents and other methods used to treat disorders of the integumentary system.

LO 3.7 Apply your knowledge of medical terms relating to the integumentary system to documentation, medical records, and medical reports.

LO 3.8 Translate the medical terms relating to the integumentary system into everyday language in order to communicate clearly with patients and their families.

Case Report 3.1

You are . . .

. . . a dermatology technologist working with dermatologist Laura Echols, MD, a member of the Fulwood Medical Group.

You are communicating with . . .

. . . Mr. Rod Andrews, a 60-year-old man, who shows you three skin lesions—two on his left forearm and one on the back of his left hand. You learn that he has been living in Arizona for the past 10 years but has recently returned to this area in order to live near his daughter and young grandchildren. You find no other skin lesions on his body.

The health professionals involved in the diagnosis and treatment of problems with the integumentary system include the following:

- **Dermatologists** are medical doctors who are specialists in skin disorders.

- **Dermatology technologists** are medical assistants who have an additional year of training in dermatology.

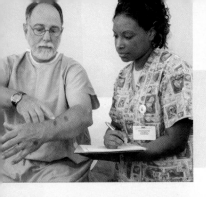

Lesson 3.1
Functions and Structure of the Skin

Objectives

*Your skin is your largest organ—it covers your entire body. The three lesions on Mr. Andrews' arm and hand developed in the outer layer of the skin, the **epidermis**. This lesson looks at the structure and function of the skin so that you will be able to use correct medical terminology to:*

3.1.1 Describe the functions of the skin.

3.1.2 Name the tissues in the different layers of the skin.

3.1.3 Specify the functions of the different layers of the skin.

Your skin's nerves allow you to feel heat, cold, pain, and comfort. Your skin wards off infections and protects your body from harmful environmental elements. Your skin is constantly shedding old cells in order to make room for new skin growth.

The **integumentary system** consists of your skin and its associated organs. **Dermatology** is the study and treatment of the integumentary system. A **dermatologist** is a medical specialist in the disorders of the skin.

Case Report 3.1 (continued)

When Dr. Echols examined Mr. Andrews, she determined that two of his lesions were basal cell **carcinomas** and treated them with **cryosurgery**, an approach that involves freezing cancerous tissue. She believed that the third lesion was a **squamous cell** carcinoma and performed a biopsy removal of the **cutaneous** (skin) lesion. You sent this to the laboratory with a request for a pathologic diagnosis and determination of whether the lesion had been completely removed.

Functions of the Skin (LO 3.1, 3.2, and 3.4)

Your skin functions in several ways to keep you healthy and safe. These important functions include the following:

- **Protection:** Your skin is a physical barrier against injury, chemicals, ultraviolet rays, microbes, and toxins and is not easily breached *(Figure 3.1)*. Bacteria and other pathogens, called normal **flora**, populate your skin's surface.

- **Water resistance:** You don't swell up every time you take a bath because your skin is water resistant. It also prevents water from leaking out of body tissues.

- **Temperature regulation:** A network of capillaries in your skin opens up or dilates **(vasodilation)** when your body is too hot. When your body is cold, this capillary network narrows **(vasoconstriction),** blood flow decreases, and your body retains heat.

- The structure of the skin to enable these functions to take place is detailed in the next section.

- **Vitamin D synthesis:** As little as 15 to 30 minutes of sunlight each day allow your skin cells to initiate the metabolism of vitamin D, which is essential for bone growth and maintenance.

- **Sensation:** Nerve endings that detect touch, pressure, heat, cold, pain, vibration, and tissue injury are particularly numerous in the skin of your face, fingers, palms, soles, nipples, and genitals.

- **Excretion and secretion:** Water and small amounts of waste products from cell metabolism are lost through your skin by **excretion** and **secretion** from your sweat glands.

- **Social functions:** The skin reflects your emotions: it blushes when you are self-conscious, goes pale when you are frightened, and wrinkles when you register disgust.

◀ **FIGURE 3.1**
Integumentary System.
The skin provides protection, contains sensory organs, and helps control body temperature.

Word Analysis and Definition

S = Suffix   P = Prefix   R = Root   R/CF = Combining Form

WORD	PRONUNCIATION	ELEMENTS		DEFINITION
biopsy	BI-op-see	S/ R/	-opsy *to view* bi- *life*	Removing tissue from a living person for laboratory examination
carcinoma	kar-sih-NOH-mah	S/ R/	-oma *tumor, mass* carcin- *cancer*	A malignant and invasive epithelial tumor
cryosurgery	cry-oh-SUR-jer-ee	S/ R/CF R/	-ery *process of* cry/o- *icy cold* -surg- *operate*	Use of liquid nitrogen or argon gas in a probe to freeze and kill abnormal tissue
cutaneous	kyu-TAY-nee-us	S/ R/CF	-ous *pertaining to* cutan/e- *skin*	Pertaining to the skin
dermatology	der-mah-TOL-oh-jee	S/ R/CF	-logy *study of* dermat/o- *skin*	Medical specialty concerned with disorders of the skin
dermatologist	der-mah-TOL-oh-jist	S/	-logist *one who studies, specialist*	Medical specialist in diseases of the skin
dermatologic (adj)	der-mah-toh-LOJ-ik	S/	-ic *pertaining to*	Pertaining to the skin and dermatology
etiology	ee-tee-OL-oh-jee	S/ R/CF	-logy *study of* eti/o- *cause*	The study of the causes of a disease
excrete (verb)	eks-KREET	P/ R	ex- *out of, away from* -crete *separate*	To pass waste products of metabolism out of the body
excretion (noun)	eks-KREE-shun	S/	-ion *action*	Removal of waste products of metabolism out of the body
flora	FLO-rah		Latin *flower*	The population of microorganisms covering the exterior and interior surfaces of healthy animals
integument	in-TEG-you-ment		Latin *a covering*	Organ system that covers the body, the skin being the main organ within the system
integumentary (adj)	in-TEG-you-MENT-ah-ree	S/ R/	-ary *pertaining to* integument- *covering of the body*	Pertaining to the covering of the body
prognosis	prog-NO-sis	P/ R/	pro- *projecting forward* -gnosis *knowledge*	Forecast of the probable future course and outcome of a disease
secrete (verb)	seh-KREET	R/	secret- *produce*	To produce a chemical substance in a cell and release it from the cell
secretion (noun)	seh-KREE-shun	S/	-ion *action*	Production by a cell(s) of a physiologically active substance and its movement out of the cell.
squamous cell	SKWAY-mus SELL		squamous Latin *scaly*	Flat, scale-like epithelial cell
synthesis	SIN-the-sis	P/ R/	syn- *together* -thesis *to organize, arrange*	The process of building a compound from different elements
synthetic (adj)	sin-THET-ik	S/ R/	-ic *pertaining to* -thet- *arrange, organize*	Built up or put together from simpler compounds
vasoconstriction	VAY-soh-con-STRIK-shun	S/ R/CF R/	-ion *action* vas/o- *blood vessel* -constrict- *narrow*	Reduction in diameter of a blood vessel
vasodilation	VAY-soh-die-LAY-shun	R/	-dilat- *widen, open up*	Increase in diameter of a blood vessel

EXERCISE

A. *Name three suffixes that mean "pertaining to":* _____ **LO 3.1** *Remember*

B. Review *the Case Report on this spread before answering the questions.*   **LO 3.2 and 3.8** *Understand*

1. Mr. Andrews' skin lesions were two different types. What were they? _____

2. What different types of treatment did Dr. Echols use to remove these lesions? _____

3. What two questions does Dr. Echols need the pathologist to answer?

_____ *and* _____

4. What treatment approach involves freezing cancerous tissue? _____

5. *Cutaneous* means: _____

Lesson 3.1 (cont'd) **Structure of the Skin**
(LO 3.1, 3.2, and 3.4)

Epidermis (LO 3.1, 3.2, and 3.4)

Mr. Andrews' three lesions were present in his **epidermis,** the most superficial layer of his skin.

The outer layer of your epidermis *(Figure 3.2)* is a keratin-packed cover of compact, dead cells that you continually shed. **Keratin**—a tough, scaly protein that is also the basis for your hair and nails—shields your body from harmful elements like chemicals and bacteria. **Dandruff** is essentially clumps of these dead keratin cells stuck together with **sebum** (oil) from **sebaceous glands.**

In the lower layers of your epidermis, cells are filled with a protein that becomes keratin. Other cells produce a brown/black pigment called **melanin,** which determines the color of your skin and protects it from **ultraviolet (UV)** light damage.

Dermis (LO 3.1, 3.2, and 3.4)

Figure 3.3 shows that the **dermis** is a much thicker connective tissue layer than the epidermis. Your dermis is the middle layer of your skin between your epidermis and **hypodermis.** It consists mostly of collagen fibers. Your dermis is well supplied with blood vessels and nerves. It contains your other skin organs: sweat glands, sebaceous glands, hair **follicles,** and nail roots.

Abbreviations

IM	intramuscular
SC	subcutaneous
TB	tuberculosis
UV	ultraviolet

Hypodermis or Subcutaneous Tissue Layer (LO 3.1, 3.2, and 3.4)

This layer beneath your dermis is the site of **subcutaneous** fat (**adipose** tissue), nerves, and blood vessels. Also called the subcutaneous tissue layer, it regulates your body's temperature and helps protect your vital organs. When this layer becomes thinner or deteriorates, as with the aging process, your skin begins to sag.

Clinical Applications
(LO 3.1, 3.2, and 3.4)

Injections are given into the three areas of the skin using the following approaches:

- **Intradermal,** in which a short, thin needle is introduced into the epidermis, raising a small **wheal** on the skin. This site is used for allergy testing or a tuberculosis (**TB**) test.

- **Subcutaneous (SC),** in which a longer needle pierces the epidermis and dermis to reach the hypodermis (subcutaneous) layer. This site is used for insulin injections and immunizations.

- **Intramuscular (IM),** in which a long needle penetrates the epidermis, dermis, and hypodermis to reach into the muscles underneath. Some antibiotics and immunizations are given this way.

In addition, there are **transdermal** applications. Here, medications are administered through the skin by an adhesive transdermal patch applied to the skin. The medication diffuses across the epidermis and enters the blood vessels in the dermis. Contraceptive hormones, **analgesics,** and antinausea/antiseasickness medications are examples of transdermal applications.

▼ **FIGURE 3.2**
 Epidermis.

▼ **FIGURE 3.3**
 Dermis and Its Organs.

Word Analysis and Definition

WORD	PRONUNCIATION	ELEMENTS		DEFINITION
adipose	ADD-ih-pose	S/ R/	-ose *full of* adip- *fat*	Containing fat
analgesic (adj)	an-al-JEE-sic	S/ P/ R/	-ic *pertaining to* an- *without* -alges- *sensation of pain*	Substance that reduces or relieves the response to pain without producing loss of consciousness
analgesia	an-al-JEE-zee-ah	S/	-ia *condition*	State in which pain is reduced or relieved
dandruff	DAN-druff		Source unknown	Scales in hair from shedding of the epidermis
dermis dermal	DER-miss DER-mal	S/ R/	Greek *skin* -al *pertaining to* derm- *skin*	Connective tissue layer of the skin beneath the epidermis Pertaining to the skin
epidermis epidermal (adj)	ep-ih-DER-miss ep-ih-DER-mal	P/ R/ S/ R/	epi- *above, upon* -dermis *skin* -al *pertaining to* -derm- *skin*	Top layer of the skin Pertaining to the epidermis
follicle	FOLL-ih-kull		Latin *small sac*	Spherical mass of cells containing a cavity or a small cul-de-sac, such as a hair follicle
hypodermis hypodermic (adj) (same as subcutaneous)	high-poh-DER-miss high-poh-DER-mik	P/ R/ S/ R/	hypo- *below* -dermis *skin* -ic *pertaining to* -derm- *skin*	Loose connective tissue layer of skin below the dermis Pertaining to the hypodermis
intradermal	in-trah-DER-mal	S/ P/ R/	-al *pertaining to* intra- *within* -derm- *skin*	Within the epidermis
intramuscular	in-trah-MUSS-kew-lar	S/ P/ R/	-ar *pertaining to* intra- *within* -muscul- *muscle*	Within the muscle
keratin	KER-ah-tin	S/ R/	-in *substance* kerat- *hard protein*	Protein present in skin, hair, and nails
melanin	MEL-ah-nin	S/ R/	-in *substance* melan- *black pigment*	Black pigment found in skin, hair, and the retina
sebaceous glands sebum	seh-BAY-shus GLANZ SEE-bum	S/ R/CF	-ous *pertaining to* sebac/e- *wax* Latin *tallow*	Glands in the dermis that open into hair follicles and secrete a waxy fluid called sebum Waxy secretion of the sebaceous glands
subcutaneous (same as hypodermic)	sub-kew-TAY-nee-us	S/ P/ R/CF	-ous *pertaining to* sub- *below* -cutan/e- *skin*	Below the skin
transdermal	trans-DER-mal	S/ P/ R/	-al *pertaining to* trans- *across, through* -derm- *skin*	Going across or through the skin
ultraviolet	ul-trah-VIE-oh-let	P/ R/	ultra- *beyond* -violet *violet, bluish purple*	Light rays at a higher frequency than the violet end of the spectrum
wheal (same as hives)	WHEEL		Old English *wheal*	Small, itchy swelling of the skin (wheals raised by an injection do not itch)

EXERCISES

A. Review *the Case Report on the previous two-page spread before answering the questions.*   **LO 3.5** *Understand*

1. What role did sunlight play in Mr. Andrews' skin cancer? _____

2. What treatments were given for Mr. Andrews' skin cancer? _____

3. What future precautions should Mr. Andrews take? _____

B. Practice *using your medical terminology in the following exercise. When possible, be sure to deconstruct the term using the slashes provided.*

   Fill in the blanks.   **LO 3.1, 3.4, and 3.5** *Apply*

1. This pigment is responsible for skin color: _____ / _____ / _____

                                                P   R/CF   S

2. Skin needs protection from this type of light: _____ / _____ / _____

                                                P   R/CF   S

Lesson 3.2
Disorders of the Skin

Objectives

*Your skin provides your body's first line of defense against injury, disease, **allergens,** and pollutants. Because your skin is continually exposed to the elements, it's susceptible to various problems and disorders. The skin shows the same types of disease as most organs— infections, tumors, cancers—but because of its protective covering, it's the first responder to many irritant and **allergenic** agents. The information in this lesson will enable you to use correct medical terminology to:*

3.2.1 Name common disorders of the skin.

3.2.2 Describe the effects of these disorders on health.

Case Report 3.2

You are . . .

. . . a medical assistant working with dermatologist Dr. Lenore Echols in Fulwood Medical Center.

You are communicating with . . .

. . . Ms. Cheryl Fox, a 37-year-old nursing assistant working in a surgical unit in Fulwood Medical Center.

Recently, Ms. Fox's fingers have become red and itchy, with occasional **vesicles.** She has also noticed irritation and swelling of her earlobes and **pruritus.** Over the weekends, both the itching and the **rash** on her hands worsen. A patch test by Dr. Echols showed that Ms. Fox is **allergic** to nickel, which is present in the rings she wears on both hands and in her earrings. She only wears this jewelry on the weekends, not during her workdays.

Dermatitis (LO 3.5)

Dermatitis is an inflammation that produces swollen, red, itchy skin. Ms. Fox has a dermatitis *(Figure 3.4)* resulting from direct exposure to an irritating agent.

The different types of dermatitis and their related causes are as follows:

- **Contact dermatitis** results from direct contact with irritants or allergens, including soaps, detergents, cleaning products, and solvents.

- **Atopic** or **allergic dermatitis** is due to allergens that include nickel in jewelry (as with Ms. Fox), perfume, cosmetics, poison ivy, and latex.

- **Eczema** is a general term used for inflamed and itchy skin conditions. When the itchy skin is scratched, it becomes **excoriated** and produces the dry, red, scaly patches characteristic of eczema. The atopic dermatitis that Ms. Fox developed is a common form of eczema.

- **Seborrheic dermatitis** produces a red rash overlaid with a yellow, oily scale and is common in people with oily skin or hair.

- **Stasis dermatitis** occurs in the lower leg when varicose veins slow the return of blood and the accumulation of fluid interferes with the nourishment of the skin.

Case Report 3.2 *(continued)*

For Ms. Fox, the **allergy** is not just a local reaction to an irritant. Her form of **atopic** or allergic dermatitis develops when the whole body becomes sensitive to an allergen. This whole-body involvement is shown by her systemic symptoms of pruritus distant from the local irritant site. Ms. Fox has stopped wearing rings and earrings that contain nickel. Her dermatitis was treated with topical steroids (see *Lesson 3.4*).

▲ **FIGURE 3.4**
Dermatitis of the Ear.

Word Analysis and Definition

S = Suffix   P = Prefix   R = Root   R/CF = Combining Form

WORD	PRONUNCIATION	ELEMENTS		DEFINITION
allergen *(The duplicate "g" is deleted.)*	**AL**-er-jen	S/ R/ R/	-gen- *produce* all- *strange, other* -erg- *work, activity*	Substance producing a hypersensitivity (allergic) reaction
allergenic (adj)	al-er-**JEN**-ik	S/	-ic *pertaining to*	Pertaining to the capacity to produce an allergic reaction
allergy allergic (adj)	**AL**-er-jee ah-**LER**-jik			Hypersensitivity to an allergen Pertaining to being hypersensitive
atopy atopic (adj)	**AT**-oh-pee ay-**TOP**-ik		Greek *strangeness*	State of hypersensitivity to an allergen—allergic
dermatitis	der-mah-**TYE**-tis	S/ R/	-itis *inflammation* dermat- *skin*	Inflammation of the skin
eczema	**EK**-zeh-mah		Greek *to boil* or *ferment*	Inflammatory skin disease, often with a serous discharge
eczematous (adj)	ek-**ZEM**-ah-tus	S/ R/CF	-tous *pertaining to* eczem/a- *eczema*	Pertaining to or marked by eczema
excoriate (verb)	eks-**KOR**-ee-ate	S/ P/ R/	-ate *pertaining to* ex- *away from* -cori- *skin*	To scratch
excoriation (noun)	eks-**KOR**-ee-**AY**-shun	S/	-ation *process*	Scratch mark
pruritus pruritic (adj)	proo-**RYE**-tus proo-**RIT**-ik	S/ R/	Latin *to itch* -ic *pertaining to* prurit- *itch*	Itching Itchy
antipruritic	**AN**-tee-proo-**RIT**-ik	P/	anti- *against*	Medication against itching
rash	**RASH**		French *skin eruption*	Skin eruption
seborrhea	seb-oh-**REE**-ah	S/ R/CF	-rrhea *flow* seb/o- *sebum*	Excessive amount of sebum
seborrheic (adj) *(The "a" is deleted to enable the word to flow.)*	seb-oh-**REE**-ik	S/	-ic *pertaining to*	Pertaining to seborrhea
stasis	**STAY**-sis		Greek *staying in one place*	Stagnation in the flow of any body fluid
vesicle	**VES**-ih-kull		Latin *blister*	Small sac containing liquid; e.g., a blister

EXERCISES

A. Review *the Case Report on this two-page spread before answering the questions.*   **LO 3.4 and 3.5** *Understand*

1. What two parts of Ms. Fox's body were exhibiting symptoms? _____

2. What were the symptoms? _____

3. Why are the symptoms confined to those two areas? _____

4. What is Ms. Fox allergic to? _____

5. Why do her symptoms worsen on the weekends? _____

B. Medical documentation *should always be neat, legible, and spelled correctly for patient safety. Also remember that the patient record is a legal document. The WAD above contains some medical terms that are difficult to spell and pronounce. After you finish this exercise, you can hear terms pronounced correctly by visiting the audio glossary contained in your Connect® course (http://connect.mheducation.com) and practice them yourself. Below, insert the correct spelling of the term on the line.*   **LO 3.5, 3.6, and 3.7** *Apply*

1. Medication has been prescribed for this patient's case of _____ dermatitis.

   seborheic   seborrheic

2. The _____ rash on the patient's face is slowly clearing after she tried the new medication.

   eczematous   exzematous

3. Ms. Fox's _____ is an allergic reaction to her jewelry, which contains nickel.

   purritis   pruritus

Lesson 3.2(cont'd)

▲ **FIGURE 3.5**
Basal Cell Carcinoma.

▲ **FIGURE 3.6**
Malignant Melanoma.

▲ **FIGURE 3.7**
Decubitus (Pressure)
Ulcer on the Heel.

Skin Cancers (LO 3.5)

The two basal cell carcinomas *(Figure 3.5)* on Mr. Andrews' arm arose from the basal (bottom) layer of his epidermis. This is the most common and the least dangerous form of skin cancer because it does not **metastasize** (spread to elsewhere in the body).

The squamous cell carcinoma on Mr. Andrews' hand arose from cells in the middle layers of the epidermis. This skin cancer responds well to surgical removal but can metastasize to lymph glands if neglected.

Malignant melanoma *(Figure 3.6)* is the least common but most dangerous skin cancer. It arises in melanin-producing cells in the basal layer of the epidermis and metastasizes quickly. If neglected, this cancer is fatal.

Excess **sunlight** can also be an irritant to the skin. Too much sun can burn the skin and may lead to cancer, as it did for Mr. Andrews.

Pressure Ulcers (LO 3.5)

When a patient lies in one position for a long period, the pressure between the bed and the body's bony projections, such as the lower spine or heel, cuts off the blood supply to the skin. Under these circumstances, **pressure** or **decubitus ulcers** can appear *(Figure 3.7)*. When this happens, the skin's protective function is compromised, making it easy for germs to enter the body. The elderly are often at risk for pressure ulcers because their skin is usually thin and dry. In addition, poor nutritional status can deplete the fatty protective layer in the hypodermis under the skin, making the body more susceptible to pressure ulcers.

Congenital Lesions (LO 3.5)

A birthmark caused by abnormal pigmentation or proliferation of blood vessels is called a nevus. Vascular nevi produce the port-wine stain or stork bite on the back of the neck and face; they resolve spontaneously in the first few years of life. The blue-gray, benign, flat Mongolian spot on the lower back of blacks, Native Americans, and Latin Americans usually fades by two years of age.

Infections of the Skin (LO 3.5)

The skin can be susceptible to many different types of infections, including viral, fungal, parasitic, and bacterial infections.

Viral Infections (LO 3.5)

Warts (verrucas) are skin growths caused by the human **papillomavirus** invading the epidermis *(Figure 3.8).*

Varicella-zoster virus causes chickenpox in unvaccinated people. Here, **macules** (small, flat spots different in color from the surrounding skin), **papules** (small, solid elevations), and **vesicles** (small sacs containing fluid) form. The virus can then remain dormant in the peripheral nerves (near the skin's surface) for decades before erupting as the painful vesicles of **herpes zoster,** also called **shingles** *(Figure 3.9).*

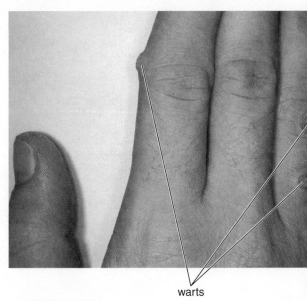

warts

▲ **FIGURE 3.8**
Warts on Hands.

▲ **FIGURE 3.9**
Shingles.

Word Analysis and Definition

S = Suffix   P = Prefix   R = Root   R/CF = Combining Form

WORD	PRONUNCIATION		ELEMENTS	DEFINITION
congenital	con-**JEN**-ih-tal	S/ P/ C/	-al *pertaining to* con- *with* -genit- *bring forth*	Present at birth
decubitus ulcer (pressure ulcer)	deh-**KYU**-bit-us **UL**-ser	P/ R/ R/	de- *from* -cubitus *lying down* ulcer *sore*	Sore caused by lying down for long periods of time
herpes zoster (shingles)	**HER**-peez **ZOS**-ter		herpes Greek *to creep or spread* zoster Greek *belt, girdle*	Painful eruption of vesicles that follows a nerve root on one side of the body
macule	**MACK**-yul		Latin *spot*	Small, flat spot or patch on the skin
malignant	mah-**LIG**-nant	S/ R/	-ant *forming, pertaining to* malign- *harmful, bad*	Tumor that invades surrounding tissues and metastasizes to distant organs
malignancy	mah-**LIG**-nan-see	S/	-ancy *state of*	State of being malignant
melanin melanoma	**MEL**-ah-nin mel-ah-**NO**-mah	S/ R/	Greek *black* -oma *tumor, mass* melan- *black pigment*	Black pigment found in skin, hair, and retina Malignant neoplasm formed from cells that produce melanin
metastasis (noun) metastasize (verb) metastatic (adj)	meh-**TAS**-tah-sis meh-**TAS**-tah-size meh-tah-**STAT**-ik	P/ R/ S/ R/ S/	meta- *beyond, subsequent to* -stasis *stagnate, stay in one place* -ize *affect in a specific way* -stat- *stationary* -ic *pertaining to*	Spread of a disease from one part of the body to another To spread to distant parts Pertaining to the character of cells that can metastasize
nevus nevi (pl)	**NEE**-vus **NEE**-veye		Latin *mole, birthmark*	Congenital lesion of the skin
papillomavirus	pap-ih-**LOH**-mah-vi-rus	S/ R/CF	-oma *mass, tumor* papill/o- *papilla, pimple* virus Latin *poison*	Virus that causes warts and is associated with cancer
papule	**PAP**-yul		Latin *pimple*	Small, circumscribed elevation on the skin
verruca	ver-**ROO**-cah		Latin *wart*	Wart caused by a virus

EXERCISES

A. Identify *the italicized element* in the first column of the chart, define it, and use it to determine the meaning of the medical term.

LO 3.1 and 3.5 *Remember*

Medical Term	Identity of Element (P, S, R, or CF)	Meaning of Element	Meaning of Medical Term
meta*stasis*	1.	2.	3.
*malign*ant	4.	5.	6.
melan*oma*	7.	8.	9.
*de*cubitus	10.	11.	12.

B. Use any two terms *from the chart above in sentences of your choice that are* not *definitions.*   **LO 3.5 and 3.7** *Apply*

Sentence:

1. _____

_____

_____

_____

2. _____

_____

_____

_____

Lesson 3.2(cont'd)

Fungal Infections (LO 3.5)

Tinea is a general term for a group of related skin infections caused by different species of **fungi.**

Tinea pedis, or athlete's foot, causes itching, redness, and peeling of the skin of the foot, particularly between the toes *(Figure 3.10)*. **Tinea capitis** describes an infection of the scalp (ringworm). **Tinea corporis** refers to ringworm infections of the body's skin and hands. **Tinea cruris,** or jock itch, is the name for infections of the groin. The fungus spreads from animals, from the soil, and by direct contact with infected individuals.

A yeast-like fungus, *Candida albicans,* can produce recurrent infections of the skin, nails, and mucous membranes. The first sign can be a frequent diaper rash or oral **thrush** in infants. Older children can show repeated or persistent lesions on the scalp. In adults, chronic **mucocutaneous candidiasis** can affect the mouth (thrush) *(Figure 3.11)*, vagina, and skin. It can also occur with diseases of the immune system *(see Chapter 7)*, as those with a compromised immune system are more susceptible to chronic infections, including fungal infections.

Parasitic Infestations (LO 3.5)

A **parasite** is an organism that lives in contact with and feeds off another organism or host. This process is called an **infestation** and is different from an **infection.**

Lice *(Figure 3.12)* are small, wingless, blood-sucking parasites that produce the disease **pediculosis** by attaching their nits (eggs) to hair and clothing.

▲ **FIGURE 3.10**
Tinea Pedis between the Toes.

▲ **FIGURE 3.11**
Thrush.

Body Louse.

▲ **FIGURE 3.12**

Itch mites *(Figure 3.13)* produce an intense, itching rash called **scabies,** which generally occurs in the genital area or near the waist, breasts, and armpits. These mites lay eggs under the skin.

Bacterial Infections (LO 3.5)

Staphylococcus aureus (commonly called "staph") is the most common bacterium to invade the skin. Staph causes pimples, boils, **carbuncles,** and **impetigo** *(Figure 3.14)*. It can also produce a **cellulitis** of the epidermis and dermis. *Group A Streptococcus* (strep) can also cause cellulitis.

Occasionally, some strains of both staph and strep can be extremely **toxic,** especially when their enzymes digest the connective tissues and spread into the muscle layers. This condition is called **necrotizing fasciitis** and requires highly aggressive surgical and antibiotic treatment.

▲ **FIGURE 3.13**
The Itch Mite of Scabies.

▲ **FIGURE 3.14**
Impetigo.

Word Analysis and Definition

S = Suffix   P = Prefix   R = Root   R/CF = Combining Form

WORD	PRONUNCIATION	ELEMENTS		DEFINITION
Candida candidiasis *Candida albicans* thrush	KAN-did-ah kan-dih-**DIE**-ah-sis KAN-did-ah **AL**-bih-kanz **THRUSH**	S/ R/	Latin *dazzling white* -iasis *state of, condition* candid- *Candida* albicans *Latin white*	A yeastlike fungus Infection with the yeastlike fungus The most common form of *Candida* Another name for infection with *Candida*
carbuncle	KAR-bunk-ul		Latin *carbuncle*	Infection of many hair follicles in a small area, often on the back of the neck
cellulitis	sell-you-**LIE**-tis	S/ R/	-itis *inflammation* cellul- *cell*	Infection of subcutaneous connective tissue
contagious	kon-**TAY**-jus		Latin *touch closely*	Can be transmitted from person to person or from a person to a surface to a person
fungus fungi (pl)	FUN-gus FUN-jee or FUN-gee		Latin *mushroom*	General term used to describe yeasts and molds
impetigo	im-peh-**TIE**-go		Latin *scabby eruption*	Infection of the skin producing thick, yellow crusts
infection infectious (adj)	in-**FECK**-shun in-**FECK**-shus	S/ R/ S/	-ion *action* infect- *internal invasion, infection* -ious *pertaining to*	Invasion of the body by disease-producing microorganisms Capable of being transmitted, or a disease caused by the action of a microorganism
infestation	in-fes-**TAY**-shun	S/ R/	-ation *process* infest- *invade*	Act of being invaded on the skin by a troublesome other species, such as a parasite
louse lice (pl)	LOWSE LISE		Old English *louse*	Parasitic insect
mucocutaneous	MYU-koh-kyu-**TAY**-nee-us	S/ R/CF R/CF	-ous *pertaining to* muc/o- *mucous membrane* -cutan/e- *skin*	Junction of skin and mucous membrane; e.g., the lips
necrotizing fasciitis (Note the spelling.)	NEH-kroh-**TIZE**-ing fash-eh-**EYE**-tis	S/ S/ R/CF S/ R/CF	-ing *quality of* -tiz- *pertaining to* necr/o- *death* -itis *inflammation* fasc/i *fascia*	Inflammation of fascia producing death of the tissue
parasite parasitic (adj)	PAR-ah-site par-ah-**SIT**-ik	S/ R/	Greek *guest* -ic *pertaining to* parasit- *parasite*	An organism that attaches itself to, lives on or in, and derives its nutrition from another species Pertaining to a parasite
pediculosis	peh-dick-you-**LOH**-sis	S/ R/	-osis *condition* pedicul- *louse*	An infestation with lice
scabies	SKAY-beez		Latin *to scratch*	Skin disease produced by mites
tinea	TIN-ee-ah		Latin *worm*	General term for a group of related skin infections caused by different species of fungi
toxin toxic (adj) toxicity (Contains two suffixes)	TOK-sin TOK-sick tok-**SIS**-ih-tee	S/ R/ S/	Greek *poison* -ic *pertaining to* tox- *poison* -ity *state, condition*	Poisonous substance formed by a cell or organism Pertaining to a toxin The state of being poisonous

EXERCISES

A. Terminology challenge. *Employ the language of dermatology to answer the following questions.*   **LO 3.1 and 3.5** *Understand*

1. Demonstrate your understanding of the terms *infection* and *infestation* by explaining how they are different.

Infection: _____

Infestation: _____

2. What are lice eggs called? _____

B. Proofread your documentation. *The following sentence has either an error in fact or an error in spelling. Correct the sentence.*   **LO 3.2 and 3.7** *Apply*

1. An infection of lice can be troublesome to eliminate. _____

Lesson 3.2 (cont'd)

▲ **FIGURE 3.15**
Systemic Lupus Erythematosus.

▲ **FIGURE 3.16**
Scleroderma.

Abbreviations

HIV   human immunodeficiency virus

SLE   systemic lupus erythematosus

Collagen Diseases (LO 3.5)

Collagen, a fibrous protein, comprises 30% of your total body protein. Because your body contains so much of this protein, collagen diseases can have a dramatic effect throughout the body and in the skin.

Systemic lupus erythematosus (SLE) is an **autoimmune** disease that occurs most commonly in women. It produces characteristic skin lesions like a butterfly-shaped, red rash on both cheeks that is joined across the bridge of the nose *(Figure 3.15)*. This disease also affects multiple organs, including the kidneys, brain, heart, and joints.

Rosacea produces a similar facial rash to that of SLE, but there are no systemic complications.

Scleroderma is a chronic, persistent autoimmune disease that also occurs more often in women. It's characterized by a hardening and shrinking of the skin that makes it feel leathery *(Figure 3.16)*. Joints show swelling, pain, and stiffness. Internal organs, including the heart, lungs, kidneys, and digestive tract, are involved in a similar process. The etiology is unknown, and there is no effective treatment.

Other Skin Diseases (LO 3.5)

Psoriasis *(Figure 3.17)* is marked by itchy, flaky, red patches of skin of various sizes covered with white or silvery scales. It appears most commonly on the scalp, elbows, and knees, and its cause is unknown.

Skin Manifestations of Internal Disease
(LO 3.1, 3.2 3.3 and 3.5)

The presence of cancer inside the body is often shown by skin lesions visible on the body's surface, even before the cancer or other disease has produced **symptoms** or been diagnosed.

Dermatomyositis *(Figure 3.18)* is often associated with ovarian cancer, which can appear within 4 to 5 years after the skin disease is diagnosed. This skin disease presents with a reddish-purple rash around the eyes. Muscle weakness commonly follows weeks or months after the appearance of the rash.

Kaposi sarcoma mostly develops in association with **HIV** infection. Raised red or brown blotches or bumps in tissues occur below the skin's surface and eventually spread throughout the body.

Herpes zoster, referred to earlier in this chapter, is common in immunocompromised patients, including the elderly, individuals with HIV, and patients on chemotherapy *(see Chapter 7).*

Breast cancer can often occur in a patient with scleroderma.

▲ **FIGURE 3.17**
Psoriasis Patch on the Elbow.

▲ **FIGURE 3.18**
Periorbital Rash of Dermatomyositis.

Word Analysis and Definition

S = Suffix   P = Prefix   R = Root   R/CF = Combining Form

WORD	PRONUNCIATION	ELEMENTS		DEFINITION
autoimmune	awe-toe-im-**YUNE**	P/ R/	auto- *self* -immune *protected from*	Diseases in which the body makes antibodies directed against its own tissues
dermatomyositis	**DER**-mah-toe-**MY**-oh-site-is	S/ R/CF R/	-itis *inflammation* dermat/o- *skin* -myos- *muscle*	Inflammation of the skin and muscles
Kaposi sarcoma	kah-**POH**-see sar-**KOH**-mah		Moritz Kaposi, Hungarian dermatologist, 1837–1902	A form of skin cancer seen in AIDS patients
psoriasis	so-**RYE**-ah-sis		Greek *the itch*	Rash characterized by reddish, silver-scaled patches
rosacea	roh-**ZAY**-she-ah		Latin *rosy*	Persistent erythematous rash of the central face
scleroderma	sklair-oh-**DERM**-ah	S/ R/CF	-derma *skin* scler/o- *hard*	Thickening and hardening of the skin due to new collagen formation
symptom *(subjective)*	**SIMP**-tum		Greek *event or feeling that has happened to someone*	Departure from normal health experienced by the patient
symptomatic (adj)	simp-toe-**MAT**-ik	S/ R/	-atic *pertaining to* symptom *symptoms*	Pertaining to the symptoms of a disease
sign *(objective)*	SINE		Latin *mark*	Physical evidence of a disease process
systemic lupus erythematosus	sis-**TEM**-ik **LOO**-pus er-ih-**THEE**-mah-**TOE**-sus	S/ R/	-ic *pertaining to* system- *the body as a whole* lupus Latin *wolf*	Inflammatory connective tissue disease affecting the whole body
		S/ R/	-osus *condition* erythemat- *redness*	

EXERCISES

A. Document *using the language of dermatology by inserting the correct term in the space provided. Always review the above WAD before you start any exercise.*   **LO 3.5 and 3.7** *Apply*

1. According to the patient's symptoms, the physician diagnosed (body attacks its own tissues) _____ disease.

2. What we thought was originally a localized problem has now spread, and the patient's final diagnosis is (inflammatory connective tissue disease affecting the whole body) _____.

3. Because of this patient's past history of HIV, his new skin lesions have been diagnosed by the pathologist as (a form of skin cancer seen in AIDS patients) _____.

4. Patients with (rash with reddish, silver-scaled patches) _____ often wear long sleeves to hide their elbows.

B. Critical thinking *and the language of dermatology will help you answer the following questions.*   **LO 3.2, 3.5, and 3.7** *Evaluate*

1. *Using the two medical terms symptom and sign from the WAD, explain which term is objective and which term is subjective, and what that means to the patient.* _____

_____

_____

_____

2. Briefly describe an immunocompromised patient. _____

_____

3. What is the role of skin lesions as a precursor to cancer? _____

_____

Lesson 3.3

Accessory Skin Organs

Case Report 3.3

You are . . .

. . . a pharmacist working in the pharmacy at Fulwood Medical Center.

You are communicating with . . .

. . . Mr. Wayne Winter, an 18-year-old man who will be starting college in a few months. Mr. Winter has had **acne** since the age of 15. He has tried several over-the-counter products, all of which have been unsuccessful in treating his acne. He's even tried retinoic acid. He has numerous **comedones**, papules, **pustules**, and **scars** on his face and forehead and has severe **cystic** lesions and scars on his back. His social life is nonexistent, and his peers frequently tease him. He wishes to change all this before he gets to college.

Your role is to explain to him how to use the medications Dr. Echols, a dermatologist, has prescribed, what their effects will be, and what possible complications may occur.

Objectives

Hair follicles, sebaceous glands, sweat glands, and **nails** *are accessory organs located in your skin. Each of these skin organs has specific anatomical and physiological characteristics. This lesson will enable you to use correct medical terminology to:*

3.3.1 Distinguish the different accessory skin organs.

3.3.2 Identify the structure and functions of the accessory skin organs.

3.3.3 Describe certain disorders affecting the accessory skin organs.

Hair Follicles and Sebaceous Glands (LO 3.4 and 3.5)

Each hair follicle on your face has a sebaceous gland opening into it *(Figure 3.19)*. This gland secretes into the follicle oily, acidic sebum, which mixes with broken-down keratin cells from the base of the follicle.

Around puberty, **androgens,** male sex hormones, are thought to trigger an excessive production of sebum from the sebaceous glands. Sebum brings with it excessive numbers of broken-down keratin cells. This blocks the hair follicle, forming a **comedo** (whitehead or blackhead). Comedones can stay closed, leading to papules, or can rupture, allowing bacteria to get in and produce **pustules.** These are the classic signs of **acne.** Acne affects about 85% of people between the ages of 12 and 25 years *(Figure 3.20)*.

Another skin problem involving the sebaceous glands is seborrheic dermatitis. Here, the glands are thought to be inflamed and to produce a different sebum. The skin around the face and scalp is reddened and covered with yellow, greasy scales. In infants, this condition is called "cradle cap." Seborrheic dermatitis of the scalp produces dandruff.

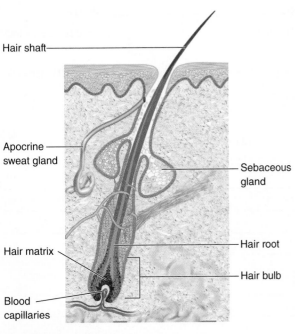

FIGURE 3.19
Hair Follicle and Sebaceous Gland.

Hair shaft

Apocrine sweat gland

Hair matrix

Blood capillaries

Sebaceous gland

Hair root

Hair bulb

FIGURE 3.20
Acne –showing pustules and papules.

Word Analysis and Definition

S = Suffix   P = Prefix   R = Root   R/CF = Combining Form

WORD	PRONUNCIATION	ELEMENTS		DEFINITION
acne	AK-nee		Greek *point*	Inflammatory disease of sebaceous glands and hair follicles
androgen	AN-droh-jen	S/ R/CF	-gen *to produce, create* andr/o- *male*	Hormone that promotes masculine characteristics
comedo (whitehead or blackhead) comedones (pl)	KOM-ee-doh kom-ee-**DOH**-nz		Latin *eat up*	Too much sebum and too many keratin cells block the hair follicle to produce the comedo
cyst	SIST		Greek *sac, bladder*	Abnormal fluid-filled sac surrounded by a membrane
cystic (adj)	SIS-tik	S/	-ic *pertaining to*	Pertaining to a cyst
pustule	PUS-tyul		Latin *pustule*	Small protuberance on the skin containing pus
scar	SKAR		Greek *scab*	Fibrotic seam that forms when a wound heals

EXERCISES

A. Review *the Case Report on this spread before answering the questions.*   **LO 3.4, 3.5, and 3.6** *Understand*

1. What does it mean if a medication is "over the counter" (OTC) in a pharmacy? _____

_____

2. Name one medication you can buy OTC in a pharmacy: _____

3. What types of skin eruptions does Mr. Winter have on his face? _____

4. What type of eruption does he have on his back that he does not have on his face? _____

5. Why does severe acne make it difficult for Mr. Winter to have an active social life? _____

6. What type of specialist did Mr. Winter consult? _____

B. Patient communication: *Rewrite the following sentences from the above Case Report and text in language Mr. Winter can understand. Substitute layperson's language for medical terms.*   **LO 3.5 and 3.8** *Apply*

1. "He has numerous comedones, papules, pustules, and scars on his face and forehead and has severe cystic lesions and scars on his back."

_____

_____

2. "Around puberty, androgens are thought to trigger excessive production of sebum from the sebaceous glands, and sebum brings with it excessive numbers of broken-down cells."

_____

_____

3. "Comedones can stay closed, leading to papules, or can rupture, allowing bacteria to get in and produce pustules."

_____

_____

C. List *the plural term of the following:*   **LO 3.2** *Remember*

1. scar _____

2. cyst _____

3. comedo _____

Lesson 3.3(cont'd) Accessory Skin Organs (LO 3.4 and 3.5)

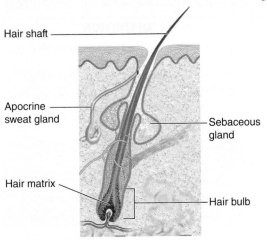

Hair shaft

Apocrine sweat gland

Sebaceous gland

Hair matrix

Hair bulb

▲ **FIGURE 3.21**
Hair Follicle.

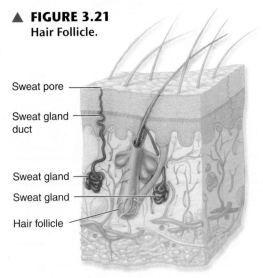

Sweat pore

Sweat gland duct

Sweat gland

Sweat gland

Hair follicle

▲ **FIGURE 3.22**
Sweat Glands.

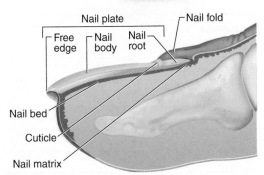

Free edge

Nail body

Nail fold

Nail groove

Cuticle

Nail plate

Nail fold

Free edge

Nail body

Nail root

Nail bed

Cuticle

Nail matrix

◀ **FIGURE 3.23**
Anatomy of a Fingernail.

Hair (LO 3.4 and 3.5)

Every hair on your body or scalp originates from epidermal cells at the base (**matrix**) of a hair follicle. As these cells divide and grow, they push older cells upward, away from the source of nutrition in the hair papilla *(Figure 3.21)*. The older cells become keratinized and die.

In most people, aging causes **alopecia,** thinning of the hair, and baldness as the follicles shrink and produce thin, wispy hairs.

Sweat Glands (LO 3.4 and 3.5)

You have 3 million to 4 million sweat glands scattered all over your skin, with clusters on your palms, soles, and forehead *(Figure 3.22)*. Their main function is to produce the watery perspiration (sweat) that cools your body. Some sweat glands open directly onto the surface of your skin. Others open into your hair follicles *(Figure 3.22)*.

In the dermis, the sweat gland is a coiled tube lined with epithelial, sweat-secreting cells. In your armpits (axillae), around your nipples, in your groin, and around your anus, different sweat glands produce a thick, cloudy secretion. This interacts with your normal skin bacteria to produce a distinct, noticeable smell. The ducts of these glands lead directly into your hair follicles *(see Figure 3.21)*.

Nails (LO 3.4 and 3.5)

Your nails consist of closely packed, thin, dead skin cells that are filled with parallel fibers of hard keratin. On the average, your fingernails grow about 1 millimeter (mm) per week. New cells are added by cell division in the nail matrix, which is protected by the nail fold of skin and the **cuticle** at the base of your nail *(Figure 3.23)*.

Diseases of Nails
(LO 3.4 and 3.5)

Fifty percent of all nail disorders are caused by fungal infections and are called **onychomycosis** *(Figure 3.24)*. With these infections, the fungus grows under the nail and leads to yellow, brittle, cracked nails that separate from the underlying nail bed.

Paronychia *(Figure 3.25)* is a bacterial infection, usually staphylococcal, of the nail base. The nail fold and cuticle become swollen, red, and painful, and pus forms under the nail.

With an **ingrown toenail,** the nail grows into the skin at the side of the nail, particularly if pressured by tight, narrow shoes. An infection can then grow underneath this ingrown toenail.

▲ **FIGURE 3.24**
Onychomycosis (Fungal Infection).

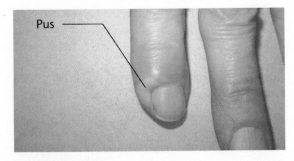

Pus

▲ **FIGURE 3.25**
Paronychia.

S = Suffix   P = Prefix   R = Root   R/CF = Combining Form

WORD	PRONUNCIATION		ELEMENTS	DEFINITION
alopecia	al-oh-**PEE**-shah		Greek *mange*	Partial or complete loss of hair, naturally or from medication
cuticle	**KEW**-tih-cul		Diminutive of cutis *skin*	Nonliving epidermis at base of fingernails and toenails
matrix	**MAY**-tricks		Latin *mother*	The formative portion of a hair, nail, or tooth
onychomycosis	oh-nih-koh-my-**KOH**-sis	S/ R/CF R/	-osis *condition* onych/o- *nail* -myc- *fungus*	Condition of a fungus infection in a nail
paronychia (**Note:** *The vowel "a" at the end of para is dropped to make the composite word flow more easily.*)	par-oh-**NICK**-ee-ah	S/ P/ R/	-ia *condition* para- *alongside* -onych- *nail*	Infection alongside the nail

EXERCISES

A. Elements *are clues to the meaning of a medical term. Identify each given element in the following chart and list its meaning. Then answer the questions below.*   **LO 3.1** *Remember*

Element	Identity of Element (P, R, CF, or S)	Meaning of Element
para	1.	2.
ia	3.	4.
myc	5.	6.
onycho	7.	8.
osis	9.	10.
onych	11.	12.

B. Construct terms *from the elements in the WAD.*   **LO 3.1, 3.2, 3.5, and 3.7** *Apply*

1. The elements in the chart above form which two terms in the WAD?

_____ and _____

2. Use the two medical terms from question 1 in different sentences that would appear in patient documentation.

Sentence:

a. _____

_____

_____

b. _____

_____

_____

3. The root form of the element meaning *nail* is _____

4. Make the root form in question 3 above into a combining form: _____

Lesson 3.4

Diagnosis and Treatment of Skin Disorders (LO 3.5 and 3.6)

Objectives

In your documentation of patient care, it is essential that you understand and communicate clearly the methods, procedures and agents used to diagnose and treat skin problems. You must be able to use correct medical terminology to:

3.4.1 Define methods and instruments used to diagnose skin disorders.

3.4.2 Describe method and pharmacologic agents used to treat skin disorders.

Keynote

Skin cancer cannot be diagnosed without a biopsy or complete removal (excision) for laboratory examination

Keynotes

- Creams are water-based emulsions with a cooling and soothing effect and are cosmetically well tolerated.
- Ointments contain no water and are oil-based to provide an occlusive layer to retain water in the skin; they are used to treat chronic, dry, scaly conditions.
- Lotions are water-based suspensions with a drying, cooling effect.
- Gels are a jelly-like watery suspension using a chemical gelling agent for insoluble drugs such as corticosteroids and retinoids

Diagnostic Procedures (LO 3.5 and 3.6)

Many skin **lesions** can be diagnosed accurately by examining the **lesion.** To highlight the lesion, the dermatologist can use a **dermascope.** This instrument shines a light on the skin and magnifies the lesion.

A **biopsy** of part of the lesion or its complete removal can be performed, particularly if cancer is suspected. The **specimen** is then sent to the laboratory for examination by a **pathologist.** Suspected fungal infections can be scraped and the scales examined under a microscope.

Therapeutic Methods and Pharmacologic Agents (LO 3.5 and 3.6)

Topical therapies are the most commonly used methods of treating skin disorders.

Cleansing agents—soaps, shampoos, and detergents—are used to clean wounds and **abrasions** and to remove crusts and scales. Normal saline can be used to clean **ulcers** and weeping and oozing lesions.

Anti-inflammatory agents are mostly **corticosteroids** as lotions, gels, creams, or ointments (*see Keynote*). Examples are hydrocortisone, triamcinalone, and betamethasone. Non-corticosteroid anti-inflammatory agents are mostly tar-based for use in **psoriasis.**

Topical antibiotics are seldom indicated. Clindamycin and erythromycin are used to treat acne and impetigo. **OTC antibiotics** such as bacitracin and polymyxin can prevent infection in scrapes and **excoriations,** but neomycin frequently causes contact dermatitis.

Antifungal agents that are effective can be bought OTC and include 1% clotrimazole (Lomotrin, Mycelex) and 1% terbinafine (Lamisil). **Antipruritics** such as diphenhydramine and hydrocortisone treat itching. **Calamine** lotion is soothing but not specifically antipruritic. **Retinoids** are applied for psoriasis, acne, and photodamage.

Systemic therapies are given orally, by injection, or intravenously, and affect the entire body. **Chemotherapy** with such drugs as methotrexate and cyclosporine is used for skin melanomas and squamous cell cancers that have metastasized and can be used for widespread psoriasis. **Systemic antibiotics** can be used for severe skin infections and **systemic antifungal agents** can be used for severe fungal infections.

WORD	PRONUNCIATION	ELEMENTS		DEFINITION
abrasion	ah-**BRAY**-shun		Latin *to scrape*	Area of skin or mucous membrane that has been scraped off
antibiotic	**AN**-tih-bye-**OT**-ik	S/ P/ R/	-tic *pertaining to* anti- *against* -bio- *life*	A substance that inhibits the growth of or destroys bacteria and other microorganisms
anti-inflammatory (Note two prefixes)	**AN**-tih-in-**FLAM**-ah-tor-ee	S/ P/ P/ R/	-ory *having the function of* anti- *against* -in- *in* -flammat- *flame*	To prevent or reduce inflammation
antifungal	**AN**-tih-**FUN**-gal	S/ R/	-al *pertaining to* -fung- *fungus*	To prevent or reduce fungal infections
chemotherapy (Note root and combining form)	**KEY**-moh-**THAIR**-ah-pee	R/CF R/	chem/o- *chemical* -therapy *medical treatment*	Treatment using chemical agents
dermascope	**DER**-mah-scope	S/ R/	-scope *instrument for viewing* derma- *skin*	An instrument to assist in examining skin lesions
excision	ek-**SIZH**-un	S/ R/	-ion *action* excis- *cut out*	Surgical removal of part or all of a structure
lesion	**LEE**-zhun		Latin *injury*	A wound, injury, or pathological change in a tissue
systemic	sis-**TEM**-ik	S/ R/	-ic *pertaining to* system- *whole body*	Pertaining to the body as a whole
ulcer	**UL**-sir		Latin *sore, ulcer*	A loss of tissue of the epidermis, usually with inflammation

EXERCISES

A. Show *three terms that are pertaining to different roots:*   **LO 3.1 and 3.2** *Understand*

1. _____

2. _____

3. _____

B. Demonstrate *your knowledge of the use of medications:*   **LO 3.6 and 3.7** *Apply*

1. If I use a lotion, its action will be _____.

2. If I give an intramuscular injection, its action will be _____.

3. If I take a medicine orally, its action will be _____.

C. Describe the different treatments for an abrasion and a laceration: **LO 3.4 and 3.5** *Understand*

_____

_____

Lesson 3.5

Burns and Injuries to the Skin

Objectives

Your role is to participate in patient care as a member of the Burn Unit team. You will be communicating with family members about the extent of the patient's injuries, the necessary and available treatment options, and the patient's prognosis. You need to be able to use correct medical terminology to:

3.5.1 Distinguish the four classes of burns.

3.5.2 Describe the **inflammatory** and repair process of the skin when it is injured.

3.5.3 Identify local and systemic complications of burns.

Keynotes

- Sunburn causes a first-degree burn.
- Scalds can cause second-degree burns.
- House fires with prolonged flame contact can cause third-degree burns.
- High-voltage electrical injury can cause fourth-degree burns.

Case Report 3.5

You are . . .

. . . a burn technologist employed in the Burn Unit at Fulwood Medical Center.

You are communicating with . . .

. . . the son and daughter of Mr. Steven Hapgood, a 52-year-old man.
Mr. Hapgood has been admitted to the Fulwood Burn Unit with severe burns over his face, chest, and abdomen. After an evening of drinking, he began smoking in bed and fell asleep. His next-door neighbors smelled smoke and called 911. In the Burn Unit, his initial treatment included large volumes of intravenous fluids to prevent **shock.**

Burns (LO 3.4 and 3.5)

Burns are the leading cause of accidental death. The immediate threats to life are from fluid loss, infection, and the systemic effects of burned dead tissue. Burn injury to the lungs through damage from heat or smoke inhalation is responsible for 60% or more of burn-related fatalities.

Burns are classified according to the depth of burnt tissue involved *(Figure 3.26):*

First-degree (superficial) burns involve only the epidermis and produce superficial **inflammation,** with redness, pain, and slight edema. Healing takes 3 to 5 days without scarring.

Second-degree (partial-thickness) burns involve the epidermis and dermis but leave some of the dermis intact. They produce redness, blisters, and more severe pain. Healing takes 2 to 3 weeks, with minimal scarring.

Third-degree (full-thickness) burns involve the epidermis, dermis, and subcutaneous tissues, which are often completely destroyed. Healing takes a long time and involves skin **grafts.**

Fourth-degree burns destroy all layers of the skin and involve underlying tendons, muscles, and, sometimes, bones.

(a)

(b)

(c)

▲ **FIGURE 3.26**
Partial- and Full-Thickness Burns.
(a) First degree (superficial thickness). (b) Second degree (partial thickness). (c) Third degree (full thickness).

Word Analysis and Definition

S = Suffix   P = Prefix   R = Root   R/CF = Combining Form

WORD	PRONUNCIATION	ELEMENTS		DEFINITION
inflammation	in-flah-**MAY**-shun	S/ P/ R/ S/	-ion *action, condition* in- *in* -flammat- *flame* -ory *having the function of*	A complex of cell and chemical reactions occurring in response to an injury or chemical or biologic agent
inflammatory (adj)	in-**FLAM**-ah-tor-ee			Causing or affected by inflammation
scald	SKAWLD		Latin *wash in hot water*	Burn from contact with hot liquid or steam
shock	SHOCK		German *to clash*	Sudden physical or mental collapse or circulatory collapse

EXERCISES

A. Review *the Case Report on this spread before answering the questions.*   **LO 3.5 and 3.7** *Understand*

1. Why is Mr. Hapgood in the Burn Unit and not on a regular surgical unit in the hospital?

_____

2. What areas of his body have the most severe burns? _____

3. How did Mr. Hapgood sustain these burns? _____

4. How do intravenous fluids get into the body? _____

5. What is the fluid treatment designed to prevent in Mr. Hapgood's case? _____

B. Lesson objectives: *Meet the lesson objectives with this exercise on burns. Employ your knowledge of medical terms from the integumentary system.*
   Fill in the blanks.   **LO 3.2, 3.5, and 3.7** *Apply*

1. Hit by lightning:

Degree of burn: _____   Signs: _____

_____

Layers of skin involved: _____

What other specific type of injury/accident could produce this burn? _____

2. Scald:

Degree of burn: _____   Signs: _____

_____

Layers of skin involved: _____

What is a scald? _____

How quickly does this heal? _____

3. Prolonged flame contact in a house fire:

Degree of burn: _____   Signs: _____

_____

Layers of skin involved: _____

What specific surgical procedure is used to promote healing for this type of burn? _____

4. Sunburn:

Degree of burn: _____   Signs: _____

_____

Layers of skin involved: _____

Why is this burn only superficial? _____

Lesson 3.5 (cont'd)

Keynote

• In third- and fourth-degree burns, there is no dermal tissue left for regeneration, and skin grafts are necessary.

Burns (continued) (LO 3.4 and 3.5)

In full-thickness burns, because there is no dermal tissue left for **regeneration,** skin grafts are necessary. The ideal graft is an **autograft,** taken from another location on the patient's body, because it is not rejected by the immune system. Mr. Hapgood had autografts taken from his unburned legs and back.

If the patient's burns are too extensive, **allografts**—grafts from another person—are used. **Homograft** is another name for allograft. These grafts are provided by skin banks, which acquire them from deceased people (**cadavers**).

A **xenograft** or **heterograft** is a graft from another species, such as a pig for heart valves.

In addition, artificial skin is being developed commercially and can stimulate the growth of new connective tissues from the patient's underlying tissue.

Case Report 3.5 (continued)

Mr. Hapgood's burns were mostly third-degree. The burned, dead tissue formed an **eschar** that can have toxic effects on the digestive, respiratory, and cardiovascular systems. The eschar was surgically removed by **debridement.**

Rule of Nines (LO 3.4 and 3.5)

The treatment and prognosis for a burn patient also depend on how much of the body surface is affected. This is estimated by subdividing the skin's surface into regions, each one of which is a fraction of or multiple of 9% of the total surface area (*Figure 3.27*). To give you a clearer idea of how these numbers come into play, the body's surface areas are assigned the following percentages:

• Head and neck = 9% (4½% anterior and 4½% posterior).

• Each arm = 9% (4½% anterior and 4½% posterior).

• Each leg = 18% (9% anterior and 9% posterior).

• The anterior trunk = 18%.

• The posterior trunk = 18%.

• Genitalia = 1%.

Aging in Skin (LO 3.4 and 3.5)

With aging, the epidermis thins and the number of melanocytes decreases, but the remaining melanocytes increase in size. Aging skin, therefore, appears thinner, paler, and more translucent, and large pigmented spots (**lentigos**) appear in sun-exposed areas. The blood vessels of the dermis become fragile, leading to bruising and bleeding under the skin. Sebaceous glands produce less oil, leading to dryness and itching. Sweat glands produce less sweat, making it harder to keep cool. The subcutaneous fat layer thins, connective tissue becomes less elastic, and the skin wrinkles and tears easily. Aging skin repairs slowly and wound healing takes up to 4 times longer. Most of these skin changes are hastened and increased by sun exposure.

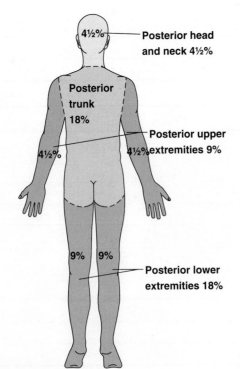

Anterior head and neck 4½%
4½%
Anterior trunk 18%
Anterior upper extremities 9%
4½%
4½%
Genitalia 1%
9% 9%
Anterior lower extremities 18%

4½%
Posterior head and neck 4½%
Posterior trunk 18%
4½%
4½%
Posterior upper extremities 9%
9% 9%
Posterior lower extremities 18%

◀ **FIGURE 3.27**
Rule of Nines.

Word Analysis and Definition

S = Suffix   P = Prefix   R = Root   R/CF = Combining Form

WORD	PRONUNCIATION	ELEMENTS		DEFINITION
allograft	AL-oh-graft	P/ R/	allo- *other* -graft *transplant*	Skin graft from another person or a cadaver
autograft	AWE-toe-graft	P/ R/	auto- *self, same* -graft *transplant*	A graft removed from the patient's own skin
cadaver	kah-DAV-er		Latin *dead body*	A dead body or corpse
debridement	day-BREED-mon (French pronunciation of -ment)	S/ P/ R/	-ment *resulting state* de- *take away* -bride- *rubbish*	The removal of injured or necrotic tissue
eschar	ESS-kar		Greek *scab of a burn*	The burnt, dead tissue lying on top of third-degree burns
heterograft *(same as xenograft)*	HET-er-oh-graft	P/ R/	hetero- *different* -graft *transplant*	A graft from another species (not human)
homograft *(same as allograft)*	HOH-moh-graft	P/ R/	homo- *same, alike* -graft *transplant*	Skin graft from another person or a cadaver
lentigo	len-TIH-go		Greek *lentil*	Age spot; small, flat, brown-black spot in the skin of older people
regenerate (verb)	ree-JEN-eh-rate	S/ P/ R/	-ate *composed of* re- *again* -gener- *produce*	Reconstitution of a lost part
regeneration (noun)	ree-JEN-eh-RAY-shun	S/	-ation *process*	The process of reconstitution
xenograft *(same as heterograft)*	ZEN-oh-graft	P/ R/	xeno- *foreign* -graft *transplant*	A graft from another species (not human)

EXERCISES

A. Review *the Case Report on this spread before answering the questions.*   **LO 3.2, 3.5, and 3.7** *Understand*

1. What is *dermal tissue?* _____

2. What degree of burns did Mr. Hapgood suffer? _____

3. The burned, dead tissue is referred to as: _____

4. What is the surgical procedure called that removes burned, dead tissue? _____

5. Why are grafts necessary for Mr. Hapgood? _____

6. What is the ideal type of graft for Mr. Hapgood? _____

7. Why? _____

B. Employ *medical language in written communication. Insert the correct term from the spread on the appropriate blank; then proofread your paragraph for spelling errors.*   **LO 3.2, 3.5, and 3.7** *Apply*

1. If the burn is deep enough, the tissue cannot _____ itself, and a skin graft is needed. This graft can come from the patient, _____, or from another person, _____, or even from another species _____. Grafts may also come from skin banks or _____.

2. An _____ is taken from the patient; an _____ can come from another person. Donor skin comes from skin banks, which acquire skin from _____. A _____ is from a different species, not human. An example of this would be a _____ for the heart.

3. Two of the terms in question 2 are also known by another name. Write them below.

_____ is the same as _____

_____ is the same as _____

4. What other body systems can be affected by severe burns? _____

Lesson 3.5 (cont'd) Wounds and Tissue Repair (LO 3.5 and 3.6)

(a)

(b)
Scab

clot

▲ **FIGURE 3.28**
Wound Healing.
(a) Bleeding into the wound. (b) Scab formation.

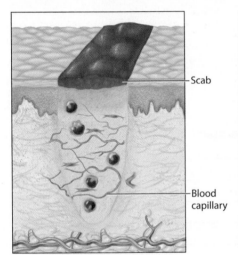
Scab

Blood capillary

▲ **FIGURE 3.29**
Formation of Granulation Tissue.

Epidermal growth

Scar tissue (fibrosis)

▲ **FIGURE 3.30**
Scar Formation.

▲ **FIGURE 3.31**
Keloid of the Earlobe—resulting from piercing of the earlobe.

If you cut yourself when shaving and produce a superficial **laceration** in the epidermis, the epithelial (surface tissue) cells along the laceration's edges will split rapidly and fill in the gap to heal it.

If you cut yourself more deeply, creating a **wound** in the dermis or hypodermis, blood vessels in the dermis break and blood escapes into the wound *(Figure 3.28a)*. The same happens when a surgeon makes an **incision.** On the other hand, a surgeon would perform an **excision** if he or she removed a lesion from the skin or any other tissue.

Escaped blood from a wound or surgical procedure forms a **clot** in the wound. The clot consists of the protein fibrin together with platelets, blood cells, and dried tissue fluids trapped in the fibers. Cells that digest and clean up the tissue debris enter the wound *(see Chapter 7)*. The surface of the clot dries and hardens in the air to form a **scab.** The scab seals and protects the wound from becoming infected *(Figure 3.28b)*.

New capillaries from the surrounding dermis then invade the clot. Three or four days after the injury, other cells migrate into the wound. These cells form new collagen fibers that pull the wound together. This soft tissue in the wound is called **granulation** tissue *(Figure 3.29)*, which is later replaced by a scar *(Figure 3.30)*.

Suturing brings together the edges of the wound to enhance tissue healing.

In some patients, there is excessive fibrosis and scar tissue, producing raised, irregular, lumpy, shiny scars called **keloids** *(Figure 3.31)*. Keloids, most commonly found on the upper body and earlobes, can extend beyond the edges of the original wound and often return if they are surgically removed.

A superficial scraping of the skin, a mucous membrane, or the cornea *(Chapter 11)* is called an **abrasion.**

Surgery on the skin is now being performed using focused light beams called lasers. These lasers remove lesions like birthmarks and tattoos and create a fresh surface over which new skin can grow.

Cosmetic Procedures (LO 3.1, 3.2, 3.5, 3.6, and 3.8)

Surgical procedures that cosmetically alter or improve the appearance of your face or body are becoming more and more common. These cosmetic procedures include:

Abdominoplasty: a "tummy tuck."

Blepharoplasty: the correction of defects in the eyelids.

Dermabrasion: the removal of upper layers of skin using a high-powered rotating brush.

Lipectomy: the surgical removal of fatty tissue by excision.

Liposuction: the surgical removal of fatty tissue using suction.

Mammoplasty: the surgical procedure to alter the size or shape of the breasts.

Rhinoplasty: the surgical procedure to alter the size or shape of the nose.

Word Analysis and Definition

S = Suffix   P = Prefix   R = Root   R/CF = Combining Form

WORD	PRONUNCIATION	ELEMENTS		DEFINITION
abdominoplasty (tummy tuck)	ab-**DOM**-ih-noh-plas-tee	S/ R/CF	-plasty *surgical repair* abdomin/o- *abdomen*	Surgical removal of excess subcutaneous fat from abdominal wall
abrasion	ah-**BRAY**-zhun		Latin *to scrape*	Area of skin or mucous membrane that has been scraped off
blepharoplasty	**BLEF**-ah-roh-plas-tee	S/ R/CF	-plasty *surgical repair* blephar/o- *eyelid*	Surgical repair of an eyelid
clot	**KLOT**		German *to block*	The mass of fibrin and cells that is produced in a wound
dermabrasion	der-mah-**BRAY**-zhun	S/ R/ R/	-ion *action* derm- *skin* -abras- *scrape off*	Removal of upper layers of skin by rotary brush
granulation	gran-you-**LAY**-shun	S/ R/	-ation *process* granul- *small grain*	New fibrous tissue formed during wound healing
incision	in-**SIZH**-un	S/ R/	-ion *action, condition* incis- *cut into*	A cut or surgical wound
excision	ek-**SIZH**-un	R/	excis- *cut out*	Surgical removal of part or all of a structure
keloid	**KEY**-loyd		Greek *stain*	Raised, irregular, lumpy scar due to excess collagen fiber production during healing of a wound
laceration	lass-eh-**RAY**-shun	S/ R/	-ation *process* lacer- *to tear*	A tear or jagged wound of the skin caused by blunt trauma; not a cut
lipectomy	lip-**ECK**-toe-me	S/ R/	-ectomy *surgical excision* lip- *lipid, fat*	Surgical removal of adipose tissue
liposuction	**LIP**-oh-suck-shun	S/ R/CF R/	-ion *action* lip/o- *fat* -suct- *suck*	Surgical removal of adipose tissue using suction
mammoplasty	**MAM**-oh-plas-tee	S/ R/CF	-plasty *surgical repair* mamm/o- *breast*	Surgical procedure to change the size or shape of the breast
rhinoplasty	**RYE**-no-plas-tee	S/ R/CF	-plasty *surgical repair* rhin/o- *nose*	Surgical procedure to change the size or shape of the nose
scab	**SKAB**		Old English *crust*	Crust that forms over a wound or sore during healing
suture (noun) suture (verb)	**SOO**-chur		Latin *seam*	Stitch to hold the edges of a wound together To stitch the edges of a wound together
wound	**WOOND**		Old English *wound*	Any injury that interrupts the continuity of skin or a mucous membrane

EXERCISES

A. Wounds: *Use your knowledge of the meaning of the following medical terms to put them in the correct order of their appearance and give a brief description of each term. Fill in the chart.* **LO 3.2, 3.5, and 3.7** *Understand*

keloid   scab   clot   laceration   wound   granulation

Medical Term	Brief Description
1.	2.
3.	4.
5.	6.
7.	8.
9.	10.
11.	12.

B. Terminology challenge: *Precision in communication is using the correct medical term for the appropriate meaning.* **LO 3.2 and 3.5** *Apply*

1. What is the difference between *abrasion* and *incision?* _____

_____

2. Which term in the WAD is an accepted treatment for acne? _____

3. Consider the terms *clot* and *scab*. Which is inside the wound and which is outside the wound? Inside: _____ Outside: _____

Chapter Review exercises, along with additional practice items, are available in Connect!

The Skeletal System
The Essentials of the Language of Orthopedics

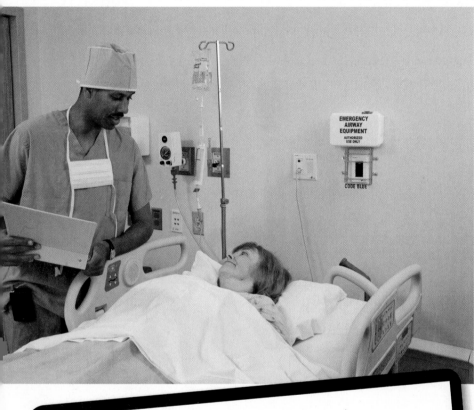

CHAPTER 4

Learning Outcomes

In order for you to work with Dr. Stannard to give optimal care to Mrs. Vargas, and to help her and her family understand the significance of her bone disorder and injury, you will need to be able to use correct medical terminology to:

LO 4.1 Use roots, combining forms, suffixes, and prefixes to construct and analyze (deconstruct) medical terms related to the skeletal system.

LO 4.2 Spell and pronounce correctly medical terms related to the skeletal system to communicate them with accuracy and precision in any health care setting.

LO 4.3 Define accepted abbreviations related to the skeletal system.

LO 4.4 Relate the different types of bones and their structure to their functions.

LO 4.5 Describe the causes, appearances, methods of diagnosis, and treatment of bone and joint disorders and bone fractures, and their methods of healing.

LO 4.6 Identify the structures of the axial skeleton and their disorders and treatments.

LO 4.7 Describe the bones and joints of the shoulder girdle and upper limb and their disorders and treatments.

LO 4.8 Relate the structure of the pelvic girdle, hip joint, and thigh bone to their functions and disorders and treatments.

LO 4.9 Relate the structures of the knee joint, ankle, and foot to their functions and disorders and treatments.

LO 4.10 Apply your knowledge of the medical terms of the skeletal system to documentation, medical records, and medical reports.

LO 4.11 Translate the medical terms of the skeletal system into everyday language in order to communicate clearly with patients and their families.

Case Report 4.1

You are . . .

. . . an orthopedic technologist working for Kenneth Stannard, MD, an orthopedist in the Fulwood Medical Group.

You are communicating with . . .

. . . Mrs. Amy Vargas, a 70-year-old housewife, who tripped while walking down the front steps of her house. She has severe pain in her right hip and is unable to stand. An X-ray shows a hip fracture and marked osteoporosis. Dr. Stannard examined her in the Emergency Department, and Mrs. Vargas is being admitted for a hip replacement.

Without your bones, you'd be shapeless—unable to sit, stand, walk, or move your fingers and toes. Your skeleton supports and protects your organ systems, and it's the foundation for much of the medical terminology you will learn in this book. For example, the radial artery (used for taking a pulse) is so named because it travels beside the radial bone of the forearm.

Understanding the surface anatomy of bones and their markings will enable you to describe and document the sites of symptoms, signs, and diagnostic and therapeutic procedures. The information in this lesson will provide you with the confidence and skills for using correct medical terminology to:

4.1.1 Recognize the different health professionals involved in the diagnosis and treatment of skeletal problems.

4.1.2 Identify the tissues that form the skeletal system.

4.1.3 Discuss the structures and functions of the skeletal system.

4.1.4 Differentiate the types of bones in the skeletal system.

4.1.5 Evaluate the major problems and diseases that occur in the skeletal system.

Abbreviations

DO	Doctor of Osteopathy
MD	Doctor of Medicine
DC	Doctor of Chiropractic
PT	Physical Therapist

Many health professionals are involved in the diagnosis and treatment of problems in the skeletal system. You may work directly and/or indirectly with one or more of the following:

- **Orthopedic surgeons (orthopedists)** are medical doctors **(MDs)** who deal with the prevention and correction of injuries of the skeletal system and associated **muscles,** joints, and ligaments.

- **Osteopathic physicians** have earned a doctor of osteopathy **(DO)** degree and receive additional training in the **musculoskeletal system** and how it affects the whole body.

- **Chiropractors (DC)** focus on the manual adjustment of joints—particularly the spine—in order to maintain and restore health.

- **Physical therapists** evaluate and treat pain, disease, or injury by physical therapeutic measures, as opposed to medical or surgical measures.

- **Physical therapist assistants** work under the direction of a physical therapist to assist patients with their physical therapy.

- **Orthopedic technologists** and **technicians** assist orthopedic surgeons in treating patients.

- **Podiatrists** are practitioners in the diagnosis and treatment of disorders and injuries of the foot.

Lesson 4.1

Bones of the Skeletal System

Tissues and Functions of the Skeletal System (LO 4.1, 4.2, and 4.4)

There are four components of the skeletal system *(Figure 4.1):*

1. **bones,**
2. **cartilage,**
3. **tendons,** and
4. **ligaments.**

Each plays an important role in the way your tissues and skeletal system function. Your skeletal system provides:

- **Support:** The bones of your vertebral column, pelvis, and legs hold up your body. The jawbone supports your teeth.

- **Protection:** The skull protects your brain. The vertebral column protects your spinal cord. The rib cage protects your heart and lungs.

- **Blood formation:** Bone marrow in many bones is the major producer of blood cells, including most of those in your immune system *(see Chapter 7).*

- **Mineral storage and balance:** The skeletal system stores calcium and phosphorus and releases them when your body needs them for other purposes.

- **Detoxification:** Bones remove metals like lead and radium from your blood, store them, and slowly release them for excretion.

- **Endocrine regulation:** Bone cells release a hormone called **osteocalcin,** which increases insulin secretion and reduces stores of fat.

▶ **FIGURE 4.1**
Adult Skeletal System, Anterior View.

WORD	PRONUNCIATION		ELEMENTS	DEFINITION
cartilage	KAR-tih-laj		Latin *gristle*	Nonvascular, firm connective tissue found mostly in joints
chiropractic	kye-roh-**PRAK**-tik	S/ R/CF R/	-ic *pertaining to* chir/o- *hand* -pract- *efficient, practical*	Diagnosis, treatment, and prevention of mechanical disorders of the musculoskeletal system
chiropractor	kye-roh-**PRAK**-tor	S/	-or *a doer*	Practitioner of chiropractic
detoxification (**Note:** *Same as detoxication*)	dee-**TOKS**-ih-fih-**KAY**-shun	S/ P/ R/	-fication *remove* de- *from, out of* -toxi- *poison*	Removing poison from a tissue or substance
ligament	**LIG**-ah-ment		Latin *band, sheet*	Band of fibrous tissue connecting two structures
muscle musculoskeletal	**MUSS**-el **MUSS**-kyu-loh-**SKEL**-eh-tal	S/ R/CF R/	Latin *muscle* -al *pertaining to* muscul/o- *muscle* -skelet- *skeleton*	A tissue consisting of cells that can contract Pertaining to the muscles and the bony skeleton
orthopedic	or-tho-**PEE**-dik	S/ R/CF R/	-ic *pertaining to* orth/o- *straight* -ped- *child*	Pertaining to the correction and cure of deformities and diseases of the musculoskeletal system; originally, most of the deformities treated were in children
orthopedist	or-tho-**PEE**-dist	S/	-ist *specialist*	Specialist in orthopedics
osteocalcin	**OSS**-tee-oh-**CAL**-sin	S/ R/CF R/	-in *chemical compound* oste/o- *bone* -calc- *calcium*	A hormone produced by bone cells
osteopath	**OSS**-tee-oh-path	S/ R/CF	-path *disease* oste/o- *bone*	Practitioner of osteopathy Medical practice based on maintaining the balance of the body
osteopathy	**OSS**-tee-**OP**-ah-thee	S/	-pathy *disease*	
tendon	**TEN**-dun		Latin *sinew*	Fibrous band that connects muscle to bone

EXERCISES

A. Review *the Case Report on this spread before answering the questions.*   **LO 4.2, 4.8, and 4.10** *Understand*

1. What kind of accident sent Mrs. Vargas to the ER? _____

2. What are her symptoms when she gets to the ER? _____

3. What diagnostic test did she have? _____

4. What did the test in question #3 above show? _____

5. What is the treatment plan for Mrs. Vargas? _____

B. Orthopedic vocabulary: *This exercise can be answered entirely by using medical terms that appear on the two pages open in front of you. Mastering these terms will start you on your way to learning the language of orthopedics. From the description, identify the correct medical terminology. Fill in the blanks.*   **LO 4.1 and 4.2** *Remember*

Description	Medical Term(s)
In addition to bones, which three terms are components of this chapter's body system?	1. 2. 3.
Which three terms refer to medical occupations?	4. 5. 6.
Which term represents a medical practice based on maintaining balance of the body?	7.
Which term has an element meaning poison?	8.
What is the name of the body system in this chapter?	9.

Lesson 4.1 (cont'd)   Bones (LO 4.2 and 4.4)

(a)

(b)

▲ FIGURE 4.2
Femur: Long Bone of the Thigh.
(a) Anterior view. (b) Interior view.

▲ FIGURE 4.3
Blood Supply to Bone.

Classification of Bones (LO 4.2 and 4.4)

The bones of your skeletal system are classified by their shape. Each falls into one of the following four shape categories:

- **Long** (considerably longer than they are wide), like the main bones of the limbs, palms, soles, fingers, and toes;

- **Short** (nearly as long as they are wide), like the patella (kneecap) and the bones of the wrists and ankles;

- **Flat,** like the bones of the skull and the ribs; or

- **Irregular,** like the vertebrae.

Structure of Bones
(LO 4.2 and 4.4)

Think about how long your arms and legs are, and then consider how few bones make up all that length. In that context, it's likely no surprise that **long bones** are the most common bones in your body *(Figure 4.2)*. The shaft (**diaphysis**) of a long bone contains compact bone (also called **cortical** bone), while each end of the bone (the **epiphysis**) is composed of spongy bone. Sandwiched between the diaphysis and epiphysis are thin layers of cartilage cells in the **epiphysial plate** or **line** that allow your bones to grow longer.

A tough, connective tissue sheath called **periosteum** covers the outer surface of all bones; it protects the bone and anchors blood vessels and nerves to the bone's surface. Strong collagen fibers attach the periosteum to the cortical bone.

Inside the diaphysis is a hollow cylinder called the **medulla** *(Figure 4.2b)*, which contains bone **marrow**, a fatty tissue in adults. Red bone marrow with blood cells in varying stages of development can be found in the epiphyseal ends of the bone and in the flat bones of the skull, the sternum, and the hip bones. Because red bone marrow is normally concentrated here, the medulla of the sternum and hip bone is the ideal source for bone marrow aspiration, a procedure where a needle is inserted into the bone to withdraw a sample of bone marrow fluid and cells to be checked for abnormalities.

Most bones have a strong blood supply *(Figure 4.3)* because of the blood vessels that travel through them in a system of small **Haversian canals.** The good supply of blood through your bones promotes healing.

Word Analysis and Definition

S = Suffix   P = Prefix   R = Root   R/CF = Combining Form

WORD	PRONUNCIATION		ELEMENTS	DEFINITION
cortex cortical (adj)	KOR-teks KOR-tih-cal	S/ R/	Latin *bark* -al *pertaining to* cortic- *cortex*	Outer portion of an organ, such as bone Pertaining to a cortex
diaphysis	die-AF-ih-sis		Greek *growing between*	The shaft of a long bone
epiphysis	ep-ih-FI-sis	P/ R/	epi- *upon, above* -physis *growth*	Expanded area at the proximal and distal ends of a long bone to provide increased surface area for attachment of ligaments and tendons
epiphysial (adj) (**Note:** *The part "is" is deleted to enable the word to flow.*)	ep-ih-FIZ-ee-al	S/	-ial *pertaining to*	Pertaining to an epiphysis
Haversian canals	hah-VER-shan ka-NALS		Clopton Havers, English physician, 1655–1702	Vascular canals in bone
marrow	MAH-roe		Old English *marrow*	Fatty, blood-forming tissue in the cavities of long bones
medulla medullary (adj)	meh-DULL-ah meh-DULL-ah-ree	S/ R/	Latin *marrow* -ary *pertaining to* medulla- *medulla*	Central portion of a structure surrounded by cortex Pertaining to a medulla
periosteum	PER-ee-OSS-tee-um	S/ P/ R/	-um *structure* peri- *around* -oste- *bone*	Strong membrane surrounding a bone
periosteal (adj)	PER-ee-OSS-tee-al	S/	-al *pertaining to*	Pertaining to the periosteum

EXERCISES

A. Elements *remain your best clue for understanding a medical term. In this exercise, the meaning of each element is given below the line—this is your clue to constructing the term. Write the correct element on the line above its meaning. After you have constructed the term, give its definition in the space provided.* **LO 4.1 and 4.2** *Apply*

1. _____ / _____ / _____

                              cortex   pertaining to

    The term is _____ and means _____.

2. _____ / _____ / _____

         around   bone   structure

    The term is _____ and means _____.

3. _____ / _____ / _____

      upon, above   growth   pertaining to

    The term is _____ and means _____.

4. _____ / _____ / _____

                           medulla   pertaining to

    The term is _____ and means _____.

B. Use this exercise *to review what you've learned about bones.* **LO 4.2 and 4.4** *Remember*

1. Bones in the skeletal system are classified by their _____.

2. What are the most common types of bones in the body? _____.

3. What is another name for "compact" bone? _____.

4. Where can you find bone marrow? _____.

5. The strong blood supply in bones is provided by the _____.

6. The shaft of a long bone is called the _____.

Lesson 4.1 (cont'd)

Keynote

- Osteomalacia occurs in some developing nations and occasionally in this country when children drink soft drinks instead of milk fortified with vitamin D.

Abbreviations

BMD	bone mineral density
DEXA	dual energy x-ray absorptiometry
FDA	Food and Drug Administration
IU	international unit(s)
mg	milligram

Diseases of Bone
(LO 4.2 and 4.5)

One of the major bone diseases is **osteoporosis,** which results from a loss of bone density *(Figure 4.4)*. More common in women than in men, the incidence of osteoporosis increases with age. In the United States alone, 10 million people are living with osteoporosis and 18 million more have low bone density **(osteopenia).** Osteopenia puts people at risk for developing osteoporosis.

In women, production of the hormone estrogen decreases after menopause, weakening the body's protection against bone loss and potentially resulting in fragile, brittle bones. In men, lower levels of testosterone have a similar but less noticeable effect.

Women at risk for osteoporosis should have a bone mineral density **(BMD)** screening using a **DEXA** scan, which is a measuring device that uses low-energy radiation beams. Men and women over 50 are often advised to follow a daily regimen of 1,200 milligrams **(mg)** of calcium, 400 to 600 international units **(IU)** of vitamin D, and 15 minutes of real sun exposure. In addition, there are several **FDA**-approved medications available for treating osteoporosis.

Other bone diseases that may not be as prevalent or publicized as osteoporosis are the following:

Osteomyelitis: an inflammation of bone and bone marrow caused by a bacterial infection, such as staphylococcus.

Osteomalacia: a disease (known as **rickets** in children) caused by vitamin D deficiency where the calcium-lacking bones become soft and flexible, lose their ability to bear weight, and become bowed.

Achondroplasia: a very rare condition where the long bones stop growing in childhood, but the axial skeleton bones are not affected *(Figure 4.5)*. People with this condition are short in stature, with the average adult measuring about 4 feet tall. Although intelligence and life span are normal, the disease is caused by a spontaneous gene mutation that then becomes a dominant gene for succeeding generations.

Osteogenesis imperfecta (OI): a rare genetic disorder producing very brittle bones that are easily fractured or broken, often **in utero** (while inside the uterus).

Primary bone cancer is found in three forms:

1. **Osteogenic sarcoma** occurs most often in bone cells around the knee in adolescents.
2. **Ewing sarcoma** occurs most often in children and adolescents.
3. **Chondrosarcoma** arises in cartilage cells, often in the pelvises of older people.

Case Report 4.1 (continued)

On questioning, Amy Vargas demonstrated many of the risk factors for osteoporosis, including family history, lack of exercise, cigarette smoking, inadequate diet, postmenopause, and increasing age.

Normal bone   Osteoporotic bone

LM 5×

▲ **FIGURE 4.4**
Normal Bone and Osteoporotic Bone.

▶ **FIGURE 4.5**
Achondroplastic Dwarf with College Roommate.

Word Analysis and Definition

S = Suffix   P = Prefix   R = Root   R/CF = Combining Form

WORD	PRONUNCIATION	ELEMENTS		DEFINITION
achondroplasia	a-kon-droh-**PLAY**-zee-ah	S/ P/ R/CF	-plasia *formation* a- *without* -chondr/o- *cartilage*	Condition with abnormal, early conversion of cartilage into bone, leading to dwarfism
osteogenesis imperfecta	OSS-tee-oh-**JEN**-eh-sis im-per-**FEK**-tah	S/ R/CF	-genesis *creation, formation* oste/o- *bone* imperfecta, Latin *unfinished*	Inherited condition in which bone formation is incomplete, leading to fragile, easily broken bones
osteomalacia	OSS-tee-oh-mah-**LAY**-she-ah	S/ R/CF	-malacia *abnormal softness* oste/o- *bone*	Soft, flexible bones lacking in calcium (rickets)
osteomyelitis	OSS-tee-oh-my-eh-**LIE**-tis	S/ R/CF R/	-itis *inflammation* oste/o- *bone* -myel- *bone marrow*	Inflammation of bone and bone marrow
osteopenia	OSS-tee-oh-**PEE**-nee-ah	S/ R/CF	-penia *deficient* oste/o- *bone*	Decreased calcification of bone
osteoporosis	OSS-tee-oh-poh-**ROE**-sis	S/ R/CF R/CF	-sis *condition* oste/o- *bone* -por/o- *opening*	Condition in which the bones become more porous, brittle, and fragile and more likely to fracture
rickets	**RICK**-ets		Old English *to twist*	Disease due to vitamin D deficiency, producing soft, flexible bones
sarcoma	sar-**KOH**-mah	S/ R/	-oma *tumor, mass* sarc- *flesh*	Malignant tumor originating in connective tissue
chondrosarcoma	CHON-droh-sar-**KOH**-mah	R/CF	chondr/o *cartilage*	Malignant tumor originating in cartilage cells
osteogenic sarcoma	OSS-tee-oh-**JEN**-ik sar-**KOH**-mah	S/ R/CF R/	-ic *pertaining to* oste/o- *bone* -gen- *creation*	Malignant tumor originating in bone-producing cells

EXERCISES

A. Review *the Case Report on this spread before answering the questions.*   **LO 4.2 and 4.5** *Understand*

1. What is a *risk factor?* _____

2. What does *post menopause* mean? _____

3. What bone disease is Mrs. Vargas at risk to develop? _____

4. What does it mean if this diagnosis is *in her family history?* _____

5. How can Mrs. Vargas alter her lifestyle to improve her health? _____

6. Name the disease that puts people at risk to develop osteoporosis. _____

B. Suffixes: *The combining form* oste/o *means bone, and it is the main element in each of the following terms. You choose the correct suffix to complete the term. Fill in the blanks.*   **LO 4.1 and 4.5** *Remember*

genesis   **genic**   **sarcoma**   **penia**   **malacia**   **porosis**   **myelitis**

1. Disease caused by vitamin D deficiency   osteo/ _____

2. Low bone density   osteo/ _____

3. Porous, brittle, fragile bones   osteo/ _____

4. Most common malignant bone tumor   osteo/ _____

5. Rare genetic disorder producing easily fractured bones, often in utero   osteo/ _____

6. Inflammation of bone and bone marrow   osteo/ _____

Note: *The meaning of the combining form never changes. The addition of six different suffixes has helped you learn six new terms in orthopedic vocabulary!*

Lesson 4.1 (cont'd) Bone Fractures (FXs) (LO 4.2 and 4.5)

Comminuted

Incomplete

Complete

Transverse

(a)

(b)

Impacted

Spiral

Oblique

(c)

(d)

Open, displaced

Linear

(e)

(f)

Greenstick

(g)

▲ **FIGURE 4.6**
Bone Fractures.

▼ **TABLE 4.1**

CLASSIFICATION AND DEFINITION OF BONE FRACTURES

Name	Description	Reference
Closed (also called **simple** fracture)	A bone is broken, but the skin is not broken.	*Figure 4.6g*
Open (also called **compound** fracture)	A fragment of the fractured bone breaks the skin, or a wound extends to the site of the fracture.	*Figure 4.6e*
Displaced	The fractured bone parts are out of line.	*Figure 4.6e*
Complete	A bone is broken into at least two fragments.	*Figure 4.6a*
Incomplete	The fracture does not extend completely across the bone. It can be hairline, as in a stress fracture in the foot, when there is no separation of the two fragments.	*Figure 4.6a*
Comminuted	The bone breaks into several pieces, usually two major pieces and several smaller fragments.	*Figure 4.6b*
Transverse	The fracture is at right angles to the long axis of the bone.	*Figure 4.6b*
Impacted	The fracture consists of one bone fragment driven into another, resulting in shortening of a limb.	*Figure 4.6c*
Spiral	The fracture spirals around the long axis of the bone.	*Figure 4.6d*
Oblique	The fracture runs diagonally across the long axis of the bone.	*Figure 4.6d*
Linear	The fracture runs parallel to the long axis of the bone.	*Figure 4.6f*
Greenstick	This is a partial fracture. One side breaks, and the other bends.	*Figure 4.6g*
Pathologic	The fracture occurs in an area of bone weakened by disease, such as cancer.	—
Compression	The fracture occurs in a vertebra from trauma or pathology, leading to the vertebra being crushed.	—
Stress	This is a fatigue fracture caused by repetitive, local stress on a bone, as occurs in marching or running.	—

Healing of Fractures (LO 4.2 and 4.5)

When a bone is fractured, blood vessels bleed into the fracture site, forming a hematoma *(Figure 4.7a)*. After a few days, bone-forming cells called **osteoblasts** move in and start to produce new bone cells (osteocytes), which form a **callus** *(Figure 4.7b)*. Osteblasts continue to produce bone cells, which form **cancellous** (spongy) bone to replace the callus *(Figure 4.7c)*. As more bone cells form, the spongy bone structure is replaced by compact bone, which fuses together the bone segments *(Figure 4.7d)*. Uncomplicated fractures take 8 to 12 weeks to heal. (Surgical procedures to help fractures heal are shown in Lesson 4.4.)

Medullary cavity

Hematoma

Compact bone

(a)

Soft callus

New blood vessels

(b)

Hard callus

Cancellous (spongy) bone

(c)

(d)

▶ **FIGURE 4.7**
Healing of Bone Fracture.

Word Analysis and Definition

WORD	PRONUNCIATION	ELEMENTS		DEFINITION
callus	KAL-us		Latin *hard skin*	Bony tissue that forms at a fracture site early in healing
cancellous	KAN-sell-us		Latin *lattice*	Bone that has a spongy or lattice-like structure
comminuted	KOM-ih-nyu-ted	S/ R/	-ed *pertaining to* comminut- *break into pieces*	A fracture in which the bone is broken into pieces
hematoma	he-mah-TOH-mah	S/ R/	-oma *tumor, mass* hemat- *blood*	Collection of blood that has escaped from blood vessels into tissue
osteoblast	OSS-tee-oh-blast	S/ R/CF	-blast *immature cell* oste/o- *bone*	A bone-forming cell
osteocyte	OSS-tee-oh-site	R/	-cyte *cell*	A bone-maintaining cell
pathologic fracture	path-oh-LOJ-ik FRAK-chur	S/ R/CF R/ S/ R/	-ic *pertaining to* path/o- *disease* -log- *to study* -ure *result of* fract- *to break*	Fracture occurring at a site already weakened by a disease process, such as cancer

EXERCISES

A. Deconstruct *the following medical terms into their basic elements. Then provide a brief definition for each term. Fill in the chart.*

LO 4.1 and 4.2 *Apply*

Medical Term	Prefix	Root/CF	Suffix	Definition of Medical Term
pathologic	1.	2.	3.	4.
osteoblast	5.	6.	7.	8.
comminuted	9.	10.	11.	12.

B. Demonstrate *your understanding of the terms by finishing this exercise.*   **LO 4.2, 4.5, and 4.10** *Understand*

1. What is the difference between an *osteoblast* and an *osteocyte*?

_____

_____

2. What is the difference between an open and a closed fracture?

_____

_____

3. What type of preexisting condition might likely cause a pathologic fracture to occur?

_____

_____

Lesson 4.2

Axial Skeleton

Case Report 4.2

You are ...

... an orthopedic technologist working in the orthopedic department of Fulwood Medical Center with Dr. Kenneth Stannard.

You are communicating with ...

... Ms. Nancy Cardenas, a 27-year-old jeweler whose car was rear-ended by another car at a traffic light 3 days ago. Ms. Cardenas suffers from severe neck pain radiating down her left arm, as well as dizziness and headaches. She is unable to go to work. Dr. Stannard has examined her and diagnosed her condition as a **whiplash** injury. An MRI shows herniation (rupture) of intervertebral discs between C5-C6 and C6-C7. Your role is to assist Dr. Stannard and document the care Ms. Cardenas receives to relieve her symptoms. Ms. Cardenas' whiplash injury caused protrusion of two cervical intervertebral discs. The centers of the discs bulge into the vertebral canal and pinch the nerves in such a way that the pain radiates to her left arm.

Objectives

In order to best evaluate, treat, and educate patients, understanding the medical terminology for the structures and functions of the vertebral column, its joints, and its ligaments is a must. The vertebral column is part of the axial skeleton, and in this lesson, information about the axial skeleton will enable you to use correct medical terminology to:

4.2.1 Identify the regions and bones of the vertebral column.

4.2.2 Describe the joints and ligaments of the vertebral column.

4.2.3 Distinguish the different bones of the skull.

4.2.4 Differentiate the major problems and diseases that affect the vertebral column and skull.

Structure of the Axial Skeleton (LO 4.2 and 4.6)

Your axial skeleton, the upright axis of your body, includes the:

1. **vertebral column,**
2. **skull, and**
3. **rib cage.**

The axial skeleton protects the brain, **spinal cord,** heart, and lungs—most of the major centers of human physiology.

Within the vertebral column, there are 26 bones divided into the following five regions *(Figure 4.8):*

- **Cervical** region, with 7 **vertebrae,** labeled C1 to C7 and curved anteriorly;

- **Thoracic** region, with 12 vertebrae, labeled T1 to T12 and curved posteriorly;

- **Lumbar** region, with 5 vertebrae, labeled L1 to L5 and curved anteriorly;

- **Sacral** region, with 5 bones that in early childhood fuse into 1 bone curved posteriorly; and

- **Coccyx** (tailbone), with 4 small bones fused together into 1 bone curved posteriorly.

The spinal cord lies protected in the vertebral canal of the vertebral column. Spinal nerves travel from the spinal cord to other parts of the body through the intervertebral **foramina.**

Intervertebral discs consisting of fibrocartilage (a form of cartilage) are also found in the axial skeleton. These discs inhabit the intervertebral space between the bodies of adjacent vertebrae and provide extra support and cushioning (acting as shock absorbers) for the vertebral column.

The vertebral column, like any other body part, is susceptible to injury and disease. One common disorder of the vertebral column is **scoliosis,** an abnormal lateral curvature of the **spine** that occurs in both children and adults. Abnormal curvature of the spine is more common in older people, particularly those with osteoporosis; in this case, the normal anteriorly concave curvature in the thoracic region **(kyphosis)** is exaggerated.

Abbreviations

C5	the fifth cervical vertebra
C5-C6	the intervertebral space between the fifth and sixth cervical vertebrae
C6	the sixth cervical vertebra
MRI	magnetic resonance imaging (diagnostic technique that produces focused slices of images of structures)

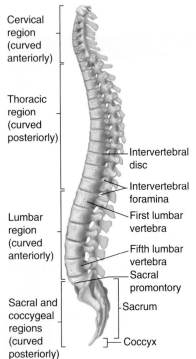

Cervical region (curved anteriorly)

Thoracic region (curved posteriorly)

Intervertebral disc

Intervertebral foramina

First lumbar vertebra

Lumbar region (curved anteriorly)

Fifth lumbar vertebra

Sacral promontory

Sacrum

Sacral and coccygeal regions (curved posteriorly)

Coccyx

◀ **FIGURE 4.8**
Vertebral Column, Lateral View.

Word Analysis and Definition

WORD	PRONUNCIATION	ELEMENTS		DEFINITION
cervical	**SER**-vih-kal	S/ R/	-al *pertaining to* cervic- *neck*	Pertaining to the neck region
coccyx	**KOK**-sicks		Greek coccyx	Small tailbone at the lowest end of the vertebral column
foramen	foh-**RAY**-men		Latin *an opening*	An opening through a structure
foramina (pl)	foh-**RAM**-in-ah			
kyphosis	ki-**FOH**-sis	S/ R/	-osis *condition* kyph- *bent, humpback*	A normal posterior curve of the spine that can be exaggerated in disease
kyphotic (adj)	ki-**FOT**-ik	S/ R/CF	-tic *pertaining to* kyph/o- *bent, humpback*	Pertaining to or suffering from kyphosis
lumbar	**LUM**-bar		Latin *loin*	The region of the back and sides between the ribs and pelvis
sacrum sacral (adj)	**SAY**-crum **SAY**-kral	 S/ R/	Latin *sacred* -al *pertaining to* sacr- *sacrum*	Segment of the vertebral column that forms part of the pelvis Pertaining to or in the region of the sacrum
scoliosis	skoh-lee-**OH**-sis	S/ R/	-osis *condition* scoli- *crooked*	An abnormal lateral curvature of the vertebral column
scoliotic (adj)	**SKOH**-lee-**OT**-ik	S/ R/CF	-tic *pertaining to* scoli/o- *crooked*	Pertaining to or suffering from scoliosis
spine	**SPINE**		Latin *spine*	Vertebral column or a short projection from a bone
spinal (adj)	**SPY**-nal	S/ R/	-al *pertaining to* spin- *spine*	Pertaining to the spine
vertebra vertebrae (pl) vertebral (adj)	**VER**-teh-brah **VER**-teh-brae **VER**-teh-bral	 S/ R/	Latin *spinal joint* -al *pertaining to* vertebr- *vertebra*	One of the bones of the spinal column Pertaining to a vertebra
whiplash	**WHIP**-lash	R/ R/	whip- *to swing* -lash *end of whip*	Symptoms caused by sudden, uncontrolled extension, and flexion of the neck, often in an automobile accident

EXERCISES

A. Review *the Case Report on this spread before answering the questions.*   **LO 4.2, 4.3, and 4.6** *Understand*

1. What are Ms. Cardenas' symptoms? _____

2. What type of accident was she involved in? _____

3. Define the abbreviation MRI in words. _____

4. Describe herniation of a disc. _____

5. What does *intervertebral* mean? _____.

6. Where does the radiating pain in her left arm originate? _____

7. The "C" in "C5–C6" means _____.

B. Apply *the correct form of the bolded similar terms appropriately in the following documentation, and you will meet a chapter objective!*

Fill in the blanks.   **LO 4.2, 4.3, and 4.6** *Apply*

vertebra   **vertebral**   **vertebrae**

1. The patient's C5 _____ was fractured in the accident.

2. A part of the axial skeleton is the _____ column.

3. The patient's C5 and C6 _____ were fractured in the accident.

Now supply the missing terms to complete the following sentence.

4. The designations C5-C6 and C6-C7 are for locations of _____.

Lesson 4.2(cont'd) **Skull and Face** (LO 4.2 and 4.6)

The Skull (LO 4.2 and 4.6)

When you glance at your face in the mirror, chances are you're not thinking about what's behind your brown eyes or your slightly crooked smile. You see one image—not its layers, pieces, or parts. However, the human skull *(Figure 4.9)* is made up of 22 separate bones. Your **cranium,** the upper part of the skull that encloses the **cranial** cavity and protects the brain, contains 8 of these 22 bones; your facial skeleton contains the rest.

Parietal bone
Sphenoid bone
Occipital bone
Temporal bone

Frontal bone
Ethmoid bone
Nasal bone
Lacrimal bone
Maxilla
Zygomatic bone
Mandible

▲ **FIGURE 4.9**
Skull, Right Lateral View.

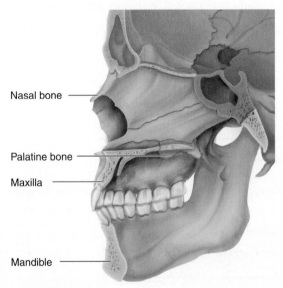

Nasal bone
Palatine bone
Maxilla
Mandible

▲ **FIGURE 4.10**
Facial Bones.

Abbreviation

TMJ   temporomandibular joint

The bones of the cranium are joined together by sutures (joints that appear as seams), which are covered on the inside and outside by a thin layer of connective tissue. These bones have the following functions:

1. The **frontal** bone forms the forehead, roofs of the (eye) orbits, and part of the floor of the cranium and contains a pair of right and left frontal sinuses above the orbits.

2. **Parietal** bones form the bulging sides and roof of the cranium.

3. The **occipital** bone forms the back of and part of the base of the cranium.

4. **Temporal** bones form the sides of and part of the base of the cranium.

5. The **sphenoid** bone forms part of the base of the cranium and the orbits.

6. The **ethmoid** bone is hollow and forms part of the nose, the orbits, and the ethmoid sinuses.

These bones of the skull provide protection for the brain and the organs of vision, taste, hearing, equilibrium, and smell.

The lower part of the skull houses the bones of the facial skeleton *(Figure 4.10)*. These bones do the following:

1. **Maxillary** bones form the upper jaw **(maxilla),** hold the upper teeth, and are hollow, forming the maxillary sinuses.

2. **Palatine** bones are located behind the maxilla and cannot be seen on a lateral view of the skull.

3. **Zygomatic** bones are the prominences of the cheeks (cheekbones) below the eyes.

4. **Lacrimal** bones form the medial wall of each orbit.

5. **Nasal** bones form the sides and bridge of the nose.

6. **The mandible** is the lower jawbone, which holds the lower teeth. The mandible articulates (joins) with the temporal bone to form the **temporomandibular joint (TMJ).**

The bones of the facial skeleton provide a frame on which the muscles and other tissues of the face facilitate eating, facial expressions, breathing, and speech.

The third component of the axial skeleton, the rib cage, is discussed in Chapter 8, "Respiratory System."

Word Analysis and Definition

S = Suffix   P = Prefix   R = Root   R/CF = Combining Form

WORD	PRONUNCIATION		ELEMENTS	DEFINITION
cranium	KRAY-nee-um		Greek *skull*	The upper part of the skull that encloses and protects the brain
cranial (adj)	KRAY-nee-al	S/ R/	-al *pertaining to* crani- *skull*	Pertaining to the skull
ethmoid	ETH-moyd	S/ R/	-oid *resembling* ethm- *sieve*	Bone that forms the back of the nose and encloses numerous air cells
lacrimal	LAK-rim-al	S/ R/	-al *pertaining to* lacrim- *tears*	Lacrimal bone forms part of the medial wall of the orbit, *or* pertaining to tears
mandible mandibular (adj)	MAN-di-bel man-DIB-you-lar	S/ R/	Latin *jaw* -ar *pertaining to* mandibul- *mandible*	Lower jaw bone Pertaining to the mandible
maxilla	mak-SILL-ah		Latin *jawbone*	Upper jawbone, containing right and left maxillary sinuses
maxillary (adj)	mak-SILL-ah-ree	S/ R/	-ary *pertaining to* maxilla- *maxilla*	Pertaining to the maxilla
occipital	ock-SIP-it-al	S/ R/	-al *pertaining to* occipit- *back of the head*	The back of the skull
palatine	PAL-ah-tine	S/ R/	-ine *pertaining to* palat- *palate*	Bone that forms the hard palate and parts of the nose and orbits
parietal	pah-RYE-eh-tal	S/ R/	-al *pertaining to* pariet- *wall*	The two bones forming the sidewalls and roof of the cranium
sphenoid	SFEE-noyd	S/ R/	-oid *resemble* sphen- *wedge*	Wedge-shaped bone at the base of the skull
temporal	TEM-pore-al	S/ R/	-al *pertaining to* tempor- *time, temple*	Bone that forms part of the base and sides of the skull
temporomandibular joint (TMJ)	TEM-pore-oh-man-DIB-you-lar JOYNT	S/ R/CF R/	-ar *pertaining to* tempor/o- *temple* -mandibul- *mandible*	The joint between the temporal bone and the mandible
zygoma zygomatic (adj)	zye-GO-mah zye-go-MAT-ik	S/ R/	French *yoke* -ic *pertaining to* zygomat- *cheekbone*	Bone that forms the prominence of the cheek Pertaining to the cheekbone

EXERCISES

A. Roots: *The following medical terms from the WAD box are alike in that they have similar suffixes, but their roots make them different terms. Define each term after you have defined the suffix. Fill in the blanks.* **LO 4.1 and 4.6** Apply

1. oid means _____.

  ethmoid: _____

  sphenoid: _____

2. al means _____.

  lacrimal: _____

  cranial: _____

B. Apply *the language of orthopedics and circle the correct answer.* **LO 4.6** Apply

1. The mandible is the:

  lower jawbone   base of the cranium   upper jawbone

2. Which of these bones is NOT in the facial skeleton?

  lacrimal   frontal   patella

3. How many bones are in the cranium?

  22   8   14

4. What does *articulate* mean?

  stretches   fractures   joins

5. What is a *suture?*

  seam   bend   sharp point

Lesson 4.3

Bones and Joints of the Shoulder Girdle and Upper Limb

Objectives

Your shoulders, arms, hands, and fingers are used nearly every time you move your body, no matter where you are—at work, at home, at the gym, in the car, or relaxing on the beach. Because these bones and joints get so much use, it's necessary to understand how they work and how to care for them. The information in this lesson will enable you to use correct medical terminology to:

4.3.1 Recognize the structures and functions of the bones and joints of the shoulder girdle.

4.3.2 Explain common disorders of the bones and joints of the shoulder girdle.

4.3.3 Identify the structures and functions of the bones and joints of the arm, elbow, and wrist.

4.3.4 Describe common disorders of the bones and joints of the arm, elbow, and wrist.

4.3.5 Specify the structures and functions of the bones and joints of the hand.

4.3.6 Define common disorders of the bones and joints of the hand.

Abbreviation

AC   acromioclavicular

Shoulder Girdle
(LO 4.2 and 4.7)

The bones and joints of your shoulder girdle connect your axial skeleton to your upper limbs.

The bones of the shoulder girdle are the **scapulae** (shoulder blades) and **clavicles** (collarbones). The scapula extends over the top of the shoulder joint to form a roof called the **acromion,** which is attached to the clavicle at the **acromioclavicular (AC)** joint. Several ligaments hold together the **articulating** surfaces of the humerus and scapula.

The shoulder joint between the scapula and the **humerus** bone of the upper arm *(Figure 4.11)* is a ball-and-socket joint, allowing the head of the humerus greater range of motion than any other joint in the body. This broad range of motion does have one drawback; because the shoulder joint is very unstable, it's prone to **dislocation.**

Disorders of the Shoulder Girdle (LO 4.2 and 4.7)

Shoulder separation is a dislocation of the acromioclavicular joint, often caused by a fall onto the point of the shoulder.

Shoulder dislocation occurs when the ball of the humerus slips out of the scapula's socket, usually anteriorly.

Shoulder subluxation occurs when the ball of the humerus slips partially out of position in the socket, and then moves back in.

Case Report 4.3

You are . . .

. . . an orthopedic technologist working with Kenneth Stannard, MD, at Fulwood Medical Center.

You are communicating with . . .

. . . James Fox, a 17-year-old male who complains of severe pain in his right wrist. While playing soccer a few hours earlier, he fell. James pushed his hand out to break his fall and heard his wrist snap. The wrist is now swollen and deformed. T 98.2, P 92, R 15, BP 110/76. On examination, his right wrist is swollen and tender and has a dinner-fork **deformity**. An IV has been started, and he has been given 3 mg of morphine IV. An X-ray of the wrist has been ordered.

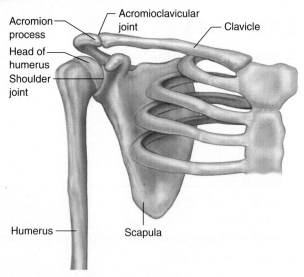

▲ **FIGURE 4.11**
Pectoral Girdle and Humerus.

Word Analysis and Definition

S = Suffix   P = Prefix   R = Root   R/CF = Combining Form

WORD	PRONUNCIATION		ELEMENTS	DEFINITION
acromion	ah-**CROW**-mee-on		Greek *tip of the shoulder*	Lateral end of the scapula, extending over the shoulder joint
acromioclavicular	ah-**CROW**-mee-oh-klah-**VICK**-you-lar	S/ R/CF R/	-ar *pertaining to* acromi/o- *acromion* -clavicul- *clavicle*	The joint between the acromion and the clavicle
articulate	ar-**TIK**-you-late	S/ R/	-ate *composed of* articul-*joint*	Two separate bones have formed a joint
articulation	ar-tik-you-**LAY**-shun	S/	-ation *process*	A joint
clavicle	**KLAV**-ih-kul		Latin *collarbone*	Curved bone that forms the anterior part of the pectoral girdle
clavicular (adj)	klah-**VICK**-you-lar	S/ R/	-ar *pertaining to* clavicul- *clavicle*	Pertaining to the clavicle
deformity	dee-**FOR**-mih-tee	S/ P/ R/	-ity *condition* de- *change of* -form- *appearance, form*	A permanent structural deviation from the normal
dislocation	dis-low-**KAY**-shun	S/ P/ R/	-ion *action, condition* dis- *apart, away from* -locat- *place*	Completely out of joint
humerus	**HYU**-mer-us		Latin *shoulder*	Single bone of the upper arm
pectoral pectoral girdle	**PEK**-tor-al **PEK**-tor-al **GIR**-del	S/ R/	-al *pertaining to* pector- *chest* girdle, Old English *encircle*	Pertaining to the chest Incomplete bony ring that attaches the upper limb to the axial skeleton
scapula scapulae (pl) scapular (adj)	**SKAP**-you-lah **SKAP**-you-lee **SKAP**-you-lar	S/ R/	Latin *shoulder blade* -ar *pertaining to* scapul- *scapula*	Shoulder blade Pertaining to the shoulder blade
subluxation	sub-luck-**SAY**-shun	S/ P/ R/	-ion *action, condition* sub- *under, below, slightly* -luxat- *dislocate*	An incomplete dislocation when some contact between the joint surfaces remains

EXERCISES

A. Review *the Case Report on this spread before answering the questions.*   **LO 4.2, 4.7, and 4.10** *Understand*

1. What are Mr. Fox's complaints when he presents at Dr. Stannard's office? _____

2. What is discovered on Mr. Fox's physical examination? _____

3. IV is the abbreviation for the medical term: _____

4. Why are they giving Mr. Fox morphine? _____

5. What diagnostic test has been ordered for Mr. Fox? _____

B. Build medical terms *using the language of orthopedics to complete this exercise. Each term is defined and partially complete. Add the rest of the elements to complete the term, and write under the line the element(s) you have used. The first one is done for you. Fill in the blanks.*
LO 4.1, 4.2, 4.7, and 4.10 *Apply*

1. incomplete dislocation _____sub_____ / _____luxat_____ / _____ion_____
                                    P   R   S

2. joint between acromion and clavicle _____ / _____ / _____ar_____

3. a joint _____ / _____ / _____ation_____

4. pertaining to the shoulder blade _____ / _____ / _____ar_____

Upper Arm and Elbow Joint
(LO 4.2 and 4.7)

Your upper arm extends from your shoulder to your elbow and contains only one bone, the **humerus** *(Figure 4.12)*. The smooth surface of the hemispherical head that articulates with the socket of the scapula is covered with articular cartilage. At the lower end of the humerus, the **trochlea** articulates with the **ulna** bone of the forearm and the **capitulum** articulates with the **radius** *(Figure 4.13)*.

Elbow Joint (LO 4.2 and 4.7)

The elbow joint has two articulations:

1. A hinge joint between the humerus and the ulna bone of the forearm, which allows flexion and extension of the elbow; and

2. A gliding joint between the humerus and the radius bone of the forearm, which allows **pronation** and **supination** of the forearm and hand.

Disorders of the Elbow Joint
(LO 4.2 and 4.7)

When you bend your elbow, you can easily feel the bony prominence (the **olecranon** *Figure 4.13*) that extends from the ulna. The olecranon can be easily fractured by a direct blow to the elbow or by a fall on a bent elbow.

The olecranon **bursa** is a thin, slippery sac between the skin and the prominence of the olecranon bone. It contains a small amount of fluid to enable the skin to move freely over the bone. If the bursa becomes irritated or inflamed, fluid accumulates and **bursitis** occurs. Treatment is **aspiration** and an antibiotic if indicated by laboratory investigation of the aspirated fluid.

Tennis elbow is caused by overuse of the elbow joint or poor form when playing tennis or golf. The pain occurs when ligaments and muscle tendons around the joint tear. Treatment is rest, ice, pain medication, massage, and stretching exercises.

When a child falls on an outstretched arm, the force of hitting the ground can be transmitted up the arm to cause a fracture of the elbow joint. This accounts for about 10% of all fractures in children.

Anterior surface

— Head

Lateral epicondyle — — Medial epicondyle

▶ **FIGURE 4.12**
Humerus.

— Humerus

Gliding joint

Radius

Olecranon —

Hinge

Ulna

▲ **FIGURE 4.13**
Elbow Joint.

Word Analysis and Definition

WORD	PRONUNCATION	ELEMENTS		DEFINITION
aspiration	as-pih-**RAY**-shun	S/	-ion *process*	Removal by suction of fluid or gas from a body cavity
aspirate (verb)	**AS**-pih-rate	R/	aspirat- *to breathe on*	
bursa	**BURR**-sah		Latin *purse*	A closed sac containing synovial fluid
bursae (pl)	**BURR**-see			
bursitis	burr-**SIGH**-tis	S/ R/	-itis *inflammation* burs- *bursa*	Inflammation of a bursa
capitulum	kah-**PIT**-you-lum	S/ R/CF	-lum *small structure* capit/u *small head*	A small head or rounded extremity of a bone
olecranon	oh-**LECK**-rah-non		Greek *point of elbow*	Prominent, proximal extremity of ulna
pronation pronate (verb) prone	pro-**NAY**-shun **PRO**-nate **PRONE**	S/ R/	-ion *action, condition* pronat- *bend down* Latin, *lying down*	Process of lying face down or of turning a hand or foot with the volar (palm or sole) surface down Lying face down, flat on your belly
radius radial (adj)	**RAY**-dee-us **RAY**-dee-al	S/ R/	Latin *spoke of a wheel* -al *pertaining to* radi- *radius*	The forearm bone on the thumb side Pertaining to the radius or to any of the structures (artery, vein, nerve) named after it
supination supine	soo-pih-**NAY**-shun soo-**PINE**	S/ R/	-ion *action, condition* supinat- *bend backward* Latin *bend backward*	Process of lying face upward or of turning a hand or foot so that the palm or sole is facing up Lying face up, flat on your spine
trochlea trochlear	**TROHK**-lee-ah **TROHK**-lee-ar	S/ R/	Latin *pulley* -ar *pertaining to* trochle- *pulley*	Smooth articular surface of bone on which another glides Pertaining to a trochlea
ulna ulnar (adj)	**UL**-nah **UL**-nar	S/ R/	Latin *elbow, arm* -ar *pertaining to* uln- *ulna*	The medial and larger bone of the forearm Pertaining to the ulna or to any of the structures (artery, vein, nerve) named after it

EXERCISES

A. Meet lesson *and chapter objectives by answering these questions using the language of orthopedics.*   **LO 4.2, 4.7, and 4.10** *Remember*

1. What two types of articulations exist in the elbow?

_____

2. The upper arm has only one bone—the _____

3. What type of joint allows flexion and extension? _____

4. List the common disorders of the elbow joint: _____

5. What does the trochlea articulate with? _____

6. What is the bone of your upper arm that extends from the shoulder to the elbow? _____

7. Based on its shape, what kind of bone is #6? _____

8. What are the two opposite terms in this WAD? _____ and _____

9. Is the radius a forearm bone or an upper arm bone? _____

10. Which is the bigger bone: the radius or the ulna? _____

B. The statement *is either true or false. Circle the correct answer.* **LO 4.7** *Understand*

1. The opposite of pronation is supination.   T   F

2. The capitulum articulates with the scapula.   T   F

3. A sports-related injury is very common in the elbow.   T   F

4. The radius is on the thumb side of the hand.   T   F

5. A hinge joint allows pronation of the hand and forearm.   T   F

Forearm, Wrist, and Hand (LO 4.2 and 4.7)

The Wrist (LO 4.2 and 4.7)

In your forearm, the radius bone on the thumb side and the larger ulna bone on the little-finger side articulate at your wrist joint with the small **carpal** bones *(Figure 4.14)*.

Disorders of the Wrist (LO 4.2 and 4.7)

A **Colles fracture** is a common fracture of the radius just above the wrist joint *(Figure 4.15)* that occurs when a person tries to break a fall with an outstretched hand.

Case Report 4.3 (continued)

The X-ray of James Fox's wrist showed a **Colles fracture** of the radius, 1 inch above the end of the bone. Dr. Stannard applied a cast with the **distal** fragment of the fracture in palmar flexion and ulnar deviation. Mr. Fox was sent home with Vicodin 500 mg **po, prn,** for pain, and an appointment to return to the clinic in a week.

Fracture of the scaphoid bone *(Figure 4.14)*—the most common fracture of a carpal bone—also results from breaking a fall with an outstretched hand, but poor blood supply here makes healing slow and difficult.

Carpal tunnel syndrome is inflammation of the tendon synovial sheaths on the back of the wrist arising from repetitive movements such as computer keyboard operation.

The Hand (LO 4.2 and 4.7)

The five fingers of your single hand have 14 bones called **phalanges.** The thumb has two phalanges, and each of the remaining four fingers has three *(Figure 4.14)*. In your palm, the five bones closest to the fingers are **metacarpals;** these connect to the phalanges at the **metacarpophalangeal** joints. The metacarpals connect at the wrist to eight small carpal bones, which then connect the hand to the bones of the forearm. All of these bones require numerous joints with ligaments to connect and stabilize them.

Disorders of the Hand (LO 4.2 and 4.7)

Osteoarthritis (OA) in the hand joints occurs from wear and tear leading to deterioration of joint cartilage. Small bony spurs called **Heberden nodes** form over the joint *(Figure 4.16)*.

Rheumatoid arthritis (RA), with destruction of joint surfaces, joint capsules, and ligaments, leads to noticeable deformity and joint instability *(Figure 4.17)*. RA occurs mostly in women, between ages 40 and 60, and affects the synovial membrane lining the joints and tendons. Lumps known as **rheumatic** nodules form over the small joints of the hand and wrist.

Radius
Ulna
Scaphoid
Carpals
Metacarpals
1
2 3 4 5
Phalanges
Proximal phalanx
Middle phalanx
Distal phalanx

▲ **FIGURE 4.14**
Bones of the Wrist and Hand.

▲ **FIGURE 4.15**
X-Ray of Colles Fracture.

Heberden nodes

▲ **FIGURE 4.16**
Hand with Osteoarthritis.

▲ **FIGURE 4.17**
Hands with Rheumatoid Arthritis.

Word Analysis and Definition

S = Suffix   P = Prefix   R = Root   R/CF = Combining Form

WORD	PRONUNCIATION		ELEMENTS	DEFINITION
arthritis	ar-**THRI**-tis	S/ R/	-itis *inflammation* arthr- *joint*	Inflammation of a joint or joints
carpus carpal (adj) metacarpal	**KAR**-pus **KAR**-pal **MET**-ah-**KAR**-pal	 S/ R/ P/	Greek *wrist* -al *pertaining to* carp- *wrist bones* meta- *after, subsequent to*	The eight carpal bones of the wrist Pertaining to the wrist The five bones between the carpus and the fingers
Colles fracture	**KOL**-ez **FRAK**-chur		Abraham Colles, Irish surgeon, 1773–1843	Fracture of the distal radius at the wrist
eponym	**EH**-po-nim		Greek *epõnymos, meaning eponymous*	A procedure or a diagnosis with a name derived from the name of the person who discovered it (if it is a disease or condition) or originated it (if it is a procedure)
Heberden node	**HEH**-ber-den **NOHD**		William Heberden, English physician, 1710–1801	Bony lump on the terminal phalanx of the fingers in osteoarthritis
metacarpophalangeal	**MET**-ah-**KAR**-poh-fay-**LAN**-jee-al	S/ P/ R/CF R/CF	-al *pertaining to* meta- *after, subsequent to* -carp/o- *bones of the wrist* -phalang/e- *phalanx, finger or toe*	The joints between the metacarpal bones and the phalanges
osteoarthritis	**OSS**-tee-oh-ar-**THRI**-tis	S/ R/CF R/	-itis *inflammation* oste/o- *bone* arthr- *joint*	Chronic inflammatory disease of joints
phalanx phalanges (pl)	**FAY**-lanks fay-**LAN**-jeez		Latin *bone of finger* or *toe*	One of the bones of the digits (fingers or toes)
rheumatism rheumatic (adj) rheumatoid arthritis	**RU**-ma-tizm ru-**MA**-tik **RU**-mah-toyd ar-**THRI**-tis	S/ R/ S/ S/	-ism *condition* rheumat- *a flow* -ic *pertaining to* -oid *resembling*	Pain in various parts of the musculoskeletal system Pertaining to or characterized by rheumatism Systemic disease affecting many joints

EXERCISES

A. Deconstruct *the following terms by filling in the blanks:*   **LO 4.1, 4.7, and 4.10** *Analyze*

1. Metacarpophalangeal: _____ / _____ / _____
                                        P   R, R/CF   S

2. Osteoarthritis: _____ / _____ / _____
                                   P   R/CF   S

   Give their meanings: 1. _____ 2. _____

B. Review *the Case Report on this spread before answering the questions.*   **LO 4.7 and 4.10** *Understand*

1. What specific type of Fx does Mr. Fox have? _____

2. Describe the fracture's location. _____

3. What is the difference between a cast and a splint? _____

4. What is the opposite of *distal?* _____

5. What pain medication was prescribed for Mr. Fox? _____

C. Review Figure 4.14 *on this spread to formulate your answers to the following questions.*   **LO 4.2, 4.7, and 4.10** *Remember*

1. What is the difference between the distal and the proximal phalanx? _____

2. What is the only finger with two phalanges instead of three? _____

3. What term can be applied to both fingers and toes? _____

4. What is the most common cause of a Colles fracture? _____

Lesson 4.4

Pelvic Girdle and Lower Limb

Objectives

You use your legs and feet constantly, every day of your life, whether you are standing, walking, or changing positions. The information in this lesson will enable you to use correct medical terminology to:

4.4.1 Identify the structures and functions of the bones and joints of the pelvic girdle.

4.4.2 Describe common disorders of the bones and joints of the pelvic girdle.

4.4.3 Identify the structures and functions of the bones and joints of the leg, knee, and ankle.

4.4.4 Recognize common disorders of the hip joint, knee, and ankle.

4.4.5 Identify the structures and functions of the bones and joints of the foot.

4.4.6 Name common disorders of the bones and joints of the foot.

The Pelvic Girdle (LO 4.2 and 4.8)

Your pelvic girdle consists of your two hip bones that articulate anteriorly with each other at the **symphysis pubis** and posteriorly with the **sacrum** (a triangular-shaped bone in your lower back). This forms the bowl-shaped **pelvis.** The two joints between your hip bones and the sacrum are called **sacroiliac joints.**

The pelvic girdle has these functions:

1. Supports the axial skeleton;
2. Transmits the upper body's weight to the lower limbs;
3. Provides attachments for the lower limbs; and
4. Protects the internal reproductive organs, urinary bladder, and distal segment of the large intestine.

Each of your hip bones is actually a fusion of three bones: the **ilium, ischium, and pubis** *(Figure 4.18a).* This fusion occurs in the region of the **acetabulum,** a cup-shaped cavity on the lateral surface of the hip bone that receives the head of the **femur,** or thigh bone *(Figure 4.18b).*

The lower part of the pelvis is formed by the lower ilium, ischium, and pubic bones that surround a short canal-like pelvic cavity, through which the rectum, vagina, and urethra pass. In females, the infant passes down this canal during childbirth.

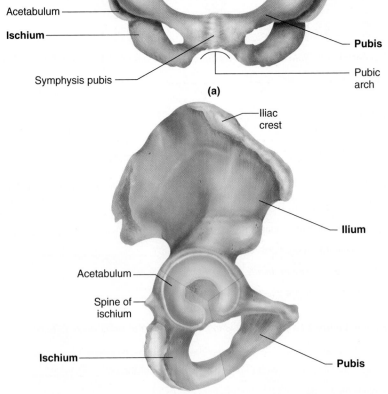

▶ **FIGURE 4.18**
Pelvic Girdle.
(a) Front view. (b) Side view.

Word Analysis and Definition

WORD	PRONUNCIATION	ELEMENTS		DEFINITION
acetabulum	ass-eh-**TAB**-you-lum		Latin *vinegar cup*	The cup-shaped cavity of the hip bone that receives the head of the femur to form the hip joint
femur	**FEE**-mur		Latin *thigh*	The thigh bone
femoral (adj)	**FEM**-oh-ral	S/ R/	-al *pertaining to* femor- *femur*	Pertaining to the femur
ilium	**ILL**-ee-um		Latin *groin*	Large wing-shaped bone at the upper and posterior part of the pelvis
ischium ischia (pl) ischial (adj)	**IS**-kee-um **IS**-kee-ah **IS**-kee-al	 S/ R/	Greek *hip* -al *pertaining to* ischi- *ischium, hip bone*	Lower and posterior part of the hip bone Pertaining to the ischium
pelvis	**PEL**-viss		Latin *basin*	Basin-shaped ring of bones, ligaments, and muscles at the base of the spine. Also, any basin-shaped cavity, like the pelvis of the kidney
pelvic (adj)	**PEL**-vik	S/ R/	-ic *pertaining to* pelv- *pelvis*	Pertaining to the pelvis
pubis pubic (adj)	**PYU**-bis **PYU**-bik	 S/ R/	Latin *pubis* -ic *pertaining to* pub- *pubis*	Alternative name for the pubic bone Pertaining to the pubic bone
sacroiliac joint	say-kroh-**ILL**-ih-ak **JOINT**	S/ R/CF R	-ac *pertaining to* sacr/o- *sacrum* -ili- *ilium*	The joint between the sacrum and the ilium
symphysis symphyses (pl)	**SIM**-feh-sis **SIM**-feh-seez		Greek *grow together*	Two bones joined by fibrocartilage; in this case, the two pubic bones

EXERCISES

A. Demonstrate your knowledge *of the precise medical term to answer the following questions. Every answer can be found in the above WAD.*

   Write the term that is: **LO 4.8 and 4.10** *Apply*

1. another name for the thigh bone _____

2. a basin-shaped ring of bones _____

3. the joint between the sacrum and the ilium _____

4. the lower posterior part of the hip bone _____

5. the wing-shaped bone in the pelvis _____

B. Meet lesson objectives *and circle the correct medical term based on the statement.*   **LO 4.8** *Remember*

1. The hip bone is a fusion of three bones: the ilium, the ischium, and the

   femur   pubis   acetabulum

2. The pelvis is shaped like a

   bowl   box   basket

3. One function of the pelvic girdle is to:

   support the cranium   attach lower limbs   transport waste products

4. What organs does the pelvic girdle protect?

   lungs   pancreas and gallbladder   bladder, intestines, reproductive

5. A triangular-shaped bone in the lower back is the

   scapula   sacrum   symphysis

Keynote

• The sciatic nerve lies directly behind the lower third of the SI joint. Many patients with SI joint strain will have pain radiating down the back of the leg.

Case Report 4.4

You are . . .

. . . a physical therapist assistant working in the physical therapy department of Fulwood Medical Center.

You are communicating with . . .

. . . Sandra Halpin, a 38-year-old female who is complaining of persistent low back pain on her left side. The pain began about two years previously, when she and her husband were moving and she was lifting heavy boxes. Her family physician has prescribed rest, back exercises, muscle relaxants, and painkillers, but she has had no relief.

On examination, she exhibits tenderness over the left sacroiliac joint, and when she presses her left knee to her chest, she experiences considerable pain over the **SI** joint. X-rays of the pelvis and hips, and an angle study of the SI joints, showed narrowing of the left SI joint space. A diagnosis of left sacroiliac joint strain has been made.

Right sacroiliac joint

Narrowing of left sacroiliac joint

▲ **FIGURE 4.19**
X-ray of the Sacroiliac (SI) joints—showing narrowing of the joint space in the left SI joint.

Sacroiliac (SI) joint strain is a common cause of lower back pain. Unlike most joints, the SI joint *(Figure 4.19)* is designed to move only 1/4 of an inch during weight-bearing and forward-bending movements. Its main function is to provide shock absorption for the spine.

Because stretching in the SI joint ligaments makes this joint overly mobile, it's susceptible to wear and tear, including painful arthritis. Another cause of pain in the SI joint is trauma, when tearing of the joint ligaments allows too much motion.

A clinical examination, joint X-ray **(radiology),** and CT scan may be used to diagnose the presence of sacroiliac strain. For temporary pain relief, a local anesthetic can be injected into the joint. Standard treatment involves **stabilizing** the joint with a **brace** and strengthening the lower back muscles with physical therapy. Occasionally, **arthrodesis** of the joint is necessary.

Diastasis symphysis pubis sometimes occurs during pregnancy. It is caused by excessive stretching of pelvic ligaments, which widens the joint between the two pubic bones. This leads to pain and difficulty in walking, climbing stairs, and turning over in bed. During pregnancy, however, hormones generally enable connective tissue in the SI joint area to relax so the pelvis can expand enough to allow birth without causing SI joint strain.

Abbreviation

SI   sacroiliac

Word Analysis and Definition

WORD	PRONUNCIATION	ELEMENTS		DEFINITION
arthrodesis	ar-**THROW**-dee-sis	S/ R/CF	-desis *to fuse together* arthr/o- *joint*	Fixation or stiffening of a joint by surgery
brace	BRACE		Old English *to fasten*	Appliance to support a part of the body in its correct position
diastasis	die-**ASS**-tah-sis		Greek *separation*	Separation of normally joined parts
radiology	ray-dee-**OL**-oh-jee	S/ R/CF	-logy *study of* radi/o- *radiation, X-rays*	The study of medical imaging
radiologist	ray-dee-**OL**-oh-jist	S/	-logist *one who studies, specialist*	Medical specialist in the use of X-rays and other imaging techniques
stable	**STAY**-bell		Latin *steady*	Steady, not varying
stabilize	**STAY**-bill-ize	S/ R/	-ize *action* stabil- *steady, fixed*	To make or hold firm and steady

EXERCISES

A. Review *the Case Report on this spread before answering the questions.*   **LO 4.8 and 4.10** *Understand*

1. What is Sandra Halpin's chief complaint? _____

2. How did she injure herself? _____

3. What has *not* helped Ms. Halpin's pain? _____

4. What other specialist besides an orthopedist has seen Ms. Halpin? _____

5. What is Ms. Halpin's final diagnosis? _____

B. Every answer *you need can be found on the two-page spread open in front of you. Fill in the blanks.*   **LO 4.8 and 4.11** *Remember*

1. What is a common cause of low back pain? _____

2. What two bones form the SI joint? _____ and _____

3. What is the main function of the SI joint? _____

4. Name one cause of pain in the SI joint. _____

5. What diagnostic tests are used to diagnose SI strain? _____

C. Read *the answer choices for each question and immediately discard the ones you know are not correct. Circle the correct answer in the remaining possibilities.*   **LO 4.8 and 4.10** *Understand*

1. What can provide temporary pain relief from SI joint strain?
  a. stretching
  b. a brace
  c. PT
  d. heat application
  e. local anesthetic injected into the joint

2. The expertise of a radiologist is in:
  a. skin diseases
  b. tissue study
  c. disorders of the brain
  d. interpreting X-rays
  e. lung conditions

3. Fixation or stiffening of a joint by surgery is called
  a. arthroscopy
  b. arthroplasty
  c. arthrodesis
  d. arthrotomy
  e. none of these

4. What substance allows the SI joint to relax enough for delivery of a baby?
  a. lymph
  b. blood
  c. enzymes
  d. synovial fluid
  e. hormones

Bones and Joints of the Hip and Thigh (LO 4.2 and 4.8)

Your **hip joint** is a ball-and-socket mechanism formed by the head of your femur (thigh bone) and the acetabulum (cup-shaped hip socket) of your hip bone *(Figure 4.20)*. The **labrum** is the articular cartilage that forms a rim around the hip joint socket, cushioning the joint and helping to keep your femoral head in place in the socket. Finally, the hip joint is secured by a thick joint capsule reinforced by strong ligaments that connect the neck of the femur to the rim of the hip socket.

Disorders and Injuries of the Hip Joint (LO 4.2 and 4.8)

Hip pointer, often a football-related injury, is a blow to the rim of the pelvis that leads to bruising of the bone and surrounding tissues.

Osteoarthritis is common in the hip as a result of aging, weight bearing, and repetitive use of the joint. The cartilage on both the acetabulum and the head of the femur deteriorates, causing friction between the bones of the femoral head and the acetabulum that leads to pain and loss of mobility.

Rheumatoid arthritis can also affect the hip, beginning in the synovial membrane and progressing to destroy cartilage and bone.

Avascular necrosis of the femoral head is the death (necrosis) of bone tissue when the blood supply is cut off (avascular), usually as a result of trauma.

Fractures of the neck of the femur occur as a result of a fall, most commonly in elderly women with osteoporosis.

Surgical Procedures of the Hip Joint (LO 4.2 and 4.8)

There are two standard surgical procedures for replacing or repairing the hip joint. **Arthroplasty,** a total replacement of the hip joint with a metal **prosthesis,** is the most common hip surgery today. Here, the diseased parts of the joint are removed and replaced with artificial parts made of titanium and other metals, ceramics, and plastics *(Figure 4.21)*.

Arthrodesis is a surgical procedure that fixates or stiffens a joint.

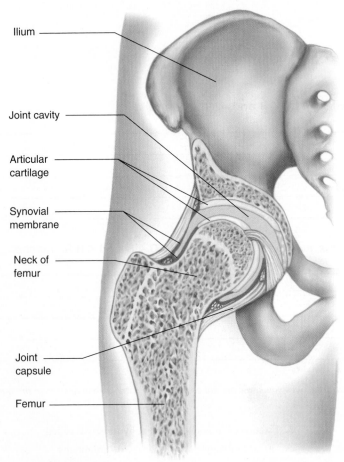

Ilium

Joint cavity

Articular cartilage

Synovial membrane

Neck of femur

Joint capsule

Femur

▲ **FIGURE 4.20**
Hip Joint.
Right frontal view of a section of the hip joint.

▲ **FIGURE 4.21**
Total Hip Replacement.
Colored x-ray of prosthetic hip.

Word Analysis and Definition

S = Suffix   P = Prefix   R = Root   R/CF = Combining Form

WORD	PRONUNCIATION	ELEMENTS		DEFINITION
arthrodesis	ar-**THROW**-dee-sis	S/ R/CF	-desis *to fuse together* arthr/o- *joint*	Fixation or stiffening of a joint by surgery
arthroplasty	**AR**-throw-plas-tee	S/ R/CF	-plasty *reshaping by surgery* arthr/o- *joint*	Surgery to repair, as far as possible, the function of a joint
avascular	a-**VAS**-cue-lar	S/ P/ R/	-ar *pertaining to* a- *without* -vascul- *blood vessel*	Without a blood supply
labrum	**LAY**-brum		Latin *lip-shaped*	Cartilage that forms a rim around the socket of the hip joint
necrosis necrotic (adj)	neh-**KROH**-sis neh-**KROT**-ik	S/ R/CF	Greek *death* -tic *pertaining to* necr/o- *death*	Pathologic death of cells or tissue Pertaining to or affected by necrosis
prosthesis prosthetic (adj)	**PROS**-thee-sis pros-**THET**-ik	S/ R/CF	Greek *addition* -ic *pertaining to* prosthet- *prosthesis*	An artificial part to remedy a defect in the body Pertaining to a prosthesis

EXERCISES

A. Proofread *the following sentences for errors in fact or spelling. Circle the error, then rewrite the sentence correctly.* **LO 4.2 and 4.10** *Apply*

1. Rheumatoid arthritis can destroy muscle and bone.

_____

2. Avascular necrosis is the death of cartilage when the blood supply is cut off.

_____

3. Arthrodesis is a total replacement of the hip joint.

_____

4. A joint is replaced with a metal prothesis.

_____

5. The labrum is a mucous membrane that forms a rim around the hip joint socket.

_____

B. Match *the correct medical term in column one with its meaning in column two.* **LO 4.2 and 4.5** *Understand*

1. _____ synovial   **A.** artificial body part

2. _____ arthroplasty   **B.** bloodless

3. _____ prosthesis   **C.** death of cells

4. _____ avascular   **D.** lubricating

5. _____ necrosis   **E.** joint repair

C. Circle *the best choice after you have discounted the answers you know are not correct.* **LO 4.2 and 4.5** *Remember*

1. What is the purpose of synovial fluid?

  a. balance   **d.** weight bearing

  b. alignment   **e.** mobility

  c. lubrication

2. What is the purpose of a prosthesis?

  a. restore well being   **d.** support the skeleton

  b. remedy a defect in the body   **e.** repair a joint

  c. maintain balance

Lesson 4.4 (cont'd)

Abbreviations

ACL anterior cruciate ligament
PCL posterior cruciate ligament

The Knee Joint
(LO 4.2 and 4.9)

Your knees do plenty of bending, whether you're climbing the stairs, exercising, sitting cross-legged, or squatting down to collect something from the floor. Each of your knees is a hinged joint formed with these four bones:

1. **The lower end of the femur,** shaped like a horseshoe;

2. **The flat upper end of the tibia;**

3. **The flat triangular patella** (kneecap), embedded in the **patellar** tendon and articulating with the femur *(Figure 4.22a);* and

4. **The fibula,** which forms a separate joint—the **tibiofibular joint** *(Figure 4.22b)*—by articulating with the tibia.

Case Report 4.5

You are . . .

. . . an Emergency Technician working in the Emergency Department of Fulwood Medical Center.

You are communicating with . . .

. . . Gail Griffith, a 17-year-old high school student and her mother, Mrs. Cindy Griffith. Gail landed awkwardly after jumping for a ball during a basketball game.

Gail: "My knee kinda popped as I landed."

Gail had to be assisted off the court. In the Emergency Department, the knee was swollen and unstable. An MRI showed a partial tear of the medial **collateral** ligament, a complete **rupture** of the anterior **cruciate** ligament, and a partial tear of the medial **meniscus**. Gail decided to have surgery, even though full recovery would take 6 months to 1 year of rehabilitation.

Mechanically, the patella's role is to provide a 30% strength increase in the extension of the knee joint.

Within the knee joint, two crescent-shaped pads of cartilage—the **medial** and **lateral menisci**—lie on top of the tibia and articulate with the femur. This cartilage helps to distribute weight more evenly across the joint surface to minimize wear and tear.

The knee joint has a fibrous capsule, lined with synovial membrane that secretes synovial fluid to lubricate the joint. Four ligaments hold the knee joint together: the **medial** and **lateral collateral ligaments** located outside the joint and the **anterior cruciate ligament (ACL)** and **posterior cruciate ligament (PCL)** located inside the joint cavity, crossing over each other to form an "X" *(Figure 4.22b)*.

The thigh muscles which move the knee joint are described in Lesson 5.3 of the next chapter.

▼ **FIGURE 4.22**
Knee Joint.
(a) Section of knee joint.
(b) Right knee joint, anterior view.

(a)

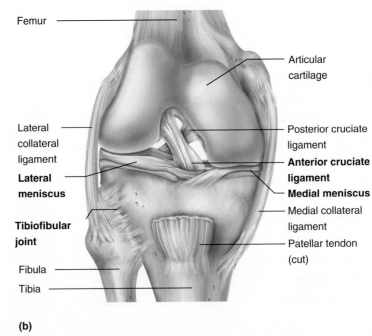

(b)

WORD	PRONUNCIATION	ELEMENTS		DEFINITION
collateral (**Note:** *An extra "l" has been inserted.*)	koh-**LAT**-er-al	S/ P/ R/	-al *pertaining to* co- *together* -later- *side*	Situated at the side, often to bypass an obstruction
cruciate	**KRU**-she-ate		Latin *cross*	Shaped like a cross. In this case, the two internal ligaments of the knee joint cross over each other to form an "X"
fibula fibular (adj)	**FIB**-you-lah **FIB**-you-lar	S/ R/	Latin *clasp* or *buckle* -ar *pertaining to* fibul- *fibula*	The smaller of the two bones of the lower leg Pertaining to the fibula
meniscus menisci (pl)	meh-**NISS**-kuss meh-**NISS**-key		Greek *crescent*	Disc of cartilage between the bones of a joint, in this case, the knee joint
patella (kneecap) patellae (pl) patellar (adj)	pah-**TELL**-ah pah-**TELL**-ee pah-**TELL**-ar	S/ R/	Latin *small plate* -ar *pertaining to* patell- *patella*	Thin, circular bone in front of the knee joint, embedded in the patellar tendon Pertaining to the patella bone or the tendon
rupture	**RUP**-tyur		Latin *break*	Break or tear of any body part
tibia tibial (adj)	**TIB**-ee-ah **TIB**-ee-al	S/ R/	Latin *large shinbone* -al *pertaining to* tibi- *tibia*	The larger bone of the lower leg Pertaining to the tibia

EXERCISES

A. Review *the Case Report on this spread before answering the questions.*   **LO 4.2, 4.9, and 4.10** *Understand*

1. What are Gail's symptoms when she presents to the ER?

    _____

2. What does MRI mean? _____

3. As a diagnostic test, what did the MRI show? _____

4. What is the meaning of the term "collateral"? _____

5. In her treatment plan, what will Gail be doing after her surgery?

    _____

6. What is the most severe of the injuries to Gail's knee?

    _____

7. Why do you think Gail opted for the surgery?

    _____

B. Spelling: *A medical term must be spelled correctly. Work with a fellow student on this exercise. Cover the WAD box with a sheet of paper while your partner dictates any 5 terms in the above WAD box to you. Write them in the "Test" column, and do your best to spell them correctly. When you are finished, remove the cover and check your spelling. If you have made any errors, rewrite the correct spelling in the "corrections" column.*   **LO 4.2, 4.9, and 4.10** *Remember*

Test   **Corrections**

1. _____   _____

2. _____   _____

3. _____   _____

4. _____   _____

5. _____   _____

Lesson 4.4 (cont'd)

Anterior cruciate
ligament (torn)

Medial collateral
ligament (torn)

Medial
meniscus (torn)

Patellar
ligament (cut)

Operative Report: Fulwood Medical Center

Patient: Gail Griffith, aged 17.
Preoperative Diagnosis: Traumatic **ACL** tear, medial collateral ligament tear, and tear of medial meniscus, right knee.

Case Report 4.5 (continued)

Postoperative Diagnosis: Same.
Procedure Performed: Arthroscopy, repair of medial collateral ligament, **ACL** reconstruction, repair of torn medial meniscus, right knee.
Operative Findings: An avulsed anterior cruciate ligament **(ACL)** of the femur with a tear of the posterior horn of the medial meniscus and tear of medial collateral ligament.

▲ **FIGURE 4.23**
Gail Griffith's Knee Injuries.

▲ **FIGURE 4.24**
Colored X-ray of Total Knee
Replacement.

The Knee Joint (continued) (LO 4.2 and 4.9)

Injuries to the Knee Joint (LO 4.2 and 4.9)

The **anterior cruciate ligament (ACL)** is the most commonly injured ligament in the knee *(Figure 4.23)*, particularly in football players and female athletes. The injury is often caused by a sudden **hyperflexion** of the knee joint when landing awkwardly on flat ground, as in Gail Griffith's case. Because of its poor vascular (blood) supply, the torn ligament does not heal and has to be surgically mended.

Other commonly injured major ligaments are the medial and lateral collateral ligaments and the posterior cruciate ligament.

Meniscus injuries result from a twist to the knee that tears the meniscus. The torn meniscus flips in and out of the joint as it moves, locking the knee and creating pain. Losing a meniscus leads to arthritic changes, so repair of the meniscus, as in Ms. Griffith's case, instead of removal (a **meniscectomy**) is preferred.

Patellar subluxation or dislocation produces an unstable, painful kneecap.

Prepatellar bursitis ("housemaid's knee") produces painful swelling over the **bursa** at the front of the knee and is seen in people who kneel for extended periods of time, like carpet layers.

Tendinitis of the patellar tendon results from overuse during activities like cycling, running, or dancing. Pain is felt where the tendon is inserted into the tibia, and this is treated with R.I.C.E (rest, ice, compression, elevation).

Surgical Procedures of the Knee Joint (LO 4.2 and 4.9)

There are several procedures and surgery options for those who sustain knee injuries. **Arthrocentesis** is the aspiration of knee joint fluid, which is examined to establish a diagnosis. Infected fluid may be drained off or medication, such as local corticosteroids, may be inserted.

Arthrography is an X-ray of a joint after injection of a contrast medium (harmless dye) into the joint to make the inside details of the joint visible.

Diagnostic arthroscopy is an exploratory procedure performed using an arthroscope to examine the internal compartments of the knee joint.

Surgical arthroscopy is performed through an arthroscope. This can be a **debridement** or removal of torn tissue like a meniscus or a ligament. It can also be a repair of a torn ligament by suturing, or tendon autograft, or repair of a torn meniscus.

Arthroplasty involves a total replacement of the knee joint *(Figure 4.24)*, usually because of osteoarthritis. The damaged cartilage and bone from the knee joint's surface are removed and replaced with metal and plastic.

Femur

Tibia

Word Analysis and Definition

S = Suffix   P = Prefix   R = Root   R/CF = Combining Form

WORD	PRONUNCIATION	ELEMENTS		DEFINITION
arthrocentesis	AR-throw-sen-TEE-sis	S/ R/CF	-centesis *puncture* arthr/o- *joint*	Aspiration of fluid from a joint
arthrography	ar-THROG-rah-fee	S/ R/CF	-graphy *process of recording* arthr/o- *joint*	X-ray of a joint taken after the injection of a contrast medium into the joint
arthroscopy	ar-THROS-koh-pee	S/	-scopy *the process of using an instrument to examine visually*	Visual examination of the interior of a joint
arthroscope	AR-thro-skope	R/CF S/	arthr/o- *joint* -scope *instrument to examine visually*	Endoscope used to examine the interior of a joint
bursa bursitis	BURR-sah burr-SIGH-tis	S/ R/	Latin *purse* -itis *inflammation* burs- *bursa*	A closed sac containing synovial fluid Inflammation of a bursa
debridement	day-BREED-mon ("Mon" is the French pronunciation of *ment*.)	S/ P/ R/	-ment *action* de- *removal, out of* -bride- *rubble, rubbish*	The removal of injured or necrotic tissue
hyperflexion	high-per-FLEK-shun	S/ P/ R/	-ion *action, condition* hyper- *excessive* -flex- *bend*	Flexion of a limb or part beyond the normal limits
meniscectomy	men-ih-SEK-toh-me	S/ R/	-ectomy *surgical excision* menisc- *crescent, meniscus*	Excision (cutting out) of all or part of a meniscus
prepatellar	pree-pah-TELL-ar	S/ P/ R/	-ar *pertaining to* pre- *before, in front of* -patell- *patella*	In front of the patella
tendinitis *(also spelled tendonitis)*	ten-dih-NYE-tis	S/ R/	-itis *inflammation* tendin- *tendon*	Inflammation of a tendon

EXERCISES

A. Review *the Case Report on this spread before answering the questions.*   **LO 4.2, 4.9, and 4.10** *Understand*

1. What was torn in Gail's knee? _____

2. What does "traumatic" mean? _____

3. Define the procedure performed: _____

4. Which part of Gail's knee has poor blood supply? _____

5. Which terms in the operative report are directional terms? _____

B. Elements: *Recognition of word elements will help you understand a medical term. For each of the following terms, identify the type of element shown in bold italics, and then define that element. Fill in the chart, and answer the questions below it.*   **LO 4.1, 4.2, and 4.9** *Remember*

Remember: An element that begins a term is not necessarily a prefix!

Medical Term	Type of Element (P, R/CF, or S)	Meaning of Element	Meaning of Term
tendin*itis*	1.	2.	3.
*pre*patellar	4.	5.	6.
de*bride*ment	7.	8.	9.
*burs*itis	10.	11.	12.
arthro*centesis*	13.	14.	15.

Lesson 4.4(cont'd)   Bones and Joints of the Lower Leg, Ankle, and Foot

(LO 4.2 and 4.9)

Your lower leg has two differently sized bones: the large medial tibia and the thin lateral fibula. The lower end of your tibia on its medial border forms a prominent process called the medial malleolus. The lower end of your fibula forms the lateral malleolus *(Figure 4.25)*. You can palpate (feel) both these prominences at your own ankle, which has two joints:

- One between the lateral malleolus of the fibula and the talus; and

- One between the medial malleolus of the tibia and the talus.

The **talus** is the most superior of the seven **tarsal** bones of the ankle *(Figure 4.25)*, and its upper surface articulates with the tibia. The heel bone is called the **calcaneus.** The tarsal bones help the ankle bear the body's weight. Strong ligaments on both sides of the ankle joint hold the joint together.

Attached to the tarsal bones are the five parallel **metatarsal** bones *(Figure 4.26)*. These bones form the instep and the ball of the foot, where they bear weight. Each toe has three phalanges, except for the big toe, which has only two. This configuration is identical to the thumb and its relation to the hand.

Disorders and Injuries of the Ankle and Foot (LO 4.2 and 4.9)

Podiatry is a health care specialty concerned with the diagnosis and treatment of disorders and injuries of the foot and toenails. A **podiatrist** is not an MD but is a doctor of podiatric medicine (DPM).

Bunions, deformities that appear as swollen bones, often occur at the base of the big toe. A bunion is also called a **hallux valgus,** and it causes the metatarsophalangeal joint to misalign and stick out.

Pott fracture is a fracture of the fibula near the ankle, often accompanied by a fracture of the medial malleolus of the tibia.

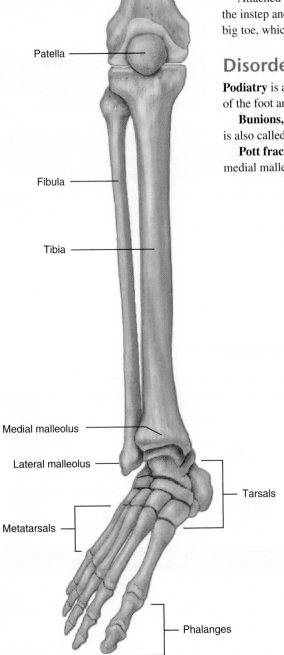

▲ **FIGURE 4.25**
Bones of the Lower Leg and Foot.

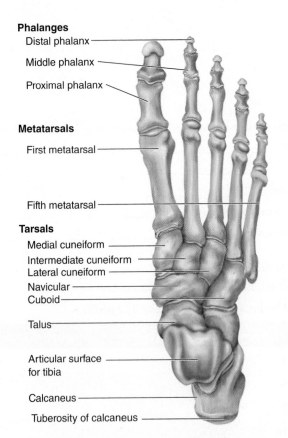

▲ **FIGURE 4.26**
Twenty-Six Bones and 33 Joints of Right Foot.

Word Analysis and Definition

WORD	PRONUNCIATION		ELEMENTS	DEFINITION
bunion	BUN-yun		French *bump*	A swelling at the base of the big toe
calcaneus	kal-KAY-knee-us		Latin *heel*	Bone of the tarsus that forms the heel
calcaneal (adj)	kal-KAY-knee-al	S/	-eal *pertaining to*	Pertaining to the calcaneus
		R/	calcan- *calcaneus*	
hallux valgus	HAL-uks VAL-gus	R/	hallux *big toe*	Deviation of the big toe toward the medial side
		R/	valgus *turn out*	of the foot
metatarsus	MET-ah-TAR-sus	S/	-us *pertaining to*	The five parallel bones of the foot between the
		P/	meta- *after, subsequent to*	tarsus and the phalanges
		R/	-tars- *ankle*	
metatarsal (adj)	MET-ah-TAR-sal	S/	-al *pertaining to*	Pertaining to the metatarsus
podiatry	poh-DIE-ah-tree	S/	-iatry *treatment*	The diagnosis and treatment of disorders and
		R/	pod- *foot*	injuries of the foot
podiatrist	poh-DIE-ah-trist	S/	-iatrist *practitioner*	Practitioner of podiatry
Pott fracture	POT FRAK-shur		Percival Pott, London surgeon, 1714–1788	Fracture of the lower end of the fibula, often with fracture of the tibial malleolus
talus	TAY-luss		Latin *heel bone*	The tarsal bone that articulates with the tibia to form the ankle joint
tarsus	TAR-sus		Latin *ankle*	The collection of seven bones in the foot that form the ankle and instep
tarsal (adj)	TAR-sal	S/	-al *pertaining to*	Pertaining to the tarsus
		R/	tars- *ankle*	

EXERCISES

A. Challenge your knowledge *of the language of orthopedics. Fill in the blanks with the correct medical terms.*   **LO 4.2, 4.9, and 4.10** *Remember*

1. Name 3 eponyms that have appeared in this chapter. _____,
_____, and _____.

2. Metatarsal bones appear in the foot; what are the similar bones called in the hand? _____

3. Another name for a bunion is _____.

4. What is another name for the heel bone? _____

5. The big toe is similar in construction to the _____ of the hand.

6. What is the prominent process called at the lower end of the tibia on its medial border? _____.

7. Describe the location for the *lateral malleolus.* _____
_____

8. What bones form the instep? _____

9. Write all the suffixes you know from this and previous chapters that all mean *pertaining to.* _____
_____

10. What is the only term in the WAD that has a prefix? _____

11. What element means *foot?* _____

12. Where do bunions frequently occur? _____

13. Why can't a podiatrist write a prescription for pain pills? _____

B. Identify the medical term *based on the brief meaning given to you below. Be sure to check your spelling when you are finished! Fill in the blanks.*
LO 4.2, 4.9, and 4.10 *Remember*

1. swelling at the base of the big toe _____

2. bone of the tarsus that forms the heel _____

Lesson 4.5

Diagnostic and Therapeutic Procedures for Bone Disorders (LO 4.5, 4.6, 4.7, 4.8, and 4.9)

Objectives

The procedures and methods, other than clinical examination, that are used to assess, diagnose, and treat bone disorders, particularly bone cancer, can be complicated and expensive and have to be used with discretion. The treatments can also cause unpleasant side effects. In order to understand and relate to this arena, you need to be able to:

4.5.1 Discuss the types of procedures used in diagnosing metabolic bone disorders.

4.5.2 Describe the types of procedures used to diagnose primary and metastatic bone cancer.

4.5.3 Define the types of chemicals used to treat metabolic bone disorders.

4.5.4 Identify the types of treatments used for primary and metastatic bone cancer.

Keynotes

- Malignant tumors that begin in bone tissue are called primary bone cancer.
- Cancer that spreads to the bones from other organs and sites of the body, such as the lung, breast, or prostate, is called metastatic cancer.
- Primary bone cancer is uncommon.

Abbreviations

BMD	bone mineral density
CAT (CT)	computed tomography scan
DEXA (DXA)	dual-energy X-ray absorptiometry
ERT	estrogen replacement therapy
MRI	magnetic resonance imaging
PET	positron emission tomography
SERM	selective estrogen receptor modulator

Diagnostic Procedures for Metabolic Bone Disorders (LO 4.5, 4.6, 4.7, 4.8, and 4.9)

- **Bone mineral density (BMD)** screening using dual-energy X-ray absorptiometry (**DEXA or DXA scan**) is used to diagnose and follow osteoporosis.
- **Nuclear bone scan** involves a radioactive substance injected into the bloodstream. From there, it travels into the bones and is detected by a special camera. It can show a bone infection, a fracture not clearly seen on X-ray, arthritis, and primary or metastatic cancer.
- **Blood tests** examine serum calcium, serum alkaline phosphate, and serum phosphate, which can be abnormal in metabolic bone disorders.
- **Bone biopsy** is the ultimate way to establish a diagnosis of osteomalacia.

Diagnostic Procedures for Bone Cancer (LO 4.5, 4.6, 4.7, 4.8, and 4.9)

- **X-ray** shows the location, shape, and size of a bone tumor.
- **Nuclear bone scan** (described above).
- **Computed tomography (CAT or CT) scan** provides a series of detailed pictures of parts of the body, taken from different angles, that are created by an X-ray machine linked to a computer.
- **Magnetic resonance imaging (MRI)** uses a magnet linked to a computer to create detailed pictures of body parts without using X-rays.

- **Positron emission tomography (PET) scan** uses radioactive **glucose** that is injected into the bloodstream and a scanner that makes a computerized picture of body parts where the glucose is being used. Cancer cells can use more glucose than normal cells and can be detected by the scan.
- **Biopsy** can be a **needle** or **incisional** biopsy.

Therapeutic Procedures for Bone Disorders (LO 4.5, 4.6, 4.7, 4.8, and 4.9)

- **Surgery** is a common treatment for many bone disorders. In bone cancer, the surgeon removes the entire tumor with margins that are negative for cancer cells. Modern surgical techniques have reduced the need for **amputation** in limb bone cancer. Surgical techniques used for specific bones, joints, and their disorders have been discussed previously in this chapter.
- **Chemotherapy** is the use of anticancer drugs, often in combinations, to kill cancer cells. Numerous drugs are available.
- **Radiotherapy** uses high-energy X-rays to kill cancer cells and is often used with surgery.
- **Cryosurgery** uses liquid nitrogen to freeze and kill cancer cells.
- **Drug therapy** for metabolic bone disorders includes, for osteoporosis, **estrogen replacement therapy (ERT),** anti-estrogens (**SERMs),** or bone-preserving medications such as calcitonin. A class of drugs called **bisphosphonates** prevents the loss of bone mass and is used in the treatment of osteoporosis, Paget disease, osteogenesis imperfecta, and any condition that features bone fragility.

WORD	PRONUNCIATION	ELEMENTS		DEFINITION
amputation (noun)	am-pyu-**TAY**-shun	S/ R/	-ation *a process* amput- *to prune, top off*	Process of removing a limb, part of a limb, a breast, or other projecting part
biopsy *(one of the "o"s is not pronounced)*	**BI**-op-see	S/ R/	-opsy *to view* bio- *life*	Process of removing tissue from a living person for laboratory examination
biphosphonate	bi-**PHOS**-fon-ate	S/ P/ R/ R/	-ate *composed of* bi- *two* -phos- *phosphate* -phon- *sound*	A class of drugs used to prevent and treat fragile bones
chemotherapy	**KEY**-moh-**THAIR**-ah-pee	R/ R/CF	-therapy *medical treatment* chem/o- *chemical*	Treatment using chemical agents
cryosurgery	cry-oh-**SUR**-jer-ee	S/ R/CF R/	-ery *process of* cry/o- *icy cold* -surg- *operate*	Use of liquid nitrogen or argon gas in surgery to freeze and kill abnormal tissue
estrogen	**ESS**-troh-jen	S/ R/CF	-gen *produce, create* estr/o- *woman*	Generic term for hormones that stimulate female secondary sex characteristics
glucose	**GLUE**-kose	S/ R/	-ose *full of* gluc- *sugar, glucose*	The final product of carbohydrate digestion and the main sugar in blood
incision	in-**SIZH**-un	S/ R/	-ion *action, condition* incis- *cut into*	A cut or surgical wound
incisional (adj)	in-**SIZH**-un-al	S/	-al *pertaining to*	Pertaining to an incision
radiotherapy	**RAY**-dee-oh-**THAIR**-ah-pee	R/CF R/	radi/o- *x-ray, radiation* -therapy *medical treatment*	Treatment using radiation

EXERCISES

A. List three terms *in this chapter that have the combining form* radi/o *in them and give their meanings:*   **LO 4.1, 4.2, and 4.10** *Remember*

1. _____

2. _____

3. _____

B. Deconstruct the following *medical terms and give their meanings:*   **LO 4.1 and 4.5** *Apply*

1. Chemotherapy: _____/ _____/ _____

                     P   R, R/CF   S

    Meaning _____

2. Cryosurgery: _____/ _____/ _____

                     P   R, R/CF   S

    Meaning _____

3. Biopsy: _____/ _____/ _____

                  P   R, R/CF   S

    Meaning _____

Chapter Review exercises, along with additional practice items, are available in Connect!

Muscles and Tendons

The Essentials of the Languages of Orthopedics and Rehabilitation

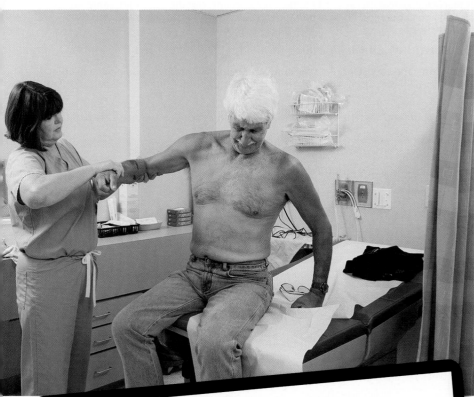

CHAPTER 5

Case Report 5.1

You are . . .

. . . an orthopedic technologist working with orthopedist Kenneth Stannard, MD, in Fulwood Medical Center.

You are Communicating with . . .

Mr. Bruce Adams, a 55-year-old construction worker who presents with severe pain in his right shoulder.

Mr. Adams' pain began 3 or 4 months ago; it is worse at the end of the workday and when he lifts his arm above his head. During the past week, the pain has woken him from sleep. Mr. Adams' primary care physician has given him pain medication, advised him to stop working, and referred him to Dr. Stannard for diagnosis and treatment. A physical examination shows that Mr. Adams' pain is noticeably limiting all the **passive** and **active** movements of his right shoulder, including his ability to lift weight.

Learning Outcomes

The **appendicular skeleton,** which includes the bones of the upper and lower limbs, is attached to the **axial skeleton** through joints and muscles. Understanding the terminology that identifies and describes the muscles and tendons of the limbs and trunk is vital to your knowledge of the human body. Information in this chapter provides correct medical terminology to:

LO 5.1 Use roots, combining forms, suffixes, and prefixes to construct and analyze (deconstruct) medical terms related to muscles and tendons and rehabilitation medicine.

LO 5.2 Spell and pronounce correctly medical terms related to muscles and tendons and rehabilitation medicine in order to communicate them with accuracy and precision in any health care setting.

LO 5.3 Define accepted abbreviations related to muscles and tendons and rehabilitation medicine.

LO 5.4 Relate the three different types of muscle to their structures, functions, and disorders.

LO 5.5 Identify diagnostic and therapeutic methods for disorders of the muscles and tendons.

LO 5.6 Describe the muscles and tendons of the trunk, shoulder girdle, and upper limbs and their disorders.

LO 5.7 Describe the muscles and tendons of the pelvic girdle and lower limbs and their disorders.

LO 5.8 Identify the goals of rehabilitation medicine and the health professionals involved in a rehabilitation program.

LO 5.9 Apply your knowledge of the medical terms of the muscles and tendons, their disorders and rehabilitation medicine to documentation, medical records, and medical reports.

LO 5.10 Translate the medical terms of the muscles and tendons and their disorders and rehabilitation medicine into everyday language in order to communicate clearly with patients and their families.

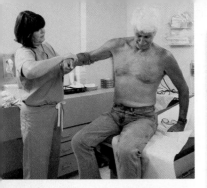

Rehabilitation programs involve a **multidisciplinary** team approach where each team member manages different rehabilitation activities. The members of a rehabilitation team include the following health professionals and their respective roles (see the WADs in this chapter for these terms):

- A **physiatrist**, often the team leader, is a physician specializing in physical medicine and rehabilitation.
- **Medical specialists** manage acute or chronic illnesses and pain.
- **Occupational therapists** practice occupational therapy **(OT)** to help improve a patient's activities of daily living **(ADLs)** and adapt to visual and other perceptual deficits.
- **Occupational therapy assistants (OTAs)** assist occupational therapists.
- **Physical therapists** practice **physical therapy (PT)** to help patients improve their strength, **range of motion (ROM)**, balance, and endurance. Physical therapists are assisted by **restorative aids** and teach patients how to use these devices.
- **Physical therapy assistants (PTAs)** assist physical therapists.
- **Rehabilitation psychologists** and counselors are specialists who help patients undergoing rehabilitation and those with resulting disabilities to reclaim their sense of belonging, contributing to, and participating in the world around them.
- **Social workers** provide support and assistance with social issues, such as health insurance, care facilities, and employment.
- **Speech therapists** evaluate and treat communication, speech, and swallowing disorders.
- **Orthotists** make and fit orthopedic appliances **(orthotics)**.
- **Nutritionists** evaluate and improve a patient's nutritional status.

Objectives

In Chapter 4, you learned how the bones of your skeleton support your body and how your joints provide mobility throughout your body. However, neither of these functions can occur without your **muscles,** *which provide posture and movement. Information in this lesson will enable you to use correct medical terminology to:*

5.1.1 Identify the functions of skeletal muscle and tendons.

5.1.2 Describe the structure of skeletal muscle and tendons.

5.1.3 Demonstrate an understanding of the major problems and diseases that occur in muscles and tendons.

5.1.4 Discuss diagnostic and therapeutic methods used to diagnose muscle disorders.

Abbreviations

ADL	activities of daily living
DC	Doctor of Chiropractic
DO	Doctor of Osteopathy
OT	occupational therapy
PT	physical therapy
ROM	range of motion
MD	Doctor of Medicine

Lesson 5.1

Muscles and Tendons

Types, Functions and Structure of Skeletal Muscle

Types of Muscle (LO 5.4)

There are three types of **muscle: skeletal, cardiac,** and **smooth.** Skeletal muscles contract on demand to provide posture and locomotion. Cardiac and smooth muscle contract without conscious thought, cardiac muscle to power the heart contractions and smooth muscle to power the movement of food through the digestive system via **peristalsis.**

Functions and Structure of Skeletal Muscle (LO 5.4)

Functions of Skeletal Muscle (LO 5.4)

Skeletal muscles, which are attached to one or more bones, are also called **voluntary** muscles. This means that you have conscious control of your muscles, which perform your movements. Each muscle consists of bundles of muscle cells (often called **fibers** because of their length), blood vessels, and nerves. Connective tissue sheets hold your muscle fibers together and connect the muscles to your bones.

Your skeletal muscle has the following functions:

1. **Movement.** All skeletal muscles are attached to bones so when a muscle **contracts,** your bones move, too *(Figure 5.1)*. This allows you to walk, run, and work with your hands.

2. **Posture.** The **tone** of your skeletal muscles holds you straight when sitting, standing, or moving.

3. **Body heat.** When skeletal muscles contract, they produce the heat needed to maintain your body temperature.

4. **Respiration.** Skeletal muscles move the chest wall as you breathe.

5. **Communication.** Skeletal muscles enable you to speak, write, type, gesture, and smile.

Word Analysis and Definition

S = Suffix   P = Prefix   R = Root   R/CF = Combining Form

WORD	PRONUNCIATION		ELEMENTS	DEFINITION
active activity	ACK-tiv ack-TIV-ih-tee	 S/ R/	Latin *movement* -ity *condition, state* activ- *movement*	Causing action or change The state of being active
contract	kon-TRAKT	P/ R/	con- *with, together* -tract *draw*	Draw together or shorten
fiber	FIE-ber		Latin *fiber*	A strand or filament
multidisciplinary	mul-tee-DIS-ih-plih-NAR-ee	S/ P/ R/	-ary *pertaining to* multi- *many* -disciplin- *instruction*	Involving health care providers from more than one profession
muscle	MUSS-el		Latin *muscle*	A tissue consisting of cells that can contract
passive	PASS-iv		Latin *to endure*	Not active
peristalsis	pear-ih-STAL-sis	P/ R/	peri- *around* -stalsis *constrict*	Waves of alternate constriction and relaxation in a tube
skeletal (adj)	SKEL-eh-tal	S/ R/	-al *pertaining to* skelet- *skeleton*	Pertaining to the skeleton
tone	TONE		Greek *tone*	Tension present in resting muscles
voluntary muscle	VOL-un-tare-ee MUSS-el	S/ R/	-ary *pertaining to* volunt- *free will*	Muscle that is under the control of the will

EXERCISES

A. Review *the Case Report on the previous spread before answering the questions. As with any Case Report exercise in this text, first read the report aloud if possible. Read it a second time and underline any medical terms you see in the report. Then answer the questions.*   **LO 5.2, 5.8, and 5.9** *Understand*

1. In your own words, explain what an orthopedist specializes in. _____

2. What motivated the patient to see the doctor? _____

3. What makes his pain worse? _____

4. Is there anything about his occupation that may have contributed to his condition? _____

5. Write all the medical terms you have identified in the case report. _____

B. Deconstruct *the following medical terms from the WAD into their basic elements; then define each element. Fill in the chart.*   **LO 5.1 and 5.4** *Analyze*

Medical Term	Prefix	Meaning of Prefix	Root(s)/CF	Meaning of Root(s)/CF	Suffix	Meaning of Suffix
contract	1.	2.	3.	4.	5.	6.
voluntary	7.	8.	9.	10.	11.	12.
skeletal	13.	14.	15.	16.	17.	18.

C. Meet lesson and chapter objectives *and use the correct medical terminology to answer the questions.*   **LO 5.2 and 5.4** *Apply*

1. Describe the structure of a muscle. _____
   _____

2. List the functions of skeletal muscle. _____

3. What connects the appendicular skeleton to the axial skeleton? _____

4. What are the three components of a muscle? _____, _____, and _____

5. What is another name for *skeletal muscle?* _____

Functions of Skeletal Muscle (continued) (LO 5.4)

▶ **FIGURE 5.1**
Muscle Contraction to Flex the Elbow Joint.

Structure of Skeletal Muscle (LO 5.4)

Your skeletal muscle fibers are narrow and measure up to 1½ inches long. Bundles of these fibers create separate muscles, which are held in place by **fascia** (*Figure 5.2*), a thick layer of connective tissue. Fascia extends beyond the muscle to form a **tendon,** which attaches to a bone's periosteum at the origin and insertion of the muscle.

Because skeletal muscle fibers contain **striations** (alternating dark and light bands of protein filaments responsible for muscle contraction), skeletal muscle can also be called **striated muscle.**

You have the same number of muscle fibers as an adult that you had in late childhood. Exercise and/or weightlifting will enlarge (**hypertrophy**) your muscles, increasing the thickness of your muscle fibers. If you neglect these muscles, they will shrink (**atrophy**).

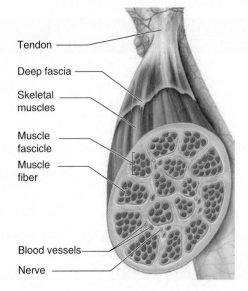

▶ **FIGURE 5.2**
Structure of Skeletal Muscle.

Disorders of Skeletal Muscles (LO 5.4)

Because you use so many different muscles for various activities, the likelihood of experiencing some form of skeletal muscle disorder in your lifetime is almost certain. **Muscle soreness** can result from vigorous exercise, particularly if your muscles are not used to it. Exercise increases the lactic acid in your muscle fibers, causing inflammation, and produces soreness in the muscles and nearby connective tissue.

Muscle cramps are sudden, short, painful contractions of a muscle or group of muscles. The cause of these cramps is unknown. A poor diet that leads to low blood potassium, calcium, and magnesium levels; caffeine and tobacco use; and reduced blood supply may contribute to muscle cramps. There are no effective medications available.

Muscle strains range from a simple stretch to a partial or complete tear in the muscle, tendon, or muscle-tendon combination. Most strains heal with RICE (*Figure 5.3*), followed by basic exercises to relieve pain and restore mobility. A complete tear may require surgery.

A **sprain** is a stretch or tear of a ligament, often in the ankle, knee, or wrist, and is also treated by RICE.

Anabolic steroids are related to testosterone but altered to make skeletal muscle hypertrophy. Used illegally in many sports to boost muscle strength, steroids have noticeable, often irreversible side effects. These include stunted growth in adolescents, shrinking testes and reduced sperm counts, masculinization of women's bodies and voices, delusions, and paranoid jealousy. Long-term effects may be increased risk of heart attack and stroke, kidney failure, and liver tumors.

Fibromyalgia affects muscles and tendons all over the body, causing chronic pain, fatigue, and depression. Its cause is unknown and there are currently no laboratory tests for it. The only treatment options are pain management, physiotherapy, and stress reduction.

▲ **FIGURE 5.3**
RICE Treatment.

Word Analysis and Definition

S = Suffix   P = Prefix   R = Root   R/CF = Combining Form

WORD	PRONUNCIATION	ELEMENTS		DEFINITION
atrophy	A-troh-fee	P/ R/	a- *without* -trophy *nourishment*	The wasting away or diminished volume of tissue, an organ, or a body part
hypertrophy	high-**PER**-troh-fee	P/ R/	hyper- *above, excessive* -trophy *nourishment*	Increase in size, but not in number, of an individual tissue element
fascia	**FASH**-ee-ah		Latin *a band*	Sheet of fibrous connective tissue
fibromyalgia	fie-broh-my-**AL**-jee-ah	S/ R/CF R/	-algia *pain* fibr/o- *fiber* -my- *muscle*	Pain in the muscle fibers
sprain	**SPRAIN**		root unknown	A wrench or tear in a ligament
strain	**STRAIN**		Latin *to bind*	Overstretch or tear in a muscle or tendon
tendon tendinitis (*also spelled* tendonitis)	**TEN**-dun ten-dih-**NYE**-tis	S/ R/	Latin *sinew* -itis *inflammation* tendin- *tendon*	Fibrous band that connects muscle to bone Inflammation of a tendon

EXERCISES

A. The following elements *are all contained in the WAD above. Circle the best answer.*   **LO 5.1** *Understand*

1. The suffix -*itis* means: condition   disease   inflammation

2. Hyper is a: suffix   prefix   root

3. The root *trophy*- means: condition   procedure   nourishment

4. *Fibro* is a: combining form root   suffix

5. The root *my*- means: tendon   ligament   muscle

6. The suffix -*algia* means: inflammation   pain   swelling

B. Terminology challenge.   **LO 5.1 and 5.4** *Analyze*

1. What term in the WAD has a root and a prefix but no suffix and means "increase in size of muscle tissue"? _____

_____

_____

2. What is the difference between a *sprain* and a *strain?*

   Sprain: _____

   Strain: _____

3. What term in the WAD has two acceptable spellings? _____ _____

- Treatment for tenosynovitis is rest, immobilization, nonsteroidal anti-inflammatory drugs (NSAIDs), local corticosteroid injections, and, occasionally, surgery.
- Thymectomy—removal of the thymus gland—is the usual treatment for myasthenia gravis.
- Toxic myopathies can be caused by alcohol, narcotics, corticosteroids, and statins.

Abbreviations

CK	creatine kinase
CT (CAT)	computed tomography scan
DMD	Duchenne muscular dystrophy
EMG	electromyography
ESR	erythrocyte sedimentation rate
ICD-10	International Statistical Classification of Diseases and Related Health Problems, version 10
MRI	magnetic resonance imaging
MSA	myositis specific antibody
PCP	phencyclidine (angel dust)
PT	physical therapy

Disorders of Skeletal Muscles (continued)
(LO 5.3 and 5.4)

Myasthenia gravis is a chronic autoimmune disease (*see Chapter 7*) characterized by varying degrees of weakness of the skeletal muscles. The weakness increases with activity and decreases with rest. Facial muscles are often involved, causing problems with eye and eyelid movements, chewing, and talking. Antibodies produced by the immune system block the passage of stimuli from motor nerves to muscles, making movements limited.

Myopathy is any muscular disease resulting in muscle weakness. The **ICD-10** lists 15 codes for different types of myopathy.

Dermatomyositis is a myopathy producing muscle weakness and skin changes around the eyes and over the knuckles.

Polymyositis is a myopathy producing muscle weakness.

Muscular dystrophy is a general term for a group of hereditary, progressive disorders affecting skeletal muscles. **Duchenne muscular dystrophy (DMD)** is the most common in boys, beginning with difficulty walking around the age of 3. Generalized muscle weakness and atrophy progress, and few live beyond 20 years of age. There is no effective treatment.

Rhabdomyolysis is the breakdown of muscle fibers, which releases a protein pigment (**myoglobin**) into the bloodstream. Myoglobin breaks down into toxic compounds that cause kidney failure. Muscle trauma, severe exertion (marathon running), alcoholism, and use of cocaine, heroin, amphetamines, or phencyclidine (**PCP**) can cause this disorder.

Tenosynovitis is an inflammation of the sheath that surrounds a tendon, often in the wrist and hands. Repetitive use of these tendons can produce pain, tenderness in the tendon, and difficulty in related joint movement.

Diagnostic Methods for Disorders of Muscles and Tendons (LO 5.3 and 5.4)

A **medical history** and **physical examination** are essential components of a diagnostic examination. Additional diagnostic tests include:

- **Blood tests.** Damaged muscles release **enzymes** such as **creatine kinase (CK)** and **aldolase** into the blood, and their levels can be measured. An **erythrocyte sedimentation rate (ESR or sed rate)** is not specific for any type of disease but indicates the presence of **inflammation,** and

serial readings can be used to measure changes in the severity of an inflammatory process.

- **Electromyography (EMG),** which involves inserting an electrode needle into the muscle to be tested to measure its electrical activity as the muscle is relaxed and contracted.
- **Magnetic resonance imaging (MRI)** and **computed tomography scan (CT or CAT scan),** which can show detailed images of damage or disease in muscles.
- **Muscle biopsy,** which allows a small piece of muscle to be removed through a hollow needle or small incision and sent to the laboratory for examination and analysis.
- **Genetic testing** of blood or other samples, which can show mutations in some of the genes that cause the different types of muscular dystrophy.
- **Myositis specific antibodies (MSA),** which can assist in confirming a diagnosis of dermatomyositis or polymyositis. Dozens of myositis-specific and myositis-associated antibodies have been identified, and research is ongoing to define their significance.

Therapeutic Methods of Disorders of Muscles and Tendons (LO 5.3 and 5.5)

RICE (rest, ice, compression, and elevation) is used in the acute phase for muscle and tendon strains and sprains.

- **Physical therapy (PT)** and **exercise** are important in the treatment of muscle diseases and involve **range of motion** exercises to prevent **contracture** of joints and exercises and resistance training to restore muscle mass and strength.
- **Medications** are used frequently in muscle diseases. Acetaminophen (paracetamol) and hydrocodone can be used for pain in the acute stages following injury. For the inflammatory myopathies, **oral corticosteroids** are often the first line of treatment, sometimes with the **antimetabolite** drugs methotrexate or azathioprine. For patients who do not respond to standard treatments, **immunosuppressive** drugs can be used.
- **Surgical** treatments include **tendon reconstruction,** in which the two ends of a ruptured or torn tendon are **sutured** back together. In ligament injuries of the elbow joint in high-level, overhead-throwing athletes, such as baseball pitchers, reconstruction techniques and tendon grafting are often used with success.
- **Orthopedic appliances** such as braces and walkers are used during recovery from muscle and tendon injury.

Word Analysis and Definition

S = Suffix   P = Prefix   R = Root   R/CF = Combining Form

WORD	PRONUNCIATION	ELEMENTS		DEFINITION
antimetabolite	AN-teh-meh-**TAB**-oh-lite	S/ P/ R/	-ite *pertaining to* anti- *against* -metabol- *change*	A substance that replaces or inhibits a specific part of a cell's normal metabolism
contracture	kon-**TRAK**-chur	S/ R/	-ure *result of* contract- *pull together*	Muscle shortening due to spasm or fibrosis
corticosteroid	**KOR**-tih-koh-**STEHR**-oyd	S/ R/CF	-steroid *steroid* cortic/o *from the cortex*	A hormone produced by the adrenal cortex
Duchenne muscular dystrophy	**DOO**-shen **MUSS**-kyu-lar **DISS**-troh-fee	P/ R/	Guillaume Benjamin Duchenne, French neurologist, 1806–1875 dys- *bad, difficult* -trophy *nourishment*	A condition with symmetrical weakness and wasting of pelvic, shoulder, and proximal limb muscles
immunosuppressive	IM-you-noh-suh-**PRESS**-iv	S/ R/CF R/	-ive *nature of* immune/o *immune response* -suppress- *press under*	Substance that causes failure of the immune system
myoglobin	**MY**-oh-**GLOW**-bin	S/ R/CF R/	-in *substance* my/o- *muscle* -glob- *globe*	Protein of muscle that stores and transports oxygen
rhabdomyolysis	**RAB**-doh-my-oh-**LIE**-sis	S/ R/CF R/CF	-lysis *destruction* rhabd/o- *rod-shaped* -my/o- *muscle*	Destruction of muscle to produce myoglobin
myopathy	my-**OP**-ah-thee	S/ R/CF	-pathy *disease* my/o- *muscle*	Any disease of muscle
myositis	my-oh-**SI**-tis	S/	-sitis *inflammation*	Inflammation of muscle tissue
statinç	**STAH**-tin		Greek *stationary*	A class of drug used to lower blood cholesterol levels
tenosynovitis	**TEN**-oh-sine-oh-**VIE**-tis	S/ R/CF R/	-itis *inflammation* ten/o- *tendon* - synov- *synovial membrane*	Inflammation of a tendon and its surrounding synovial sheath
thymectomy	thigh-**MEK**-toe-me	S/ R/	-ectomy *surgical excision* thym- *thymus gland*	Surgical removal of the thymus gland

EXERCISES

A. The following statements *are written in your medical record. Explain their meaning to your patient.*   **LO 5.2, 5.5, and 5.10** *Analyze*

1. In order to diagnose the cause of Mrs. Patricia Keene's muscle weakness, an EMG and MRI will be performed.

   Explanation _____

   _____

   _____

2. Mrs. Keene has polymyositis, which is not responding to corticosteroids. An immunosuppressive will be added to her drug regimen.

   Explanation _____

   _____

   _____

B. Deconstruct *the following medical terms and give their meanings:*   **LO 5.2 and 5.5** *Analyze*

1. Corticosteroid: _____ / _____ / _____

                   P   R, R/CF   S

   Meaning _____

   _____

2. Antimetabolite: _____ / _____ / _____

                  P   R, R/CF   S

   Meaning _____

   _____

Lesson 5.2

Muscles and Tendons of the Shoulder Girdle, Trunk, and Upper Limb

Shoulder Girdle
(LO 5.6)

Your **pectoral** (shoulder) **girdle** connects your axial skeleton to your upper limbs and helps you to move these limbs. Without your shoulder girdle, you wouldn't be able to throw a ball, drive a car, or reach that top shelf of your closet or kitchen cabinet. In fact, you wouldn't be able to move your upper limbs.

The muscles and tendons in your shoulder girdle get plenty of use. Four muscles that **originate** on your scapula wrap around the shoulder joint and fuse together. This fusion forms one large tendon (the **rotator cuff**), which is **inserted** into the humerus *(Figure 5.4)*. Your rotator cuff keeps the ball of the humerus tightly in the scapula's socket and provides the kind of strength needed by baseball pitchers.

Case Report 5.1 (continued)

When Dr. Stannard evaluated Mr. Adams, an MRI revealed a full-thickness tear of his rotator cuff. Mr. Adams has been scheduled for **ambulatory** surgery to repair the tear.

Common Disorders of the Shoulder Girdle (LO 5.7)

Rotator cuff tears (a frequent injury to the shoulder girdle) are caused by wear and tear from overuse in work situations or in certain sports, such as baseball, football, and golf. These tears can be partial or complete.

Tendonitis of the shoulder joint is caused when the rotator cuff and/or biceps tendon becomes inflamed from overuse.

Bursitis, inflammation of the lubricating sac of the rotator cuff, can also be produced by overuse.

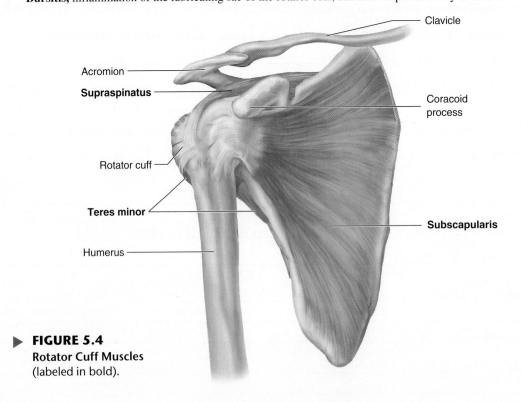

▶ **FIGURE 5.4**
Rotator Cuff Muscles
(labeled in bold).

Word Analysis and Definition

WORD	PRONUNCIATION	ELEMENTS		DEFINITION
ambulatory	AM-byu-LAY-tor-ee	S/ R/	-ory *having the function of* ambulat- *walking*	Surgery or any other care provided without an overnight stay in a medical facility
insertion insert (verb)	in-SIR-shun in-SIRT	S/ R/	-ion *action, condition* insert- *put together*	The insertion of a muscle is the attachment of a muscle to a more movable part of the skeleton, as distinct from the origin
origin	OR-ih-gin		Latin *source of*	Fixed source of a muscle at its attachment to bone
pectoral	PEK-tor-al	S/ R/	-al *pertaining to* pector- *chest*	Pertaining to the chest
pectoral girdle	PEK-tor-al GIR-del		girdle, Old English *encircle*	Incomplete bony ring that attaches the upper limb to the axial skeleton
rotator cuff	roh-TAY-tor CUFF	S/ R/	-or *one who does* rotat- *rotate* cuff, Old English *band*	Part of the capsule of the shoulder joint

EXERCISES

A. Review *the Case Report on this spread before answering the questions. Apply your knowledge of medical language to fill in the correct answers.*
LO 5.2, 5.5, and 5.6 *Understand*

1. What type of diagnostic test did Mr. Adams have? _____

2. What did the test in question #1 reveal? _____

3. Define *full thickness tear.* Use the glossary or a dictionary. _____

_____

4. Why does the tear have to be repaired surgically? _____

5. How do you think Mr. Adams may have injured himself? _____

B. Meet *lesson objectives by answering the following questions. Fill in the blanks.*   **LO 5.2 and 5.6** *Understand*

1. A frequent sports injury to the shoulder girdle is _____.

2. The four muscles that originate on the scapula fuse together into the _____.

3. The pectoral girdle connects the axial skeleton to _____.

4. Is the rotator cuff a tendon, ligament, or muscle? _____

5. Where is the insertion point of the rotator cuff? _____

C. Review the WAD *for answers to the questions below.*   **LO 5.1, 5.2, 5.4, and 5.6** *Understand*

1. Explain the terms *origin* and *insertion* in relation to muscles:

   Origin: _____

   Insertion: _____

2. Which suffix means *one who does?* _____

3. If a patient is checked into the hospital as *ambulatory,* what does that mean?

_____

4. The axial skeleton connects to the limbs, which facilitates what body function? _____

Lesson 5.2(cont'd) Upper Arm and Elbow Joint (LO 5.6)

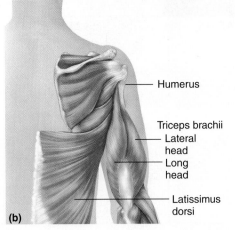

▲ FIGURE 5.5
Muscles Joining Arm to Body.
(a) Anterior view.
(b) Posterior view.

Your muscles connect your humerus (upper arm bone) to your shoulder girdle, vertebral column, and ribs. These muscles enable your arm to move freely at the shoulder joint. Your major anterior muscles (those at the front of your body) are the **deltoid** (shoulder muscle) and **pectoralis major** (chest muscle) *(Figure 5.5a)*. Among the major posterior muscles is the **latissimus dorsi,** found in your back *(Figure 5.5b)*.

Muscles that move your elbow joint and forearm originate on the upper arm bone or shoulder girdle and are inserted into the bones of your forearm. On the front of the arm, you have a group of three muscles *(Figure 5.5a)*—**biceps brachii, brachialis,** and **brachioradialis.** These muscles flex your forearm at the elbow joint and rotate your forearm and hand sideways or laterally (supination). A single muscle on the back of your arm (the **triceps brachii**) extends your elbow joint and forearm *(Figure 5.5b)*.

Common Disorder of the Elbow (LO 5.6)

Tennis elbow is a common injury. Upper arm and forearm muscle tendons are inserted into the upper arm bone just above the elbow joint. Small tears in these tendons at their attachments can be caused by trauma or overuse of the elbow joint. Treatment is rest, ice, pain medication, massage, and stretching exercises.

Forearm, Wrist, and Hand (LO 5.6)

The muscles of your forearm are responsible for various movements. These muscles supinate and pronate your forearm (turning it upward and downward), flex and extend your wrist joint and hand, and move your hand medially and laterally (back and forth crossways). These terms of movement are detailed in Chapter 2.

Your forearm is bigger near the elbow because the forearm muscles are fleshy and bulky. Your wrist is much thinner because these muscles have become tendons that pass over your wrist on the way to being inserted into your finger bones.

Abbreviation

CTS   carpal tunnel syndrome

Common Disorders of the Wrist (LO 5.6)

Because you use your hands and wrists almost constantly, your wrists can be prone to disorders and injuries.

Ganglion cysts are fluid-filled cysts on the back of the wrist, which result from irritation or inflammation of the synovial tendon sheaths in this area. These cysts usually disappear on their own.

Stenosing tenosynovitis is a painful inflammation of the synovial sheaths on the back of the wrist.

Carpal tunnel syndrome (CTS) develops on the front of the wrist and results from inflammation and swelling of overused tendon sheaths. Repetitive movements, like typing on a computer keyboard, can lead to CTS. A feeling of "pins and needles" or pain and loss of muscle power in the thumb side of the hand are common.

▲ FIGURE 5.6
Palmar Surface of the Hand.

The Hand (LO 5.6)

When you look at the palm of your hand, you'll see a prominent pad of muscles (the **thenar eminence**) at the base of your thumb *(Figure 5.6)*. A smaller pad of muscles (the **hypothenar eminence**) is located at the base of your little finger. The back of your hand is called the **dorsum.**

Word Analysis and Definition

WORD	PRONUNCIATION	ELEMENTS		DEFINITION
biceps brachii	BYE-sepz BRAY-key-eye	P/ R/ R/CF	bi- *two* -ceps *head* brachi/i *of the arm*	A muscle of the arm that has two heads or points of origin on the scapula
brachialis	BRAY-kee-al-is	S/ R/	-alis *pertaining to* brachi- *arm*	Muscle that lies underneath the biceps and is the strongest flexor of the forearm
brachioradialis	BRAY-kee-oh-RAY-dee-al-is	S/ R/CF R/	-alis *pertaining to* brachi/o- *arm* -radi- *radius*	Muscle that helps flex the forearm
cyst	SIST		Greek *fluid-filled sac*	An abnormal, fluid-containing sac
deltoid	DEL-toyd	S/ R/	-oid *resembling* delt- *triangle*	Large, fan-shaped muscle connecting the scapula and clavicle to the humerus
dorsum	DOOR-sum		Latin *back*	The back of any part of the body, including the hand
dorsal (adj)	DOOR-sal	S/ R/	-al *pertaining to* dors- *back*	Pertaining to the back of any part of the body
ventral *(opposite of* **dorsal***)*	VEN-tral	R/	ventr- *belly*	Pertaining to the belly or situated nearer to the surface of the belly
ganglion	GANG-lee-on		Greek *swelling*	Fluid-containing swelling attached to the synovial sheath of a tendon
latissimus dorsi	lah-TISS-ih-muss DOOR-sigh	S/ R/ R/	-imus *most* latiss- *wide* dorsi *of the back*	The widest (broadest) muscle in the back
stenosis	steh-NOH-sis		Greek *narrowing*	Narrowing of a passage
thenar eminence	THAY-nar EM-in-ens	R/	eminence, Latin *stand out* thenar *palm*	The fleshy mass at the base of the thumb
hypothenar eminence	high-poh-THAY-nar EM-in-ens	P/	hypo- *below, smaller*	The fleshy mass at the base of the little finger
triceps brachii	TRY-sepz BRAY-key-eye	P/ R/ R/CF	tri- *three* -ceps *head* brachi/i *of the arm*	Muscle of the arm that has three heads or points of origin

EXERCISES

A. Analyze *the underlined word or part of a word as your clue for the element in the correct term.*
LO 5.2 and 5.6 *Analyze*

1. arm muscle with <u>three</u> heads _____

2. <u>triangular</u>-shaped muscle _____

3. <u>widest</u> muscle in the back _____

4. arm muscle with <u>two</u> heads _____

5. strongest flexor of the fore<u>arm</u> _____

B. Elements *can have more than one meaning and must be applied differently to specific medical terms. Fill in the blanks.*
LO 5.1 and 5.2 *Understand*

1. Give an example of a medical term (other than *hypothenar*), from any chapter, that begins with *hypo* and in which *hypo* means *below*.

   Term: _____ means _____.

2. Give an example of a medical term, from any chapter, that begins with *hypo* and in which *hypo* means *deficient* or *less than* (in the sense of location).

   Term: _____ means _____.

> ## Study Hint
>
> To help remember the difference between the *thenar* eminence and the *hypothenar* eminence, focus on the prefix *hypo,* which can mean below or smaller. If you hold the hand open, palm facing you, with the thumb straight up, the *hypothenar* eminence is the fleshy mass at the base of the little finger, which is the smallest one on the hand.

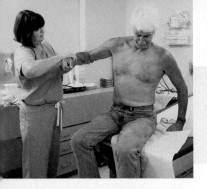

Lesson 5.3

Pelvic Girdle, Thigh, Leg, and Foot

Muscles of the Hip and Thigh (LO 5.4 and 5.7)

Some of your body's most powerful muscles support your hip joint and move your thigh. These muscles originate on the pelvic girdle and are inserted into the femur. Among these prominent muscles are your three **gluteus** muscles—**maximus, medius,** and **minimus** *(Figure 5.7)*—and the **adductor** muscles that run down your inner thigh.

Thigh Muscles (LO 5.4 and 5.7)

Your thigh muscles move your knee joint and lower leg. Your anterior thigh (the front of your thigh) contains your large **quadriceps femoris** muscle. This muscle has four heads: the rectus femoris, vastus lateralis, vastus medialis, and the vastus intermedius (which lies beneath the rectus femoris). These four muscle heads join into the **quadriceps tendon** (which contains the patella) and continue as the patellar tendon to be inserted into the tibia *(Figure 5.8)*. The quadriceps muscle **extends** (straightens) the knee joint and, because of the lower leg's weight, it has to be a very strong muscle.

Your posterior (rear) thigh is composed mostly of your three **hamstring muscles**—the **biceps femoris, semimembranosus,** and **semitendinosus** *(Figure 5.9)*. These muscles flex (bend) your knee joint and rotate your leg. The hollow area at the back of your knee between your hamstring tendons is the **popliteal fossa.**

Muscles and Tendons of the Lower Leg, Ankle, and Foot (LO 5.4 and 5.7)

The muscles of your lower leg move your ankle, foot, and toes. Your front leg muscles bend your foot backward at the ankle and extend your toes. The side or lateral leg muscles turn your foot outward or evert it. Your back leg muscles plantar-flex your foot at the ankle, flex your toes, and turn in or invert your foot. The **gastrocnemius** muscle *(Figure 5.10(a))*, located at the back of your leg, forms a large part of your calf. The distal end of this muscle joins the tendon of the smaller calf (soleus) muscle to create the **Achilles (calcaneal) tendon,** which is attached to the heel bone **(calcaneus)** *(Figure 5.10(b))*. Together, your gastrocnemius muscle and Achilles tendon make it possible for you to "push off" when jumping or running. For more detailed foot movement descriptions, you may review the terms in Chapter 2.

▼ **FIGURE 5.7**
Hip Joint.
Muscles of the hip and thigh, lateral view.

Gluteus medius
Gluteus maximus
Biceps femoris
Tensor fasciae latae
Sartorius
Rectus femoris
Vastus lateralis
Iliotibial band (fascia)

◄ **FIGURE 5.8**
Anterior Muscles of the Thigh.

Rectus femoris
Vastus lateralis
Vastus medialis
Quadriceps femoris tendon
Patella
Patellar tendon

◄ **FIGURE 5.9**
Posterior Thigh Muscles.

Hamstring group
Biceps femoris long head
Biceps femoris short head
Semitendinosus
Semimembranosus
Popliteal fossa

Tibia
Gastrocnemius
Tibialis anterior
Soleus

Gastrocnemius
Medial head
Lateral head

Tendon of gastrocnemius

Achilles (calcaneal) tendon

Calcaneus

▲ **FIGURE 5.10**
Muscles of Lower Leg and Foot.
(a) Muscles of the front of the right leg.
(b) Muscles of the back of the right leg.

Word Analysis and Definition

WORD	PRONUNCIATION	ELEMENTS		DEFINITION
abduction abduct (verb)	ab-**DUCK**-shun ab-**DUKT**	S/ P/ R/	-ion *process, action* ab- *away from* -duct- *lead*	Action of moving away from the midline
adductor	ah-**DUCK**-tor	S/ P/ R/	-or *that which does something* ad- *toward* -duct- *lead*	Muscle that moves the thigh toward the midline
adduction	ah-**DUCK**-shun	S/	-ion *action, condition*	Action of moving toward the midline
calcaneus	cal-**KAY**-knee-us		Latin *the heel*	The heel bone
calcaneal tendon (*same as* Achilles tendon) Achilles	kal-**KAY**-knee-al ah-**KILL**-eeze	S/ R/	-eal *pertaining to* calcan- *calcaneus* mythical Greek warrior	The tendon of the heel formed from gastrocnemius and soleus muscles and inserted into the calcaneus
gastrocnemius	gas-trok-**KNEE**-me-us	S/ R/	-ius *pertaining to* gastrocnem- *calf of leg*	Major muscle in back of the lower leg (the calf)
gluteus gluteal (adj)	**GLUE**-tee-us **GLUE**-tee-al	 S/ R/	Greek *buttocks* -eal *pertaining to* glut- *buttocks*	Refers to one of three muscles in the buttocks Pertaining to the buttocks
maximus	**MAKS**-ih-mus		Latin *the biggest* or *the greatest*	The gluteus maximus muscle is the largest muscle in the body, covering a large part of each buttock
medius	**MEE**-dee-us		Latin *middle*	The gluteus medius muscle is partly covered by the gluteus maximus
minimus	**MIN**-ih-mus		Latin *smallest*	The gluteus minimus is the smallest of the gluteal muscles and lies under the gluteus medius
popliteal fossa	pop-**LIT**-ee-al **FOSS**-ah	S/ R/CF	-al *pertaining to* poplit/e- *ham, back of knee* fossa, Latin *trench, ditch*	The hollow at the back of the knee
quadriceps femoris	**KWAD**-rih-seps **FEM**-or-is	P/ R/ S/ R/	quadri- *four* -ceps *head* -is *belonging to, pertaining to* femor- *femur*	An anterior thigh muscle with four heads (origins)

EXERCISES

A. Spelling: *A medical term must be spelled correctly. Work with a fellow student on this exercise. Cover the WAD with a sheet of paper while your partner dictates any 5 terms in the above WAD to you. Write them in the "Test" column, and do your best to spell them correctly. When you are finished, remove the cover and check your spelling. If you have made any errors, rewrite the correct spelling in the "Corrections" column. After you have corrected your exercise, dictate the remaining 5 terms to your partner.*   **LO 5.2 and 5.7** *Apply*

Test   Corrections

1. _____   _____

2. _____   _____

3. _____   _____

4. _____   _____

5. _____   _____

B. Identify *the medical term, based on the brief meaning given to you. Be sure to check your spelling when you are finished! Fill in the blanks.*
LO 5.2 and 5.7 *Remember*

1. Which terms relate to size? _____

2. Another name for the calcaneal tendon is: _____

3. Where is the popliteal fossa? _____

Lesson 5.4

Physical Medicine and Rehabilitation (PM&R)

Objectives

As a health professional, you may be directly involved in helping a patient through the rehabilitation and recovery process after an illness, surgery, or medical procedure. The information in this lesson will enable you to use correct medical terminology to:

5.4.1 Identify the members of the rehabilitation team.

5.4.2 Discuss the purposes of rehabilitation medicine.

5.4.3 Define the goals for a restorative rehabilitation program for specific common problems.

5.4.4 Define the different types of rehabilitation.

5.4.5 Use the activities of daily living as a measure to assess therapy needs and effectiveness.

Case Report 5.2

You are . . .

. . . a **certified occupational therapist assistant** working in the Rehabilitation Unit at Fulwood Medical Center.

You are communicating with . . .

. . . Mr. Hank Johnson, a 65-year-old print shop owner.

One year ago, Mr. Johnson had an elective left total-hip replacement for osteoarthritis. Four months later, he had a myocardial infarction. Two weeks ago, while on his exercise bike, he had a stroke. His right arm and leg were paralyzed, he lost his speech, and he had difficulty swallowing. He arrived in the Emergency Department within 3 hours of the stroke and received thrombolytic **therapy** *(see Chapter 6)*. Mr. Johnson is now receiving **physical therapy, occupational therapy,** and speech therapy in the inpatient Rehabilitation Unit. He is able to say some simple words and has begun to have voluntary movements in the arm and leg. Your roles are to help him regain function in his arm and leg and to monitor and record his progress.

Physical Medicine and Rehabilitation (PM&R)
(LO 5.5 and 5.8)

PM&R health professionals are listed and defined at the beginning of this chapter.

Physical medicine and rehabilitation is also called **physiatry.** Its goal is to develop a comprehensive program to put together the different pieces of a person's life—medical, social, emotional, and **vocational**—after injury or disease. PM&R programs cover a wide spectrum, from prevention of injury in athletes to treating sports-related injuries in sports medicine to coping with complicated multiple trauma.

Mr. Hank Johnson *(see Case Report 5.2)* will need a program designed specifically to get him back on his feet literally and in so many other ways.

Stroke Rehabilitation
(LO 5.5 and 5.8)

The goals of Mr. Johnson's **rehabilitation** program are to enable him to:

- Walk safely using an **assistive device.**
- Use his hands with accuracy.
- Restore his speech abilities.
- Prevent a second stroke.

Because he received thrombolytic therapy *(see Chapter 6)* within 3 hours of his stroke's onset, he has a 50% chance of being left with little or no residual difficulty, compared to a 35% chance had he not received the therapy.

Social workers are helping Mr. Johnson's wife to make their home safe for his return, including obtaining **adaptive equipment.** Raised toilet seats, handrails in the bath and shower, eating devices, and other adaptive equipment will help Mr. Johnson perform activities of daily living during his recovery. Social workers will also help Mrs. Johnson to work with Medicare to obtain the maximum allowable benefits. Anyone who has had one stroke is at high risk for having a second stroke. Therefore, during this rehabilitative period, Mr. Johnson will be evaluated for such risk factors as narrowing of the carotid arteries with plaque, thrombosis *(see Chapter 6)*, and the presence of atrial fibrillation *(see Chapter 6)*.

Abbreviation

PM&R physical medicine and rehabilitation

Word Analysis and Definition

S = Suffix   P = Prefix   R = Root   R/CF = Combining Form

WORD	PRONUNCIATION	ELEMENTS		DEFINITION
assistive device	ah-**SIS**-tiv de-**VICE**	S/ R/ R/	-ive *nature of* assist- *aid, help* device *an appliance*	Tool, software, or hardware to assist in performing daily activities
occupational therapy	**OCK**-you-**PAY**-shun-al **THAIR**-ah-pee	S/ R/ R/	-al *pertaining to* occupation- *work* therapy *treatment*	Use of work and recreational activities to increase independent function
orthotic	or-**THOT**-ik	S/ R/	-ic *pertaining to* orthot- *correct*	Orthopedic appliance to correct an abnormality
orthotist	or-**THOT**-ist	S/	-ist *specialist*	Specialist who makes and fits orthopedic appliances
physiatry physiatrist	fih-**ZIE**-ah-tree fih-**ZIE**-ah-trist	 S/ R/ R/	Greek *science of nature* -ist *specialist* phys- *nature* -iatr- *treatment*	Physical medicine Specialist in physical medicine
physical medicine	**FIZ**-ih-cal **MED**-ih-sin	S/ R/	-al *pertaining to* physic- *body*	Diagnosis and treatment by means of remedial agents, such as exercises, manipulation, heat, etc.
physical therapy *(also known as physiotherapy)* physiotherapy (syn)	**FIZ**-ih-cal **THAIR**-ah-pee **FIZ**-ee-oh-**THAIR**-ah-pee	S/ R/ R/ R/CF	-al *pertaining to* physic- *body* therapy *treatment* physi/o- *body*	Use of remedial processes to overcome a physical defect Another term for physical therapy
rehabilitation	**REE**-hah-bill-ih-**TAY**-shun	S/ P/ R/	-ion *action, condition* re- *again* -habilitat- *restore*	Therapeutic restoration of an ability to function as before
therapy	**THAIR**-ah-pee		Greek *medical treatment*	Systematic treatment of a disease, dysfunction, or disorder
therapeutic (adj)	**THAIR**-ah-**PYU**-tik	S/ R/	-ic *pertaining to* therapeut- *treatment*	Relating to the treatment of a disease or disorder
therapist	**THAIR**-ah-pist	S/ R/	-ist *specialist* therap- *treatment*	Professional trained in the practice of a particular therapy

EXERCISES

A. Review *the Case Report on this spread before answering the questions. Apply your knowledge of medical language to fill in the correct answers.*
LO 5.2, 5.5, and 5.9 *Apply*

1. Why did Mr. Johnson need a hip replacement? _____

2. What is a *myocardial infarction?* _____

3. What does it mean if you are an *inpatient?* _____

4. What two major medical events has Mr. Johnson suffered recently? _____

5. What are the goals of Mr. Johnson's rehabilitation program? _____
_____

B. Deconstruct *the following medical terms into their word elements. Some terms will not have every element present. Then use any one term in a sentence of patient documentation. Fill in the blanks.* **LO 5.1, 5.2, and 5.8** *Analyze*

Medical Term	Prefix	Root/CF	Suffix	Meaning of Term
physiatrist	1.	2.	3.	4.
rehabilitation	5.	6.	7.	8.
orthotic	9.	10.	11.	12.
multidisciplinary	13.	14.	15.	16.
orthotist	17.	18.	19.	20.
physiotherapy	21.	22.	23.	24.

Sentence: _____
_____.

Lesson 5.4(cont'd)

Definitions (LO 5.2, 5.3, and 5.8)

The following definitions of terms or phrases specific to rehabilitation will help you to understand more precisely the different kinds of rehabilitation in which you may be involved as a health professional.

Rehabilitation medicine focuses on function. Being able to function is essential to an individual's independence and ability to have a good quality of life.

Restorative rehabilitation restores a function that has been lost, such as after a hip fracture, hip replacement, or stroke. This process can be intense, but it's also usually short term.

Maintenance rehabilitation strengthens and maintains a function that is gradually being lost. It is less intense than restorative rehabilitation but often long term. Problems of senescence (old age), like difficulty with balance or flexibility, require this long-term approach.

Rehabilitation medicine is also involved with the **prevention** of function loss and the prevention of injury. In sports medicine, an example is the prevention of shoulder and elbow injuries often experienced by baseball pitchers.

Activities of daily living (ADLs) are the routine activities of personal care. The six basic ADLs are eating, bathing, dressing, grooming, toileting, and transferring. Assistive devices are designed to make ADLs easier to perform and help maintain the patient's independence. Examples of these devices include reachers and grabbers, easy-pull sock aids, long shoehorns, jar openers, and eating aids *(Figure 5.11).* ADLs are also a measurement to assess therapy needs and monitor its effectiveness.

Instrumental activities of daily living (IADLs) relate to independent living. These activities include managing money, using a telephone, cooking, driving, shopping for groceries and personal items, and doing housework.

Amputations (LO 5.2, 5.3, and 5.8)

Seventy-five percent of all amputations are performed on people over 65 years of age with **peripheral vascular disease (PVD).** This includes complications from arteriosclerosis and diabetes. Most of these cases involve **below-the-knee amputations (BKAs).**

On the other hand, the wars in Iraq and Afghanistan led to soldiers losing their arms and legs from have the detonation of explosive devices. In some of these cases, amputations are also required, depending on the level of damage an explosion has caused to the soldier's body.

Rehabilitation after amputation is an increasingly important component in rehabilitation programs. Immediately after surgery, the objectives of the rehabilitation team are to:

- Promote healing of the stump;
- Strengthen the muscles above the site of the amputation;
- Strengthen arm muscles to assist in ambulation or help with walking using a cane, crutches, or other assistive devices;
- Prevent **contractures** or **tightening** of the joints above the amputation (knee and hip for BKAs);
- Shrink the post-amputation stump with elastic cuffs or bandages to fit the socket of a temporary **prosthesis** *(Figure 5.12);* and
- Provide emotional, psychological, and family support.

▲ **FIGURE 5.11**
Assistive Device for Dressing.

Abbreviations

ADLs	activities of daily living
BKA	below-the-knee amputation
COTA	certified occupational therapist assistant
IADLs	instrumental activities of daily living
PVD	peripheral vascular disease

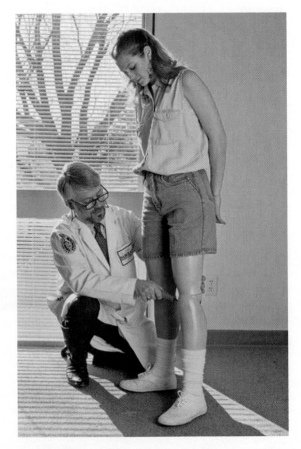

▲ **FIGURE 5.12**
Sixteen-Year-Old Being Fitted with Prosthesis.

Word Analysis and Definition

S = Suffix   P = Prefix   R = Root   R/CF = Combining Form

WORD	PRONUNCIATION	ELEMENTS		DEFINITION
amputation	am-pyu-**TAY**-shun	S/ R/	-ation *a process* amput- *prune*	Removal of a limb, part of a limb, or other projecting body part
contracture	kon-**TRAK**-chur	S/ R/	-ure *result of* contract- *pull together*	Muscle shortening due to spasm or fibrosis
prevention	pree-**VEN**-shun	S/ R/	-ion *action, condition* prevent- *prevent*	Process to prevent occurrence of a disease or health problem
prosthesis	**PROS**-thee-sis		Greek *an addition*	An artificial part to remedy a defect in the body
restorative rehabilitation	ree-**STOR**-ah-tiv **REE**-hah-bill-ih-**TAY**-shun	S/ R/	-ative *quality of* restor- *renew*	Therapy that promotes renewal of health and strength

EXERCISES

A. Deconstruct *the following terms and give their meanings:*   **LO 5.1, 5.2, and 5.8** *Analyze*

1. Rehabilitation: _____ / _____ / _____

   P   R, R/CF   S

   Meaning: _____

2. Therapeutic: _____ / _____ / _____

   P   R, R/CF   S

   Meaning: _____

3. Restorative: _____ / _____ / _____

   P   R, R/CF   S

   Meaning: _____

B. Rehabilitation *medicine has its own specific goals and terminology. Apply the language of rehabilitation medicine to answer the following questions.*
LO 5.2, 5.3, and 5.8

1. Each of these three types of rehabilitation medicine has a specific focus. Explain what they are.

   a. rehabilitation: _____

   b. restorative rehabilitation: _____

   c. maintenance rehabilitation: _____

2. What does the abbreviation *ADL* stand for? _____

3. List the basic ADLs: _____

   _____

4. What do the IADLs relate to? _____

5. Give an example of an IADL: _____

C. Utilize *the correct language of rehabilitation in the following paragraph. The word bank contains more terms than you need to use—some terms you may use more than once. When you have finished the exercise, proofread it again to see if it makes sense. Fill in the blanks.*   **LO 5.2, 5.8, and 5.9** *Apply*

adapt	**contracture**	**amputation(s)**	**prosthesis**
amputee	**adaptive equipment**	**elective**	**amputate**
residual	**PVD**	**assistive**	**protocol**

Seventy-five percent of all (1) _____ are performed on patients over 65 years of age with (2) _____ complicating arteriosclerosis and diabetes. Loss of blood flow to a limb area produces necrotic tissue, which in time can become infected or gangrenous and makes the need for this procedure urgent, rather than (3) _____. A traumatic (4) _____ can occur in an industrial accident, motor vehicle accident, or household accident. The decision to (5) _____ is a serious one and must be undertaken by a qualified surgeon. The (6) _____ will require postoperative training in how to (7) _____ to the use of a (8) _____ and/or (9) _____. Hopefully, there will be no muscle (10) _____ or (11) _____ pain after the surgery.

Additional exercises available in **connect**

Chapter Review exercises, along with additional practice items, are available in Connect!

The Cardiovascular and Circulatory Systems

The Essentials of the Language of Cardiology

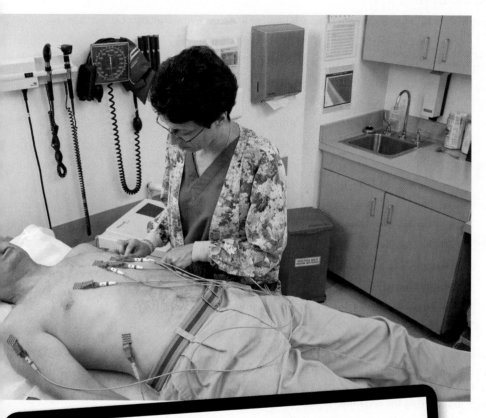

CHAPTER 6

Learning Outcomes

The health of a patient's heart—in fact, the entire cardiovascular system—will always be a factor in the diagnosis and treatment of any condition, no matter what discipline or setting you find yourself working in as a health professional. From routine blood pressure checks to ultrasounds to surgical procedures, the condition of a patient's cardiovascular system must be carefully monitored. In order to best understand, communicate, and document conditions affecting the heart, blood vessels, and blood, you need to be able to:

LO 6.1 Use **roots, combining forms, suffixes, and prefixes** to construct and analyze (deconstruct) medical terms related to the cardiovascular and circulatory systems.

LO 6.2 Spell and pronounce correctly medical terms and their plurals related to the cardiovascular and circulatory systems to communicate them with accuracy and precision in any health care setting.

LO 6.3 Define accepted abbreviations related to the cardiovascular and circulatory systems.

LO 6.4 Relate the anatomical structure of the heart to its functions, the blood flow through it, and disorders of its wall and valves.

LO 6.5 Describe the blood supply to the heart, the electrical properties of the heart, and their related diagnostic tests and therapeutic procedures.

LO 6.6 Identify the different circulatory systems and the disorders of arteries and veins.

LO 6.7 Apply your knowledge of the medical terms of the cardiovascular and circulatory systems to documentation, medical records, and medical reports.

LO 6.8 Translate the medical terms of the cardiovascular and circulatory systems into everyday language in order to communicate clearly with patients and their families.

Case Report 6.1

You are . . .

. . . a cardiovascular technologist (CVT) employed by the **Cardiology** Department at Fulwood Medical Center. You have been called to the Emergency Department (ED) to perform an **electrocardiogram (ECG** or **EKG)**, STAT.

You are communicating with . . .

. . . Mr. Hank Johnson, a 64-year-old owner of a printing company. Eight months ago, he had a left total hip replacement. In the past 3 months, Mr. Johnson has returned to his daily workouts. This morning, while riding his exercise bike, he felt a tightness in his chest, but continued cycling. He developed pain in the center of his chest, radiating down his left arm and up into his jaw, and became **diaphoretic.** His personal trainer called 911. You perform the ECG and the automatic report describes abnormalities in the chest leads. As you remove the **electrodes,** Mr. Johnson complains that he is feeling faint and having difficulty breathing (DOB). You are the only person in the room.

The health professionals involved in the diagnosis and treatment of problems with the cardiovascular system include the following:

- **Cardiologists** are medical doctors who specialize in disorders of the cardiovascular system.
- **Cardiovascular surgeons** are surgeons who specialize in surgery of the heart and the peripheral blood vessels.
- **Cardiovascular technologists** and technicians assist physicians in the diagnosis and treatment of cardiovascular disorders.
- **Vascular technologists** are practitioners who assist physicians by performing diagnostic and monitoring procedures using ultrasound.
- **Cardiac sonographers** or echocardiographers are technologists who use ultrasound to observe the heart chambers, valves, and blood vessels.
- **Phlebotomists** or phlebotomy technicians assist physicians by drawing patient blood samples for laboratory testing.
- **Perfusionists** are highly trained health care professionals who use the heart-lung machine during cardiac and other surgeries that require cardiopulmonary bypass.

▶ **FIGURE 6.1**
Position of Heart in Thoracic Cavity.
(a) Position of heart in mediastinum.
(b) Relationship of heart to sternum.

Lesson 6.1

The Heart

Location of the Heart (LO 6.4)

It is important to know precisely where the heart is located so that you can perform effective **cardiopulmonary resuscitation (CPR).** The heart is located in the **thoracic cavity** between the lungs, in an area called the **mediastinum** *(Figure 6.1a).* The heart is shaped like a blunt cone, pointing down and to the left. It rests at an angle with the majority of its mass to the left of the **sternum** *(Figure 6.1b).*

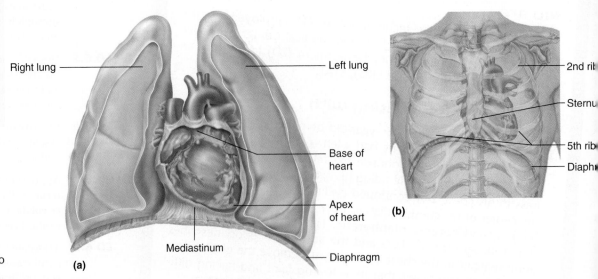

Word Analysis and Definition

S = Suffix   P = Prefix   R = Root   R/CF = Combining Form

WORD	PRONUNCIATION	ELEMENTS		DEFINITION
cardiac	**KAR**-dee-ak	S/ R/	-ac *pertaining to* cardi- *heart*	Pertaining to the heart
cardiologist	kar-dee-**OL**-oh-jist	S/ R/CF	-logist *one who studies,* *specialist* cardi/o- *heart*	A medical specialist in the diagnosis and treatment of the heart (cardiology)
cardiology	kar-dee-**OL**-oh-jee	S/	-logy *study of*	Medical specialty of diseases of the heart
cardiopulmonary resuscitation (CPR)	**KAR**-dee-oh-**PUL**-mo-nar-ee ree-sus-ih-**TAY**-shun	S/ R/CF R/ S/ R/-	-ary *pertaining to* cardi/o- *heart* -pulmon- *lung* -ation *a process* resuscit- *revive from appar-* *ent death*	The attempt to restore cardiac and pulmonary function
cardiovascular	**KAR**-dee-oh-**VAS**-kyu-lar	S/ R/CF R/	-ar *pertaining to* cardi/o- *heart* -vascul- *blood vessel*	Pertaining to the heart and blood vessels
diaphoresis (noun)	**DIE**-ah-foh-**REE**-sis	S/ R/	-esis *condition* diaphor- *sweat*	Sweat, perspiration, or sweaty
diaphoretic (adj)	**DIE**-ah-foh-**RET**-ic	S/	-etic *pertaining to*	Pertaining to sweat or perspiration
electrocardiogram (ECG, EKG)	ee-lek-troh-**KAR**-dee-oh-gram	S/ R/CF R/CF	-gram *a record* electr/o- *electricity* -cardi/o- *heart*	Record of the electrical signals of the heart
electrocardiograph electrocardiography	ee-lek-troh-**KAR**-dee-oh-graf ee-**LEK**-troh-kar-dee-**OG**-rah-fee	S/ S/	-graph *to record* -graphy *process of* *recording*	Machine that produces the electrocardiogram The method of recording and the interpretation of electrocardiograms
electrode	ee-**LEK**-trode	S/ R/	-ode *way, road* electr- *electricity*	A device for conducting electricity
mediastinum	**ME**-dee-ass-**TIE**-num	S/ P/ R/	-um *structure* media- *middle* -stin- *partition*	Area between the lungs containing the heart, aorta, venae cavae, esophagus, and trachea
perfusion	per-**FYU**-zhun	S/ R/	-ion *action* perfus- *to pour*	The act of forcing blood to flow through a lumen or a vascular bed
phlebotomist	fleh-**BOT**-oh-mist	S/ R/CF R/	-ist *specialist in* phleb/o- *vein* -tom- *incise, cut*	Person skilled in taking blood from veins
phlebotomy	fleh-**BOT**-oh-me	S/	-tomy *surgical incision*	Withdrawing blood from a vein through a needle or catheter
sternum	**STIR**-num		Latin *the chest*	Long, flat bone forming the center of the anterior wall of the chest
thoracic cavity	**THOR**-ass-ik **KAV**-ih-tee	S/ R/	-ic *pertaining to* thorac- *chest* cavity, Latin *hollow*	Space within the chest containing the lungs, heart, esophagus, trachea, aorta, venae cavae, and pulmonary vessels

EXERCISES

A. Review *the Case Report on the opening two-page spread before answering the questions.*   **LO 6.3 and 6.7** *Remember*

1. The following abbreviations all appear in the Case Report. Demonstrate your understanding of the abbreviations by writing out the terms they represent.

   a. EKG _____

   b. ED _____

   c. CVT _____

   d. SOB _____

   e. ECG _____

B. Apply the language *of cardiology in the following documentation. Be sure to use the correct form (noun, adjective) of the term. There is only one best answer for each blank.*   **LO 6.2 and 6.7** *Apply*

cardiologist   **cardiovascular**   **cardiology**   **cardiopulmonary**

1. The _____ Department sent a specialist to examine the patient in the Emergency Room because of his symptoms. The _____ ordered an angioplasty, which found that the patient had three obstructed arteries in his heart, so the _____ surgeon prepared to operate immediately. Before surgery could begin, the patient suffered a heart attack and _____ resuscitation was needed.

Functions and Structure of the Heart (LO 6.4)

Functions of the Heart (LO 6.4)

In order to keep your body alive, your heart must work all the time, without stopping. Its three most important functions are to:

1. **Pump blood.** As your heart contracts, it generates pressure that moves your blood through your blood vessels.

2. **Route blood.** Your heart essentially has two pumps: one on the right side that sends blood through the **pulmonary** circulation of your lungs and back to the second pump on your left side, which sends blood through the **systemic** circulation of your body. Your heart valves make this one-way flow of blood possible.

3. **Regulate blood supply.** The changing metabolic needs of your tissues and organs—for example, when you exercise—are met by changes in the rate and force of your heart's contractions.

Case Report 6.1 (continued)

A **myocardial infarction** (heart attack) is what was happening to Mr. Johnson at the beginning of this chapter. The changes on the ECG showed this event.

Structure of the Heart (LO 6.4)

The heart wall consists of three layers *(Figure 6.2):*

1. **Endocardium:** Connective tissue lining the inside of your heart.

2. **Myocardium:** Cardiac muscle cells that contract to enable your heart to pump blood.

3. **Epicardium:** An outer single layer of cells overlying a thin layer of connective tissue.

The **pericardium** is a double-layered connective tissue sac that surrounds and protects your heart.

Blood Supply to Heart Muscle (LO 6.5)

Because your heart beats continually and forcefully, it requires an abundant supply of oxygen and nutrients. To meet this need, your cardiac muscle has its own blood circulation called the **coronary circulation** *(Figure 6.3).* This system of arteries arises directly from the **aorta.**

If any of your coronary arteries become blocked, the blood supply to a part of your cardiac muscle is cut off **(ischemia)** and the cells supplied by that artery die **(necrosis)** within minutes. This is a **myocardial infarction (MI)** or a "heart attack."

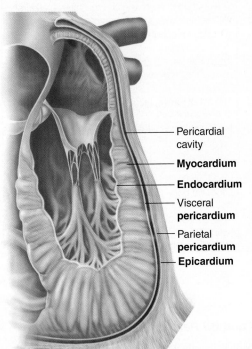

Pericardial cavity
Myocardium
Endocardium
Visceral **pericardium**
Parietal **pericardium**
Epicardium

▲ **FIGURE 6.2**
Heart Wall.

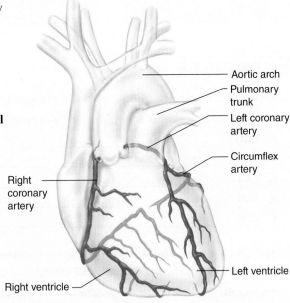

Aortic arch
Pulmonary trunk
Left coronary artery
Circumflex artery
Right coronary artery
Left ventricle
Right ventricle

▲ **FIGURE 6.3**
Coronary Arterial Circulation.

Abbreviation

MI   myocardial infarction

Word Analysis and Definition

WORD	PRONUNCIATION	ELEMENTS		DEFINITION
aorta aortic (adj)	a-**OR**-tuh a-**OR**-tik	 S/ R/	Greek *lift up* -ic *pertaining to* aort- *aorta*	Main trunk of the systemic arterial system Pertaining to the aorta
coronary circulation	**KOR**-oh-nair-ee **SER**-kyu-**LAY**-shun	S/ R/ S/ R/	-ary *pertaining to* coron- *crown, coronary* -ion *action, condition* circulat- *circular route*	Blood vessels supplying the heart muscle
endocardium endocardial (adj)	EN-doh-**KAR**-dee-um EN-doh-**KAR**-dee-al	S/ P/ R/ S/	-um *structure* endo- *inside* -cardi- *heart* -al *pertaining to*	The inside lining of the heart Pertaining to the endocardium
epicardium epicardial (adj)	EP-ih-**KAR**-dee-um EP-ih-**KAR**-dee-al	S/ P/ R/ S/	-um *structure* epi- *upon, above* -cardi- *heart* -al *pertaining to*	The outer layer of the heart wall Pertaining to the epicardium
infarct infarction	in-**FARKT** in-**FARKT**-shun	P/ R/ S/	in- *in* -farct- *area of dead tissue* -ion *action, condition*	Area of cell death resulting from an infarction Sudden blockage of an artery
ischemia ischemic (adj)	is-**KEY**-me-ah is-**KEY**-mik	S/ R/ S/	-emia *a blood condition* isch- *to keep back* -emic *a condition of the blood*	Lack of blood supply to a tissue Pertaining to or affected by the lack of blood supply to a tissue
myocardium myocardial (adj)	**MY**-oh-**KAR**-dee-um my-oh-**KAR**-dee-al	S/ R/CF R/ S/	-um *structure* my/o- *muscle* -cardi- *heart* -al *pertaining to*	Muscular layer of the heart Pertaining to heart muscle
necrosis necrotic (adj)	neh-**KROH**-sis neh-**KROT**-ik	S/ R/ S/ R/CF	-osis *condition* necr- *death* -tic *pertaining to* necr/o- *death*	Pathologic death of cells or tissue Pertaining to or affected by necrosis (death)
pericardium (noun) pericardial (adj)	per-ih-**KAR**-dee-um per-ih-**KAR**-dee-al	S/ P/ R/ S/	-um *structure* peri- *around* -cardi- *heart* -al *pertaining to*	A double layer of membranes surrounding the heart Pertaining to the pericardium
pulmonary	**PULL**-moh-**NAR**-ee	S/ R/	-ary *pertaining to* pulmon- *lung*	Pertaining to the lungs and their blood supply

EXERCISES

A. Review *the Case Report on this two-page spread before answering the questions.*   **LO 6.1, 6.2, 6.3, and 6.5** *Analyze*

1. Based on the patient's ECG, what was his final diagnosis? _____

2. What is the abbreviation for this condition? _____

3. Deconstruct the medical terms in #1 above. _____/_____/_____

                               P   R/CF   S

                    _____/_____/_____

                               P   R/CF   S

B. Elements: *Solid knowledge of elements will help increase your medical vocabulary. Many of the elements in the WAD above will appear throughout later chapters. Learn these elements now, and you will recognize them later. Put a ✓ in the appropriate column to identify the type of element, and then fill in the last two columns.*   **LO 6.1 and 6.5** *Apply*

Element	Prefix	Root	CF	Suffix	Meaning of Element	Medical Term with This Element
um	1.				2.	3.
emia	4.				5.	6.
isch	7.				8.	9.
myo	10.				11.	12.

Blood Flow through the Heart (LO 6.4)

Your heart *(Figure 6.6)* has four chambers through which your blood flows. These chambers are the:

1. Right **atrium**
2. Right **ventricle**
3. Left atrium
4. Left ventricle

Your right and left atria are separated by a thin muscle wall called the **interatrial septum.** Your right and left ventricles are divided by a thicker muscle wall called the **interventricular septum.**

Your left ventricle pumps blood to all the parts of your body (except the lungs) through the **systemic circulation.** Oxygen (O_2) and nutrients are delivered to your body's cells, and carbon dioxide (CO_2) and metabolic waste products are removed from the cells. This **deoxygenated** blood, via the veins, returns to the heart where the right ventricle pumps blood into the **pulmonary circulation** to the lungs. In the lungs, the carbon dioxide waste material is exchanged for oxygen from inhaled air *(Figure 6.5)*. This oxygenated blood then travels through the pulmonary veins back to the left side of the heart.

You have four valves that work together to ensure the correct flow of blood through your heart; on the right side are the **tricuspid** and **pulmonary** valves, and on the left side are the **mitral (bicuspid)** and **aortic** valves *(Figure 6.4)*.

▲ **FIGURE 6.4**
Anatomy of the Heart.

▲ **FIGURE 6.6**
External Anatomy of the Heart: Frontal View.

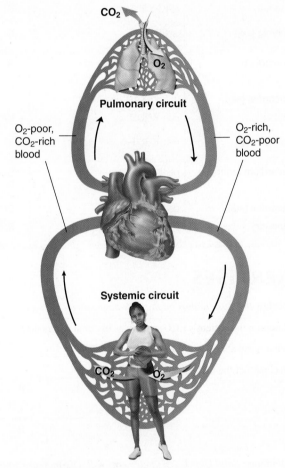

▲ **FIGURE 6.5**
Schematic of Cardiovascular System.

Word Analysis and Definition

WORD	PRONUNCIATION	ELEMENTS		DEFINITION
atrium atria (pl) atrial (adj)	A-tree-um A-tree-ah A-tree-al	S/ R/ S/	-um *structure* atri- *entrance, atrium* -al *pertaining to*	Chamber where blood enters the heart on both the right and left sides Pertaining to the atrium
bicuspid	by-**KUSS**-pid	S/ P/ R/	-id *having a particular quality* bi- *two* -cusp- *point*	Having two points; a bicuspid heart valve has two flaps
interatrial	IN-ter-**AY**-tree-al	S/ P/ R/	-al *pertaining to* inter- *between* -atri- *atrium*	Between the atria of the heart
interventricular (IV)	IN-ter-ven-**TRIK**-you-lar	S/ P/ R/	-ar *pertaining to* inter- *between* -ventricul- *ventricle*	Between the ventricles of the heart
mitral	**MY**-tral		Latin *turban*	Shaped like the headdress of a Catholic bishop
septum septa (pl)	**SEP**-tum **SEP**-tah		Latin *partition*	A thin wall dividing two cavities
tricuspid	try-**KUSS**-pid	S/ P/ R/	-id *having a particular quality* tri- *three* -cusp- *point*	Having three points; a tricuspid heart valve has three flaps
ventricle	**VEN**-trih-kel		Latin *small belly*	Chamber of the heart (pumps blood) or a cavity in the brain (produces cerebrospinal fluid)

Study Hint

Try to relate these same prefixes to common English words. It will help you remember the meaning of the prefix in the medical terms.

EXERCISES

A. Prefixes *can generally answer a question: Where is it? What color is it? How big is it? How many are there? This exercise groups some prefixes from the WAD and asks you to identify what makes them similar. Studying elements in similar groups will make them easier to remember. Fill in the chart.*

LO 6.1 and 6.2 *Apply*

Prefix	Meaning of Prefix	Medical Term with This Prefix	Meaning of Medical Term
bi	1.	2.	3.
tri	4.	5.	6.

These prefixes are similar because: _____

B. This chart has the same prefixes *but is asking for an English word where the prefix means the same as it does in the medical word.*   **LO 6.1 and 6.2** *Apply*

_____

Prefix	Meaning of Prefix	English Term with This Prefix	Meaning of English Term
bi	1.	2.	3.
tri	4.	5.	6.

C. Meet lesson objectives *and use the language of cardiology to answer the following questions.*   **LO 6.2, 6.4, and 6.6** *Remember*

1. Name the four chambers in the heart. _____

2. List the four valves in the heart. _____

3. What is the function of a valve? _____

4. What is the purpose of the systemic circulation? _____

Lesson 6.1 (cont'd)

Keynotes

- Vital signs (VS) measure temperature (T), pulse (P), respiration (R), and blood pressure (BP) to assess cardiorespiratory function.
- A heart rate slower than 60 is called bradycardia. *(Figure 6.9)* A heart rate faster than 100 is called tachycardia *(Figure 6.10)*.

Abbreviations

AV	atrioventricular
BP	blood pressure
P	pulse
R	respiration
SA	sinoatrial
T	temperature
VS	vital signs

The Heartbeat (LO 6.4 and 6.5)

The actions of the four heart chambers are coordinated. When the atria contract (atrial **systole**), the ventricles relax (ventricular **diastole**). When the atria relax (atrial diastole), the ventricles contract (ventricular systole). Then the atria and ventricles all relax briefly. This series of events is a complete cardiac cycle, or heartbeat.

The "lub-dub, lub-dub" sounds heard through the stethoscope are made by the heart valves snapping as they close. If there is an abnormality in valve closure, it will produce an extra, abnormal sound called a **murmur.**

Electrical Properties of the Heart (LO 6.4 and 6.5)

As your heart muscles contract, they generate a small electrical current that sustains your heartbeat rhythm through a conduction system *(Figure 6.7)*. Here is how this conduction system works:

1. A small region of specialized muscle cells in the right atrium's **sinoatrial (SA) node** initiates your heartbeat. The SA node is the **pacemaker** of your heart's rhythm.

2. Electrical signals from the SA node spread out through the atria and rejoin at the **atrioventricular (AV) node.** The AV is the electrical gateway to the ventricles.

3. Electrical signals leave the AV node and travel to the ventricular myocardium where they stimulate the ventricular myocardium to contract, creating your heartbeat.

Sinus rhythm is the term used to describe a normal heartbeat, where normal electrical conduction leads to a ventricular rate of about 60 to 80 beats per minute. An abnormal cardiac rhythm is called an **arrhythmia** or a **dysrhythmia.**

An **electrocardiograph** is a device that picks up the heart muscle's electrical changes and amplifies them to record an electrocardiogram in the form of waves *(Figure 6.8)*.

▲ **FIGURE 6.7**
Cardiac Conduction System.

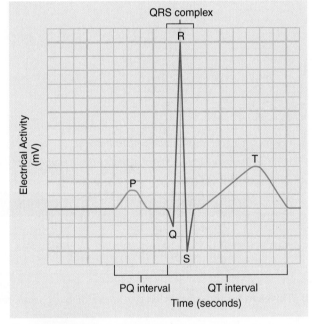

▲ **FIGURE 6.8**
Normal Electrocardiogram.

▲ **FIGURE 6.9**
Bradycardia.

▲ **FIGURE 6.10**
Tachycardia.

Word Analysis and Definition

WORD	PRONUNCIATION	ELEMENTS		DEFINITION
arrhythmia (Note: *double "rr"*)	a-**RITH**-me-ah	S/ P/ R/	-ia *condition* a- *without* -rrhythm- *rhythm*	Condition when the heart rhythm is abnormal
atrioventricular (AV)	A-tree-oh-ven-**TRICK**-you-lar	S/ R/CF R/	-ar *pertaining to* atri/o- *entrance, atrium* -ventricul- *ventricle*	Pertaining to both the atrium and the ventricle
diastole (noun)	die-**AS**-toe-lee		Greek *dilation*	Dilation of heart cavities, during which they fill with blood
diastolic (adj)	die-as-**TOL**-ik	S/ R/	-ic *pertaining to* diastol- *diastole*	Pertaining to diastole
dysrhythmia (Note: *single "r"*)	dis-**RITH**-me-ah	S/ P/ R/	-ia *condition* dys- *bad, difficult* -rhythm- *rhythm*	An abnormal heart rhythm
murmur	**MUR**-mur		Latin *low voice*	Abnormal heart sound heard with a stethoscope when a valve closes or opens abnormally
sinoatrial (SA) node	sigh-noh-**AY**-tree-al NODE	S/ R/CF R/	-al *pertaining to* sin/o- *sinus* -atri- *atrium*	The center of modified cardiac muscle fibers in the wall of the right atrium that acts as the pacemaker for the heart rhythm
sinus rhythm	**SIGH**-nus **RITH**-um		sinus Latin *channel, cavity* rhythm Greek *to flow*	The normal (optimal) heart rhythm arising from the sinoatrial node
systole (noun) systolic (adj)	**SIS**-toe-lee sis-**TOL**-ik	S/ R/	Greek *contraction* -ic *pertaining to* systol- *systole, contraction*	Contraction of the heart muscle Pertaining to systole
vital signs	**VI**-tal SIGNS		vital Latin *life* signs Latin *mark*	A procedure during a physical examination in which temperature (T), pulse (P), respirations (R), and blood pressure (BP) are measured to assess general health and cardiorespiratory function

EXERCISES

A. Match *the correct element to its meaning.*   **LO 6.1** *Understand*

_____ **1.** atrio
a. without

_____ **2.** ar
b. contraction

_____ **3.** ia
c. bad, difficult

_____ **4.** systol
d. entrance

_____ **5.** dys
e. condition

_____ **6.** a
f. pertaining to

B. Spelling: *The terms in the WAD can be particularly difficult to spell, yet they occur all the time in a cardiologist's dictation. Circle the correct choice for the documentation.*   **LO 6.4, and 6.5** *Apply*

1. An (arhythmia/arrhythmia) has been confirmed with the EKG.

2. Her (sysstolic/systolic) blood pressure is dangerously high.

3. The (murrmur/murmur) was detected during ventricular (dyastole/diastole).

4. Cardiac (dysrrhythmia/dysrhythmia) can be a symptom of a serious underlying condition.

5. The (sinoatrial/synoatrial) node is the pacemaker for the heart rhythm.

Lesson 6.2
Disorders of the Heart

Objectives

Any loss of consciousness precipitated by exertion can be due to a cardiac arrhythmia or a **cardiomyopathy**. *In this lesson, the information will enable you to:*

6.2.1 Name common cardiac arrhythmias.

6.2.2 Discuss common disorders of the heart and heart valves.

6.2.3 Describe coronary heart disease.

6.2.4 Explain hypertensive heart disease.

6.2.5 Define the term *cardiomyopathy*.

Case Report 6.2

You are . . .

. . . an EMT-P called to the gymnasium of Fulwood University.

You are communicating with . . .

. . . Danny Gitlin, a 21-year-old guard on the university basketball team. Danny lost consciousness during a strenuous practice. He had no pulse but was revived by the coach, who used an automatic external **defibrillator (AED)**. Danny has never lost consciousness before, but he has noticed episodes of rapid **palpitations** after games. On examination, he is fully conscious and appears to be fit. His pulse is 70 but irregular in rate and force. His blood pressure is 110/65 mmHg. He has no known family history of heart disease.

Disorders of the Heart

(LO 6.4, and 6.5)

Abnormal Heart Rhythms (LO 6.5)

Arrhythmias are abnormal or irregular heartbeats, and six types are commonly seen:

1. **Premature beats** occur most often in elderly people and are usually associated with caffeine and stress.

2. **Atrial fibrillation (A-fib)** occurs when the two atria quiver rather than contract correctly to pump blood. This causes blood to pool in the atria and sometimes clot.

3. **Ventricular tachycardia (V-tach)** is a rapid heartbeat occurring in the ventricles.

4. **Ventricular arrhythmias** include:

   a. **Premature ventricular contractions (PVCs),** which result when extra impulses arise from a ventricle; and

▶ **FIGURE 6.11**
Automatic External Defibrillator.

Abbreviations

AED	automatic external defibrillator
A-fib	atrial fibrillation
EMT-P	Emergency Medical Technician–Paramedic
ICD	implantable cardioverter/defibrillator
PVC	premature ventricular contraction
V-fib	ventricular fibrillation
V-tach	ventricular tachycardia

   b. **Ventricular fibrillation (V-fib),** which occurs when the ventricles lose control, quivering instead of pumping.

5. **Heart block** occurs when interference in cardiac electrical conduction prevents the atria's contractions from coordinating with the ventricles' contractions.

6. **Palpitations** are brief but unpleasant sensations of a rapid or irregular heartbeat. They can be brought on by exercise, anxiety, and stimulants like caffeine.

Arrhythmias can be treated with medications, but some patients require mechanical **pacemakers.** Pacemakers consist of a battery, electronic circuits, and computer memory to generate electronic signals. These signals are carried along thin, insulated wires to the heart muscle. Pacemakers are ideal for patients with a very slow heart rate (bradycardia).

In emergency situations, external **defibrillation** is performed through **automatic external defibrillators,** or **AEDs** (*Figure 6.11*). AEDs send an electric shock to the heart in order to stop the heart temporarily so that a normal contraction rhythm can resume. This procedure was used for Danny Gitlin.

People with life-threatening arrhythmias may need an **implantable defibrillator (ICD),** which senses abnormal rhythms. An ICD gives the heart a small electric shock to return its rhythm to normal.

Defibrillation is the nonsynchronized delivery of energy to the heart during any phase of the cardiac cycle used in emergency situations. **Cardioversion** is the delivery of lower levels of energy synchronized to the large R waves of the QRS complex and is mostly used for A-fib or flutter and V-tach.

Word Analysis and Definition

WORD	PRONUNCIATION	ELEMENTS		DEFINITION
cardioversion	KAR-dee-oh-VER-zhun	S/ R/CF	-version *change* cardi/o- *heart*	Restoration of a normal heart rhythm by electric shock or medications
defibrillation	dee-fib-rih-LAY-shun	S/ P/ R/	-ation *process* de- *from, out of* -fibrill- *small fiber*	Restoration of normal cardiac activity in life-threatening cardiac arrhythmias
defibrillator	dee-FIB-rih-lay-tor	S/	-ator *instrument*	Instrument for defibrillation
fibrillation	fi-brih-LAY-shun	S/ R/	-ation *a process* fibrill- *small fiber*	Uncontrolled quivering or twitching of the heart muscle
implantable	im-PLAN-tah-bul	S/ P/ R/	-able *capable* im- *in* -plant- *insert*	A device that can be inserted into tissues
pacemaker	PACE-may-ker	S/ R/	-maker *one who makes* pace- *step*	Device that regulates cardiac electrical activity
palpitation	pal-pih-TAY-shun	S/ R/	-ation *a process* palpit- *throb*	Forcible, rapid beat of the heart felt by the patient

EXERCISES

A. Review *the Case Report on this spread before answering the questions.*   **LO 6.3, 6.4, and 6.7** *Understand*

1. What does it mean to *lose consciousness?* _____

2. Danny "had no pulse." What does that mean? _____

3. Where do you see AEDs in public areas? _____

4. What symptom is Danny having? _____

5. What brought on Danny's loss of consciousness? _____

B. Construct *the correct medical terms to match the definitions given. Notice, in particular, that some terms do not have prefixes or suffixes but every term must have a root and/or combining form. Fill in the blanks.*   **LO 6.1, 6.4, and 6.5** *Apply*

1. Forceful, rapid beat of the heart

    _____ / _____ / _____

    P   R/CF   S

2. Uncontrolled heart muscle twitching

    _____ / _____ / _____

    P   R/CF   S

3. Device that restores uncontrolled twitching of cardiac muscle to normal rhythm

    _____ / _____ / _____

    P   R/CF   S

4. Implanted device that regulates cardiac electrical activity

    _____ / _____ / _____

    P   R/CF   S

5. Terminology challenge: Find the medical term on this spread that means *slow heart rate*. What element in the term makes you sure it relates to the heart?

    Term: _____   Element: _____

- Cor pulmonale is failure of the right ventricle to pump properly. Almost any chronic lung disease causing low blood oxygen (hypoxia) can cause this disorder.
- Malfunctions of the valves on the right side of the heart are much less common than those on the left side.

Disorders of the Heart
(continued)

Disorders of Heart Valves
(LO 6.4)

The heart valves can malfunction in two basic ways. Malfunctions most often occur in the heart's left side.

1. **Stenosis:** The valve cannot open fully, and its opening is narrowed (constricted). Because blood cannot flow freely through the valve, it accumulates in the chamber behind the valve.

2. **Incompetence** or **insufficiency** is a condition where the heart valve cannot close fully, allowing blood to leak or **regurgitate** (flow back) through the valve to the heart chamber from which it came.

   Mitral valve stenosis can occur following rheumatic fever. Because the blood cannot flow freely through the valve, the left atrium becomes dilated (enlarged). Eventually, chronic heart failure results.
   Mitral valve prolapse (MVP) occurs when the cusps of the valve bulge back into the left atrium when the left ventricle contracts. This allows blood to flow back into the atrium.
   Aortic valve stenosis is common in the elderly when the valves become calcified due to atherosclerosis. Blood flow into the systemic circulation is diminished, leading to dizziness and fainting. The left ventricle dilates, **hypertrophies,** ceases to beat strongly, and ultimately fails.
   Aortic valve incompetence initially produces few symptoms other than a murmur. Eventually the left ventricle is unable to cope with the excess volume of blood and fails. (*Figure 6.12* enables you to review the locations of the valves and chambers.)
   When a valve replacement is necessary, there are two types of artificial valves available:

1. Mechanical or **prosthetic** valves, which are made from metal alloys and plastics; or

2. **Tissue** valves, which can come from a pig or cow, a human cadaver (dead person), or a patient's own pericardium.

Disorders of the Heart Wall
(LO 6.4)

Endocarditis is an inflammation of the heart's lining, which is usually secondary to an infection elsewhere. Intravenous drug users and people with damaged heart valves are at high risk for endocarditis.

Case Report 6.2 (continued)

The physical findings on Danny Gitlin suggested a cardiomyopathy, which was confirmed by echo-cardiography. Exercise testing (a cardiac stress test), with close medical supervision, produced a ventricular arrhythmia that returned to normal on cessation of the test. Danny was treated with beta blockers and restricted to nonstrenuous sports.

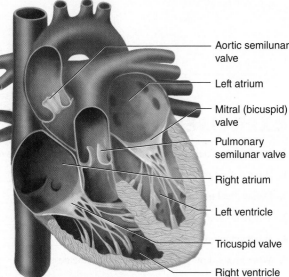

▲ **FIGURE 6.12**
Heart Valves.

Labels: Aortic semilunar valve; Left atrium; Mitral (bicuspid) valve; Pulmonary semilunar valve; Right atrium; Left ventricle; Tricuspid valve; Right ventricle

Myocarditis is an inflammation of the heart muscle. It can be bacterial, viral, or fungal in origin, or can arise as a complication of other diseases like influenza.
   Pericarditis is inflammation of the covering of the heart. The inflammation causes an **exudate** (pericardial effusion) to be released into the pericardial space between the two layers of the pericardium. This interferes with the heart's ability to contract and expand normally, which reduces cardiac output (**CO**) and leads to a life-threatening condition called **cardiac tamponade.**
   Cardiomyopathy is a weakening of the heart muscle that makes it pump inadequately. This causes the heart to enlarge (**cardiomegaly**) and leads to heart failure.

WORD	PRONUNCIATION	ELEMENTS		DEFINITION
cardiomegaly	KAR-dee-oh-MEG-ah-lee	S/ R/CF	-megaly *enlargement* cardi/o- *heart*	Enlargement of the heart
cardiomyopathy	KAR-dee-oh-my-OP-ah-thee	S/ R/CF R/CF	-pathy *disease* cardi/o -*heart* -my/o- *muscle*	Disease of the heart muscle, the myocardium
cor pulmonale	KOR pul-moh-NAH-lee	S/ R/	cor Latin *heart* -ale *pertaining to* pulmon- *lung*	Right-sided heart failure arising from chronic lung disease
endocarditis (Note: The extra "i" from the root *cardi* is dropped when joined to the suffix -*itis*.)	EN-doh-kar-DIE-tis	S/ P/ R/	-itis *inflammation* endo- *within* -cardi- *heart*	Inflammation of the lining of the heart
exudate	EKS-you-date	S/ P/ R/	-ate *pertaining to* ex- *out of* -sud- *sweat*	Fluid that has passed out of a tissue or capillaries as a result of inflammation or injury
hypertrophy (can be a noun or a verb)	high-PER-troh-fee	P/ R/	hyper- *above, excessive* -trophy *development*	Increase in size, but not in number, of an individual tissue element
incompetence	in-KOM-peh-tense	S/ P/ R/	-ence *quality of* in- *not* -compet- *strive together*	Failure of a valve to close completely
insufficiency	in-suh-FISH-en-see	S/ P/ R/CF	-ency *quality of* in- *not* -suffic/i- *enough*	Lack of completeness of function; e.g., a heart valve that fails to close properly
myocarditis (Note: The extra "i" from the root *cardi* is dropped when joined to the suffix -*itis*.)	MY-oh-kar-DIE-tis	S/ R/CF R/	-itis *inflammation* my/o- *muscle* -cardi- *heart*	Inflammation of the heart muscle
pericarditis (Note: The extra "i" from the root *cardi* is dropped when joined to the suffix -*itis*.)	PER-ih-kar-DIE-tis	S/ P/ R/	-itis *inflammation* peri- *around* -cardi- *heart*	Inflammation of the pericardium, the covering of the heart
prolapse	pro-LAPS		Latin *a falling*	An organ slips out of its normal position
prosthesis (noun)	pros-THEE-sis		Greek *an addition*	A manufactured substitute for a missing or diseased part of the body
prosthetic (adj)	pros-THET-ik	S/ R/	-ic *pertaining to* prosthet- *artificial part*	Pertaining to a prosthesis
regurgitate	ree-GUR-jih-tate	S/ P/ R/	-ate *pertaining to* re- *back* -gurgit- *flood*	To flow backward; e.g., blood through a heart valve
stenosis	ste-NOH-sis	S/ R/CF	-sis *abnormal condition* sten/o- *narrow*	Narrowing of a canal or passage, e.g., of a heart valve
tamponade	tam-poh-NAID	S/ R/	-ade *a process* tampon- *plug*	Pathologic compression of an organ, such as the heart

EXERCISES

A. Review *the Case Report on this spread before answering the questions.*   **LO 6.4, 6.5, and 6.8** *Apply*

1. Translate into layman's language: "The physical findings suggested a cardiomyopathy, which was confirmed by echocardiography." _____

_____

2. The cardiac stress test produced *ventricular arrhythmia* for Danny Gitlin. What made it go away? _____

_____

B. Demonstrate *that you can use the term below correctly. Write a sentence of patient documentation for each of the term's meanings.*
LO 6.2, 6.4, and 6.7 *Apply*

1. *Prosthesis* is a term that appears in Chapter 9 relating to orthopedic surgery. Give an example of a heart prosthesis, and another example of an orthopedic prosthesis.

   a. Heart prosthesis: _____

   _____

   b. Orthopedic prosthesis: _____

   _____

Coronary Artery Disease (CAD) (LO 6.5)

Coronary artery disease occurs when the coronary arteries supplying blood to the myocardium are constricted by **atherosclerotic plaques** called **atheroma** (compare *Figure 6.13(a)* to *6.13(b))*. This reduces the blood supply to the cardiac muscle. Platelet clumping can occur on the plaque and form a blood clot (**coronary thrombosis**). **Atherosclerosis** is the most common form of **arteriosclerosis** (hardening of the arteries), and it can lead to **arteriosclerotic** heart disease (**ASHD**).

Angina pectoris (pain in the chest on exertion) is often the first symptom of a reduced oxygen supply to the myocardium. **Myocardial infarction (MI)** is the death of myocardial cells, caused by the lack of blood supply (**ischemia**) when an artery eventually becomes blocked (**occluded**). If the ischemia is not reversed within 4 to 6 hours, the myocardial cells die (**necrosis).**

- Risk factors for CAD include:
  - Heredity
  - Age
  - Obesity
  - Lack of exercise
  - Tobacco
  - Diabetes mellitus
  - Stress
  - High blood pressure
  - Elevated serum cholesterol

- All these risk factors—except heredity and age—can be reduced by lifestyle changes.

Case Report 6.2 (continued)

For Mr. Johnson in the Emergency Department, the ECG (EKG) indicated that he was having an MI affecting the anterior wall of his left ventricle. The cardiovascular technician, who did not want to leave the patient alone, used the call system to obtain nursing and medical help.

Shock is a life-threatening condition that occurs when the body is not getting sufficient blood flow; this can damage multiple organs. A classification of shock includes:

- **Cardiogenic shock** occurs when the heart fails to pump blood effectively through the body's organs and tissues.

- **Hypovolemic shock** occurs from a loss of blood volume, often due to excessive bleeding (hemorrhage) or dehydration.

- **Anaphylactic shock** is caused by a severe allergic reaction.

- **Septic shock** is caused by a severe infection.

- **Neurogenic shock** is associated with damage to the nervous system.

Cardiac arrest is the sudden cessation of cardiac activity that results from **anoxia** (lack of oxygen in the body tissues). Most patients show **asystole** (no heartbeat) on the cardiac monitor *(Figure 6.14).* A person in cardiac arrest has no pulse, is not breathing, and can be referred to as a **pulseless nonbreather (PNB).**

(a) Lumen — — Artery wall

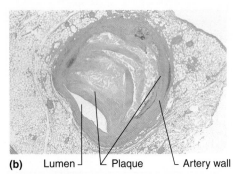

(b) Lumen — — Plaque — Artery wall

▲ **FIGURE 6.13**
Arterial Structure.
(a) Normal coronary artery.
(b) Advanced atherosclerosis.

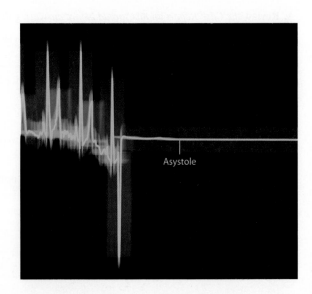

Asystole

ASHD	arteriosclerotic heart disease
CAD	coronary artery disease
MI	myocardial infarction
PNB	pulseless nonbreather

▶ **FIGURE 6.14**
Electrocardiogram (ECG) Showing Asystole.

Word Analysis and Definition

S = Suffix   P = Prefix   R = Root   R/CF = Combining Form

WORD	PRONUNCIATION	ELEMENTS		DEFINITION
anoxia (noun)	an-**OCK**-see-ah	S/ P/ R/	-ia *condition* an- *without* -ox- *oxygen*	Without oxygen
anoxic (adj)	an-**OCK**-sik	S/	-ic *pertaining to*	Pertaining to or suffering from lack of oxygen
arteriosclerosis	ar-**TIER**-ee-oh-skler-**OH**-sis	S/ R/CF R/CF	-sis *abnormal condition* arteri/o- *artery* -scler/o- *hardness*	Hardening of the arteries
arteriosclerotic (adj)	ar-**TIER**-ee-oh-skler-**OT**-ik	S/	-tic *pertaining to*	Pertaining to or affected by arteriosclerosis
asystole	a-**SIS**-toe-lee	P/ R/CF	a- *without* -systol/e *contraction*	Absence of contractions of the heart
atheroma (plaque)	ath-er-**ROE**-mah	S/ R/	-oma *tumor, mass* ather- *porridge, gruel*	Fatty deposit in the lining of an artery
atherectomy atherosclerosis	ath-er-**EK**-toe-me **ATH**-er-oh-skler-**OH**-sis	S/ S/ R/CF R/CF	-ectomy *surgical excision* -sis *abnormal condition* ather/o- *porridge, gruel* -scler/o- *hardness*	Surgical removal of the atheroma Hardening of the arteries due to atheroma (plaque)
cardiogenic	**KAR**-dee-oh-**JEN**-ik	S/ R/CF R/	-ic *pertaining to* cardi/o- *heart* -gen- *produce*	Of cardiac origin
hypovolemia hypovolemic	**HIGH**-poh-vo-**LEE**-me-ah **HIGH**-poh-vo-**LEE**-mik	S/ S/ P/ R/	-emia *a blood condition* -emic *a condition in the blood* hypo- *below* -vol- *volume*	Decreased blood volume in the body Pertaining to a decreased blood volume in the body
occlude (verb) occlusion (noun)	oh-**KLUDE** oh-**KLU**-zhun		Latin *to close*	To close, plug, or completely obstruct A complete obstruction
substernal	sub-**STER**-nal	S/ P/ R/	-al *pertaining to* sub- *under* -stern- *chest*	Under (behind) the sternum or breastbone

EXERCISES

A. Review *the Case Report on this spread before answering the questions.*   **LO 6.2, 6.5, and 6.7** *Understand*

1. What specific place in Mr. Johnson's heart was affected by his MI?

    _____

2. What does an MI do to the living tissue in Mr. Johnson's heart?

    _____

3. What is the medical term for this condition in question #2? _____

4. What is the function of the part of the heart that is the answer in question #1 above?

    _____

5. What indicated Mr. Johnson was having a heart attack? _____

B. Recall *the use of the prefix in the following terms. You have seen this prefix before, and you will see it again—same prefix, different elements, more terms. Fill in the blanks.*   **LO 6.1 and 6.2** *Remember*

1. The prefix *sub* means _____.

2. *Substernal* means _____.

3. *Sublingual* means _____.

4. *Subcutaneous* means _____.

5. *Submandibular* means _____.

Disorders of the Heart *(continued)*

Hypertensive Heart Disease (LO 6.4, and 6.5)

Hypertension (HTN), the most common cardiovascular disorder in this country, affects more than 20% of the adult population. It results from a prolonged elevated blood pressure in the vascular system, which forces the ventricles to work harder to pump blood.

High blood pressure is indicated by a blood pressure reading of 140/90 mmHg (millimeters of mercury) or higher. A normal blood pressure is below 120/80 mmHg. The first number, or **systolic** reading, reflects the blood pressure when the heart is contracting. The second number, or **diastolic** reading, reflects the blood pressure when the heart is relaxed between contractions.

Primary or **essential hypertension** is the most common type of hypertension. Its etiology is **idiopathic** (unknown).

Secondary hypertension results from other diseases like kidney disease, atherosclerosis, and hyperthyroidism.

Malignant hypertension is a rare, severe, life-threatening form of hypertension that involves a blood pressure reading of greater than 200/120 mmHg. Aggressive intervention is mandatory to reduce the blood pressure.

Congestive Heart Failure (CHF) (LO 6.4, and 6.5)

CHF occurs when the heart is unable to supply enough cardiac output to meet the body's metabolic needs, and the blood backs up to congest the lungs. The most common conditions leading to CHF are:

- Cardiac ischemia
- Severe hypertension
- Valvular regurgitation
- Aortic stenosis
- Cardiomyopathy

Congenital Heart Disease (CHD) (LO 6.4)

CHD is the result of an abnormal development of the heart in the fetus. Common **congenital** defects or abnormalities can usually be surgically repaired, and can include the following:

1. **Atrial septal defect (ASD)** is a hole in the interatrial septum *(Figure 6.15).*

2. **Ventricular septal defect (VSD)** is a gap in the interventricular septum *(Figure 6.15).*

3. **Patent ductus arteriosus (PDA)** arises from a failure of the ductus arteriosus (a normal blood vessel in the fetus) to close within 24 hours of birth.

4. **Coarctation of the aorta** is a narrowing of the aorta anywhere along its length. This causes **hypertension** in the arms behind the narrowing and **hypotension** in the lower limbs and organs (like the kidney) below the narrowing.

5. **Tetralogy of Fallot (TOF)** is a **syndrome** in which four congenital heart defects prevent enough blood from reaching the lungs. TOF occurs in about 5 out of every 10,000 newborns. Babies and children with TOF have episodes of cyanosis and are often called "blue babies." Treatment is with open heart surgery soon after birth or in infancy.

Right atrium
Blood flow
Left atrium
Atrial septal defect
Ventricular septal defect
Left ventricle
Interventricular septum
Right ventricle

▲ **FIGURE 6.15**
Atrial and Ventricular Septal Defects.

Word Analysis and Definition

WORD	PRONUNCIATION	ELEMENTS		DEFINITION
coarctation	koh-ark-**TAY**-shun	S/ R/	-ation *process* coarct- *press together, narrow*	Constriction, stenosis, particularly of the aorta
congenital	kon-**JEN**-ih-tal	S/ P/ R/	-al *pertaining to* con- *together, with* -genit- *bring forth*	Present at birth, either inherited or due to an event during gestation up to the moment of birth
cyanosis	sigh-ah-**NO**-sis	S/ R/	-osis *condition* cyan- *dark blue*	Blue discoloration of the skin, lips, and nail beds due to low blood oxygen
hypertension	**HIGH**-per-**TEN**-shun	S/ P/ R/	-ion *condition, action* hyper- *excessive* -tens- *pressure*	Persistent high arterial blood pressure
hypotension	**HIGH**-poh-**TEN**-shun	P/	hypo- *low*	Persistent low arterial blood pressure
idiopathic	**ID**-ih-oh-**PATH**-ik	S/ R/CF R/	-ic *pertaining to* idi/o- *unknown* -path- *disease*	Pertaining to a disease of unknown etiology
patent ductus arteriosus (PDA) (Note: *This term is composed only of roots.*)	**PAY**-tent **DUK**-tus ar-ter-ee-**OH**-sus		patent Latin *lie open* ductus Latin *leading* arteriosus Latin *artery*	An open, direct channel between the aorta and the pulmonary artery in the newborn
syndrome	**SIN**-drohm	P/ R/	syn- *together* -drome *running*	Combination of signs and symptoms associated with a particular disease process
tetralogy of Fallot (TOF)	te-**TRA**-loh-jee of fah-**LOW**	P/ R/	tetra- *four* -logy *study of* Etienne-Louis Fallot, French physician, 1850–1911	Set of four congenital heart defects occurring together

EXERCISES

A. Abbreviations *need to be used carefully so that you communicate exactly what is necessary. The following sentences contain abbreviations—translate the abbreviations into their correct medical terms. Rewrite the sentences without the abbreviations and convey the same message. Fill in the blanks.*
LO 6.2, 6.3, and 6.4 *Understand*

1. ASD, TOF, VSD, and PDA are all examples of CHD.

_____

_____

2. The patient's symptoms were HTN and DOB.

_____

_____

3. Aortic stenosis and cardiac ischemia are common conditions leading to CHF.

_____

_____

B. Language: *Answer the questions below.*   **LO 6.2, 6.4, and 6.8** *Understand*

1. Translate for your patient from medical to layman's language: "hypertension's etiology is idiopathic."

_____

2. What is the difference between primary and secondary hypertension?

_____

3. Which type of hypertension is life-threatening?

_____

4. Why is it considered life-threatening?

_____

Lesson 6.2 (cont'd)

▲ **FIGURE 6.16**
Holter monitor.

Cardiologic Investigations and Procedures
(LO 6.3, and 6.5)

Blood Tests (LO 6.2, 6.3, and 6.5)

A **lipid profile** helps determine the risk of CAD and comprises:

- Total cholesterol;
- High-density **lipoprotein (HDL)** ("good cholesterol");
- Low-density lipoprotein (**LDL**) ("bad cholesterol"); and
- **Triglycerides.**

Troponin I and **T** are part of a protein complex in muscle that is released into the blood during a muscle injury. Troponin I is found in heart muscle but not in skeletal muscle, which makes it a highly-sensitive indicator of a recent MI.

Diagnostic Tests (LO 6.3, and 6.5)

Several diagnostic tests are used to measure heart health.

An **electrocardiogram (ECG** or **EKG)** is a paper record of the electrical signals of your heart.

Cardiac stress testing is an exercise tolerance test that raises your heart rate through exercise (like jogging on a treadmill) and monitors its effect on cardiac function. **Nuclear imaging** of the heart, which involves the injection of a radioactive substance, can be used with the stress test.

Echocardiography uses ultrasound waves to study cardiac function.

Magnetic resonance imaging (MRI) can produce detailed images of the heart and identify sections of cardiac muscle that are not receiving an adequate blood supply.

Cardiac catheterization detects pressure and blood flow patterns in the heart. A thin tube is inserted into a vein or artery and is then threaded into the heart under X-ray guidance.

A **coronary angiogram** uses a contrast dye injected during cardiac catheterization to identify coronary artery blockages.

Treatment Procedures (LO 6.3, and 6.5)

The most immediate need in the treatment of MI is to get blood and oxygen to the affected myocardium. This can be attempted in several ways:

1. **Injection of clot-busting (thrombolytic) drugs:** These drugs are injected within 3½ hours of the MI to dissolve the **thrombus.**

2. **Artery-cleaning angioplasty (percutaneous transluminal coronary angioplasty, or PTCA):** A balloon-tipped **catheter** is guided to the blockage site and inflated. The inflated balloon expands the artery from the inside by compressing the plaque against the artery's walls.

3. **Stent placement:** To reduce the likelihood that the artery will close up again (occlude), a wire-mesh tube, or **stent,** is placed inside the vessel. **Drug-eluting** stents are covered with a special medication to help keep the artery open.

4. **Cardioversion** and **defibrillation** have been discussed earlier.

5. **Radiofrequency ablation** uses a catheter with an electrode in its tip that is guided into the heart to destroy cells from which abnormal cardiac rhythms are originating.

6. **Coronary artery bypass surgery (CABG):** Healthy blood vessels harvested from the leg, chest, or arm are used to bypass (detour) the blood around blocked coronary arteries.

7. **Heart transplant:** The heart of a recently deceased person (donor) is transplanted into the recipient after the recipient's diseased heart has been removed.

Abbreviations

CABG	coronary artery bypass graft
ECG or EKG	electrocardiogram
HDL	high-density lipoprotein
LDL	low-density lipoprotein
MI	myocardial infarction
MRI	magnetic resonance imaging
PTCA	percutaneous transluminal coronary angioplasty

Word Analysis and Definition

S = Suffix   P = Prefix   R = Root   R/CF = Combining Form

WORD	PRONUNCIATION	ELEMENTS		DEFINITION
ablation	ab-**LAY**-shun	S/ R/	-ion *process* ablat- *take away*	Removal of a tissue to destroy its function
angiogram	**AN**-jee-oh-gram	S/ R/CF	-gram *a record* angi/o- *blood vessel*	Radiograph obtained after injection of radiopaque contrast material into blood vessels
angiography	**AN**-jee-**OG**-rah-fee	S/	-graphy *process of recording*	Radiography of blood vessels after injection of contrast material
angioplasty	**AN**-jee-oh-**PLAS**-tee	S/ R/CF	-plasty *surgical repair* angi/o- *blood vessel*	Recanalization of a blood vessel by surgery
catheter	**KATH**-eh-ter		Greek *to send down*	Hollow tube to allow passage of fluid into or out of a body cavity, organ, or vessel
catheterize (verb)	**KATH**-eh-teh-**RIZE**	S/ R/	-ize *action* catheter- *catheter*	To introduce a catheter
catheterization (noun)	**KATH**-eh-ter-ih-**ZAY**-shun	S/	-ization *process of inserting*	Introduction of a catheter
echocardiography	**EK**-oh-kar-dee-**OG**-rah-fee	S/ R/CF R/CF	-graphy *process of recording* ech/o- *sound wave* -cardi/o- *heart*	Ultrasound recording of heart function
lipoprotein	**LIE**-poh-pro-teen	R/CF R/	lip/o- *fat* -protein *protein*	Bonding of molecules of fat and protein
percutaneous	**PER**-kyu-**TAY**-nee-us	S/ P/ R/	-ous *pertaining to* per- *through* -cutane- *skin*	Passage through the skin, in this case, by needle puncture
stent	STENT		Charles Stent, English dentist, 19th century	Wire-mesh tube used to keep arteries open
thrombus thrombi (pl) thrombolytic (adj) thrombolysis	**THROM**-bus **THROM**-bee throm-boh-**LIT**-ik throm-**BOH**-lih-sis	 S/ R/CF R/	Latin *clot* -lytic *pertaining to destruction* thromb/o- *blood clot* -lysis *dissolve*	A clot attached to a diseased blood vessel or heart lining Able to dissolve or break up a blood clot Dissolving of a thrombus (clot)
triglyceride	try-**GLISS**-eh-ride	S/ P/ R/	-ide *having a particular quality* tri- *three* -glycer- *sweet, glycerol*	Lipid containing three fatty acids

EXERCISES

A. Elements *are your best clue to understanding a medical term. Test yourself on the elements in column 1: Write the meaning of the element in its appropriate column. The first one is done for you.*   **LO 6.1, 6.2, and 6.4** *Apply*

Element	Meaning of Prefix	Meaning of Root/CF	Meaning of Suffix
per	through		
1. cardio			
2. cutane			
3. tri			
4. lipo			

B. Explain in your own words *each of the medical terms represented by these abbreviations.*   **LO 6.3 and 6.7** *Understand*

1. PTCA

P _____

T _____

C _____

A _____

2. CABG

C _____

A _____

B _____

G _____

Cardiac Pharmacology (LO 6.4 and 6.5)

Clinically, there are eight types of cardiac drugs in use:

1. **Anticoagulants** are drugs that reduce susceptibility to blood clot formation *see Chapter 7*. This can help prevent deep vein thrombosis (**DVT**), pulmonary embolism, myocardial infarction (**MI**), and stroke.

   Coumadin (warfarin, a rat poison) and heparin are anticoagulants in frequent use. Dabigatran (Pradaxa) and related drugs are newer anticoagulants. Aspirin prevents platelets from clumping together as part of clot formation and is used to help prevent heart or artery diseases and strokes.

2. **Chronotropic drugs** alter the heart rate. Positive chronotropic drugs such as epinephrine (adrenaline), norepinephrine, and atropine increase the heart rate. Negative chronotropic drugs, such as quinidine, procainamide, lidocaine, and propranalol, slow the heart.

3. **Inotropic drugs** can also be positive and negative. Positive inotropic drugs increase the force of the ventricular contraction to increase cardiac output when the function is impaired, as in congestive heart failure, cardiogenic shock, and cardiomyopathy. Digitalis and its derivatives, digoxin and digitoxin, are the most effective positive inotropic drugs.

   Negative inotropic drugs decrease the strength of the ventricular contraction and are used for treating hypertension, angina, and heart attacks. Beta blockers (beta-adrenergic-blocking agents) and calcium-channel blockers are examples of negative inotropic drugs.

4. **Antiarrhythmic drugs** change the electrical properties of the myocardial cells to restore a normal rate and rhythm to the heart beat. Beta blockers, which can reduce the strength and rate of myocardial contractions, are used in treating arrhythmias.

5. **Vasoconstrictor drugs** contract the smooth muscle in blood vessels, which increases both arterial and venous blood pressures—hence, they are also called **pressor drugs.** These drugs are used to help resuscitate seriously ill patients and for the treatment of hypotension in the **operating room (OR).**

6. **Vasodilator drugs** relax smooth muscle in arterioles, which leads to a drop in blood pressure. Therefore, they are used in treating hypertension, angina, and congestive heart failure. Organic nitrates dilate coronary arteries. An example is nitroglycerin, which can be given **sublingually** for rapid action lasting for 30 minutes or via transdermal patches, which last 12 hours. There are a number of types of vasodilators, including ACE inhibitors, angiotensin II receptor blockers, and calcium-channel blockers.

7. **Diuretics** indirectly affect the heart by stimulating urine production, thus reducing the fluid volume with which the heart has to cope. Examples include **Lasix** and **thiazides.**

8. **Lipid-regulating drugs** inhibit the progression of atherosclerosis by lowering "bad cholesterol," or low-density lipoprotein (**LDL**), and/or increasing "good cholesterol," or high-density lipoprotein (**HDL**). Statins also lower LDL but carry a risk of muscle damage. Fibrates and niacin lower triglycerides.

Abbreviations

ACE	angiotensin-converting enzyme
DVT	deep vein thrombosis
OR	operating room

Word Analysis and Definition

WORD	PRONUNCIATION	ELEMENTS		DEFINITION
antiarrhythmic	AN-tee-a-RITH-mik	S/ P/ R/	-ic *pertaining to* anti- *against* -rrhythm- *rhythm*	Pertaining to restoring a normal cardiac rhythm
anticoagulant	AN-tee-koh-AG-you-lant	S/ P/ R/	-ant *forming* anti- *against* -coagul- *clump*	Substance that prevents clotting
chronotropic	KRONE-oh-TROH-pic	S/ R/CF	-tropic *change* chron/o- *time*	Affecting the rate of rhythmic movements—in this case, the heart rate
diuretic	die-you-RET-ic	S/ P/ R/	-ic *pertaining to* di- *through* -uret- *urination*	Agent that increases urine output
inotropic	IN-oh-TROH-pic	S/ R/	-tropic *change* ino- *sinew*	Affecting the contractility of cardiac muscle
lipid	LIP-id		Greek *fat*	General term for fatty compounds
pressor	PRESS-or		Latin *to press*	Producing increased blood pressure
sublingual	sub-LING-wal	S/ P/ R/	-al *pertaining to* sub- *beneath* -lingu- *tongue*	Underneath the tongue
vasoconstrictor	VAY-so-con-STRIK-tor	S/ R/CF R/	-or *that which does something* vas/o *blood vessel* -constrict- *narrow*	Agent that reduces the diameter of a blood vessel
vasodilator	VAY-so-die-LAY-tor	R/	-dilat- *widen, open up*	Agent that increases the diameter of a blood vessel

EXERCISES

A. Deconstruct *the medical terms in this chart into their basic elements and give the meaning of the term. Fill in the blanks.*   **LO 6.1 and 6.5** *Analyze*

Medical Term	Prefix	Root, Root/CF	Suffix	Meaning
inotropic	1.	2.	3.	4.
diuretic	5.	6.	7.	8.
anticoagulant	9.	10.	11.	12.
sublingual	13.	14.	15.	16.
vasodilator	17.	18.	19.	20.

B. Choose *any two terms from the table in Exercise A above and use each in a sentence that is not a definition.*   **LO 6.2, 6.5, and 6.7** *Remember*

1. _____

   _____

2. _____

   _____

Lesson 6.3
Circulatory Systems

In order to understand the **etiologies** *and effects of Mrs. Jones' problems (see Case Report 6.3), and to clearly communicate with her and Dr. Bannerjee, you first need to have the medical terminology and knowledge to be able to:*

6.3.1 Specify the functions of the systemic and pulmonary circulations.

6.3.2 Identify the major **arteries** and **veins** in the body.

6.3.3 Explain the **hemodynamics** and control of blood flow.

6.3.4 Describe common disorders of the circulatory system.

Abbreviations

BP	blood pressure
CMA	certified medical assistant
H/O	history of
NKA	no known allergies
OA	osteoarthritis
P	pulse rate

Case Report 6.3

You are . . .

. . . a certified medical assistant **(CMA)** working for Dr. Lokesh Bannerjee, a cardiologist in Fulwood Medical Center.

You are communicating with . . .

. . . Mrs. Martha Jones. You are documenting her medical record after Dr. Bannerjee interviewed and examined her.

Fulwood Medical Center
Consultation Request and Report Form

Patient's Name: Jones, MARTHA   Age: 52
To: Dr. LOKESH BANNERJEE   Department: Cardiology
From: Dr. Susan Lee   Department: Primary Care
Patient's Location: FULWOOD MEDICAL CENTER
Type of Consultation Desired:
☐ Consultation Only
☐ Consulation and follow Jointly
☒ Accept in Transfer
Referring Diagnoses: CLAUDICATION, POSSIBLE DVT
Reason for Consultation: severe pain in both legs on walking

Signature: _____   Date: 2/21/09   Time 1105 hrs
Consultation Report: by Lokesh Bannerjee
Chief complaint: Pt. c/o severe pain in both legs on walking about 100 yards or climbing a flight of stairs. Pain is so severe she must stop and wait 5 mins. before she can go on. For the past two weeks she has noticed soreness and hardness along a vein in her left calf.
Past medical history: Known type 2 diabetic with hypertension, CAD, diabetic retinopathy, and OA of her hips and knees. Several episodes of ketoacidosis and one of pulmonary edema. Bariatric surgery performed 8 months prior at 275 lbs.
Medications: metformin, verapamil, propanolol, Mevacor
Allergies: NKA
Physical examination: Ht: 5'2"   Wt: 110 lbs.   BP: 170/100 sitting. P: 80, regular. Both feet show slight pitting edema and skin is pale, cold, and dry. Small ulcer on lateral margin of each big toe. Varicosities, both legs. Tender cord in superficial vein of left calf. Flexion of left foot produces pain in left calf. Chest clear. Heart sounds unremarkable. No loss of sensation in legs or feet.
Impression: 1. varicose veins, both legs.
             2. severe claudication, both legs.
             3. probable deep vein thrombosis, left leg
             4. possible peripheral neuropathy
             5. H/O diabetes type 2, CAD, hypertension, retinopathy, OA
Plan: Admit patient to cardiology unit stat for IV heparin and conversion to oral anticoagulant therapy with Coumadin. Doppler studies, venogram, and angiogram have been ordered.

Signature: _____   Date 2/21/09   Time 1250 hrs

ORDER # **267116** ANDRUS CLINI-REC ® PRIMARY CARE CHARTING SYSTEM • © BIBBERO SYSTEMS, INC. • PETALUMA, CA
TO REORDER CALL TOLL FREE: (800) BIBBERO (800-242-9330)   MFG IN U.S.A.

Word Analysis and Definition

WORD	PRONUNCIATION	ELEMENTS		DEFINITION
artery	AR-ter-ee		Greek *artery*	Thick-walled blood vessel carrying oxygenated blood away from the heart
claudication	klaw-dih-**KAY**-shun	S/	-ation *a process*	Intermittent leg pain and limping
		R/	claudic- *limping*	
Doppler	DOP-ler		Johann Doppler, Austrian mathematician and physician, 1803–1853	Diagnostic instrument that sends an ultrasonic beam into the body
hemodynamics	HE-mo-die-**NAM**-iks	S/	-ics *knowledge*	The science of the blood flow through the circulation
		R/CF	hem/o- *blood*	
		R/	-dynam- *power*	
varix	**VAIR**-iks		Latin *dilated vein*	Dilated, tortuous vein
varices (pl)	**VAIR**-ih-seez			
varicose (adj)	**VAIR**-ih-kose	S/	-ose *full of*	Characterized by or affected with varices
		R/	varic- *varicosity; dilated, tortuous vein*	
vein	VANE		Latin *vein*	Blood vessel carrying blood toward the heart
venous (adj)	VEE-nuss	S/	-ous *pertaining to*	Pertaining to a vein
		R/	ven- *vein*	
venogram	VEE-noh-gram	S/	-gram *recording*	Radiograph of veins after injection of radiopaque contrast material
		R/CF	ven/o- *vein*	

EXERCISES

A. **Review** *the Case Report on this spread before answering the questions.*   **LO 6.2, 6.6, and 6.7** *Understand*

1. What are Mrs. Jones' symptoms? _____

2. List here Mrs. Jones' other diseases/conditions. _____

3. Why did Mrs. Jones have bariatric surgery? _____

4. What's the purpose of anticoagulant therapy? _____

5. Of all the studies ordered for Mrs. Jones, which one uses ultrasound? _____

6. What is *pitting edema?* _____

7. What diagnosis in Mrs. Jones' past medical history relates to her episodes of ketoacidosis? _____

8. What does *peripheral* mean? _____

9. If Mrs. Jones had pulmonary edema, what organs would be involved? _____

10. Describe what a varicose vein might look like. _____

B. **Singulars and plurals,** *nouns and adjectives: Terms from the WAD can all be correctly inserted into the following paragraph of radiology documentation. Fill in the blanks.*   **LO 6.2, 6.6, and 6.7** *Apply*

veins   varicosities   varix   vein   varicose   varices   venogram   venous

1. The _____ performed on this patient's left saphenous and popliteal _____ shows the following: One slightly engorged and dilated _____ at the midpoint of the saphenous _____ and several _____ at the terminal end of the popliteal vein where _____ blood is pooling.

Diagnosis: _____ veins. These _____ need immediate attention by a vascular surgeon.

Lesson 6.3 (cont'd)

- All arteries of the systemic circulation arise either directly or indirectly from the aorta.
- Blood flows from arteries to veins through capillary beds.

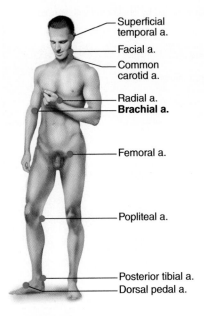

▲ **FIGURE 6.17**
Arterial Pulses—9 locations.
(a. = artery).

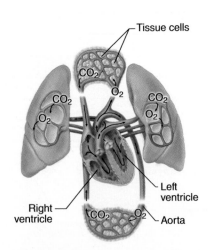

▲ **FIGURE 6.18**
Systemic and Pulmonary
Circulations.

Circulatory System
(LO 6.6)

The term **circulatory system** refers to your heart and blood vessels. It has two major divisions *(see Figure 6.18):*

1. The **pulmonary circulation,** which carries deoxygenated blood from the heart to the lungs, and returns oxygenated blood to the heart; and

2. The **systemic circulation,** which supplies oxygenated blood to every organ except the lungs, and then returns deoxygenated blood to the heart, which pumps it into the pulmonary circulation.

Functions of the Circulatory System (LO 6.6)

The circulatory system has the following three functions:

- **Transportation.** It carries oxygen, nutrients, hormones, and enzymes that **diffuse** from the blood into the cells. Waste products and carbon dioxide diffuse back from the cells into the system and are carried to the lungs, liver, and kidney for excretion.

- **Homeostasis maintenance.** The systemic circulation directs blood flow to the tissues to enable them to meet their metabolic needs.

- **Blood pressure regulation.** In the systemic circulation, the arteries' ability to expand and contract in coordination with the systole and diastole of the heartbeat maintains a steady flow of blood and blood pressure to the tissues.

Arterial Pulses (LO 6.6)

The pulse is always part of a clinical examination because it can provide information about heart rate, heart rhythm, and the state of the arterial wall by **palpation** *(Figure 6.17).* The most easily accessible artery is the radial artery at the wrist, where the pulse is usually taken.

Blood Pressure (BP) (LO 6.6)

Blood pressure is the force the blood exerts on arterial walls as it is pumped around the circulatory system by the left ventricle. The pressure is measured using a **sphygmomanometer** and a **stethoscope,** usually at the **brachial** artery *(Figure 6.17).*

Arterioles, Capillaries, and Venules (LO 6.6)

As the arteries branch farther away from the heart and distribute blood to specific organs, they become smaller, muscular vessels called **arterioles.** By contracting and relaxing, these arterioles are the primary controllers that help the body direct the amount of blood that the organs and structures receive.

From the arterioles, the blood flows into **capillaries** and **capillary beds** *(Figure 6.19).* Red blood cells flow in single file through the small capillaries.

From the capillaries, tiny **venules** accept the blood and merge to form veins. The veins form reservoirs for blood. At any moment, 60% to 70% of the total blood volume is contained in the venules and veins.

Systemic Venous Circulation (LO 6.6)

There are three major types of veins:

1. **Superficial,** such as those you can see under the skin of your arms and hands;

2. **Deep,** which run parallel to arteries and drain the same tissues that the arteries supply; and

3. **Venous sinuses,** which are in the head and heart and have specific functions.

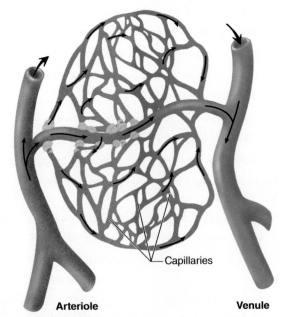

▲ **FIGURE 6.19**
Capillary Bed.

Word Analysis and Definition

WORD	PRONUNCIATION	ELEMENTS		DEFINITION
arteriole	ar-**TER**-ee-ole	S/ R/	-ole *small* arteri- *artery*	Small terminal artery leading into the capillary network
brachial	**BRAY**-kee-al	S/ R/	-al *pertaining to* brachi- *arm*	Pertaining to the arm
capillary capillaries	**KAP**-ih-lair-ee **KAP**-ih-lair-eez	S/ R/	-ary *pertaining to* capill- *hairlike structure*	Minute blood vessel between the arterial and venous systems
diffuse	di-**FUZE**		Latin *to pull in different directions*	To disseminate or spread out
homeostasis	hoh-mee-oh-**STAY**-sis	S/ R/CF	-stasis *stand still* home/o- *the same*	Maintaining the stability, or equilibrium, of a system or the body's internal environment
palpate (verb) palpation (noun)	**PAL**-pate pal-**PAY**-shun	S/ R/	Latin *touch, stroke* -ion *action, condition* palpat- *touch, stroke*	To examine with the fingers and hands Examination with the fingers and hands
sphygmomanometer	**SFIG**-moh-mah-**NOM**-ih-ter	S/ R/CF R/CF	-meter *instrument to measure* sphygm/o- *pulse* -man/o- *pressure*	Instrument for measuring arterial blood pressure
stethoscope	**STETH**-oh-skope	S/ R/CF	-scope *instrument to examine* steth/o- *chest*	Instrument for listening to respiratory and cardiac sounds
vena cava venae cavae (pl)	**VEE**-nah **KAY**-vah **VEE**-nee **KAY**-vee	R/CF R/	ven/a *vein* cava *cave*	One of the two largest veins in the body The two largest veins in the body (superior and inferior venae cavae)
venule	**VEN**-yule or **VEEN**-yule	S/ R/	-ule *small* ven- *vein*	Small vein leading from the capillary network

EXERCISES

A. Build *your knowledge of the elements and terms that make up the language of the cardiovascular system. All your answers can be found in the WAD. Fill in the blanks.*   **LO 6.1, 6.2, and 6.6** *Understand*

1. The two suffixes in the WAD that both mean *small* are _____ and _____.

2. List the three general terms in the WAD that are small *blood vessels:* _____, _____, and _____

3. Name two instruments found in an internal medicine practice: _____ and _____

4. State of equilibrium in the body is called _____.

5. The two largest veins in the body are the _____.

B. Construct *the correct medical term to match the definition.*   **LO 6.1, 6.2, and 6.6** *Apply*

1. minute blood vessel between the arterial and venous systems:

_____ / _____ / _____
  P   R/CF   S

2. instrument for listening to respiratory and cardiac sounds:

_____ / _____ / _____
  P   R/CF   S

3. pertaining to the arm:

_____ / _____ / _____
  P   R/CF   S

4. instrument for measuring arterial blood pressure:

_____ / _____ / _____
  P   R/CF   S

5. small terminal artery leading into the capillary network:

_____ / _____ / _____
  P   R/CF   S

Lesson 6.3 (cont'd)

Keynote

- All the disorders of the systemic arterial and venous systems are grouped under the term peripheral vascular disease (PVD).

Abbreviations

DVT deep vein thrombosis
PVD peripherial vascular disease

▲ **FIGURE 6.20**
Varicose Veins of the Leg.

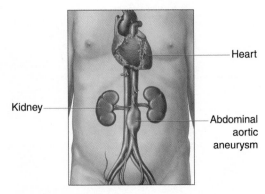

▲ **FIGURE 6.21**
Diagram of an Abdominal Aneurysm.

Case Report 6.3 (continued)

Mrs. Martha Jones, who had been referred to Dr. Bannerjee's cardiovascular clinic, has several circulatory problems related to her diabetes and obesity. She was diagnosed previously with hypertension, CAD, and diabetic retinopathy. She now has severe pain in her legs when walking. Doppler studies and angiograms showed significant blockage of blood flow due to arteriosclerosis of the large arteries in her legs. This blockage produces the pain when walking (intermittent claudication) and is part of her peripheral vascular disease **(PVD).**

The ulcers on the edges of her big toes are a result of thickening capillary walls and arterioles; this has led to poor circulation in her feet. Mrs. Jones' diabetes has caused these problems.

In addition, in her left leg's venous (vein) system, the tender cord-like lesion is due to **thrombophlebitis** of a superficial vein. A venogram showed a deep vein thrombosis **(DVT).**

Disorders of Veins (LO 6.2 and 6.6)

Our veins and arteries can be prone to certain disorders, like the DVT experienced by Mrs. Jones in the preceding case report.

Thrombophlebitis is an inflammation of the lining of a vein, allowing clots (thrombi) to form.

Deep vein thrombosis (DVT) is a thrombus formation in a deep vein. The increased pressure in the capillaries due to back pressure from the blocked blood flow in the veins creates a collection of fluid in the tissues called **edema.**

A major complication of thrombus (clot) formation is that a piece of the clot can break off **(embolus)** and be carried in the bloodstream to another organ where it can block blood flow. It often lodges in the lungs, causing a pulmonary embolus or mass *(see Chapter 8).*

Varicose veins are superficial veins that have lost their elasticity and appear swollen and tortuous *(Figure 6.20).* Their valves become incompetent, and blood flows backward and pools. Smaller, more superficial varicose veins are called spider veins. Treatments offered include laser technology and **sclerotherapy,** in which solutions that scar the veins are injected into them. **Collateral** circulations develop to take the blood through alternative routes.

A phlebotomist is a technician who draws blood (phlebotomy).

Disorders of Arteries (LO 6.2 and 6.6)

An **aneurysm** is a localized **dilation** of an artery, and this commonly occurs in the abdominal aorta *(Figure 6.21).* Aneurysms can **rupture,** leading to severe bleeding and hypovolemic shock. Surgical repair consists of excision of the aneurysm and replacement with a **synthetic** graft.

Intracranial aneurysms are an important cause of bleeds into the cranial cavity and brain tissue.

Thromboangiitis obliterans (Buerger disease) is an inflammatory disease of the arteries with clot formation, usually in the legs. The occlusion of arteries and impaired circulation lead to intermittent pain when walking, and a person will often limp to compensate.

Raynaud disease is episodes of spasm (following exposure to cold) of the small arteries supplying the fingers, hands, and feet. It can be associated with connective tissue disorders like scleroderma and lupus.

Carotid artery disease affects the carotid arteries—the two major arteries supplying the brain. They can be involved in arteriosclerosis and the deposition of plaque. This puts the patient at risk for a stroke. A carotid **endarterectomy** can be performed to surgically remove the plaque.

Labels for Figure 6.21: Heart, Kidney, Abdominal aortic aneurysm

Word Analysis and Definition

WORD	PRONUNCIATION		ELEMENTS	DEFINITION
aneurysm	**AN**-yur-izm		Greek *dilation*	Circumscribed dilation of an artery or cardiac chamber
collateral	koh-**LAT**-er-al	P/ R/	col- *with, together* -lateral *at the side*	Situated at the side, often to bypass an obstruction
dilation	die-**LAY**-shun	S/ R/	-ion *action, condition* dilat- *widen, dilate, open up*	Stretching or enlarging an opening
edema (noun) edematous (adj)	ee-**DEE**-mah ee-**DEM**-ah-tus	S/ R/	Greek *swelling* -tous *pertaining to* edema- *swelling*	Excessive accumulation of fluid in cells and tissues Pertaining to or affected by edema
endarterectomy	**END**-ar-ter-**EK**-toe-me	S/ P/ R/	-ectomy *surgical excision* end- *within* -arter- *artery*	Surgical removal of plaque from an artery
phlebitis	fleh-**BIE**-tis	S/ R/	-itis *inflammation* phleb- *vein*	Inflammation of a vein
rupture	**RUP**-tyur		Latin *break*	Break or tear of any organ or body part
sclerotherapy	**SKLEH**-roh-**THAIR**-ah-pee	S/ R/CF	-therapy *treatment* scler/o- *hardness*	Injection of a solution into a vein to thrombose it
sclerose (verb)	skleh-**ROSE**	S/ R/	-ose *full of* scler- *hardness*	To harden or thicken
sclerosis (noun)	skleh-**ROH**-sis	S/	-osis *condition*	Thickening or hardening of a tissue
synthetic	sin-**THET**-ik	S/ P/ R/	-ic *pertaining to* syn- *together* -thet- *arrange*	Built up or put together from simpler compounds
thromboembolism	**THROM**-boh-**EM**-boh-lizm	S/ R/CF R/	-ism *condition* thromb/o- *clot* -embol- *plug*	A piece of detached blood clot (embolus) blocking a distant blood vessel
thrombophlebitis	**THROM**-boh-fleh-BY-tis	S/ R/CF R/	-itis *inflammation* thromb/o- *clot* -phleb- *vein*	Inflammation of a vein with clot formation

EXERCISES

A. Review *the Case Report on this spread before answering the questions.*   **LO 6.2, 6.6, and 6.7** *Understand*

1. What diagnostic tests has Mrs. Jones had? _____

2. What other problems has the patient's diabetes caused? _____

3. Besides her diabetes what other complicating factor did Mrs. Jones have that contributed to her current problems? _____

4. Does Mrs. Jones have atherosclerosis or arteriosclerosis? _____

5. Define a *superficial* vein. _____

6. Define the difference between the two terms mentioned in question #4 above: _____

7. What skin problem(s) does Mrs. Jones have as a result of the poor blood circulation in her feet? _____

8. What is *thrombophlebitis?* _____

B. Analyze *the italicized terms and their elements to answer the following questions. Review the WAD and circle the correct term.*
   LO 6.1 and 6.6 *Analyze*

1. Its suffix tells you *thrombophlebitis* is:

    a clot   an inflammation   an excision

2. *Endarterectomy* means the plaque has been:

    incised   removed   repaired

3. The combining form *phleb/o* means:

    artery   vein   capillary

4. *Aneurysm* describes a blood vessel that is:

    dilated   constricted   collapsed

Chapter Review exercises, along with additional practice items, are available in Connect!

CHAPTER 7

The Blood, Lymphatic, and Immune Systems

The Essentials of the Languages of Hematology and Immunology

Learning Outcomes

In order to be able to communicate intelligently with Dr. Lee and to appropriately document Ms. Luisa Sosin's medical care, you first need to be familiar with the anatomy, physiology, and medical terminology of hematology. This chapter will provide you with information that enables you to:

LO 7.1 Use roots, combining forms, suffixes, and prefixes to construct and analyze (deconstruct) medical terms related to the blood, lymphatic, and immune systems.

LO 7.2 Spell and pronounce correctly medical terms and their plurals related to the blood, lymphatic, and immune systems in order to communicate them with accuracy and precision in any health care setting.

LO 7.3 Define accepted abbreviations related to the blood, lymphatic, and immune systems.

LO 7.4 Relate the functions of blood to its components.

LO 7.5 Relate the structure of red blood cells to their functions and disorders.

LO 7.6 Relate the structures of the major types of white blood cells to their functions and disorders.

LO 7.7 Explain hemostasis and its disorders.

LO 7.8 Identify the different ABO and Rh blood groups, their roles and effects.

LO 7.9 Describe the diagnostic laboratory studies, therapeutic procedures, and pharmacologic agents used in blood disorders.

LO 7.10 Relate the structure of the lymphatic system and its organs to its functions and disorders.

LO 7.11 Describe the structure and functions of the immune system, its disorders, and the roles, methods, and effects of immunization.

LO 7.12 Differentiate the major types of infection.

LO 7.13 Apply your knowledge of the medical terms of the blood, lymphatic, and immune systems to documentation, medical records, and medical reports.

LO 7.14 Translate the medical terms of the blood, lymphatic, and immune systems into everyday language in order to communicate clearly with patients and their families.

Case Report 7.1

You are . . .

. . . a medical assistant employed by Susan Lee, MD, a primary care physician at Fulwood Medical Center.

You are communicating with . . .

. . . Ms. Luisa Sosin, a 47-year-old woman who presented a week ago with fatigue, lethargy, and muscle weakness. A physical examination revealed paleness (pallor) of her skin, a pulse rate of 90, and a respiratory rate of 20. Dr. Lee referred her for extensive blood work. She also determined that Ms. Sosin had been taking aspirin and NSAIDs (nonsteroidal anti-inflammatory drugs) for the past 6 months for lower back pain. Ms. Sosin's laboratory reports show an **iron-deficiency anemia**. You are responsible for documenting her examination and care.

The health professionals involved in the diagnosis and treatment of problems with the blood, lymphatic, and immune systems include the following:

- **Hematologists** are physicians who specialize in the diagnosis, treatment, and prevention of blood and bone marrow diseases.
- **Immunologists** and **allergists** are physicians who specialize in immune system disorders, such as allergies, asthma, and immunodeficiency and autoimmune diseases.
- **Epidemiologists** are medical scientists involved in the study of epidemic diseases and how they are transmitted and controlled.
- **Medical** or **clinical laboratory technicians** perform routine testing procedures on body fluids, blood, and other tissues using microscopes, computers, and other laboratory equipment.
- **Immunology technicians** are certified laboratory technicians with a special interest in immunology who generally work alongside medical researchers.
- **Transfusion technicians** are certified technicians who deal with all phases of blood transfusions.
- **Phlebotomists** assist physicians by drawing patient blood samples for laboratory testing.

Objectives

The average-sized adult carries about 5 liters (10 pints) of blood in the body at all times. The information in this lesson relates to the composition, functions, and uses of blood, and enables you to use correct medical terminology to:

7.1.1 Identify the components of blood.

7.1.2 Describe plasma and its functions.

7.1.3 Explain the functions of blood.

Keynote

- Serum is identical to plasma except for the absence of clotting proteins.

Abbreviations

Hct   hematocrit
RBC   red blood cell
WBC   white blood cell

Lesson 7.1

Components and Functions of Blood

Components of Blood

(LO 7.3 and 7.4)

The study of the blood and its disorders—the red and white blood cells within the blood, their proportions, and overall cell health—is called **hematology.** A **hematologist** is a medical specialist who is trained in this area.

Blood is a type of connective tissue that consists of cells contained in a liquid **matrix.** If a blood specimen is collected in a tube and centrifuged, the cells of the blood separate out and fill the bottom 45% of the tube *(see Figure 7.1).* Ninety-nine percent of these cells are red blood cells **(RBCs);** white blood cells **(WBCs)** and **platelets** make up the remainder of this sample. The **hematocrit (Hct)** is the percentage of total blood volume composed of red blood cells.

Plasma—a clear, yellowish liquid that is 91% water—makes up the remaining 55% of the blood sample in the tube. Plasma is a **colloid,** a liquid that contains floating particles, most of which are plasma proteins. **Nutrients,** waste products, hormones, and enzymes are dissolved in plasma for transportation. When blood clots, and the solid clot is removed, **serum** remains. Serum is a clear, yellowish fluid that contains all the blood proteins not used in clotting and all the electrolytes, antibodies, antigens, and hormones that are carried in blood.

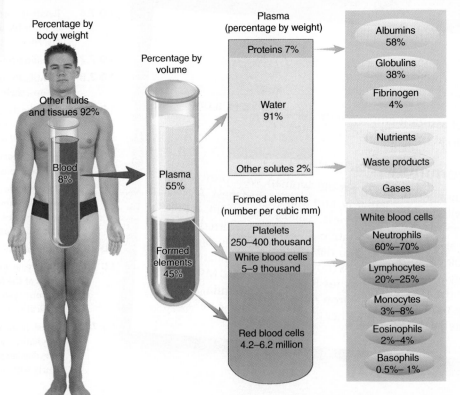

▶ **FIGURE 7.1**
Components of Blood.

S = Suffix   P = Prefix   R = Root   R/CF = Combining Form

WORD	PRONUNCIATION	ELEMENTS		DEFINITION
allergist	AL-er-jist	S/ R/ R/	-ist *specialist* all- *other, strange* -erg- *work*	Specialist in hypersensitivity reactions
anemia	ah-NEE-me-ah	P/ S/	an- *without* -emia *a blood condition*	Decreased number of red blood cells
anemic (adj)	ah-NEE-mik	S/	-emic *pertaining to a condition of the blood*	Pertaining to or suffering from anemia
colloid	COLL-oyd	S/ R/	-oid *resembling* coll- *glue*	Liquid containing suspended particles
hematocrit (Hct)	he-MAT-oh-krit	S/ R/CF	-crit *to separate* hemat/o- *blood*	Percentage of red blood cells in the blood
hematology	he-mah-TOL-oh-jee	S/ R/CF	-logy *study of* hemat/o- *blood*	Medical specialty of the blood and its disorders
hematologist	he-mah-TOL-oh-jist	S/	-logist *one who studies, specialist*	Specialist in hematology
matrix	MAY-triks		Latin mater *mother*	Substance that surrounds and protects cells, is manufactured by the cells, and holds cells together
nutrient	NYU-tree-ent		Latin *to nourish*	Constituent of food necessary for the body to function normally
nutrition	nyu-TRISH-un	S/ R/	-ion *action, condition* nutrit- *nourishment*	The study of food and liquid requirements for normal function of the human body
nutritionist	nyu-TRISH-un-ist	S/	-ist *specialist*	A person who specializes in the study of food and liquid requirements for normal function of the human body
plasma	PLAZ-mah		Greek *something formed*	Fluid, noncellular component of blood
platelet (*Also called* thrombocyte.)	PLAYT-let	S/ R/	-let *little, small* plate- *flat*	Small particle involved in the clotting process
serum	SEER-um		Latin *whey*	Fluid remaining after removal of blood cells and the formation of a clot
vitamin (**Note:** *The duplicate letter "a" is omitted. It was originally thought that all vitamins were amines.*)	VYE-tah-min	S/ R/	-amin(e) *nitrogen-containing substance* vita- *life*	Essential organic substance necessary in small amounts for normal cell function

EXERCISE

A. Review *Case Report 7.1 before answering the questions.*   **LO 7.2, 7.3, and 7.5** *Understand*

1. What are Ms. Sosin's symptoms? _____

2. What additional testing did Dr. Lee order? _____

3. What is the medical term for *paleness?* _____

4. The abbreviation NSAIDs means _____

5. What diagnosis is confirmed with Ms. Sosin's lab results? _____

B. Match *the definition in column 1 with the correct medical term in column 2. Fill in the blanks.*   **LO 7.4, and 7.5** *Understand*

_____ **1.** decreased number of RBCs	**A.** platelet
_____ **2.** study of blood disorders	**B.** plasma
_____ **3.** fluid remaining after removal of clot	**C.** anemia
_____ **4.** fluid noncellular component of blood	**D.** hematology
_____ **5.** also called a thrombocyte	**E.** serum

Lesson 7.1 (cont'd)

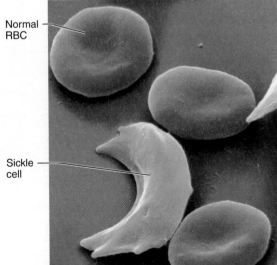

(a)

(b)

▲ **FIGURE 7.2**
Red Blood Cells.
(a) Top view. (b) Side view.

▶ **FIGURE 7.3**
Sickle Cell Disease

Functions of Blood (LO 7.4)

Your blood travels throughout your body while performing a number of important functions. Your blood:

1. **Maintains your body's homeostasis** (*see Chapter 2*).

2. **Transports nutrients, vitamins, and minerals** from your digestive system and storage areas to your organs and cells. Examples of nutrients are glucose and amino acids (*see Chapter 9*).

3. **Transports waste products** from your cells and tissues to your liver and kidney for excretion. These waste products include creatinine, urea, bilirubin, and lactic acid.

4. **Transports hormones,** like insulin and thyroxine (*see Chapter 12*), from your endocrine glands to target cells.

5. **Transports gases,** like oxygen and carbon dioxide (*see Chapter 8*), to and from your lungs and cells.

6. **Protects against foreign substances, including microorganisms and toxins.** Cells and chemicals in your blood are an important part of your immune system's protective properties.

7. **Forms clots.** Clots provide protection against blood loss. Clotting is the first step in tissue repair and restoration of normal function.

Structure, Functions, and Disorders of Red Blood Cells (Erythrocytes) (LO 7.5)

Structure of RBCs (Erythrocytes) (LO 7.5)

Each RBC is a disk with edges that are thicker than and raised above the flattened center (*Figure 7.2*). This biconcave surface area enables a more rapid flow of gases into and out of the disk.

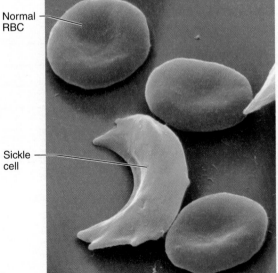

Normal RBC

Sickle cell

The main component of RBCs is **hemoglobin (Hb)**, which gives the cells and blood their red color. Hb is composed of the iron-containing pigment **heme** bound to a protein called **globin.** The rest of the red blood cell consists of the cell membrane, water, electrolytes, and enzymes. Mature RBCs do not have a nucleus.

Functions of RBCs (Erythrocytes) (LO 7.3 and 7.5)

The functions of the RBCs are to:

1. **Transport oxygen (O_2),** in combination with hemoglobin, throughout the body, from the lungs to the cells;

2. **Transport carbon dioxide (CO_2)** from the tissue cells to the lungs for excretion; and

3. **Transport nitric oxide (NO),** a gas produced by the lining cells of blood vessels that signals smooth muscle to relax, throughout the body.

Disorders of Red Blood Cells (LO 7.3 and 7.5)

Anemia is a red blood cell condition where the number of RBCs or amount of hemoglobin contained in each RBC is reduced. Both of these conditions reduce the blood's oxygen-carrying capacity, producing shortness of breath **(SOB)** and fatigue.

The different types of anemia include:

- **Iron-deficiency anemia** is the diagnosis for Ms. Sosin (*Case Report 7.1* on page 137). The cause was chronic bleeding from her gastrointestinal tract due to the aspirin and other painkillers she was taking. Her stools were positive for **occult blood.** Other causes of iron-deficiency anemia can be heavy menstrual bleeds or a diet deficient in iron.

- **Pernicious anemia (PA)** is due to vitamin B_{12} deficiency. It is caused by a shortage of intrinsic factor, which is normally secreted by cells in the stomach lining (*see Chapter 9*) and binds with B_{12}. This complex is absorbed into the bloodstream. Without B_{12}, hemoglobin cannot form. The number of red cells decreases, hemoglobin concentration decreases, and the size of the red cells increases.

- **Sickle cell anemia** is a genetic disorder found most commonly in African Americans. Here, the production of abnormal hemoglobin causes the RBCs to form a rigid sickle shape (*Figure 7.3*). The abnormal cells **agglutinate** (clump together) and block small capillaries. This creates intense pain in the **hypoxic** tissues (a sickle cell crisis) and can lead to stroke, kidney failure, and heart failure. **Sickle cell trait** is a minor form of this disease and rarely has any symptoms.

Word Analysis and Definition

WORD	PRONUNCIATION		ELEMENTS	DEFINITION
agglutinate (verb)	ah-**GLUE**-tin-ate	S/ P/ R/	-ate *composed of, pertaining to* ag- (ad-) *to* -glutin- *stick*	Stick together to form clumps
erythrocyte	eh-**RITH**-roh-site	S/ R/CF	-cyte *cell* erythr/o- *red*	Red blood cell (RBC)
heme	**HEEM**		Greek *blood*	The iron-based component of hemoglobin that carries oxygen
hemoglobin oxyhemoglobin hemoglobinopathy	HE-moh-**GLOW**-bin OCK-see-he-moh-**GLOW**-bin HE-moh-**GLOW**-bin-**OP**-ah-thee	R/CF R/ R/ S/ R/CF R/CF	hem/o- *blood* -globin *protein* oxy- *oxygen* -pathy *disease* hem/o- *blood* -globin/o- *protein*	Red-pigmented protein that is the main component of red blood cells Combination of hemoglobin and oxygen Disease caused by the presence of an abnormal hemoglobin in red blood cells
hypoxia (Note: *The duplicate letter "o" is omitted.*) hypoxic (adj)	high-**POCK**-see-ah high-**POCK**-sik	S/ P/ R/ S/	-ia *condition* hypo- *below, deficient* -ox- *oxygen* -ic *pertaining to*	Below-normal levels of oxygen in tissues, gases, or blood Deficient in oxygen
occult blood	oh-**KULT BLUD**		occult Latin *to hide*	Blood that cannot be seen in the stool but is positive on a fecal occult blood test
pallor	**PAL**-or		Latin *paleness*	Paleness of the skin
pernicious anemia	per-**NISH**-us ah-**NEE**-me-ah	S/ P/ R/ P/ R/	-ous *pertaining to* per- *through* -nici- *lethal* an- *without* -emia *a blood condition*	Chronic anemia due to lack of vitamin B$_{12}$
polycythemia	POL-ee-sigh-**THEE**-me-ah	P/ R/ R/	poly- *many, much* -cyth- *cell* -emia *blood condition*	A disease of bone marrow, excess production of RBCs
trait	**TRAYT**		Latin *an extension*	A discrete characteristic that has a known quality

EXERCISES

A. Review *the Case Report on page 140 before answering the questions.*   **LO 7.5 and 7.13** *Understand*

1. What caused Ms. Sosin's condition? _____

2. What diagnostic test was positive for the patient? _____

3. Name two other causes for the condition Ms. Sosin has. _____ and _____

B. Fill *in the correct disorder that matches the description.*   **LO 7.2, 7.3, and 7.5** *Apply*

1. numbers of RBCs reduced   _____

2. bone marrow cannot produce sufficient new cells of all types   _____

3. genetic disorder found most commonly in African Americans   _____

4. caused by excessive destruction of normal and abnormal RBCs   _____

5. disorder caused by vitamin B$_{12}$ deficiency   _____

Lesson 7.1 (cont'd)

Keynote

- Leukocytosis is too many white blood cells and often indicates the presence of an infection.

▲ **FIGURE 7.4**
Neutrophils Are Granulocytes.

▲ **FIGURE 7.5**
Eosinophils Are Granulocytes.

▲ **FIGURE 7.6**
Basophils Are Granulocytes.

Abbreviations

DIFF	differential white blood cell count
Ig	immunoglobulin
PMNL	polymorphonuclear leukocyte

Disorders of Red Blood Cells (continued)

- **Hemolytic anemia** is caused by excessive destruction of normal and abnormal RBCs. **Hemolysis** (the destruction of RBCs) can result from toxic substances, such as snake and spider venoms, mushroom toxins, and overdoses of drugs, entering the bloodstream. Trauma to RBCs by hemodialysis or heart-lung machines, or an incompatible blood transfusion, can also cause hemolysis.
- **Aplastic anemia** is a condition in which the bone marrow is unable to produce sufficient new cells of all types—red cells, white cells, and platelets. It can be associated with exposure to radiation, benzene, and certain drugs.
- **Polycythemia** is an overproduction of RBCs by the bone marrow due to unknown causes.

Types and Functions of White Blood Cells (Leukocytes) (LO 7.3 and 7.6)

The types of white blood cells (**WBCs**) can be categorized as **granulocytes** or **agranulocytes.** Granulocytes contain a granular cytoplasm, made up of granules, which are sites for enzyme and chemical production. Agranulocytes do not contain cytoplasmic granules.

Granulocytes (LO 7.3 and 7.6)

1. **Neutrophils** (*Figure 7.4*), also called **polymorphonuclear leukocytes (PMNLs),** are normally 55% to 65% of the total WBC count. These cells ingest bacteria, fungi, and some viruses. In **neutropenia,** the number of neutrophils is decreased. In **neutrophilia,** the number is increased.
2. **Eosinophils** (*Figure 7.5*) are normally 2% to 4% of the total WBC count. They leave the bloodstream to enter tissue that is undergoing an allergic response. In allergic reactions, the number and percentage of eosinophils increase.

▲ **FIGURE 7.7**
Monocytes Are Agranulocytes.

3. **Basophils** (*Figure 7.6*) are normally less than 1% of the total WBC count. Basophils migrate to damaged tissues to release histamine (which increases blood flow) and heparin (which prevents blood clotting).

Agranulocytes (LO 7.3 and 7.6)

4. **Monocytes** (*Figure 7.7*) are the largest blood cells and are normally 3% to 8% of the total WBC count. Monocytes leave the bloodstream and become **macrophages** that ingest bacteria, dead neutrophils, and dead cells in the tissues.
5. **Lymphocytes** (*Figure 7.8*) are the smallest white blood cells and comprise 25% to 35% of the total WBC count. Lymphocytes are produced in red bone marrow and migrate through the bloodstream to lymphatic tissues—lymph nodes, tonsils, spleen, and thymus—where they multiply.
   There are two main types of lymphocytes:

   a. **B cells** differentiate into plasma cells, which are stimulated by bacteria or toxins to produce antibodies or immunoglobulins (**Ig**) (*Chapter 7*).

   b. **T cells** attach directly to foreign antigen-bearing cells like bacteria, which they kill with toxins they secrete.

In a laboratory report, a **differential white blood cell count (DIFF)** lists the percentages of the different leukocytes in a blood sample.

Disorders of White Blood Cells (LO 7.3 and 7.6)

A normal cubic millimeter (mm^3) of blood contains 5,000 to 10,000 white blood cells. In **leukocytosis,** the total WBC count exceeds 10,000 per cubic millimeter. Other conditions that increase the WBC count beyond the normal range include:

- Allergic reactions, which increase the number of eosinophils;
- Typhoid fever, malaria, and tuberculosis, which increase the number of monocytes; and
- Whooping cough and infectious mononucleosis, which increase the number of lymphocytes.

▲ **FIGURE 7.8**
Lymphocytes Are Agranulocytes.

Word Analysis and Definition

WORD	PRONUNCIATION	ELEMENTS		DEFINITION
agranulocyte	a-GRAN-you-loh-site	S/ P/ R/CF	-cyte *cell* a- *without, not* -granul/o- *granule*	A white blood cell without any granules in its cytoplasm
aplastic anemia	a-PLAS-tik ah-NEE-me-ah	S/ P/ R/ P/ R/	-tic *pertaining to* a- *without* -plas- *formation* an- *without* -suffix *a blood condition*	Condition in which the bone marrow is unable to produce sufficient red cells, white cells, and platelets
basophil	BAY-so-fill	S/ R/CF	-phil *attraction* bas/o- *base*	A basophil's granules attract a basic blue stain in the laboratory
eosinophil	ee-oh-SIN-oh-fill	S/ R/CF	-phil *attraction* eosin/o- *dawn*	An eosinophil's granules attract a rosy-red color on staining
granulocyte	GRAN-you-loh-site	S/ R/CF	-cyte *cell* granul/o- *small grain*	A white blood cell that contains multiple small granules in its cytoplasm
leukocyte leucocyte (syn) (Note: *Either spelling is acceptable.*)	LOO-koh-site	S/ R/CF	-cyte *cell* leuk/o- *white*	Another term for a white blood cell
leukocytosis	LOO-koh-sigh-TOE-sis	S/	-osis *condition*	An excessive number of white blood cells
lymphocyte	LIM-foh-site	R/ R/CF	-cyte *cell* lymph/o- *lymph*	Small white blood cell with a large nucleus
hemolysis hemolytic (adj)	he-MOL-ih-sis he-moh-LIT-ik	S/ R/CF S/ R/	-lysis *destruction* hem/o- *blood* -ic *pertaining to* -lyt- *destroy*	Destruction of red blood cells so that hemoglobin is liberated Pertaining to the destruction of red blood cells
monocyte	MON-oh-site	S/ P/	-cyte *cell* mono- *single*	Large white blood cell with a single nucleus
mononucleosis	MON-oh-nyu-klee-OH-sis	S/ P/ R/	-osis *condition* mono- *single* -nucle- *nucleus*	Presence of large numbers of specific, diagnostic mono-nuclear leukocytes
neutrophil neutropenia neutrophilia	NEW-troh-fill NEW-troh-PEE-nee-ah NEW-troh-FILL-ee-ah	S/ R/CF S/ S/	-phil *attraction* neutr/o- *neutral* -penia *deficiency* -philia *attraction*	Neutrophils' granules take up purple stain equally, whether the stain is acid or alkaline A deficiency of neutrophils An increase in neutrophils
polymorphonuclear	POL-ee-more-foh-NEW-klee-ar	S/ P/ R/CF R/	-ar *pertaining to* poly- *many* -morph/o- *shape* -nucle- *nucleus*	White blood cell with a multilobed nucleus

EXERCISES

A. A suffix *completes a medical term. The element* leuk *or* leuk/o *remains the same in each term below. Review the WAD before you start the exercise.*

Fill in the blanks.   **LO 7.1 and 7.6** *Apply*

penia   **cyte**   **cytosis**   **emia**

1. An excessive number of white blood cells is: _____

2. The disease when the blood is taken over by the WBCs is: _____

3. Another term for a white blood cell is: _____

4. A deficient number of white blood cells is: _____

5. What is the difference between leuco and leuko? _____

B. Fill *in the blanks.*   **LO 7.1, 7.2, 7.4, 7.5, and 7.6** *Remember*

1. Write a medical term with the element that means "deficiency." _____ / _____ / _____

2. Which disorder causes a deficiency of all types of blood cells? _____

3. Where in the body are blood cells produced? _____

4. Name one function of blood. _____

5. What disease is a cancer of the blood-forming tissues? _____

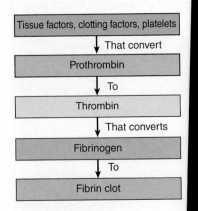

▲ FIGURE 7.9
Blood Coagulation.

Disorders of White Blood Cells (continued)

Infectious mononucleosis occurs in the 15- to 25-year-old population. Its cause—the **Epstein-Barr virus (EBV)**—is a very common virus and a member of the herpes family. The EBV is transmitted by an exchange of saliva, such as a kiss.

Leukemia is cancer of the blood-forming tissues and produces a high number of leukocytes and their precursors. The **leukemic** cells multiply, taking over the bone marrow and causing a deficiency of normal red blood cells, white blood cells, and platelets. This makes the patient anemic and vulnerable to infection and bleeding.

In **leukopenia**, the WBC count drops below 5,000 cells per cubic millimeter of blood. Leukopenia is seen in viral infections like measles, mumps, chickenpox, poliomyelitis, and AIDS.

In **pancytopenia**, the erythrocytes (red blood cells), leukocytes (white blood cells), and thrombocytes (platelets) in the circulating blood are all noticeably reduced. This can occur with cancer chemotherapy.

Hemostasis (LO 7.3 and 7.7)

Hemostasis, the control of bleeding, is a vital issue in maintaining **homeostasis,** the state of the body's equilibrium. Uncontrolled bleeding can offset the body's balance by decreasing blood volume and lowering blood pressure.

Platelets (also called **thrombocytes**) play a key role in hemostasis. They are minute fragments of large bone marrow cells and consist of a small amount of granular cytoplasm surrounded by a plasma membrane. They have no nucleus.

Hemostasis is achieved through a three-step process:

1. **Vascular spasm,** an immediate but temporary constriction of the injured blood vessels.
2. **Platelet plug formation,** an accumulation of platelets that bind themselves together and adhere to surrounding tissues. The binding and adhesion of platelets are mediated through **von Willebrand factor (vWF),** a protein produced by the cells lining the blood vessels.
3. **Blood coagulation** is the process of going through **prothrombin** and **thrombin** to the formation of a blood clot that traps blood cells, platelets, and tissue fluid in a network of **fibrin** (*Figure 7.9*).

After a blood clot forms, platelets adhere to strands of fibrin and contract to pull the fibers and the edges of the broken blood vessel together. **Fibroblasts** invade the clot to produce a fibrous connective tissue that seals the blood vessel.

Disorders of Coagulation (Coagulopathies) (LO 7.3 and 7.7)

There are several disorders that can prevent the blood from clotting properly, and these can lead to further health problems.

- **Hemophilia,** in its classical form (hemophilia A), is a disease males inherit from their mothers. It results from a deficiency of the coagulation factor named **factor VIII.**

- **Von Willebrand disease (vWD)**—the most common hereditary bleeding disorder—is a protein deficiency of the factor VIII complex (**vWF**) that is different from the factor deficiency involved in hemophilia.

Abbreviations

DIC	disseminated intravascular coagulation
EBV	Epstein-Barr virus
ITP	idiopathic thrombocytopenic purpura
vWD	von Willebrand disease
vWF	von Willebrand factor

WORD	PRONUNCIATION	ELEMENTS		DEFINITION
coagulant	koh-**AG**-you-lant	S/ R/	-ant *forming, pertaining to* coagul- *clot, clump*	Substance that causes clotting
coagulation anticoagulant	koh-ag-you-**LAY**-shun **AN**-tee-koh-**AG**-you-lant	S/ P/	-ation *process* anti- *against*	Process of blood clotting Substance that prevents clotting
fibrin	**FIE**-brin		Latin *fiber*	Stringy protein fiber that is a component of a blood clot
fibroblast	**FIE**-broh-blast	S/ R/CF	-blast *immature cell* fibr/o- *fiber*	Cell that forms collagen fibers
hematoma (*also called* bruise)	he-mah-**TOE**-mah	S/ R/	-oma *mass, tumor* hemat- *blood*	Collection of blood that has escaped from vessels into surrounding tissues
hemophilia	he-moh-**FILL**-ee-ah	S/ R/CF	-philia *attraction* hem/o- *blood*	An inherited disease from a deficiency of clotting factor VIII
hemostasis (**Note:** *Homeostasis has a very different meaning.*)	he-moh-**STAY**-sis	S/ R/CF	-stasis *control, stop* hem/o- *blood*	Control of or stopping bleeding
leukemia	loo-**KEE**-mee-ah	S/ R/	-emia *a blood condition* leuk- *white*	Disease when the blood is taken over by white blood cells and their precursors
leukemic (adj)	loo-**KEE**-mik	S/	-emic *pertaining to a blood condition*	Pertaining to or affected by leukemia
leukopenia	loo-koh-**PEE**-nee-ah	S/	-penia *deficiency*	A deficient number of white blood cells
pancytopenia	**PAN**-site-oh-**PEE**-nee-ah	S/ P/ R/CF	-penia *deficiency* pan- *all* -cyt/o- *cell*	Deficiency of all types of blood cells
prothrombin	pro-**THROM**-bin	S/ P/ R/	-in *substance* pro- *before* -thromb- *blood clot*	Protein formed by the liver and converted to thrombin in the blood-clotting mechanism
thrombocyte (*also called* platelet)	**THROM**-boh-site	S/ R/CF	-cyte *cell* thromb/o- *blood clot*	Another name for a platelet
thrombocytopenia	**THROM**-boh-site-oh-**PEE**-nee-uh	S/ R/CF	-penia *deficiency* -cyt/o- *cell*	Deficiency of platelets in circulating blood
von Willebrand	VON **WILL**-eh-brand		E.A. von Willebrand, Finnish physician, 1870–1949	

EXERCISES

A. Review *the Case Report on this spread before answering the questions.*   **LO 7.7, 7.13, and 7.14** *Understand*

1. Why is Janis Tierney in the Emergency Department at Fulwood Medical Center?

_____

2. What is causing her blood-related issues? _____

3. What are her symptoms? _____

4. What blood-related issues does she have in her past medical history? _____

5. Translate into medical language: "her blood clotting cells are unable to stick together"

_____

B. Review *the two pages open in front of you to determine the answers to the following questions. Circle the best choice.*   **LO 7.1 and 7.7** *Understand*

1. In the term *hemostasis,* the suffix means:

blood   condition   control

2. Which term relates to a color?

hemophilia   petechia   purpura

3. The process of blood clotting is called:

homeostasis   coagulation   thrombocytopenia

4. A piece of thrombus that has broken off into the circulation is called:

an embolus   a fibroblast   a coagulant

Keynote

• All blood groups are inherited.

Abbreviations

Ab	antibody
ABO	blood group system
Rh	Rhesus

Case Report 7.3

You are . . .

. . . an emergency medical technician–paramedic (EMT-P) working in the Level One Trauma Unit at Fulwood Medical Center.

You are communicating with . . .

. . . Ms. Joanne Rodi, an 18-year-old student, who has been admitted to the unit from the operating room. Ms. Rodi has had surgery for multiple fractures sustained in a car accident. She is receiving a blood **transfusion**. You document that her temperature has risen to 102.8°F, her respirations have risen to 24 per minute, and she has chills. You take her blood pressure, and it has fallen to 90/60. What is your next step?

(a)

(b)

▲ **FIGURE 7.10**
Subsurface Bleeding.
(a) Purpura. (b) Petechiae.

Disorders of Coagulation (Coagulopathies) *(continued)*

• **Disseminated intravascular coagulation (DIC)** occurs when a severe bacterial infection activates the clotting mechanism simultaneously throughout the cardiovascular system. Small clots form and obstruct blood flow into tissues and organs, particularly the kidney, leading to renal failure.

• **Thrombus** formation **(thrombosis)** is a clot that forms attached to a diseased or damaged area on the walls of blood vessels or the heart. If part of the thrombus breaks loose and moves through the circulation, it is called an **embolus.**

• **Thrombocytopenia** is a deficiency of platelets.

• **Purpura** is bleeding into the skin from small arterioles that produces a larger individual lesion than the tiny red spots or **petechiae** from capillary bleeds *(Figure 7.10a and b).* **Bruises** (or **hematomas**) are leaks of blood from all types of blood vessels.

• **Idiopathic thrombocytic purpura (ITP)** occurs when the immune system destroys the body's platelets. An acute, self-limiting form of the disease occurs in children; a chronic form affects adults.

Blood Groups and Transfusions (LO 7.3 and 7.8)

Red Cell Antigens (LO 7.3 and 7.8)

Antigens are molecules that exist on the surfaces of red blood cells. **Antibodies** are present in the plasma. Each antibody can combine with only a specific antigen. If the plasma antibodies combine with another red cell antigen, bridges form to connect these red cells together. This is called **agglutination,** or clumping, of the cells. Hemolysis (destruction) of the cells also occurs.

The antigens on the surfaces of the cells have been categorized into groups. Two of these groups—the **ABO** and **Rh** blood groups—are the most important.

Case Report 7.3 *(continued)*

In Joanne Rodi's case, she has type A blood and by mistake received type AB blood, the red cells of which agglutinated in the presence of her anti-B antibodies. Your immediate response is to stop the transfusion, replace it with a saline **infusion**, call your supervisor, and notify the doctor.

Word Analysis and Definition

S = Suffix   P = Prefix   R = Root   R/CF = Combining Form

WORD	PRONUNCIATION	ELEMENTS		DEFINITION
agglutination (noun)	ah-glue-tih-**NAY**-shun	S/ P/ R/	-ation *process* ag- *to (same as ad-)* -glutin- *glue*	Process by which cells or other particles adhere to each other to form clumps
antibody antibodies (pl)	AN-tee-body	P/ R/	anti- *against* -body *substance, body*	Protein produced in response to an antigen
antigen	AN-tee-gen	P/ R/	anti- *against* -gen *produce, create*	Substance capable of triggering an immune response
autologous	awe-**TOL**-oh-gus	P/ R/	auto- *self, same* -logous *relation*	Blood transfusion with the same person as donor and recipient—self-transfusion
embolus	**EM**-boh-lus		Greek *plug, stopper*	Detached piece of thrombus, a mass of bacteria, quantity of air, or foreign body that blocks a blood vessel
infusion	in-**FYU**-zhun	P/ R/	in- *in* -fusion *to pour*	Introduction intravenously of a substance other than blood
petechia petechiae (pl)	peh-**TEE**-kee-ah peh-**TEE**-kee-ie		Latin *spot on the skin*	Pinpoint capillary hemorrhagic spot in the skin
purpura	**PUR**-pyu-rah		Greek *purple*	Skin hemorrhages that are red initially and then turn purple
Rhesus factor	**REE**-sus **FAK**-tor		Greek *mythical king of Thrace*	Antigen on surface of red blood cells of Rh+ individuals; it was first identified in Rhesus monkeys
transfusion	trans-**FYU**-zhun	P/ R/	trans- *across* -fusion *to pour*	Transfer of blood or a blood component from donor to recipient

EXERCISES

A. Review *the Case Report on this spread before answering the questions.*   **LO 7.2, 7.8, 7.13, and 7.14** *Understand*

1. What is the difference between transfusion and infusion? _____

_____

2. What is the patient's current status regarding her surgery? _____

3. Is she experiencing hypotension or hypertension now? _____

4. Who could be involved in the error that caused this problem for the patient? _____

5. What in Ms. Rodi's type A blood caused the agglutination to occur? _____

6. What diagnosis originally put Ms. Rodi in the trauma unit? _____

7. What symptoms signify Ms. Rodi is having a bad reaction? _____

8. Why should the transfusion be stopped immediately? _____

9. What is the purpose of the saline solution? _____

10. Critical thinking: Discuss why it is a good idea to know your blood type and the blood type of members of your immediate family. _____

_____

_____

_____

B. Review *the elements in the WAD before starting this exercise. Fill in the blanks.*   **LO 7.1 and 7.8** *Apply*

_____ **1.** trans   **A.** to pour

_____ **2.** anti   **B.** glue

_____ **3.** fusion   **C.** against

_____ **4.** glutin   **D.** across

_____ **5.** gen   **E.** produce

Lesson 7.1 (cont'd) Blood Groups and Transfusions (continued)

ABO Blood Group (LO 7.3 and 7.8)

The two major antigens on the cell surface are antigen A and antigen B.

A person with only antigen A has *type A* blood.

A person with only antigen B has *type B* blood.

A person with both antigen A and antigen B has *type AB* blood.

A person with neither antigen has *type O* blood and is a universal donor, able to give blood to any other person. Specific antibodies are synthesized in the plasma during the first 8 months after birth:

- Whenever antigen A is absent, anti-A antibody is produced.
- Whenever antigen B is absent, anti-B antibody is produced.

Figure 7.11 shows the different combinations of antigens and antibodies in the different blood types.

A **transfusion** of blood or packed red blood cells replaces lost red blood cells to restore the blood's oxygen-carrying capacity. **Autologous** donation and transfusion occur when people donate their own blood ahead of time to be given back to them if necessary during a surgical procedure.

Rh Blood Group (LO 7.3 and 7.8)

If an Rh antigen is present on the red cell surface, the blood is said to be Rh-positive (Rh+). This is common, as about 85% of people are Rh-positive. If there is no Rh antigen on the surface, the blood is Rh-negative (Rh−), which is the case for the other 15% of the population.

If an Rh-negative person receives a transfusion of Rh-positive blood, anti-Rh antibodies will be produced. This can cause RBC clumping (agglutination) and destruction (hemolysis).

If an Rh-negative woman and an Rh-positive man conceive an Rh-positive child *(Figure 7.12a)*, the placenta normally prevents **maternal** and **fetal** blood from mixing. However, at birth or during a **miscarriage,** fetal cells can enter the mother's bloodstream. These Rh-positive cells stimulate the mother's tissues to produce Rh antibodies *(Figure 7.12b).*

If the mother becomes pregnant with a second Rh-positive fetus, her Rh antibodies can cross the **placenta** and agglutinate and hemolyze the fetal red cells *(Figure 7.12c)*. This causes hemolytic disease of the newborn **(HDN, or erythroblastosis fetalis).**

Hemolytic disease of the newborn due to Rh incompatibility can be prevented. The Rh-negative mother giving birth to an Rh-positive child should be given Rh-immune globulin **(RhoGAM).**

Other causes of hemolytic disease in newborns include ABO **incompatibility,** incompatibility in other blood group systems, hereditary **spherocytosis,** and infections acquired before birth.

Keynote

- Rh factor is an antigen on the surface of a red blood cell. Its presence or absence is inherited.

Abbreviations

HDN	hemolytic disease of the newborn
Rh	rhesus
RhoGAM	Rhesus immune globulin

(a)

(b)

(c)

(d)

▲ **FIGURE 7.11**
(a) Type A blood.
(b) Type B blood.
(c) Type AB blood.
(d) Type O blood.

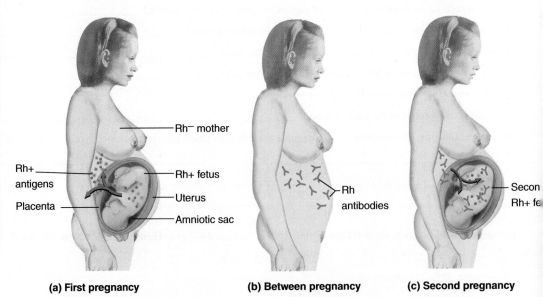

(a) First pregnancy   (b) Between pregnancy   (c) Second pregnancy

▲ **FIGURE 7.12**
Hemolytic Disease of the Newborn.
(a) First pregnancy. (b) Between pregnancies. (c) Second pregnancy.

Word Analysis and Definition

WORD	PRONUNCIATION	ELEMENTS		DEFINITION
erythroblastosis fetalis	eh-**RITH**-roh-blast-**OH**-sis fee-**TAH**-lis	S/ R/CF R/ S/ R/	-osis *condition* erythr/o- *red* -blast- *immature cell* -is *belonging to* fetal- *fetus*	Erythroblastosis fetalis is a hemolytic disease of the newborn (HDN)
fetus	**FEE**-tus		Latin *offspring*	Human organism from the end of the eighth week after conception to birth
fetal (adj)	**FEE**-tal	S/ R/	-al *pertaining to* fet- *fetus*	Pertaining to the fetus
incompatible	in-kom-**PAT**-ih-bul	S/ P/ R/	-ible *can do* in- *not* -compat- *tolerate*	Substances that interfere with each other physiologically
incompatibility	in-kom-**PAT**-ih-bil-i-tee	S/	-ibility *able to do*	The quality of being incompatible
maternal	mah-**TER**-nal	S/ R/	-al *pertaining to* matern- *mother*	Pertaining to or derived from the mother
miscarriage	mis-**KAR**-aj	P/	mis- *not, incorrect* -carriage Old English *to carry*	Spontaneous expulsion of the products of pregnancy before fetal viability
placenta	plah-**SEN**-tah		Latin *a cake*	Organ that allows metabolic exchange between the mother and the fetus
spherocyte	**SFEAR**-oh-site	R/CF R/	spher/o- *sphere* -cyte *cell*	A spherical cell
spherocytosis	**SFEAR**-oh-site-**OH**-sis	S/	-osis *condition*	Presence of spherocytes in blood

EXERCISES

A. Apply *the language of hematology and answer the following questions.*   **LO 7.2, 7.3, and 7.8** *Apply*

1. For blood to be Rh+ what must it have? _____

2. How are Rh antibodies produced? _____

3. What prevents maternal and fetal blood from mixing? _____

4. What gets destroyed in HDN? _____

5. What is the medical term for HDN? _____

B. Unscramble the letters *for the correct medical term to match the definition.*   **LO 7.2 and 7.8** *Apply*

1. Presence of spherocytes in blood: rsoyspcosheti _____

2. Substances that interfere with each other: imitlnoeacpb _____

3. Pertaining to the fetus: aetfl _____

4. Spontaneous expulsion of the products of pregnancy: riraamceisg _____

5. Pertaining to the mother: anlrmaet _____

C. Use your knowledge *of medical terminology to answer the following questions.*   **LO 7.2 and 7.8** *Remember*

1. What is the medical term for *red blood cells clumping together?* _____

2. What is more common: being Rh+ or Rh– ? _____

3. The presence or absence of Rh factor at birth is _____.

4. What follows after red blood cells clump together? _____

5. Define *spherocytosis.* _____

Diagnostic Procedures for Blood Disorders
(LO 7.3, 7.4, 7.5, 7.6, 7.7, and 7.9)

The patient's medical and family histories and physical examination are most important tools in diagnosing blood disorders.

- A **complete blood count (CBC)** gives important information about the types and numbers of cells in the blood, enabling diagnosis of the cause of such symptoms as weakness, fatigue, and bruising. Included in the CBC is the number of red blood cells; if the count is low, anemia could be present, and if the count is high, polycythemia can be the diagnosis. If the total amount of **hemoglobin** in the blood and the **hematocrit** are both low in the CBC, anemia is present. A red blood cell **index,** the **mean corpuscular volume (MCV),** shows the average size of the red blood cells. If the cells are small **(microcytic),** the most common cause is an iron-deficiency anemia. If the cells are large **(macrocytic),** a possible cause is pernicious anemia.

- A **white blood cell (WBC) count** is usually included in a CBC along with the numbers and types of the different WBCs, a **WBC differential.** These tests give the pathologists and clinicians who read the tests critical information about the body's response to infection, **toxic** medicines, chemicals, and allergens and show many other conditions, such as leukemia.

- Also included in a CBC is the number of platelets. A low platelet count can indicate **idiopathic thrombocytopenic purpura (ITP).** There are more than a dozen **coagulopathies** (bleeding disorders), and the diagnostic procedures to determine the cause of a patient's abnormal bleeding include the CBC, a **bleeding time, prothrombin time (PT), and partial thromboplastin time (PTT),** which help define where deficiencies might lie in the clotting process. The combination of all these tests is called a **coagulation panel.**

- Other diagnostic procedures for blood disorders include a **blood smear,** in which a drop of blood is smeared on a slide, stained, and examined under a microscope to determine the size and shape of RBCs, WBCs, and platelets. A **bone marrow aspiration (biopsy)** is a procedure used to define the production of the different blood cells. In disorders of the lymphatic system, the essential diagnostic procedure is biopsy of an enlarged lymph node. This can be followed by x-rays, CT scans, and MRI scans to determine the spread of a disease such as lymphoma.

Therapeutic Procedures for Blood Disorders
(LO 7.4, 7.5, 7.6, 7.7, and 7.9)

In anemia, treatment consists of replacing any deficiency in the production of hemoglobin, such as iron or vitamin B_{12}. For hemolytic and aplastic anemias, the treatment is to define and remove the toxin, drug, or radiation source that is causing the destruction of, or inability of the bone marrow to produce, red cells. A **bone marrow transplant** is the transfer of bone marrow from a healthy, compatible donor to a patient with aplastic anemia, leukemia, lymphoma, or other disease.

- Several drugs affect blood clotting. **Aspirin** is given in small 81-mg doses to reduce platelet adherence and agglutination. **Heparin,** given **parenterally,** acts quickly to prevent prothrombin and fibrin formation. **Warfarin (Coumadin),** given orally, also acts to prevent prothrombin and fibrin formation, and its effect is monitored by PT blood tests. Dabigatran etexilate (Pradaxa) and other similar compounds are given orally as anticoagulants in cases of non-valvular auricular fibrillation (see Chapter 6) to prevent blood clots from forming and **embolizing. Streptokinase** dissolves the fibrin in blood clots, and, if given intravenously within 3 to 4 hours of a heart attack, is often effective in dissolving the clot that has caused the heart attack. **Tissue plasminogen activator (TPA)** binds to fibrin and also dissolves clots that have caused heart attacks.

WORD	PRONUNCIATION		ELEMENTS	DEFINITION
aspiration	as-pih-**RAY**-shun	S/ R/	-ion *process* aspirat- *to breathe on*	Removal by suction of fluid or gas from a body cavity
coagulopathy coagulopathies (pl)	koh-ag-you-**LOP**-ah-thee	S/ R/CF	-pathy *disease* coagul/o *clotting*	Disorder of blood clotting
corpuscle	**KOR**-pus-ul	S/ R/	-cle *small* corpus- *body*	A red blood cell
corpuscular (adj)	kor-**PUS**-kyu-lar	S/	-ar *pertaining to*	Pertaining to a red blood cell
index indices (pl)	**IN**-deks **IN**-dih-seez		Latin *one that points out*	A standard indicator of measurement
macrocyte	**MACK**-roh-site	P/ S/	macro- *large* -cyte *cell*	Large red blood cell
macrocytic (adj)	mack-roh-**SIT**-ik	S/	-ic *pertaining to*	Pertaining to a large red blood cell
microcyte	**MY**-kroh-site	P/ S/	micro- *small* -cyte *cell*	Small red blood cell
microcytic (adj)	my-kroh-**SIT**-ik	S/	-ic *pertaining to*	Pertaining to a small red blood cell
parenteral	pah-**REN**-ter-al	S/ P/ R/	-al *pertaining to* par- *beside, abnormal* -enter- *intestine*	Administering medication by any other means than the GI tract
streptokinase	strep-toe-**KI**-nase	P/ R/	strepto- *curved* -kinase *enzyme*	An enzyme that dissolves clots
transplant	**TRANZ**-plant	P/ R/	trans- *across* -plant *insert, plant*	To transfer from one tissue or organ to another

EXERCISES

A. Answer *the following questions.*   **LO 7.4, 7.6, and 7.7** *Remember*

1. Define the components of a clotting panel.

_____

_____

2. What does the mean corpuscular volume show? _____

_____

3. What does a WBC differential show? _____

_____

B. Deconstruct *the following terms into their elements and give their meaning.*   **LO 7.1, 7.2, 7.5, and 7.7** *Analyze*

1. parenteral _____ / _____ / _____

                       P   R, R/CF   S

   Meaning: _____

2. coagulopathy _____ / _____ / _____

                       P   R, R/CF   S

   Meaning: _____

3. corpuscular: _____ / _____ / _____

                       P   R, R/CF   S

   Meaning: _____

Lesson 7.2

Lymphatic System

Objectives

As part of your body's defense mechanisms, the lymphatic system and its fluid provide surveillance and protection against foreign materials. In this lesson, the information provided will enable you to use correct medical terminology to:

7.2.1   Detail the anatomy of the **lymphatic** system.

7.2.2   Define the functions of the lymphatic system.

7.2.3   Identify the major cells of the lymphatic system and their functions.

7.2.4   Distinguish the anatomy and functions of the **lymph nodes, tonsils, thymus,** and **spleen.**

7.2.5   Recognize the common disorders of the lymphatic system.

Abbreviation

Ab   antibody

Case Report 7.4

You are . . .

. . . a medical assistant working with Susan Lee, MD, in her primary care clinic.

You are communicating with . . .

. . . Ms. Anna Clemons, a 20-year-old waitress, who is a new patient. She has noticed a lump in the left side of her neck. On questioning, you learn that Ms. Clemons has lost about 8 pounds in the past couple of months, has felt tired, and has had some night sweats. Her vital signs are normal. There are two firm, enlarged **lymph nodes** in her left neck in front of the sternocleidomastoid muscle (the long muscle in the side of the neck that extends up to the base of the skull behind the ear). Physical examination is otherwise unremarkable.

Lymphatic System (LO 7.10)

You live in a world that surrounds you with chemicals and disease-causing organisms waiting for a chance to enter your body and harm you. Your body has three lines of defense mechanisms against foreign organisms **(pathogens),** cells (cancer), or molecules **(pollutants** and **allergens).**

1. **Physical defense mechanisms** include your skin and mucous membranes; chemicals in your perspiration, saliva, and tears; hairs in your nostrils; and cilia and mucus to protect your lungs. The physical defense mechanisms are further discussed in the individual body system chapters.

2. **Humoral defense mechanisms** *(see Lesson 7.3),* based on antibodies **(Abs).** These are found in body fluids and bind to bacteria, toxins, and extracellular viruses, tagging them for destruction.

3. **Cellular defense mechanisms,** based on defensive cells **(lymphocytes).** These directly attack suspicious cells like cancer cells, transplanted tissue cells, or cells infected with viruses or parasites.

The lymphatic system has three functions:

1. **Absorb** excess **interstitial** fluid and return it to the bloodstream;

2. **Remove** foreign chemicals, cells, and debris from the tissues; and

3. **Absorb** dietary lipids from the small intestines *(see Chapter 9).*

Word Analysis and Definition

WORD	PRONUNCIATION	ELEMENTS		DEFINITION
absorb	ab-**SORB**		Latin *to swallow*	To take in
allergen (**Note:** *The duplicate letter "g" is omitted.*)	**AL**-er-jen	S/ R/ R/	-gen *create* all- *other, strange* -erg- *work*	Substance creating a hypersensitivity (allergic) reaction
allergic (adj) allergy	ah-**LER**-jik **AL**-er-jee	S/ S/	-ic *pertaining to* -ergy *process of working*	Pertaining to or suffering from an allergy Hypersensitivity to a particular allergen
interstitial	in-ter-**STISH**-al	S/ R/	-al *pertaining to* interstiti- *space between cells*	Pertaining to spaces between cells in an organ or tissue
lymph	LIMF		Latin *clear, spring water*	A clear fluid collected from tissues and transported by lymph vessels to the venous circulation
lymphatic (adj)	lim-**FAT**-ik	S/ R/	-atic *pertaining to* lymph- *lymph*	Pertaining to lymph or the lymphatic system
lymphoid (adj)	**LIM**-foyd	S/	-oid *resembling*	Resembling lymphatic tissue
node	NOHD		Latin *a knot*	A circumscribed mass of tissue
pathogen	**PATH**-oh-jen	S/ R/CF	-gen *produce, create, form* path/o- *disease*	A disease-causing microorganism
pollutant	poh-**LOO**-tant	S/ R/	-ant *pertaining to* pollut- *unclean*	Substance that makes an environment unclean or impure

EXERCISES

A. Review *the Case Report on this spread before answering the questions.*   **LO 7.10 and 7.13** *Understand*

1. What are Ms. Clemons' symptoms? _____

2. What is present on physical examination of the patient? _____

3. Where is the sternocleidomastoid muscle? _____

4. What was the status of the patient's VS? _____

5. What is a node? _____

B. Build *the correct medical terms that match the definitions given. Fill in the blanks.*   **LO 7.1 and 7.10** *Apply*

1. substance that makes the environment unclean or impure:

   _____ / _____ / _____

             P   R/CF   S

2. substance creating a hypersensitivity reaction:

   _____ / _____ / _____

             P   R/CF   S

3. resembling lymphatic tissue:

   _____ / _____ / _____

             P   R/CF   S

4. a disease-causing microorganism:

   _____ / _____ / _____

             P   R/CF   S

5. hypersensitivity to a particular allergen:

   _____ / _____ / _____

             P   R/CF   S

- Tissues that are the first line of defense against pathogens—for example, the airway passages—have lymphatic tissue in the submucous layers to help protect against invasion.

Lymphatic System *(continued)*
(LO 7.2 and 7.10)

The lymphatic system *(Figure 7.13)* has three components:

1. A network of thin **lymphatic capillaries and vessels,** similar to blood vessels, that penetrates the **interstitial spaces** (the spaces between tissues) of nearly every tissue in the body except cartilage, bone, red bone marrow, and the CNS;

2. A group of tissues and organs that produce **immune cells;** and

3. **Lymph,** a clear colorless fluid similar to blood plasma but with a composition that varies throughout the body. It flows through the network of lymphatic capillaries and vessels.

The **lymphatic network** begins with lymphatic capillaries that are closed-ended tubes nestled among **blood capillary networks** *(Figure 7.14)*. The lymphatic capillaries are designed to let interstitial fluid enter so it can become lymph. In addition, bacteria, viruses, cellular debris, and traveling cancer cells can enter the lymphatic capillaries with the interstitial fluid. The lymphatic capillaries converge to form the larger **lymphatic collecting vessels,** which resemble small veins and have one-way valves. They travel alongside veins and arteries.

Cervical lymph node

R. lymphatic duct

Thymus

Lymphatic vessels

Thoracic duct

Bone marrow

Lymphatic vessels

Axillary lymph node

Spleen

Inguinal lymph node

◀ **FIGURE 7.13**
The Lymphatic System.
(R. = right; L. = left)

Lymph Nodes (LO 7.2 and 7.10)

At irregular intervals, the collecting vessels mentioned above enter into the lymph nodes *(Figure 7.15)*. There are hundreds of lymph nodes stationed all over the body *(Figure 7.13)*. They are concentrated in the neck, axilla, and groin. Their functions are to filter impurities from the lymph and alert the immune system to the presence of pathogens.

The lymph moves slowly through the nodes, which filter the lymph and remove any foreign matter. Macrophages in the lymph nodes ingest and break down foreign matter and display its fragments to T cells. This alerts the immune system to the presence of an invader. Lymph leaves the nodes when it enters into the **efferent** collecting vessels. All these lymph vessels move lymph toward the thoracic cavity.

Collecting vessels merge into **lymphatic trunks** that drain lymph from a major body region. These lymphatic trunks then merge into two large **lymphatic ducts**—the thoracic duct on the left and the right lymphatic duct, which empty into the veins beneath the collarbone, the subclavian veins *(Figure 7.13)*.

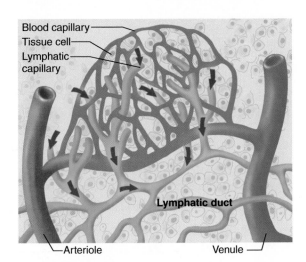

Blood capillary
Tissue cell
Lymphatic capillary

Lymphatic duct

Arteriole

Venule

▲ **FIGURE 7.14**
Lymphatic Flow.

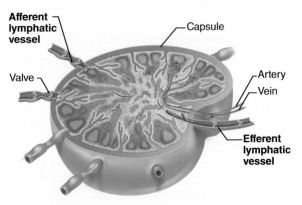

Afferent lymphatic vessel

Capsule

Valve

Artery

Vein

Efferent lymphatic vessel

▲ **FIGURE 7.15**
Lymph Node.

Word Analysis and Definition

WORD	PRONUNCIATION	ELEMENTS		DEFINITION
efferent	**EFF**-eh-rent	S/ R/	-ent *end result, pertaining to* effer- *move away from the center*	Moving away from a center
afferent (Note: *These are opposite terms.*)	**AFF**-eh-rent	R/	affer- *move toward the center*	Moving toward a center
immune	im-**YUNE**		Latin *protected from*	Protected from an infectious disease
immunity	im-**YUNE**-ih-tee	S/ R/	-ity *condition* immun- *immune*	State of being protected
immunology	im-you-**NOL**-oh-jee	S/ R/CF	-logy *study of* immun/o- *immune*	The science and practice of immunity and allergy
immunologist	im-you-**NOL**-oh-jist	S/	-logist *one who studies, specialist*	Medical specialist in immunology
immunize (verb)	**IM**-you-nize	S/ R/	-ize *affect in a specific way* immun- *immune*	To cause to be resistant to an infectious disease
immunization (noun)	**IM**-you-nih-**ZAY**-shun	S/	-ization *process of inserting or creating*	Administration of an agent to provide immunity

EXERCISES

A. Precision *in usage is important if you want to communicate correct information. These six terms all contain a common root/combining form. Insert the correct term in each sentence.*   **LO 7.2, 7.10, and 7.11** *Apply*

immune   immunology   immunity   immunologist   immunization   immunize

1. One who specializes in (the study of the science of immunity and allergy) _____ is termed an (type of specialist) _____.

2. The _____ system is a group of specialized cells in different parts of the body that recognize foreign substances and neutralize them.

3. We need to _____ young children before they start school.

4. A prior (injection) _____ obtained before she went overseas boosted her (status of being immune) _____ to the disease.

B. Review *the text on the opposite page and fill in the blanks.*   **LO 7.2 and 7.10** *Remember*

1. Meet a lesson objective and list the 3 components of the lymphatic system:

   a. _____   **b.** _____   **c.** _____

2. Based on the elements, where are the interstitial spaces? _____

3. Lymph is similar to what other body fluid? _____

4. Name the three functions of the lymphatic system.   **a.** _____   **b.** _____   **c.** _____

5. Lymphatic capillaries and vessels penetrate the interstitial spaces nearly everywhere in the body except _____
   _____.

6. Where in the body are the major concentrations of lymph nodes? _____

7. What enters lymphatic capillaries to become lymph? _____
   _____

8. Where does the lymphatic network begin? _____
   _____

9. Where do the two large lymphatic ducts empty? _____
   _____

▲ FIGURE 7.16
Position of Spleen.

(a)

(b)

▲ FIGURE 7.17
Thymus.
(a) Large thymus in infant.
(b) Adult thymus.

Abbreviation

Ig   immunoglobulin

Lymphatic Tissues and Cells (LO 7.2 and 7.10)

In some organs, lymphocytes and other cells form dense clusters called lymphatic **follicles.** These are constant features in the lymph nodes, the tonsils, and the ileum (a part of the small intestine).

Lymphatic tissues are composed of a variety of cells that include:

* **T lymphocytes (T cells):** The "T" stands for thymus, which is where these cells develop and mature. T lymphocytes make up 75% to 85% of body lymphocytes.

* **B lymphocytes (B cells):** These cells mature in the bone marrow. B lymphocytes make up 15% to 25% of lymphocytes. They respond to a specific antigen and become plasma cells to produce antibodies (**immunoglobulins, Ig**) that immobilize, neutralize, and prepare the specific antigen for destruction. Macrophages that have developed from monocytes ingest and destroy antigens, tissue debris, **bacteria,** and other foreign matter (phagocytosis).

Lymphatic Organs (LO 7.2 and 7.10)

Spleen (LO 7.2 and 7.10)

The **spleen,** a highly vascular and spongy organ, is the largest lymphatic organ. It is located in the left upper quadrant of the abdomen, below the diaphragm and lateral to the kidney *(Figure 7.16)*.

The functions of the spleen are to:

* **Phagocytose (consume)** bacteria and other foreign materials.

* **Initiate an immune response** when antigens are found in the blood.

* **Phagocytose old, defective erythrocytes** and platelets.

* **Serve as a reservoir** for erythrocytes and platelets.

Tonsils and Adenoids (LO 7.2 and 7.10)

The **tonsils** *(see Chapter 8)* are two masses of lymphatic tissue located at the entrance to the upper part of the throat (the oropharynx) that entrap inhaled and ingested pathogens. **Adenoids** are similar tissues on the posterior wall of the upper pharynx or nasopharynx *(see Chapter 8)*. The tonsils and adenoids form lymphocytes and antibodies, trap bacteria and viruses, and drain them into the tonsillar lymph nodes for elimination. Both the tonsils and the adenoids can also become infected.

Thymus (LO 7.2 and 7.10)

The thymus, a small organ of the immune system located in the center of the upper chest, has both endocrine *(see Chapter 12)* and lymphatic functions. T lymphocytes develop and mature in the thymus and are released into the bloodstream. The thymus is largest in infancy *(Figure 7.17a)* and reaches its maximum size at puberty. It then shrinks *(Figure 7.17b)* and is eventually replaced by fibrous and fatty (adipose) tissue.

Word Analysis and Definition

S = Suffix   P = Prefix   R = Root   R/CF = Combining Form

WORD	PRONUNCIATION	ELEMENTS		DEFINITION
adenoid	ADD-eh-noyd	S/	-oid *resemble*	Single mass of lymphoid tissue in the midline at the back of the throat
		R/	aden- *gland*	
adenoidectomy	ADD-eh-noy-**DEK**-toh-me	S/	-ectomy *surgical excision*	Surgical removal of the adenoid tissue
bacterium	bak-**TEER**-ee-um		Greek *a staff*	A unicellular, simple, microscopic organism
bacteria (pl)	bak-**TEER**-ee-ah			
follicle	**FOLL**-ih-kull		Latin *a small sac*	Spherical mass of cells containing a cavity; or a small cul-de-sac, such as a hair follicle
immunoglobulin	IM-you-noh-**GLOB**-you-lin	S/	-in *chemical compound, substance*	Specific protein evoked by an antigen. All antibodies are immunoglobulins
		R/CF	immun/o- *immune*	
		R/	-globul- *globular, protein*	
spleen	SPLEEN		Greek *spleen*	Vascular, lymphatic organ in left upper quadrant of abdomen
splenectomy	sple-**NECK**-toe-me	S/	-ectomy *surgical excision*	Surgical removal of the spleen
(Note: *Single "e" in* splen)		R/	splen- *spleen*	
splenomegaly	sple-noh-**MEG**-ah-lee	S/	-megaly *enlargement*	Enlarged spleen
		R/CF	splen/o- *spleen*	
thymus	**THIGH**-mus		Greek *sweetbread*	Endocrine gland located in the mediastinum
tonsil	**TON**-sill		Latin *tonsil*	Mass of lymphoid tissue on either side of the throat at the back of the tongue

EXERCISES

A. Review *all the terms and elements in the WAD above. Pay careful attention to spelling and pronunciation. Answer the following questions by circling the best choice.*   **LO 7.10** *Remember*

1. In the term *adenoid* one of the elements means:

tissue   organ   gland

2. The correct plural of bacterium is:

bacteria   bacteriae   bacteriums

3. In addition to referring to a lymph follicle, the term *follicle* can also apply to:

digits   bones   hair

4. What do *tonsil* and *adenoid* have in common?

lymphatic tissue   connective tissue   adipose tissue

5. Immunoglobulin can also be considered:

tissue collection   pathogens   antibodies

B. Review *all the terms and elements in the WAD above. Pay careful attention to spelling and pronunciation. Answer the following questions by circling the best choice.*   **LO 7.1, 7.3, and 7.10** *Remember*

1. The suffix in the term *adenoidectomy* implies:

surgical excision   surgical fixation   surgical incision

2. A microscopic organism is:

bacteria   follicle   bacterium

3. The spleen is located in the:

ABG   RLQ   LUQ

4. The specific protein evoked by an antigen is:

bacterium   enzyme   immunoglobulin

5. The element meaning *enlargement* is:

megaly   ectomy   oid

Disorders of the Lymphatic System
(LO 7.10)

Case Report 7.4 (continued)

Ms. Anna Clemons has cancerous nodes in her neck. They were caused not by metastatic cancer but by a cancer of the lymph nodes called **Hodgkin lymphoma,** which is detailed later on this page.

Physicians routinely feel the accessible lymph nodes in the neck (**cervical nodes**), axilla (armpit) (**axillary nodes**), and groin (**inguinal nodes**) for enlargement and tenderness, which indicate disease in the tissues drained by the lymph nodes.

Cancerous lymph nodes are enlarged, firm, and usually painless. Infections in the lymph nodes cause them to be swollen and tender to the touch, a condition called **lymphadenitis.** All lymph node enlargements are collectively called **lymphadenopathy.** When lymph nodes are removed, the process is called **lymphadenectomy.**

Lymphoma is a malignant growth (**neoplasm**) of the lymphatic organs, usually the lymph nodes. Associated symptoms can be fever, night sweats, fatigue, and weight loss. Lymphomas are grouped into two categories by microscopic examination of affected lymphatic tissues:

1. **Hodgkin lymphoma,** or **Hodgkin disease:** The cancer spreads in an orderly manner to adjoining lymph nodes. This enables the disease to be staged depending on how far it has spread; and

2. **Non-Hodgkin lymphomas:** These occur much more frequently than Hodgkin lymphoma. They include some 30 different disease entities in 10 different subtypes.

Diagnostic procedures used to determine lymphoma include a biopsy of an enlarged node, x-rays, CT and MRI scans, a **lymphangiogram,** and a bone marrow biopsy.

Tonsillitis, inflammation of the tonsils and adenoids, occurs mostly in infancy and childhood. The infection can be viral or bacterial, usually streptococcal. It produces enlarged, tender lymph nodes under the jaw. The infection can be recurrent, and a tonsillectomy is sometimes performed *(see Chapter 8).* If the adenoids also show recurrent infection, an adenoidectomy can be performed, often at the same time as the **tonsillectomy.**

Splenomegaly, an enlarged spleen, is not a disease in itself but the result of an underlying disorder. But when the spleen enlarges, it traps and stores an excessive number of blood cells and platelets (**hypersplenism**), reducing the number of blood cells and platelets in the bloodstream. Occasionally, a splenectomy is necessary.

Ruptured spleen is a common complication from car accidents or other trauma when the abdomen and rib cage are damaged. Intra-abdominal bleeding from the ruptured spleen can be extensive, with a dramatic fall in blood pressure. It is considered a surgical emergency requiring a splenectomy.

Lymphedema is localized, brawny (does not easily pit on finger pressure), minimally pitting fluid retention caused by a compromised lymphatic system, often after surgery or radiation therapy. It can also be primary, where the cause is unknown.

Word Analysis and Definition

S = Suffix   P = Prefix   R = Root   R/CF = Combining Form

WORD	PRONUNCIATION	ELEMENTS		DEFINITION
hypersplenism (Note: One "e" in this term)	high-per-**SPLEN**-izm	S/ P/ R/	-ism *condition* hyper- *excessive* -splen- *spleen*	Condition in which the spleen removes blood components at an excessive rate
inguinal	**IN**-gwin-al	S/ R/	-al *pertaining to* inguin- *groin*	Pertaining to the groin
lymphadenectomy	lim-**FAD**-eh-**NECK**-toe-me	S/ R/	-ectomy *surgical excision* lymphaden- *lymph node*	Surgical excision of a lymph node(s)
lymphadenitis lymphadenopathy	lim-**FAD**-eh-**NEYE**-tis lim-**FAD**-eh-**NOP**-ah-thee	S/ S/ R/CF	-itis *inflammation* -pathy *disease* lymphaden/o- *lymph node*	Inflammation of a lymph node(s) Any disease process affecting a lymph node(s)
lymphangiogram	lim-**FAN**-jee-oh-gram	S/ R/CF	-gram *recording* lymphangi/o- *lymphatic vessels*	Radiographic images of lymph vessels and nodes following injection of contrast material
lymphedema	**LIMF**-eh-**DEE**-mah	R/ R/	lymph- *lymph* -edema *edema*	Tissue swelling due to lymphatic obstruction
lymphoma	lim-**FOH**-mah	S/ R/	-oma *tumor, mass* lymph- *lymphatic system, lymph*	Any neoplasm of lymphatic tissue
Hodgkin	**HOJ**-kin		Thomas Hodgkin, British physician, 1798–1866	Hodgkin lymphoma is marked by chronic enlargement of lymph nodes spreading to other nodes in an orderly way
neoplasm (noun) neoplastic (adj) neoplasia (Note: The "m" in -plasm is removed to allow the elements to flow.)	**NEE**-oh-plazm **NEE**-oh-**PLAS**-tic **NEE**-oh-**PLAY**-zee-ah	P/ R/ S/ S/	neo- *new* -plasm *to form* -tic *pertaining to* -ia *condition*	A new growth, either a benign or malignant tumor Pertaining to a neoplasm Process that results in formation of a tumor

EXERCISES

A. Review *the Case Report on this spread before answering the questions.*   **LO 7.2, 7.10, and 7.13** *Understand*

1. What medical term in the Case Report signifies that the nodes are *malignant?* _____

2. What is the correct medical term for lymph nodes in the neck? _____

3. What is *metastatic* cancer? _____

4. Is this a primary or secondary cancer site? _____

5. What is another term for Hodgkin lymphoma? _____

6. Ms. Clemons does not have cancer anywhere else in her body. What sentence in the Case Report confirms that? _____

_____

B. Elements *remain your best tool for understanding the meaning of a term. Match the meaning of the definition in column 1 with the correct element in column 2.*   **LO 7.1 and 7.10** *Apply*

_____ **1.** groin   **A.** lymphangio

_____ **2.** lymph node   **B.** gram

_____ **3.** tumor, mass   **C.** inguin

_____ **4.** recording   **D.** oma

_____ **5.** lymph vessels   **E.** lymphadeno

C. Meet lesson objectives *and use the language of immunology to answer the following questions.*   **LO 7.2 and 7.10** *Remember*

1. Name the diagnostic procedures used to determine lymphoma. _____

2. What is a common injury from a motor vehicle accident? _____

3. What surgery is often performed at the same time as a tonsillectomy? _____

4. What is the difference between *pitting edema* and *lymphedema?* _____

Lesson 7.3

Immune System

Case Report 7.5

You are ...

... a laboratory technician working the night shift at Fulwood Medical Center.

You are communicating with ...

... Mr. Michael Cowan, a 40-year-old homeless man and drug addict, who has presented to the Emergency Department with a high fever, with no obvious cause.

You have been called to the emergency room to take blood from Mr. Cowan. You insert the needle into an **antecubital** vein, but he starts jerking his arm around and trying to get off the **gurney.** In the struggle, the needle comes out of the vein and pricks your hand through your glove.

You immediately flush and clean your wound, report the incident, seek immediate medical attention, and go through your initial medical evaluation. However, because of your possible exposure to Mr. Cowan's blood, it is essential that you have knowledge about your own immune system and its response to a potential infection. This will help you to make informed decisions about your treatment and future employment.

The Immune System (LO 7.11, and 7.13)

The immune system is a group of specialized cells in different parts of the body that recognize and neutralize foreign substances. It is the **third line of defense** listed earlier in this chapter. When the immune system is weak, it allows pathogens, including the viruses that cause common colds and flu, and cancer cells, to successfully invade the body.

Three characteristics distinguish immunity from the first two lines of defense of physical and cellular mechanisms:

1. **Specificity:** The immune response is directed against a specific pathogen. Immunity to one pathogen does not grant immunity to others. Specificity has one disadvantage; if a virus or a bacterium changes a component of its genetic code, it then becomes a new organism to the immune system. This **mutation** occurs, for example, with bacteria in response to antibiotics and in HIV's response to anti-HIV drugs (**development of resistance).**

2. **Memory:** When exposure to the same pathogen occurs again, the immune system recognizes the pathogen and has its responses ready to act quickly.

3. **Discrimination:** The immune system learns to recognize agents (antigens) that represent **"self"** and agents (antigens) that are **"nonself"** (foreign). Most of this recognition is developed prior to birth. A variety of disorders occur when this discrimination breaks down. They are known as **autoimmune disorders.**

An antigen is any molecule that triggers an immune response. Most antigens are unique in their structure. It is this uniqueness that enables your body to distinguish its own (self) molecules from foreign (nonself) molecules.

Word Analysis and Definition

WORD	PRONUNCIATION	ELEMENTS		DEFINITION
antecubital	an-teh-**KYU**-bit-al	S/ P/ R/	-al *pertaining to* ante- *in front of, before* -cubit- *elbow*	In front of the elbow
autoimmune	awe-toe-im-**YUNE**	P/ R/	auto- *self, same* -immune *protected*	Immune reaction directed against a person's own tissue
discrimination	**DIS**-krim-ih-**NAY**-shun	S/ P/ R/	-ation *process* dis- *away from* -crimin- *distinguish*	Ability to distinguish between different things
gurney	**GURR**-knee		Scottish *to grimace in pain*	A stretcher on wheels used to transport hospital patients
mutation	myu-**TAY**-shun		Latin *to change*	Change in the chemistry of a gene
specific	speh-**SIF**-ik	S/ R/	-ic *pertaining to* specif- *species*	Relating to a particular entity
specificity (Note: *Has two suffixes.*)	spes-ih-**FIS**-ih-tee	S/	-ity *condition, state*	State of having a specific, fixed relation to a particular entity
toxin toxicity	**TOK**-sin toks-**ISS**-ih-tee	S/ R/	Greek *poison* -ity *state, condition* toxic- *poison*	Poisonous substance formed by a cell or organism The state of being poisonous

EXERCISES

A. Review *the Case Report on this spread before answering the questions.*   **LO 7.2, 7.11, and 7.13** *Understand*

1. If you are taking blood from a patient, what is your occupation? _____

2. Where is the *antecubital* vein? _____

3. What is a gurney? _____

4. Why could this be a future health problem for you? _____

5. What is the main concern about Mr. Cowan's blood? _____

B. Review *the two pages spread open before you. Provide a brief answer to each of the questions below.*   **LO 7.2, 7.11, and 7.13** *Apply*

1. What happens when the immune system becomes weak?

_____

2. Does the immune system contain any specific organs?

_____

3. Describe an *autoimmune* disorder.

_____

4. Briefly describe the development of resistance.

_____

5. What occurs when discrimination of the immune system breaks down?

_____

C. Each of these questions *requires a one-word answer. Think carefully before writing the answers.*   **LO 7.2, 7.11, and 7.13** *Apply*

1. Use one word to describe the main purpose of the immune system. _____

2. Change in the chemistry of a gene produces a _____.

3. What is a molecule called that triggers a response? _____

Lesson 7.3 (cont'd)

Immunity (LO 7.11)

Immunity is the state of being able to resist a specific infectious disease. It is classified biologically into two types, although these often respond to the same antigen:

1. **Cellular (cell-mediated) immunity:** This is a direct form of defense based on the actions of lymphocytes to attack foreign and diseased cells and destroy them. The many different types of T cells, B cells, and macrophages described in the previous lesson of this chapter are involved in this style of attack (*Figure 7.18*).

2. **Humoral (antibody-mediated) immunity:** This is an indirect form of attack that employs antibodies produced by plasma cells, which have been developed from B cells. The antibodies bind to an antigen and tag it for destruction. These antibodies are called **immunoglobulins,** present in blood plasma and body secretions.

Complement Fixation (LO 7.2 and 7.11)

The complement system is a group of 20 or more proteins continually present in blood plasma. Immunoglobulins bind to foreign cells, initiating the binding of **complement** to the cell and leading to its destruction.

Immunization (LO 7.2 and 7.11)

Immunization is the preventive method of stimulating the immune system without exposing the body to an infection. An agent (**vaccine**) composed of the antigenic components of a killed or **attenuated** microorganism or its inactivated toxins is injected into the body. **Vaccination** is a crucial step in keeping our population healthy. For example, vaccination has eradicated smallpox worldwide. However, if we stop vaccinating against smallpox, our population will again be susceptible to smallpox outbreaks. The same concept applies to the diseases in childhood immunizations (*Table 7.1*).

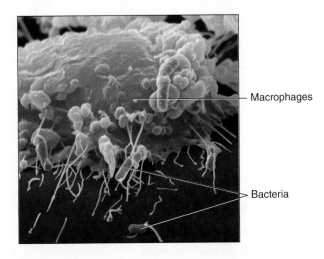

▶ **FIGURE 7.18**
Macrophage Phagocytoses Bacteria. Filamentous extensions of a macrophage cell snare the bacteria and draw them to the surface of the cell where they are engulfed into the macrophage.

▼ **TABLE 7.1**

RECOMMENDED IMMUNIZATIONS FOR PERSONS AGED 0 TO 6 YEARS

Hepatitis A (HepA)	Hepatitis B (HepB)
Rotavirus (RV)	Influenza (Yearly)
Inactivated poliovirus (IPV)	Varicella (chickenpox)
Diphtheria, tetanus, pertussis (DTaP)	Pneumococcal (PCV)
Measles, mumps, rubella (MMR)	
Hemophilus influenza type b (Hib)	

Source: Centers for Disease Control and Prevention, 2014.

Word Analysis and Definition

WORD	PRONUNCIATION	ELEMENTS		DEFINITION
attenuate	ah-**TEN**-you-ate	S/ R/	-ate *composed of, pertaining to* attenu- *weaken*	Weaken the ability of an organism to produce disease
attenuated (adj)	ah-**TEN**-you-a-ted	S/	-ated *pertaining to a condition*	Weakened
complement	**KOM**-pleh-ment		Latin *that which completes*	Group of proteins in serum that finish off the work of antibodies to destroy bacteria and other cells
humoral immunity	**HYU**-mor-al im-**YUNE**-ih-tee	S/ R/ S/ R/	-al *pertaining to* humor- *fluid* -ity *condition* immun- *immune*	Defense mechanism arising from antibodies in the blood
vaccinate (verb)	**VAK**-sin-ate	S/ R/	-ate *pertaining to, composed of* vaccin- *vaccine, giving a vaccine*	To administer a vaccine
vaccination vaccine	vak-sih-**NAY**-shun **VAK**-seen	S/	-ation *process* Latin *related to a cow*	Administration of a vaccine Preparation to generate active immunity

EXERCISES

A. Patient Education. *Explain the following in language your patient can understand.*   **LO 7.11 and 7.14** *Analyze*

1. Explain to your patient how immunization works to protect the body.

_____

_____

2. Give your patient a brief explanation of what the complement system does for the body.

_____

_____

3. Your patient has asked you what *agglutinate* means. Explain the concept to him or her.

_____

_____

4. How is *agglutinate* different from *attenuate?* _____

_____

5. What type of cells produce antibodies? _____

B. Meet lesson and chapter objectives *by using the language of the immune system to fill in the blanks.*   **LO 7.11 and 7.13** *Apply*

1. If vaccination is the process of injecting the agent, what is the injected agent called? _____

2. What is a toxin? _____

3. What disease has been eradicated worldwide? _____

4. What destroys foreign cells in the body? _____

5. Name three vaccinations a child between 0–6 years should receive. _____

Lesson 7.3 (cont'd)

Keynotes

- Common food and drug allergens are peanuts, milk, eggs, wheat, shellfish, penicillin and related antibiotics, and sulfa drugs.

- HIV is found in blood, semen, vaginal secretions, saliva, tears, and breast milk of infected mothers.

- The most common means of transmission of HIV are:
  - Sexual intercourse (vaginal, oral, anal).
  - Shared needles for drug use.
  - Contaminated blood products. (All donated blood is now tested for HIV.)
  - Transplacental transmission, from an infected mother to her fetus.

Abbreviations

AIDS	acquired immunodeficiency syndrome
HIV	human immunodeficiency virus

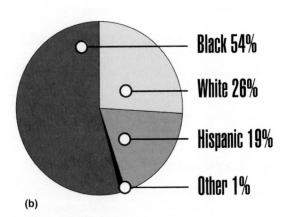

Men 70%

Women 30%

(a)

Black 54%

White 26%

Hispanic 19%

Other 1%

(b)

▲ **FIGURE 7.19**
New HIV Infections Each Year in the United States.
(a) by gender (b) by race.

Disorders of the Immune System (LO 7.11)

The immune system is prone to very serious disorders, from allergic reactions to life-threatening infections.

Hypersensitivity is an excessive immune response to an antigen that would normally be tolerated. In most allergic (hypersensitivity) reactions, allergens (antigens) stimulate the cells to produce **histamine.** The symptoms produced by these changes include edema, mucus hypersecretion and congestion, watery eyes, and hives **(urticaria).**

Hypersensitivity includes:

- **Allergies**—reactions to environmental antigens like pollens, molds, dusts, foods, and drugs.
- **Autoimmune disorders**—abnormal reactions to your own tissues.
- **Alloimmune disorders**—reactions to tissues transplanted from another person.

Anaphylaxis is an acute, immediate, and severe allergic reaction, which can be relieved by **antihistamines.**

Anaphylactic shock is more severe and is characterized by difficulty in breathing **(dyspnea)** due to bronchiole constriction, circulatory shock, and even death. It is a life-threatening medical emergency.

Asthma is triggered by allergens, listed above, and by air pollutants, drugs, and emotions. Bronchioles constrict spasmodically **(bronchospasm),** leading to the wheezing and coughing of asthma.

Autoimmune disorders are an over-vigorous response of the immune system. Here, the immune system fails to distinguish self-antigens from foreign antigens. These self-antigens produce autoantibodies that attack the body's own tissues. This type of response occurs, for example, in lupus erythematosus, type 1 diabetes, multiple sclerosis, rheumatoid arthritis, and psoriasis.

Immunodeficiency disorders are a deficient response of the immune system where it fails to respond vigorously enough. These disorders are classified into three categories:

1. **Congenital (inborn) disorders** are caused by a genetic abnormality that is often sex-linked, with boys affected more often than girls. An example is **inherited combined immunodeficiency disease,** characterized by an absence of both T cells and B cells (*Figure 7.19*). These children are very susceptible to **opportunistic** infections and must live in protective sterile enclosures.

2. **Immunosuppression** is a common side effect of corticosteroids used in treatment to prevent transplant rejection and in chemotherapy treatment for cancer.

3. **Acquired immunodeficiency** results from diseases like **acquired immunodeficiency syndrome (AIDS),** which involves a severely depressed immune system from infection with the human immunodeficiency virus **(HIV).**

HIV and AIDS (LO 7.11)

HIV is one of a group of viruses known as **retroviruses.** Like other viruses, it can replicate only inside a living host cell and it invades helper T cells and cells in the upper respiratory tract and CNS. Inside the cell, the virus can stay **dormant** for months or years. When it is activated (AIDS), the new viruses emerge from the dying host cell and attack more cells. This dormant phase **(incubation)** can range from a few months to 12 years.

As the virus destroys more and more cells, the body cannot produce antibodies. Symptoms appear, including chills, fever, night sweats, fatigue, weight loss, and lymphadenitis. Opportunistic infections by bacteria, viruses, and fungi can occur. These infections include toxoplasmosis, pneumocystitis, tuberculosis, herpes simplex, cytomegalovirus, and candidiasis. Cancers can also invade, and a form of skin cancer called **Kaposi sarcoma** (*Figure 7.20*) is common.

HIV survives poorly outside the human body. It is destroyed by laundering, dishwashing, chlorination, and the use of disinfectants, alcohol, and germicidal skin cleansers.

▲ **FIGURE 7.20**
Lesions of Kaposi sarcoma, a malignancy that is a complication of AIDS.

Word Analysis and Definition

S = Suffix   P = Prefix   R = Root   R/CF = Combining Form

WORD	PRONUNCIATION	ELEMENTS		DEFINITION
alloimmune	AL-oh-im-YUNE	P/ R/	all/o- *other, strange* -immune *immunity*	Immune reaction directed against foreign tissue
anaphylaxis	AN-ah-fih-LAK-sis	P/ R/	ana- *excessive* -phylaxis *protection*	Immediate severe allergic response
anaphylactic (adj)	AN-ah-fih-LAK-tik	S/ R/	-tic *pertaining to* -phylac- *protect*	Pertaining to anaphylaxis
asthma	AZ-mah		Greek *asthma*	Episodes of breathing difficulty due to narrowed or obstructed airways. Suffering from or pertaining to asthma.
asthmatic (adj)	az-MAT-ik	S/ R/	-atic *pertaining to* asthm- *asthma*	
dormant	DOR-mant	S/ R/	-ant *forming* dorm- *sleep*	Inactive
histamine	HISS-tah-mean	R/ R/	hist- *derived from histidine* -amine *nitrogen- containing substance*	Compound liberated in tissues as a result of injury or an immune response
antihistamine	AN-tih-HISS-tah-mean	P/	anti – *against*	Drug used to treat allergic symptoms because of its action antagonistic to histamine
hypersensitivity	HIGH-per-sen-sih-TIV-ih-tee	S/ P/ R/	-ity *condition* hyper- *excessive* -sensitiv- *feeling*	Exaggerated abnormal reaction to an allergen
immunodeficiency	IM-you-noh-dee-FISH-en-see	S/ R/CF R/	-ency *quality, state of* immun/o- *immune response* -defici- *failure, lacking*	Failure of the immune system
immunosuppression	IM-you-noh-suh-PRESH-un	S/ R/	-ion *action, condition* -suppress- *press under*	Failure of the immune system caused by an outside agent
incubation	in-kyu-BAY-shun	S/ R/	-ation *process* incub- *lie on, hatch*	Process to develop an infection
Kaposi sarcoma	Kah-POH-see sar-KOH-mah		Moritz Kaposi, Hungarian dermatologist, 1837–1902	A skin cancer often seen in AIDS patients
opportunistic	OP-or-tyu-NIS-tik	S/ R/	-istic *pertaining to* opportun- *take advantage of*	An organism or a disease in a host with lowered resistance
retrovirus	REH-troh-VIE-rus	P/ R/	retro- *backward* -virus *poison*	Virus with an RNA core
urticaria	ur-tee-KARE-ee-ah		Latin *nettle*	Rash of itchy wheals (hives)

EXERCISES

A. Build *more medical vocabulary for the language of immunology. Complete the construction of each term by using the following elements to fill in the blanks. There are more answers than you need.* **LO 7.1 and 7.11** *Apply*

defici   allo   suppress   sensitiv   ion   hyper   incub   osis   phylaxis   ic   ency   dorm

1. exaggerated, abnormal reaction to an allergen:_____ / _____ / _____ / ity

2. inactive: _____ / _____ / _____ / ant

3. process to develop an infection: _____ / _____ / _____ / ation

4. Terminology challenge: Make a study hint for yourself for dorm = sleep. _____

_____

B. Understanding. *How well do you understand the languages of hematology and immunology?* **LO 7.2 and 7.11** *Understand*

1. List every term in the WAD that could be a diagnosis. _____

2. What is the difference between *dormant* and *incubation?* _____

3. What is anaphylaxis? _____

4. What can relieve the condition in #3 above? _____

5. What term is a life-threatening emergency? _____

Lesson 7.3 (cont'd)

- When viruses spread from person to person, they are said to be **contagious.**
- Viral diseases do not respond to antibiotics.
- Nosocomial infections (hospital-acquired infections) are becoming increasingly common and lethal.
- Handwashing is the most important factor in preventing the transmission of infections.

Abbreviations

CA-MRSA	community-associated methicillin-resistant *Staphylococcus aureus*
CDC	Centers for Disease Control and Prevention
CRE	carbapenem-resistant *Enterobacteriaceae*
MRSA	methicillin-resistant *Staphylococcus aureus*
SARS	severe acute respiratory syndrome
WNV	West Nile virus

Infection (LO 7.12)

Microbes (microorganisms) are everywhere—in the air, water, and soil and all over our bodies, where they are called **normal flora.** These normal microorganisms are found on your skin, in your nose and respiratory tract, and in your mouth and digestive tract. Your brain and cardiovascular system, however, are microbe-free **(sterile).**

If microorganisms other than the normal flora invade the body, they become pathogens, which cause an **infection.** Pathogens include bacteria, viruses, fungi, and parasites. If the infection harms the body, it creates an **infectious disease.** Bacterial, viral, fungal, and parasitic infections are all caused by pathogens.

Bacterial Infections (LO 7.12)

Thousands of different bacteria can cause infections. Bacteria are single-celled microorganisms that reproduce by dividing. Frequently seen bacteria include:

- **Staphylococcus ("staph"),** which can be harmless when present on the skin's surface but causes infections in wounds or other normally sterile places, like in a joint or the peritoneum;
- **Streptococcus ("strep"),** which is a cause of sore throats;
- **Pneumococcus,** which is a cause of pneumonia; and
- **Coliform** bacteria that normally live in the GI tract but cause infections elsewhere, such as the urinary tract.

In addition, methicillin-resistant *Staphylococcus aureus* **(MRSA)** is a type of bacteria that is resistant to the antibiotics normally used to treat staph infections. MRSA infections occur most frequently in hospitals **(nosocomial** infection), but are now being seen in community health care facilities as community-associated MRSA **(CA-MRSA).**

Clostridium difficile (C.diff) infection is a growing problem in health care facilities, and the infection kills 14,000 people in America alone each year. When **broad-spectrum** antibiotics, such as **clindamycin,** have destroyed normal gut flora, *C.diff* can take over the gut and release toxins, causing severe diarrhea and abdominal pain that can be difficult to treat and can be life threatening or fatal.

Carbapenem-resistant Enterobacteriaceae **(CRE)** is a lethal "superbug" occuring in American hospitals and responsible for about 9,300 infections and 610 deaths every year. The antibiotic carbapenem is considered a last-resort antibiotic for bacteria that have not responded to other antibiotics. In several cases the CRE has been found in duodenoscopes (*see Chapter 9*), the complex design of which which makes them difficult to clean and sterilize.

Viral Infections (LO 7.12)

Viruses are the smallest of the microorganisms. They cannot be seen under an ordinary light **microscope** but are visible through electron **microscope.** Viruses spread from person to person through coughs, sneezes, and unwashed hands.

Viruses cause specific childhood diseases like measles (rubeola), German measles (rubella), chickenpox (varicella), and mumps. They cause upper respiratory infections (*see Chapter 8),* including modern respiratory infections like **severe acute respiratory syndrome (SARS), avian influenza** (bird flu), and **West Nile virus (WNV).** WNV is a seasonal **epidemic** in North America that flares up in the summer and fall.

Fungal Infections (LO 7.12)

Many fungi are "good fungi," for example, the mushrooms that you eat and the yeasts that ferment beer and bread. Penicillin is derived from a fungus. The most common pathogenic fungi are those that cause skin infections (*see Chapter 3).*

Opportunistic fungi are normally harmless, but like their name, they pounce on any opportunity to cause disease. People who are on prolonged doses of antibiotics, are receiving chemotherapy or immunosuppressive therapy, or have diabetes mellitus or AIDS are especially susceptible.

Parasitic Infections (LO 7.12)

Parasites are organisms that live on or in another organism and steal nourishment from their host. In many rural areas of the world, parasites are **endemic. Malaria** is caused by a parasite that is transmitted from person to person by a single mosquito bite.

Pinworms are the most common parasite in America. Pinworm eggs are introduced into the body through the mouth and hatch in the intestine. The young worms migrate to the anus, where the female deposits her eggs. These eggs can be transferred unknowingly by the fingers from the anus or from infected bedding, to the mouth of the same child or to another child.

Word Analysis and Definition

WORD	PRONUNCIATION	ELEMENTS		DEFINITION
broad-spectrum	broad-**SPECK**-trum		broad Latin *wide* spectrum Latin *image*	An antibiotic with a wide range of activity against a variety of organisms
Clostridium difficile	klah-**STRID**-ee-um **DIFF**-ih-seal	S/ R/	-ium *structure* clostrid- *spindle*	Gram-positive spore-forming bacteria that causes antibiotic-associated diarrhea.
contagious	kon-**TAY**-jus	S/ P/ R/	-ious *pertaining to* con- *with, together* -tag- *touch*	Infection can be transmitted from person to person or from a person to a surface to a person
endemic	en-**DEM**-ik	S/ P/ R/	-ic *pertaining to* en- *in* -dem- *the people*	Pertaining to a disease always present in a community
epidemic	ep-ih-**DEM**-ik	P/	epi- *above, upon*	Pertaining to an outbreak in a community of a disease or a health-related behavior
pandemic	pan-**DEM**-ik	P/	pan- *all*	Pertaining to a disease attacking the population of a very large area
flora	**FLO**-rah		Latin *flower*	Microorganisms covering the exterior and interior surfaces of a healthy animal
infect (verb) infection (noun) infectious (adj)	in-**FEKT** in-**FEK**-shun in-**FEK**-shus	S/ R/ S/	Latin *invade internally* -ion *condition, action* infect- *internal invasion* -ious *pertaining to*	To invade an organism by a microorganism Invasion of the body by disease-producing microorganisms Capable of being transmitted to a person; or a disease caused by the action of a microorganism
microbe microorganism	**MY**-krohb **MY**-kroh-**OR**-gan-izm	P/ R/ S/ R/	micro- *small* -be *life* -ism *process* -organ- *organ, instrument*	Short for microorganism Any organism too small to be seen by the naked eye
microscope microscopic microscopy	**MY**-kroh-skope **MY**-kroh-**SKOP**-ik my-**CROSS**-koh-pee	P/ S/ S/ S/	micro- *small* -scope *instrument for viewing* -ic *pertaining to* -scopy *to examine, to view*	Instrument for viewing something small that cannot be seen in detail by the naked eye Visible only with the aid of a microscope Investigation of minute objects through a microscope
nosocomial	noh-soh-**KOH**-mee-al	S/ R/CF R/	-ial *pertaining to* nos/o- *disease* -com- *take care of*	Acquired while in the hospital

EXERCISES

A. Correct usage *of the appropriate grammatical form of a medical term is the mark of an educated professional. Practice your language of immunology in the following sentences. Fill in the blanks.* **LO 7.2 and 7.12** *Apply*

1. infect   infection   infectious

This patient has a rarely seen (a) _____. Please refer her to the (b) _____ disease specialist.

2. bacterium   bacteria   bacterial

The (a) _____ streptococcus causes (b) _____ infections in the throat.

3. sterile   sterility   sterilize

An autoclave is used to (a) _____ instruments.

If the (b) _____ of an instrument is in question, it should not be used.

The term (c) _____ can also mean *unable* to *reproduce.*

B. Use the language of immunology *and circle the best answer.* **LO 7.2 and 7.12** *Understand*

1. What agent causes infections in wounds and joints?

    staph   pneumococcus   heme

2. What term is the same as "microbe free"?

    opportunistic   anemic   sterile

3. MRSA occurs most frequently in:

    prisons   schools   hospitals

4. Another name for microbes is:

    normal flora   bacteria   pollutants

Additional exercises available in **connect**

Chapter Review exercises, along with additional practice items, are available in Connect!

The Respiratory System

The Essentials of the Language of Pulmonology

CHAPTER 8

Case Report 8.1

You are . . .

. . . an advanced-level **registered respiratory therapist (RRT)** working with **pulmonologist** Tavis Senko, MD, in the Acute Respiratory Care unit of Fulwood Medical Center.

You are communicating with . . .

. . . Mr. Jude Jacobs, a 68-year-old white retired mail carrier, who has chronic obstructive pulmonary disease **(COPD)** and is on continual **oxygen (O₂)** by nasal prongs. He has smoked two packs of cigarettes per day throughout his adult life.

Last night, he was unable to sleep because of increased shortness of breath **(SOB)** and cough. He had to sit upright in bed in order to breathe. His cough produces yellow **sputum.**

Mr. Jacobs' vital signs are temperature **(T)** of 101.6°, pulse **(P)** of 98, respirations **(R)** of 36, and blood pressure **(BP)** 150/90. On examination, he is **cyanotic** and frightened, and he is on oxygen by nasal prongs. Air entry is diminished in both lungs, and there are **rales** (crackles) at the bases of both lungs.

You have been ordered to draw blood for arterial blood gases **(ABGs)** and to measure the amount of air entering and leaving his lungs by using **spirometry.**

Learning Outcomes

In order to provide optimal care to Mr. Jacobs, determine what is causing his symptoms and signs, and communicate with the other health professionals involved in his care, you need to be able to:

LO 8.1 Use roots, combining forms, suffixes, and prefixes to construct and analyze (deconstruct) medical terms related to the respiratory system.

LO 8.2 Spell and pronounce correctly medical terms related to the respiratory system in order to communicate with accuracy and precision in any health care setting.

LO 8.3 Define accepted abbreviations related to the respiratory system.

LO 8.4 Relate the structures of the anatomical elements of the upper respiratory tract to their functions and signs and symptoms of respiratory disorders.

LO 8.5 Use the structures of the elements of the lower respiratory tract to explain the mechanics of respiration and the functions and disorders of the lower respiratory tract.

LO 8.6 Explain the diagnostic and therapeutic procedures and pharmacologic agents used for disorders of the respiratory system.

LO 8.7 Apply your knowledge of the medical terms of the respiratory system to documentation, medical records, and medical reports.

LO 8.8 Translate the medical terms of the respiratory system into everyday language in order to communicate clearly with patients and their families.

Abbreviations

ABG	arterial blood gas
COPD	chronic obstructive pulmonary disease
O₂	oxygen
RRT	registered respiratory therapist

In your future career, being able to communicate comfortably, accurately, and effectively with the health professionals involved in the diagnosis and treatment of respiratory problems is key. You may work directly and/or indirectly with one or more of the following:

- **Pulmonologists** are physicians who specialize in the diagnosis and treatment of lung/pulmonary conditions.
- **Registered respiratory therapists (RRT) or respiratory care practitioners** assist physicians in evaluating, treating, and caring for patients who have respiratory disorders. They also supervise RT technicians.
- **Respiratory therapy (RT) technicians** assist physicians and RRTs in evaluating, monitoring, and treating patients with respiratory disorders.
- **Sleep technologists** are trained in sleep technology and sleep medicine. These technologists assist sleep specialists in the assessment, monitoring, management, and follow-up care of patients with sleep disorders.

Introduction to the Respiratory System
(LO 8.4 and 8.5)

It sounds like a good scheme. Humans and animals breathe in **oxygen** and breathe out **carbon dioxide,** while plants and trees breathe in carbon dioxide and breathe out oxygen. Unfortunately, we continue to generate increasing amounts of carbon dioxide in the air by burning coal, oil, and natural gas, and cutting down forests, thus disturbing this natural balance. In addition, humans have created organic and inorganic chemicals and small particles of solid matter, which float through the air and enter our bodies as we breathe. These **pollutants** can damage our respiratory tracts and cause cancer, brain damage, and birth defects.

The Respiratory Tract (LO 8.4 and 8.5)

The **respiratory tract** (*Figure 8.1*) has six connected elements:

1. **Nose**
2. **Pharynx**
3. **Larynx**
4. **Trachea**
5. **Bronchi** and **bronchioles**
6. **Alveoli**

Respiration has two components:

- **Ventilation,** which is the movement of air and its gases into (**inspiration**) and out of (**expiration**) the lungs; and
- The **exchange of gases** between air and blood, and between blood and interstitial fluids.

Functions of the Respiratory System (LO 8.4 and 8.5)

Your respiratory system is responsible for the following key functions:

1. **Exchange of gases:** All of your body cells need oxygen and produce carbon dioxide. Your respiratory system allows oxygen from the air to enter the blood and carbon dioxide to leave the blood and enter the air.
2. **Regulation of blood pH:** Regulation occurs by changing carbon dioxide levels in the blood.
3. **Protection:** The respiratory system protects against foreign bodies and against some microorganisms.
4. **Voice production:** Movement of air across the vocal cords makes voice and sound possible.
5. **Olfaction:** The 12 million receptor cells for smell are in a quarter-sized patch of epithelium. These are located in the **olfactory region** (*Figure 8.2*), the extreme superior region of the nasal cavity. Each cell has 10 to 20 hair-like structures called **cilia** that project into the nasal cavity in a thin mucous film.

Because the olfactory region is right at the top of your nose, you often have to sniff deeply to stimulate the sense of smell. Because dogs have 4 billion receptor cells in their noses, they can be trained to sniff for drugs, explosives, or human scent.

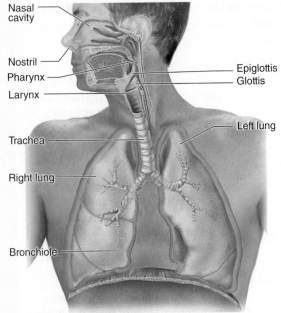

▲ FIGURE 8.1
The Respiratory System.

Labels: Nasal cavity, Nostril, Pharynx, Larynx, Trachea, Right lung, Bronchiole, Epiglottis, Glottis, Left lung

▲ FIGURE 8.2
Olfactory Region of the Nose.

Labels: Olfactory tract, Olfactory bulb, Olfactory mucosa

Word Analysis and Definition

WORD	PRONUNCIATION	ELEMENTS		DEFINITION
alveolus alveoli (pl) alveolar (adj)	al-**VEE**-oh-lus al-**VEE**-oh-lee al-**VEE**-oh-lar	 S/ R/	Latin *hollow sac* -ar *pertaining to* alveol- *air sac*	Terminal element of respiratory tract where gas exchange occurs Pertaining to the alveoli
bronchus bronchi (pl) bronchiole	**BRONG**-kuss **BRONG**-key **BRONG**-key-ole	 S/ R/CF	Greek *windpipe* -ole *small* bronch/i- *bronchus*	One of two subdivisions of the trachea Increasingly smaller subdivisions of bronchi
cilium cilia (pl)	**SILL**-ee-um **SILL**-ee-ah		Latin *eyelash*	Hairlike motile projection from the surface of a cell
expiration (**Note:** *The "s" is deleted from the root* spirat *because the prefix* ex *already has the "s" sound.*)	EKS-pih-**RAY**-shun	S/ P/ R/	-ion *action, condition, process of* ex- *out* -spirat- *breathe*	Breathe out
inspiration (**Note:** *The opposite of* expiration)	in-spih-**RAY**-shun	S/ P/ R/	-ion *action, condition, process of* in- *into* -spirat- *breathe*	Breathe in
olfaction olfactory (adj)	ol-**FAK**-shun ol-**FAK**-toh-ree	S/ R/ S/	-ion *action, condition, process of* olfact- *smell* -ory *having the function of*	Sense of smell Relating to the sense of smell
oxygen	**OCK**-si-jen	S/ R/	-gen *create* oxy- *oxygen*	The gas essential for life
pharynx pharyngeal (adj)	**FAH**-rinks fah-**RIN**-jee-al	 S/ R/	Greek *throat* -eal *pertaining to* pharyng- *pharynx*	Tube from the back of the nose to the larynx. Pertaining to the pharynx
pulmonary pulmonology pulmonologist	**PULL**-moh-**NAR**-ee **PULL**-moh-**NOL**-oh-jee **PULL**-moh-**NOL**-oh-jist	S/ R/ S/ R/CF S/	-ary *pertaining to* pulmon- *lung* -logy *study of* pulmon/o- *lung* -logist *one who studies, specialist*	Pertaining to the lungs Study of the lungs, or the medical specialty of disorders of the lungs Specialist in treating disorders of the lungs
rale rales (pl)	RAHL RAHLS		French *rattle*	Crackle heard through a stethoscope when air bubbles through liquid in the lungs
respiration respirator respiratory (adj)	RES-pih-**RAY**-shun RES-pih-**RAY**-tor RES-pih-rah-tor-ee	S/ P/ R/ S/ S/	-ation *a process, formed from* re- *again* -spir- *to breathe* -ator *person or thing that does something* -atory *pertaining to, produced by*	Process of breathing; fundamental process of life used to exchange oxygen and carbon dioxide Another name for ventilator Pertaining to respiration
sputum	**SPYU**-tum		Latin *to spit*	Matter coughed up and spat out by individuals with respiratory disorders
trachea trachealis (adj)	**TRAY**-kee-ah tray-kee-**AY**-lis	 S/ R/	Greek *windpipe* -alis *pertaining to* trache- *trachea*	Air tube from the larynx to the bronchi Pertaining to the trachea

EXERCISES

A. Review *Case Report 8.1 before answering the questions.*   **LO 8.2, 8.4, 8.5, and 8.6** *Understand*

1. A pulmonologist is a specialist in diseases of the _____.

2. Why is Mr. Jacobs receiving continual O_2 by nasal prongs? _____

3. What is *sputum?* _____

4. Which test ordered for Mr. Jacobs involves drawing his blood? _____

5. Describe the sound of rales. _____

6. What in Mr. Jacobs' medical history accounts for the COPD he has today? _____

Lesson 8.1

Upper Respiratory Tract

The Nose (LO 8.4)

When you breathe in air through your nose, the air goes through the nostrils **(nares)** into the **nasal cavity.** Internal hairs guard the nares to prevent large particles from entering your body.

The nasal **septum** divides the nasal cavity into right and left compartments. The **palate** forms the floor of the nose *(Figure 8.3)*. The **paranasal frontal** and **maxillary sinuses** *(Chapter 4)* open into the nose.

Functions of the Nose (LO 8.4)

The nose serves as an important part of the respiratory system in several ways:

1. **Passageway for air** to enter or leave the body.

2. **Air cleanser:** The nasal hairs and the mucus (secreted by the nasal mucous membrane) trap particles of dust and solid pollutants.

3. **Air moisturizer:** It adds moisture to the air. Moisture is secreted by the nasal mucosa (mucous membrane) and from tears that drain into the nasal cavity through the nasal lacrimal duct *(see Chapter 11)*.

4. **Air warmer:** The blood flowing through the nasal cavity beneath the mucous membrane lining also warms the air. This prevents damage from cold to the more fragile lower respiratory passages.

5. **Sense of smell (olfaction):** The olfactory region recognizes some 4,000 separate smells *(see previous pages)*.

Disorders of the Nose (LO 8.4)

A **common cold** is a viral upper respiratory infection **(URI).** It is contagious and easily transmitted in airborne droplets through coughing and sneezing. There is no proven effective treatment.

Rhinitis, also called **coryza,** is an inflammation of the nasal mucosa, which is usually viral.

Allergic rhinitis affects 15% to 20% of the population. The mucous membranes of the nose, pharynx, and sinuses swell and produce a clear, watery discharge. Treatment entails defining and removing the allergy-causing agent.

Sinusitis is an infection of the paranasal sinuses, often following a viral upper respiratory tract infection. It can also be part of an allergic response. It can be treated with **antibiotics** and **decongestants.**

A **deviated nasal septum** occurs when the partition between the two nostrils is pushed to one side, leading to a partially obstructed airway in one nostril. Treatment is by surgery.

Nasal polyps are benign growths arising from the mucosa of the nasal cavity or a sinus. These can be surgically removed.

Epistaxis (a nosebleed) is bleeding from the septum of the nose, usually as a result of trauma.

Most nose bleeds can be treated at home by pinching the soft part of the nose for 15 to 20 minutes. If this fails, medical treatment can consist of **cauterization,** or nasal packing with gauze strips.

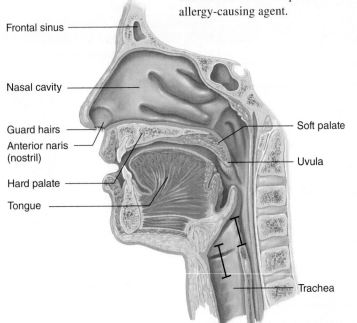

Frontal sinus

Nasal cavity

Guard hairs

Anterior naris (nostril)

Hard palate

Tongue

Soft palate

Uvula

Trachea

◀ **FIGURE 8.3**
Upper Respiratory Tract.

Word Analysis and Definition

S = Suffix   P = Prefix   R = Root   R/CF = Combining Form

WORD	PRONUNCIATION		ELEMENTS	DEFINITION
cautery	KAW-ter-ee		Greek *branding iron*	A device to scar, burn, or cut a tissue
cauterize	KAW-ter-ize	S/	-ize *action*	To apply a cautery
		R/	cauter- *to burn*	
cauterization	KAW-ter-eye-ZAY-shun	S/	ation *a process*	The act of cauterizing
coryza (*also called* **rhinitis**)	koh-RYE-zah		Greek *catarrh*	Acute inflammation of the mucous membrane of the nose
decongestant	dee-con-JESS-tant	S/	-ant *pertaining to*	Agent that reduces the swelling and fluid in the nose and sinuses
		P/	de- *take away, remove*	
		R/	-congest- *accumulation of fluid*	
epistaxis	ep-ih-STAK-sis	S/	-is *pertaining to*	Nosebleed
		P/	epi- *above, upon*	
		R/	-stax- *fall in drops*	
naris	NAH-ris		Latin *nostril*	Nostril
nares (pl)	NAH-rees			
nasal	NAY-zal	S/	-al *pertaining to*	Pertaining to the nose
		R/	nas- *nose*	
palate	PAL-at		Latin *palate*	Roof of the mouth, floor of the nose
paranasal	PAR-ah-NAY-zal	S/	-al *pertaining to*	Adjacent to the nose
		P/	para- *adjacent to*	
		R/	-nas- *nose*	
polyp	POL-ip		Latin *many feet*	Any mass of tissue that projects outward
rhinitis (*also called* **coryza**)	rye-NIE-tis	S/	-itis *inflammation*	Acute inflammation of the nasal mucosa
		R/	rhin- *nose*	
septum	SEP-tum		Latin *partition*	Thin wall separating two cavities or tissue masses
septa (pl)	SEP-tah			
sinus	SIGH-nus		Latin *cavity*	Cavity or hollow space in a bone or other tissue
sinusitis	sigh-nu-SIGH-tis	S/	-itis *inflammation*	Inflammation of the lining of a sinus
		R/	sinus- *sinus*	

EXERCISES

A. Elements: *Work with elements to build your knowledge of the language of pulmonology. One element in each of the following medical terms is boldfaced. Identify the type of element (P, R, CF, or S) in column 2; then write the meaning of that element in column 3. Finally, write the meaning of the complete term in column 4.*   **LO 8.1 and 8.4** *Apply*

Medical Term	Type of Element	Meaning of Element	Meaning of the Term
1. **nas**al	_____	_____	_____
2. decongest**ant**	_____	_____	_____
3. **rhin**itis	_____	_____	_____
4. epi**stax**is	_____	_____	_____
5. **para**nasal	_____	_____	_____
6. sinus**itis**	_____	_____	_____

B. Apply *the language of pulmonology to answer the following questions correctly.*   **LO 8.1, 8.4, and 8.7** *Apply*

1. There are two elements in the WAD that have the same meaning. Which are they? _____ and _____ both mean _____.

2. List all the terms in this WAD that are a diagnosis. _____

3. Where else in the body would the term *septa* apply? _____

4. Which elements in the WAD mean *inflammation*? _____

5. What is another term for *nostril*? _____

6. What is the difference between *rhinitis* and *sinusitis*? _____

Case Report 8.2

You are . . .

. . . a sleep technologist in the Sleep Disorders Clinic at Fulwood Medical Center. You are about to position the electrodes on your patient for an overnight **polysomnography** (sleep study).

You are communicating with . . .

. . . Mr. Tye Gawlinski, a 29-year-old professional football player, and his wife, Mrs. Helen Gawlinski states that her husband snores loudly and has 40 or 50 periods in the night when he stops breathing. The snoring is so loud that she cannot sleep, even in the adjoining bedroom. Mr. Gawlinski complains of being tired all day and not having the energy he needs for his job. The sleep study is being performed to confirm a diagnosis of obstructive sleep **apnea**.

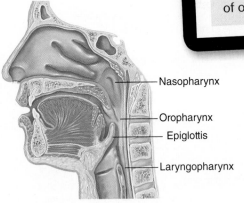

▲ **FIGURE 8.4**
Regions of the Pharynx.

The Pharynx (LO 8.4)

Your pharynx is a muscular funnel that receives air from the nasal cavity, and food and drink from the oral cavity. It is divided into three regions *(Figure 8.4)*:

1. **Nasopharynx:** Located at the back of the nose and above the soft palate and uvula. The posterior surface contains the pharyngeal **tonsil (adenoid).** Only air moves through this region;

2. **Oropharynx:** Located at the back of the mouth, and below the soft palate and above the epiglottis. It contains two sets of tonsils called the palatine and lingual tonsils. Air, food, and drink all pass through this region; and

3. **Laryngopharynx:** Located below the tip of the epiglottis. It is the pathway to the esophagus. Only food and drink pass through the laryngopharynx.

Disorders of the Pharynx (LO 8.4)

Snoring occurs regularly in 25% of normal adults and is most common in overweight males. It worsens with age. Snoring noises are made at the back of the mouth and nose where the tongue and upper pharynx meet the soft palate and uvula *(Figure 8.5).*

Obstructive sleep apnea is the condition Mr. Gawlinski has. Bulky neck tissue from his football training causes an obstruction by the soft tissues at the back of his nose and mouth. This leads to frequent episodes of gasping for breath, followed by complete cessation of breathing **(apnea).** These episodes reduce the level of oxygen in the blood **(hypoxemia),** making his heart pump harder. If this problem goes untreated for several years, it can cause hypertension and cardiac enlargement.

Pharyngitis is an acute or chronic infection involving the pharynx, tonsils, and uvula. It is usually viral in children. Increasing air humidity and getting extra rest are effective treatments.

Tonsillitis is usually a viral infection of the tonsils in the oropharynx. In less than 20% of cases, this infection is caused by a streptococcus. A rapid strep test and throat culture are used to identify the strep sore throat or pharyngitis.

Nasopharyngeal carcinoma is a rare form of cancer that occurs mostly in males between the ages of 50 and 60. Treatment includes radiation and chemotherapy.

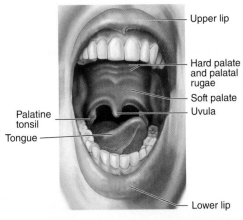

▲ **FIGURE 8.5**
Soft Tissues at the Back of the Mouth.

Case Report 8.2 (continued)

Initially, Mr. Gawlinski was instructed to sleep on his side and to use a device that, through a mask over his nose and mouth, produces a continuous positive airway pressure **(CPAP)** in his airways. He found this very uncomfortable, and it kept him awake. Instead, he chose to have the pillar procedure, in which three tiny pillars were placed in the back of his throat to support the tissues. Subsequently, Mr. Gawlinski has stopped snoring and Mrs. Gawlinski is back in the same bed.

Abbreviation

CPAP continuous positive airway pressure

Word Analysis and Definition

S = Suffix   P = Prefix   R = Root   R/CF = Combining Form

WORD	PRONUNCIATION	ELEMENTS		DEFINITION
adenoid	ADD-eh-noyd	S/ R/	-oid *resembling* aden- *gland*	Single mass of lymphoid tissue in the midline at the back of the throat
apnea	AP-nee-ah	P/ R/	a- *without* -pnea *breathe*	Absence of spontaneous respiration
hypoxemia	high-pock-**SEE**-me-ah	S/ P/ R/	-emia *condition of the blood* hyp- *below* -ox- *oxygen*	Low oxygen level in arterial blood
hypoxia (noun)	high-**POCK**-see-ah	S/	-ia *condition*	Decreased below normal levels of oxygen in tissues, gases, or blood
hypoxic (adj)	high-**POCK**-sik	S/	-ic *pertaining to*	Deficient in oxygen
laryngopharynx	lah-**RIN**-go-**FAH**-rinks	R/CF R/	laryng/o- *larynx* -pharynx *pharynx, throat*	Region of the pharynx below the epiglottis that includes the larynx
nasopharynx	NAY-zoh-**FAH**-rinks	R/CF R/	nas/o- *nose* -pharynx *pharynx, throat*	Region of the pharynx at the back of the nose and above the soft palate
nasopharyngeal (adj)	NAY-zoh-fah-**RIN**-jee-al	S/ R/CF	-eal *pertaining to* -pharyng- *pharynx, throat*	Pertaining to the nasopharynx
oropharynx	OR-oh-fah-rinks	R/CF R/	or/o- *mouth* -pharynx *pharynx, throat*	Region at the back of the mouth between the soft palate and the tip of the epiglottis.
oropharyngeal (adj)	OR-oh-fah-**RIN**-jee-al	S/ R	-eal *pertaining to* -pharyng- *pharynx, throat*	Pertaining to the oropharynx
pharyngitis	fair-in-**JIE**-tis	S/ R/	-itis *inflammation* pharyng- *pharynx, throat*	Inflammation of the pharynx
polysomnography	POLL-ee-som-**NOG**-rah-fee	S/ P/ R/CF	-graphy *process of recording* poly- *many* -somn/o- *sleep*	Test to monitor brain waves, muscle tension, eye movement, and oxygen levels in the blood as the patient sleeps
tonsil	**TON**-sill		Latin *tonsil*	Mass of lymphoid tissue on either side of the throat at the back of the tongue
tonsillitis (Note: *double "ll"*)	ton-sih-**LIE**-tis	S/ R/	-itis *inflammation* tonsill- *tonsil*	Inflammation of the tonsils
tonsillectomy	ton-sih-**LEK**-toh-me	S/	-ectomy *surgical excision*	Surgical removal of the tonsils

EXERCISES

A. Review *the Case Report on this spread before answering the questions.*   **LO 8.2, 8.4, and 8.7** *Understand*

1. What are Mr. Gawlinski's chief complaints? _____

2. What does polysomnography measure? _____

3. If apnea is complete cessation of breathing, what is dyspnea? _____

4. Hypoxia refers to the level of _____ in the blood.

5. Is the answer to question #4 above too high or too low? _____

B. Use the medical terms *from this spread to fill in the blanks.*   **LO 8.2, 8.4, 8.6, and 8.8** *Apply*

1. Two terms that mean "inflammation of" are _____
   and _____.

2. If left untreated, chronic obstructive sleep apnea could cause _____.

3. The medical term for a common sore throat is _____.

4. Surgical excision of the tonsils is _____.

5. Mr. Gawlinski underwent the diagnostic procedure of _____.

6. What is a nonmedical term for question #5 above? _____.

- On December 14, 1799, President George Washington died of an obstructed airway due to acute epiglottitis.

- Croup occurs in children aged 3 months to 5 years.

- Heavy smokers and drinkers have a 200-times greater risk of developing cancer of the larynx.

The Larynx (LO 8.4)

The flow of inhaled air moves on from your pharynx to your **larynx.** The upper opening into the larynx from the oropharynx is called the **glottis.** The spoon-shaped **epiglottis** guards the glottis. When you swallow food, your tongue pushes down the epiglottis to close the glottis and direct the food into the esophagus behind it *(Figure 8.6).* The **thyroid** cartilage, or the Adam's apple, forms the anterior and lateral walls of the larynx. Inside the larynx, two pairs of horizontal ligaments—your **vocal** cords *(Figures 8.7 and 8.8)*—stretch across the lateral walls and enable sounds to be made as air passes between them.

Functions of the Larynx (LO 8.4)

Two major roles of your larynx are:

1. Maintaining an open passage for the movement of air to and from the trachea *(Figure 8.7)* and

2. Producing sounds through the vocal cords.

Sound Production Air moving past the vocal cords makes them vibrate to produce sound. The force of the air moving past the vocal cords determines the loudness of the sound. Muscles in the cords pull them closer together with varying degrees of tautness *(Figure 8.8).* A high-pitched sound is produced by taut cords, and a low-pitched sound is made by more relaxed cords. Males' vocal cords are longer and thicker than those of females. They vibrate more slowly and produce lower-pitched sounds.

The crude sounds produced by the larynx are transformed into words by the actions of the pharynx, tongue, teeth, and lips.

Disorders of the Larynx (LO 8.4 and 8.6)

Laryngitis is an inflammation of the mucosal lining of the larynx, which produces hoarseness and sometimes progresses to a loss of voice.

Epiglottitis is an inflammation of the epiglottis. **Acute epiglottitis** is seen most commonly in children between the ages of 2 and 7 years. It can cause acute airway obstruction, which requires a tube to be inserted into the windpipe **(intubation).** It is preventable by vaccine.

Croup (laryngotracheobronchitis) is a group of viral diseases causing an inflammation and obstruction of the upper airway. It's most common in children between the ages of 3 months and 5 years. In severe cases, a child makes a high-pitched, squeaky, inspiratory noise called **stridor.** Humidity is the initial treatment.

Papillomas or polyps are benign tumors of the larynx due to overuse or irritation. These are surgically removed using a **laryngoscope.**

Carcinoma of the larynx produces a persistent hoarseness. Its incidence peaks among people in their 50s and 60s. Treatment can be radiation and/or chemotherapy.

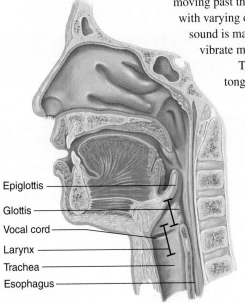

Epiglottis
Glottis
Vocal cord
Larynx
Trachea
Esophagus

▲ **FIGURE 8.6**
Larynx Location.

Epiglottis

Vestibular fold

Vocal cord

Trachea

▲ **FIGURE 8.7**
View of Larynx Using a Laryngoscope.

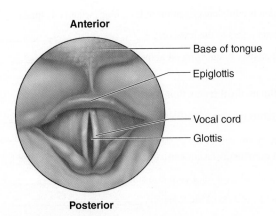

Anterior

Base of tongue

Epiglottis

Vocal cord

Glottis

Posterior

▲ **FIGURE 8.8**
Vocal Cords Pulled Close and Taut.

WORD	PRONUNCIATION		ELEMENTS	DEFINITION
croup (also called laryngotracheobronchitis)	KROOP		Old English to cry out loud	Infection of the upper airways in children characterized by a barking cough
epiglottis	ep-ih-GLOT-is	P/ R/	epi- above -glottis mouth of windpipe	Leaf-shaped plate of cartilage that shuts off the larynx during swallowing
epiglottitis	ep-ih-glot-EYE-tis	S/ R/	-itis inflammation -glott- mouth of windpipe	Inflammation of the epiglottis
glottis	GLOT-is		Greek opening of larynx	The opening from the oropharynx into the larynx
intubation	IN-tyu-BAY-shun	S/ P/ R/	-ation a process in- in -tub- tube	Insertion of a tube into the trachea
laryngotracheobronchitis (also called croup)	lah-RING-oh-TRAY-kee-oh-brong-KIE-tis	S/ R/CF R/CF R/	-itis inflammation laryng/o- larynx -trache/o -trachea -bronch- bronchus	Inflammation of the larynx, trachea, and bronchi
larynx laryngeal (adj)	LAH-rinks lah-RIN-jee-al	S/ R/	Greek larynx -eal pertaining to laryng- larynx	Organ of sound production Pertaining to the larynx
laryngitis	lah-rin-JEYE-tis	S/ R/CF	-itis inflammation laryng/o- larynx	Inflammation of the larynx
laryngoscope	lah-RING-oh-skope	S/	-scope instrument for viewing	Hollow tube with a light and camera used to visualize or operate on the larynx
papilla papillae (pl)	pah-PILL-ah pah-PILL-ee		Latin small pimple	Any small projection
papilloma	pap-ih-LOH-mah	S/ R/CF	-oma tumor, mass papill/o- pimple	Benign projection of epithelial cells
stridor	STRY-door		Latin a harsh, creaking sound	High-pitched noise made when there is a respiratory obstruction in the larynx or trachea
vocal	VOH-kal	S/ R/	-al pertaining to voc- voice	Pertaining to the voice

EXERCISES

Study Hint

Whether the term is 24 letters long or 5 letters long, *the principle is the same:* Know the meaning of the elements, and you will know the meaning of the term!

A. Deconstruction: *For long or short medical terms, deconstruction into word elements is your key to solving the meaning of the term. Follow the directions and fill in the blanks.*
LO 8.1 and 8.4 *Analyze*

1. *laryngotracheobronchitis*

   Slash all the elements of this term. _____ / _____ / _____

2. Combine the meanings of the elements, and define the term.

   _____

3. *vocal*

   Slash all the elements of this term. _____ / _____ / _____

4. Combine the meanings of the elements, and define the term.

   _____

B. Apply *the language of pulmonology to answer the following questions correctly.*   **LO 8.2, 8.4, and 8.7** *Apply*

1. What is another term meaning *croup*? _____

2. What body parts are involved in speech production? _____

3. What is the squeaky noise on *inspiration* termed? _____

4. What is the medical term for a benign tumor of the *larynx*? _____

5. To aid in breathing, what can be inserted into the windpipe? _____

Lesson 8.2

Lower Respiratory Tract

Objectives

Once the air you inhale has passed through the upper airway and many of the pollutants and impurities have been filtered out, the major needs still remain: to get oxygen (O_2) into the blood and remove carbon dioxide (CO_2) from the blood. To make this possible, the inhaled air has to travel into the alveoli of the lungs, where these exchanges can occur. In this lesson, you will learn to use correct medical terminology to:

8.2.1 Trace the passage of air from the larynx into the alveoli and back.

8.2.2 Describe the mechanics of ventilation.

8.2.3 Integrate the functions of the different elements of the lower airway with their structures.

8.2.4 Discuss the effects of common disorders of the lungs on health.

Abbreviations

CO_2	carbon dioxide
O_2	oxygen

Trachea (LO 8.5)

The flow of inhaled air now moves into your trachea (windpipe). This is a rigid tube that descends from the larynx and divides into the two main **bronchi** *(Figure 8.9)*, which serve as airways going to your right and left lungs.

The Lungs (LO 8.5)

Your two lungs are the main organs of respiration and are located in the thoracic cavity. Each lung is a soft, spongy, cone-shaped organ with its **base** resting on the **diaphragm** and its top **(apex)** above and behind the clavicle. Its outer convex, costal surface presses against the **rib cage.** Its inner concave surface presses against the chest region **(mediastinum).**

The right lung has three **lobes:** superior, middle, and inferior. The left lung has two lobes; superior and inferior *(Figure 8.9a)*. Each lobe is separated from the others by **fissures.**

Tracheobronchial Tree (LO 8.5)

The tracheobronchial tree is an upside-down, tree-like structure that conducts air in your chest. It is comprised of the trachea, bronchi, and bronchial tubes. As inhaled air continues down the respiratory tract, the main bronchi divide into a **secondary (lobar)** bronchus for each lobe. Each secondary bronchus then divides into tertiary (third) bronchi that supply **segments** of each lobe *(Figure 8.10)*. These divisions create branch-like airways.

Bronchioles and Alveoli (LO 8.5)

These tertiary bronchi further divide into **bronchioles,** which in turn divide into several thin-walled **alveoli.** Each **alveolus** is a thin-walled sac supported by a thin **respiratory membrane.** This membrane allows the exchange of gases with the surrounding pulmonary capillary network.

The Pleura (LO 8.5)

The **pleura** is a double-layered serous membrane that covers the surface of both lungs. The space between these two layers is called the **pleural cavity,** which contains a thin film of lubricant fluid. This lubricant enables the lungs to expand (inspiration) and deflate (expiration) with minimal friction.

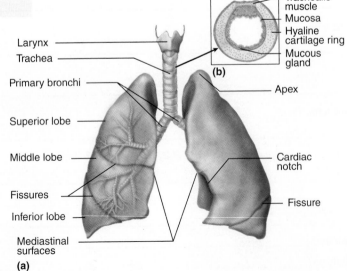

▶ **FIGURE 8.9**
Lower Respiratory Tract.
(a) Gross anatomy.
(b) C-shaped tracheal cartilage.

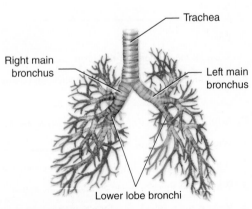

▲ **FIGURE 8.10**
Latex Cast of the Tracheobronchial Tree.

Word Analysis and Definition

WORD	PRONUNCIATION		ELEMENTS	DEFINITION
diaphragm	DIE-ah-fram		Greek *diaphragm*	The muscular sheet separating the abdominal and thoracic cavities
diaphragmatic (adj)	DIE-ah-frag-MAT-ik	S/ R/CF	-tic *pertaining to* diaphragm/a- *diaphragm*	Pertaining to the diaphragm
fissure fissures (pl)	FISH-ur	S/ R/	-ure *process, result of* fiss- *split*	Deep furrow or cleft
lobe lobar (adj)	LOBE LOW-bar	S/ R/	Greek *lobe* -ar *pertaining to* lob- *lobe*	Subdivision of an organ or other part Pertaining to a lobe
lobectomy	low-BECK-toe-me	S/	-ectomy *surgical excision*	Surgical removal of a lobe
mediastinum	ME-dee-ass-TIE-num	S/ P/ R/	-um *structure* media- *middle* -stin- *partition*	Area between the lungs containing the heart, aorta, venae cavae, esophagus, and trachea
mediastinal (adj)	ME-dee-ass-TIE-nal	S/	-al *pertaining to*	Pertaining to the mediastinum
pleura pleurae (pl) pleural (adj)	PLUR-ah PLUR-ee PLUR-al	S/ R/	Greek *rib* -al *pertaining to* pleur- *pleura*	Membrane covering the lungs and lining the ribs in the thoracic cavity Pertaining to the pleura
pleurisy	PLUR-ih-see	S/	-isy *inflammation*	Inflammation of the pleura
segment	SEG-ment		Latin *to cut*	A section of an organ or structure

EXERCISES

A. Precision *in communication means using the correct form of the medical term, as well as the correct spelling. Test your knowledge of plurals, adjectives, and spelling with this exercise. Circle the correct choice.* **LO 8.2, 8.5, and 8.7** *Remember*

1. The median partition of the thoracic cavity is the:

   mediastenum   mediasternum   mediastinum   midiasternum

2. The patient was diagnosed with _____ pneumonia.

   lobe   lobular   lobar   lumbar

3. The _____ tissue was sent to pathology for a diagnosis.

   plural   pleural   ploral   pliral

4. The muscle separating the abdominal and thoracic cavities is the:

   diaphram   diaphragm   diaphracum   diaphragmm

5. Removal of a portion of a lung is a:

   lobotomy   lobectomy   lobarectomy   lobarotomy

Study Hint

Frequent errors are made on test questions regarding the term *pleural*, meaning *pertaining to the pleura*. It is not spelled "plural," which means *more than one*. Be especially careful when dealing with this term, and always check your spelling. Both terms sound alike, are spelled differently, and have very different meanings. *The right answer (pleural) is wrong if it is spelled "plural."* Don't lose points on a test because of carelessness.

B. Meet lesson objectives *and practice the language of pulmonology with your answers below.* **LO 8.2, 8.5, and 8.7** *Apply*

1. Trace the passage of air from the nose into the alveoli. _____

   _____

2. What are the basic components of the lower respiratory tract? _____

   _____

3. Which component of the respiratory system allows exchange of gases? _____

4. What are the two gases that need to be exchanged in the respiratory system? _____

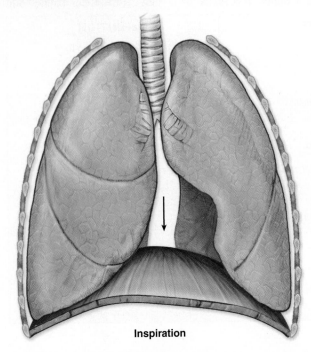

Inspiration

Diaphragm contracts; vertical
dimensions of thoracic cavity increase.

(a)

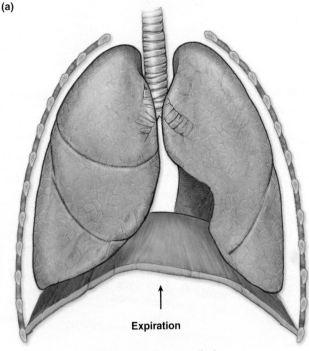

Expiration

Diaphragm relaxes; vertical
dimensions of thoracic cavity decrease.

(b)

▲ **FIGURE 8.11**
Inspiration and Expiration.

A resting adult breathes 10 to 15 times per minute and **inhales** about 500 mL of air during inspiration and **exhales** it during expiration. The mission is to get air into and out of the alveoli so that oxygen can enter the bloodstream and carbon dioxide can exit.

Your diaphragm does most of the work. In inspiration, it drops down and flattens to expand the thoracic cavity and reduce the pressure in the airways. The external intercostal muscles also help by lifting the chest wall up and out to further expand the thoracic cavity *(Figure 8.11a).*

Expiration is a process of letting go. The diaphragm and the intercostal muscles relax, and the thoracic cavity springs back to its original size *(Figure 8.11b).*

Common Signs and Symptoms of Respiratory Disorders (LO 8.4 and 8.5)

The common signs and symptoms of respiratory disorders are often visible and audible, and they include the following:

1. **Cough** is triggered by irritants in the respiratory tract. Irritants include cigarette smoke (as with Mr. Jacobs), infection, or tumors, as in lung cancer. A productive cough produces **sputum,** which can be swallowed or **expectorated.** Bloody sputum is called **hemoptysis.** Thick, yellow **(purulent)** sputum indicates infection. A **nonproductive** cough is dry and hacking.

    Abnormal amounts of mucus arising from the upper respiratory tract and expectorated or coughed up are called **phlegm.**

2. **Dyspnea,** or difficult breathing **(DOB),** can occur from exertion or, in severe disorders, during rest when all the respiratory muscles are used to exchange only a small volume of air.

3. **Cyanosis** is seen when the blood has increased levels of **unoxygenated hemoglobin** and has a characteristic dark red-blue color.

4. **Changes in the rate of breathing** may occur. **Eupnea** is the normal, easy respiration (around 15 breaths per minute) in a resting adult. Both **tachypnea** (rapid rate of breathing) and **hyperpnea** (breathing deeper and more rapidly than normal) are signs of respiratory difficulty, as is **bradypnea** (slow breathing).

5. **Sneezing** is caused by irritants in the nasal cavity.

6. **Hiccups** are reflex spasms of the diaphragm. The etiology is unknown, and there is no specific medical cure.

7. **Yawning** is a reflex that originates in the brainstem in response to hypoxia, boredom, or sleepiness. The exact mechanisms are not known.

Abbreviation

DOB   difficulty of breath

Word Analysis and Definition

S = Suffix   P = Prefix   R = Root   R/CF = Combining Form

WORD	PRONUNCIATION	ELEMENTS		DEFINITION
bradypnea (opposite of **tachypnea**)	brad-ip-**NEE**-ah	P/ R/	brady- *slow* -pnea *breathe*	Slow breathing
cyanosis	sigh-ah-**NO**-sis	S/ R/	-osis *condition* cyan- *dark blue*	Blue discoloration of the skin, lips, and nail beds due to low levels of oxygen in the blood
cyanotic (adj)	sigh-ah-**NOT**-ik	S/ R/CF	-tic *pertaining to* cyan/o *dark blue*	Pertaining to or marked by cyanosis
dyspnea	disp-**NEE**-ah	P/ R/	dys- *bad, difficult* -pnea *breathe*	Difficult breathing
eupnea	yoop-**NEE**-ah	P/ R/	eu- *normal, good* -pnea *breathe*	Normal breathing
exhale	**EKS**-hail	P/ R/	ex- *out* -hale *breathe*	Breathe out
expectorate	ek-**SPEK**-toh-rate	S/ P/ R/	-ate *pertaining to* ex- *out* -pector- *chest*	Cough up and spit out mucus from the respiratory tract
hemoptysis	he-**MOP**-tih-sis	R/CF S/	hem/o- *blood* -ptysis *spit*	Bloody sputum
hyperpnea	high-perp-**NEE**-ah	P/ R/	hyper- *excessive* -pnea *breathe*	Deeper and more rapid breathing than normal
inhale	**IN**-hail	P/ R/	in- *in* -hale *breathe*	Breathe in
phlegm	**FLEM**		Greek *flame*	Abnormal amounts of mucus expectorated from the respiratory tract
tachypnea (opposite of **bradypnea**)	tak-ip-**NEE**-ah	P/ R/	tachy- *rapid* -pnea *breathe*	Rapid breathing

EXERCISES

A. Construct terms: *Knowing just one element will enable you to build more terms with the addition of other elements. Practice building your pulmonology terms with the following root and various prefixes. Fill in the blanks.* **LO 8.1, 8.2, and 8.5** *Apply*

1. The root *pnea* means _____.

Add the following prefixes to the root pnea *to form the new terms.*

tachy   brady   dys   eu   hyper

2. difficult breathing   _____ / pnea

3. deeper breathing than normal   _____ / pnea

4. slow breathing   _____ / pnea

5. normal breathing   _____ / pnea

6. rapid breathing   _____ / pnea

Study Hint

The English word *breath* is a noun and is the air you inhale and exhale. ("Take a deep breath.") The English word *breathe* has an "e" on the end of it and is the verb meaning to *inhale and exhale*. ("She was unable to breathe.").

B. Apply *the language of pulmonology to answer the following questions correctly.* **LO 8.2, 8.4, and 8.5** *Apply*

1. Demonstrate that you can use *breath* and *breathe* correctly. Write a brief sentence for each.

1a. _____

1b. _____

2. How do *exhale* and *inhale* relate to respiration? _____

3. Respiration takes place in which body cavity? _____

Keynotes

- Worldwide, COPD is the third leading cause of death, killing over 3 million people each year.
- COPD affects 330 million people in the world, which is 5% of the population.
- 25% of chronic smokers develop COPD.
- Worldwide, COPD had an economic cost of $2.1 trillion in 2010.
- Tobacco smoking is the most common cause of COPD. Air pollution and genetics play smaller roles.

Abbreviations

CAO	chronic airway obstruction
CF	cystic fibrosis
CHF	congestive heart failure
COPD	chronic obstructive pulmonary disease

Disorders of the Lower Respiratory Tract

(LO 8.3 and 8.5)

There are a number of disorders that are specific to your lower respiratory tract. These disorders are described below.

Acute bronchitis can be viral or bacterial, leading to the production of excess mucus with some obstruction of airflow. It resolves without significant residual damage to the airway.

Chronic bronchitis is the most common obstructive disease, caused by cigarette smoking or repeated episodes of acute bronchitis. Along with excess mucus production, cilia are destroyed. A pattern develops, involving chronic cough, dyspnea, and recurrent acute infections.

In advanced chronic bronchitis, hypoxia and **hypercapnia** (excess carbon dioxide) are produced and heart failure follows.

Bronchiolitis is a viral inflammation of the small airway bronchioles. It occurs in adults as the early and often unrecognized start of airway changes in cigarette smokers or in those exposed to "secondhand smoke." Bronchiolitis also affects children under the age of 2 because their small airways become blocked very easily. In severe cases, this disease can cause noticeable respiratory distress.

Pulmonary emphysema is a disease of the respiratory bronchioles and alveoli. These airways become enlarged, and the septa between the alveoli are destroyed, forming large sacs of air **(bullae).** There is a loss of surface area for gas exchange.

Chronic airway obstruction (CAO) is also called **chronic obstructive pulmonary disease (COPD).** It is a progressive disease, as Mr. Jacobs' history shows. It involves both chronic bronchitis and emphysema. A history of heavy cigarette smoking *(Figure 8.12),* with chronic cough and sputum production, is followed by increasing dyspnea and need for oxygen. Right-sided heart failure (cor pulmonale, *see Chapter 6*) is the end result, due to pulmonary hypertension and backup of blood into the right ventricle.

Bronchiectasis is the abnormal dilation of the small bronchioles due to repeated infections. The damaged, dilated bronchi are unable to clear secretions, making them prone to further infections and increased damage.

Bronchial asthma is a disorder with recurrent acute episodes of bronchial obstruction. This results from a constriction of bronchioles **(bronchoconstriction),** a **hypersecretion** of mucus, and an inflammatory swelling of the bronchiolar lining. Between attacks, breathing can be normal. The etiology of asthma is an allergic response to substances like pollen, animal dander, or the feces of dust mites.

Cystic fibrosis (CF) is a genetic disorder caused by an increased **viscosity** (thickness and stickiness) of secretions from the pancreas, salivary glands, liver, intestine, and lungs. In the lungs, a very thick mucus obstructs the airways and causes repeated infections. Many CF patients die before the age of 30 from respiratory failure.

Pulmonary edema is the collection of fluid in the lung tissues and alveoli. It commonly results from left ventricular failure or mitral valve disease with congestive heart failure **(CHF).**

During **auscultation** (examination by stethoscope) of the chest, the air bubbling through abnormal fluid in the alveoli and small bronchioles, as in pulmonary edema, produces a noise called **rales.** When the bronchi are partly obstructed and air is being forced past the obstruction, a high-pitched noise called a **rhonchus** is heard.

(a)

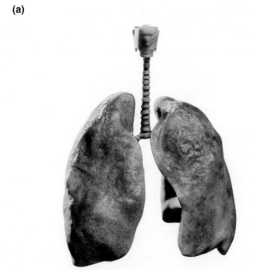

(b)

▲ **FIGURE 8.12**
Whole Lungs.
(a) Lungs of a Non-smoker.
(b) Lungs of a Smoker.

Word Analysis and Definition

WORD	PRONUNCIATION		ELEMENTS	DEFINITION
asthma	AZ-mah		Greek *asthma*	Episodes of breathing difficulty due to narrowed or obstructed airways
asthmatic (adj)	az-MAT-ik	S/ R/	-atic *pertaining to* asthm- *asthma*	Pertaining to or suffering from asthma
auscultation	aws-kul-TAY-shun	S/ R/	-ation *a process* auscult- *listen to*	Diagnostic method of listening to body sounds with a stethoscope
bronchiectasis	brong-key-ECK-tah-sis	S/ R/CF	-ectasis *dilation* bronch/i- *bronchus*	Chronic dilation of the bronchi following inflammatory disease and obstruction
bronchiolitis	brong-key-oh-LYE-tis	S/ R/CF	-itis *inflammation* bronchiol/o *bronchus*	Inflammation of the small bronchioles
bronchitis	brong-KI-tis	S/ R/	-itis *inflammation* bronch- *bronchus*	Inflammation of the bronchi
bronchoconstriction	BRONG-koh-kon-STRIK-shun	S/ R/CF R/	-ion *action, condition* bronch/o- *bronchus* -constrict- *to narrow*	Reduction in diameter of a bronchus
bulla bullae (pl)	BULL-ah BULL-ee		Latin *bubble*	Bubble-like dilated structure
cystic fibrosis	SIS-tik fie-BRO-sis	S/ R/ S/ R/	-ic *pertaining to* cyst- *cyst* -osis *abnormal condition* fibr- *fiber*	Genetic disease in which excessive viscid mucus obstructs passages, including bronchi
emphysema	em-fih-SEE-mah	P/ R/	em- *in, into* -physema *blowing*	Dilation of respiratory bronchioles and alveoli
hypercapnia	HIGH-per-KAP-nee-ah	S/ P/ R/	-ia *condition* hyper- *excessive* -capn- *carbon dioxide*	Abnormal increase of carbon dioxide in the arterial bloodstream
hypersecretion	HIGH-per-seh-KREE-shun	S/ P/ R/	-ion *action, condition* hyper- *excessive* -secret- *secrete*	Excessive secretion of mucus (or enzymes or waste products)
rhonchus rhonchi (pl)	RONG-kuss RONG-key		Greek *snoring*	Wheezing sound heard on auscultation of the lungs; made by air passing through a constricted lumen
viscosity viscous (adj) (cf. **viscus**, *any internal organ*)	viss-KOS-ih-tee VISS-kus	S/ R/	-ity *condition* viscos- *viscous, sticky*	The resistance of a fluid to flow Sticky fluid that is resistant to flow

EXERCISES

A. Elements. *The elements below all appear in the language of pulmonology. Challenge your knowledge of these elements, and make the correct match.*

Fill in the blanks.   **LO 8.1, 8.4, and 8.5** *Understand*

_____ **1.** ectasis	**A.** listen to	
_____ **2.** capn	**B.** sticky	
_____ **3.** physema	**C.** carbon dioxide	
_____ **4.** viscos	**D.** blowing	
_____ **5.** auscult	**E.** small	
_____ **6.** ole	**F.** dilation	

B. Apply *the language of pulmonology to answer the following questions correctly.*   **LO 8.2, 8.5, and 8.7** *Apply*

1. A sticky fluid that is resistant to flow: _____

2. If hypoxia and hypercapnia are both present, what condition will likely follow? _____

3. *Hypercapnia* is excessive _____.

4. *Hypoxia* is deficient _____.

Disorders of the Lower Respiratory Tract (continued)

LO 8.3 and 8.5

Pneumonia *(Figure 8.13)* is an acute infection of the alveoli and lung **parenchyma** (functional cells of the lung). Pneumonia is mostly caused by bacteria or viruses. The alveoli become filled with inflammatory fluid, decreasing the exchange of oxygen and carbon dioxide. **Lobar pneumonia** is an infection limited to one lung lobe. **Bronchopneumonia** is an infection in the bronchioles that spreads to the alveoli.

When an area of the lung **(segment)** or a lobe becomes airless as a result of the infection, the lung is **consolidated.** When an area of the lung collapses as a result of bronchial obstruction, this is called **atelectasis.**

Pleurisy, an inflammation of the pleurae, can be a complication of pneumonia. This condition makes breathing painful because the parietal pleura is very pain-sensitive. The inflammation often leads to fluid accumulating in the pleural cavity. This is a **pleural effusion.** If the pleural effusion contains pus, the condition is called **empyema.** If it contains blood, the condition is called **hemothorax.** When pleural fluid is drawn off for therapeutic reasons or for laboratory analysis, the procedure is **aspiration** or **thoracentesis.**

Lung abscess can be a complication of bacterial pneumonia or cancer. Long-term antibiotics are used, and partial surgical excision of the abscess may be necessary.

Pneumothorax is the entry of air into the pleural cavity *(Figure 8.14)*. The cause can be unknown, called a **spontaneous pneumothorax,** but it often results from trauma when a fractured rib, knife blade, or bullet lacerates the pleura.

Adult respiratory distress syndrome (ARDS) is sudden, life-threatening lung failure caused by a variety of underlying conditions from major trauma to sepsis. The alveoli fill with fluid and collapse, shutting down gas exchange. Hypoxia results. **Mechanical ventilation** is mandatory. The mortality rate is 35% to 50%.

Neonatal respiratory distress syndrome (NRDS) is seen in premature babies whose lungs have not matured enough to produce surfactant, a substance secreted in the lungs. The alveoli collapse, and mechanical ventilation is needed to keep them open.

Chronic infections of the lung parenchyma are the result of prolonged exposure to infection or to occupational irritant dusts or droplets. These disorders are called **pneumoconioses.** Levels of dust inhalation overwhelm the airways' particle-clearing abilities. The dust particles accumulate in the alveoli and parenchyma, leading to fibrosis. **Asbestosis** results from inhaling asbestos particles and can lead to a cancer in the pleura called **mesothelioma. Silicosis** from silica particles is called "stonecutters' disease." **Anthracosis** from coal dust particles is called "coal miners' disease." (**Anthrax** is a different disease, caused by toxins produced by the anthrax bacillus.) **Sarcoidosis** produces lesions and is a fibrotic (scarring) disorder of the lung parenchyma.

Pulmonary tuberculosis is a chronic, infectious disease of the lungs.

Lung cancer, related to tobacco use, was once only a male disease. Now, fatalities in women from lung cancer exceed those from breast cancer. Ninety percent of lung cancers arise in the mucous membranes of the larger bronchi and are called **bronchogenic carcinomas.** A subgroup of bronchogenic carcinomas called **adenocarcinoma** accounts for 30% to 50% of all lung cancers and is the most common in women. The lung cancer obstructs the bronchus, spreads into the surrounding lung tissues, and metastasizes to the lymph nodes, liver, brain, and bone. This disease is associated with cigarette smoking.

Abbreviations

ARDS	adult respiratory distress syndrome
NRDS	neonatal respiratory distress syndrome

▲ **FIGURE 8.13**
Chest X-ray of Patient with Pneumonia in the Lower Lobe of the Left Lung.

▲ **FIGURE 8.14**
Left Pneumothorax.
There are no lung markings seen in the area of the pneumothorax.

Word Analysis and Definition

S = Suffix P = Prefix R = Root R/CF = Combining Form

WORD	PRONUNCIATION	ELEMENTS		DEFINITION
adenocarcinoma	ADD-eh-noh-kar-sih-**NOH**-mah	S/ R/CF R/	-oma *tumor* aden/o- *gland* -carcin- *cancer*	A cancer arising from glandular epithelial cells
anthracosis	an-thra-**KOH**-sis	S/ R/	-osis *condition* anthrac- *coal*	Lung disease caused by the inhalation of coal dust
anthrax	**AN**-thraks		Greek *carbuncle*	A severe, malignant infectious disease
asbestosis	as-bes-**TOE**-sis	S/ R/	-osis *condition* asbest- *asbestos*	Lung disease caused by the inhalation of asbestos particles
aspiration	as-pih-**RAY**-shun	S/ R/	-ion *process* aspirat- *to breathe on*	Removal by suction of fluid or gas from a body cavity
atelectasis	at-el-**ECK**-tah-sis	S/ R/	-ectasis *dilation* atel- *incomplete*	Collapse of part of a lung
bronchogenic	BRONG-koh-**JEN**-ik	S/ R/CF	-genic *creation* bronch/o- *bronchus*	Arising from a bronchus
bronchopneumonia	BRONG-koh-new-**MOH**-nee-ah	S/ R/CF R/	-ia *condition* bronch/o- *bronchus* -pneumon- *air, lung*	Acute inflammation of the walls of smaller bronchioles with spread to lung parenchyma
empyema	EM-pie-**EE**-mah	S/ P/ R/	-ema *quality of, quantity of* em- *in, into* -py- *pus*	Pus in a body cavity, particularly in the pleural cavity
hemothorax	he-moh-**THOR**-ax	R/CF R/	hem/o- *blood* -thorax *chest*	Blood in the pleural cavity
parenchyma	pah-**REN**-ki-mah		Greek *to pour in*	The specific functional cells of a gland or organ (e.g., the lung) that are supported by the connective tissue framework
pneumoconiosis pneumoconioses (pl)	new-moh-koh-nee-**OH**-sis new-moh-koh-nee-**OH**-seez	S/ R/CF R/	-osis *condition* pneum/o- *lung, air* -coni- *dust*	Fibrotic lung disease caused by the inhalation of different dusts
pneumonia pneumonitis (*same as* pneumonia)	new-**MOH**-nee-ah new-moh-**NI**-tis	S/ R/ S/	-ia *condition* pneumon- *lung, air* -itis *inflammation*	Inflammation of the lung parenchyma (tissue)
pneumothorax	new-moh-**THOR**-ax	R/CF R/	pneum/o- *air, lung* -thorax *chest*	Air in the pleural cavity
sarcoidosis (**Note:** *Two suffixes*)	sar-koy-**DOH**-sis	S/ S/ R/	-osis *condition* -oid- *resembling* sarc- *flesh*	Granulomatous lesions of the lungs and other organs; cause is unknown
silicosis	sil-ih-**KOH**-sis	S/ R/	-osis *condition* silic- *silicon, glass*	Fibrotic lung disease from inhaling silica particles
thoracentesis (*same as* pleural tap)	**THOR**-ah-sen-**TEE**-sis	S/ R/	-centesis *to puncture* thora- *chest*	Insertion of a needle into the pleural cavity to withdraw fluid or air
tuberculosis	too-**BER**-kyu-**LOW**-sis	S/ R/	-osis *condition* tubercul- *nodule, swelling, tuberculosis*	Infectious disease that can infect any organ or tissue

EXERCISES

A. Suffixes: *The WAD above contains a lot of suffixes you will see again in other medical terms you will meet in later chapters. Confirm your knowledge of suffixes by filling in the chart with the correct meaning for the element.* **LO 8.1 and 8.2** *Remember*

Suffix	Meaning of Suffix	Medical Term with This Suffix
centesis	1.	2.
oma	3.	4.
osis	5.	6.
ia	7.	8.

Lesson 8.3

Diagnostic and Therapeutic Procedures

Objectives

Specific diagnostic and therapeutic procedures, as well as a wide range of pharmacologic agents, are available to help patients with lung diseases. In this lesson, the information will enable you to use correct medical terminology to:

8.3.1 Identify specific pulmonary function tests (PFTs) and other diagnostic procedures.

8.3.2 Describe common therapeutic procedures.

8.3.3 List different classes of pharmacologic agents and their effects on the lungs.

Keynotes

- Measure pulmonary function with a spirometer, a peak flow meter, and arterial blood gases.

- Bronchoscopy is a procedure for inserting a fiber optic tube into the bronchial tubes to visually examine the tubes, take a tissue biopsy, or do a washing for secretions.

- Mediastinoscopy is used to stage lung cancer and diagnose mediastinal masses. The mediastinoscope is inserted through an incision in the suprasternal notch.

- Thoracentesis is the insertion of a needle through an intercostal space to remove fluid from a pleural effusion for laboratory study or to relieve pressure. The procedure is also called a pleural tap.

Case Report 8.1 (continued)

Mr. Jacobs' forced expiratory volume was only 40% of normal because the fibrotic (scarring) effects of his repeated lung infections had reduced the volume of his airways. When he was off oxygen, his arterial oxygen levels were below 50% of normal. Even with nasal prongs and oxygen, his arterial oxygen levels were still only 75% of normal.

Diagnostic Procedures (LO 8.4, 8.5, and 8.6)

Pulmonary Function Tests (PFTs) (LO 8.4, 8.5, and 8.6)

Pulmonary function can be measured by the following PFTs to estimate the quality of a patient's respiratory function. A **spirometer** is a device for measuring the volume of air that patients move in and out of their respiratory systems. The volume of air expired at the end of the test is the patient's **forced expiratory vital capacity (FVC).** The spirometer also measures **firstflow rates.** For example, the **forced expiratory volume in 1 second (FEV1)** is the amount of air expired in the second of the test.

A **peak flow meter** records the greatest flow of air that can be sustained for 10 milliseconds on forced expiration, the **peak expiratory flow rate (PEFR).** This test is valuable in following the course of asthma, and in postoperative care to monitor the return of lung function after anesthesia.

Arterial blood gases, the measurement of oxygen and carbon dioxide levels in the blood, are good indicators of respiratory function.

A **pulse oximeter** is a sensor placed on the finger to measure the oxygen saturation of the blood.

Other Diagnostic Procedures (LO 8.4, 8.5, and 8.6)

Chest x-ray (CXR) is a radiographic image of the chest taken in **anteroposterior (AP), posteroanterior (PA),** lateral, and sometimes oblique and lateral decubitus positions.

Computed tomography (CT), angiography of the pulmonary circulation using contrast materials, **magnetic resonance angiography (MRA)** to define emboli in the pulmonary arteries, and **ultrasonography** of the pleural space are chest-imaging techniques in modern use. **Positron emission tomography (PET)** can sometimes distinguish benign from malignant lesions.

Tracheal aspiration uses a soft catheter that allows brushings and washings to be performed to remove cells and secretions from the trachea and main bronchi. The catheter can be passed through a tracheostomy or **endotracheal** (windpipe) tube, or through the mouth and nose.

Percutaneous transthoracic needle aspiration is the insertion of a needle with a cutting chamber through an intercostal space (between the ribs) to take a specimen of parietal pleura for examination.

Thoracotomy is used to obtain an open biopsy of tissue from the lung, hilum, pleura, or mediastinum. It is performed through an intercostal incision under general anesthesia.

Abbreviations

AP	anteroposterior	FVC	forced vital capacity	PEFR	peak expiratory flow rate
CT	computed tomography	MRA	magnetic resonance angiography	PET	positron emission tomography
CXR	chest x-ray	PA	posteroanterior	PFTs	pulmonary function tests
FEV1	forced expiratory volume in 1 second				

Word Analysis and Definition

S = Suffix   P = Prefix   R = Root   R/CF = Combining Form

WORD	PRONUNCIATION	ELEMENTS		DEFINITION
bronchoscopy	brong-**KOS**-koh-pee	S/ R/CF	-scopy *to examine, view* bronch/o *bronchus*	Examination of the interior of the tracheobronchial tree with an endoscope
bronchoscope	**BRONG**-koh-skope	S/	-scope *instrument for viewing*	Endoscope used for bronchoscopy
endotracheal	en-doh-**TRAY**-kee-al	S/ P/ R/	-al *pertaining to* endo- *inside* -trache- *trachea*	Pertaining to being inside the trachea
mediastinoscopy	**ME**-dee-ass-tih-**NOS**-koh-pee	S/ R/CF	-scopy *to examine, view* mediastin/o *mediastinum*	Examination of the mediastinum using an endoscope
spirometer	spy-**ROM**-eh-ter	S/ R/CF	-meter *measure* spir/o- *to breathe*	An instrument used to measure respiratory volumes
spirometry	spy-**ROM**-eh-tree	S/	-metry *process of measuring*	Use of a spirometer
thoracotomy	thor-ah-**KOT**-oh-me	S/ R/CF	-tomy *surgical incision* thorac/o *chest*	Incision through the chest wall
tomography	toe-**MOG**-rah-fee	S/ R/CF	-graphy *process of recording* tom/o- *cut, slice, layer*	Radiographic image of a selected slice of tissue
transthoracic	tranz-thor-**ASS**-ik	S/ P/ R/	-ic *pertaining to* trans- *across* -thorac- *chest*	Going through the chest wall
ultrasonography	**UL**-trah-soh-**NOG**-rah-fee	S/ P/ R/CF	-graphy *process of recording* ultra- *beyond* -son/o- *sound*	Delineation of deep structures using sound waves

EXERCISES

A. Review *the Case Report on this spread before answering the questions.*   **LO 8.2, 8.5, 8.6, and 8.7** *Understand*

1. Where can you substitute an abbreviation in the Case Report? _____

2. In what blood vessels is O_2 measured? _____

3. What is the noun form for *fibrotic?* _____

4. What has reduced the volume of Mr. Jacobs' airways? _____

5. Will supplemental oxygen improve Mr. Jacobs' condition 100%? _____

6. What is a medical term for *scarred* tissue? _____

7. Reference a keynote and define the location of the suprasternal notch. _____

_____

B. Abbreviations *are helpful only if you know how to interpret them. This exercise asks questions about the abbreviations in the Abbreviations box on this*
   spread. Your knowledge of the language of pulmonology will assist you. Fill in the blanks.   **LO 8.2, 8.3, and 8.6** *Apply*

1. Insert the abbreviations that are directional terms.

_____

2. List the abbreviations that stand for diagnostic radiological procedures.

_____

3. Name the abbreviations that are measurements of PFTs.

_____

4. Write a sentence (that is not directly out of the text) using any of the abbreviations listed on the left-hand page.

_____

_____

Lesson 8.3(cont'd) Therapeutic Procedures
(LO 8.6)

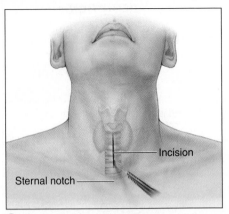

① Tracheotomy incision is made superior to sternal notch.

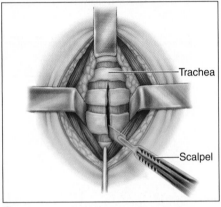

② Retractors separate the tissue, and an incision is made through the third and fourth tracheal rings.

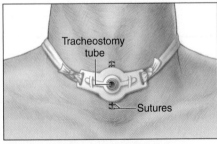

③ A tracheostomy tube is inserted, and the remaining incision is sutured closed.

▲ **FIGURE 8.15**
Tracheostomy Procedure.

Abbreviations

CPAP	continuous positive airway pressure
PDT	postural drainage therapy
PEEP	positive end expiratory pressure

Many effective therapeutic procedures are available for successfully treating pulmonary function disorders. These procedures are outlined below.

Pulmonary rehabilitation includes education, breathing exercises and retraining, exercises for the upper and lower extremities, and psychosocial support.

Nutritional support is critical for patients who have difficulty breathing, or who need to lose or have lost a lot of weight.

Immunizations are available against influenza and the pneumococcus bacterium—the most common cause of bacterial pneumonia.

Postural drainage therapy (PDT) uses gravity (by positioning and tilting the patient) to promote the drainage of secretions from lung segments. Chest **percussion** (tapping) on the chest wall can help loosen, mobilize, and drain any retained secretions. These two procedures are part of **chest physiotherapy.**

Constant positive airway pressure (CPAP) is an attempt to keep alveoli open by maintaining a positive pressure in the airways. A mask is fitted over the patient's nose and mouth and attached to a **ventilator.** This can be used at night when sleeping or for acute situations in COPD.

Positive end expiratory pressure (PEEP) is a ventilation technique to keep the alveoli from collapsing in ARDS and neonatal respiratory distress syndrome.

An **oropharyngeal airway** is used in the unconscious patient during bag and mask ventilation to maintain an open airway. A tube is inserted to prevent the tongue from falling back and obstructing the airway and to facilitate suctioning the airway. An **endotracheal intubation** involves the placement of a tube into the trachea. This allows the patient to be placed on a ventilator so his or her breathing can be controlled.

Pulmonary resection is the surgical removal of lung tissue.

- **Wedge resection** is the removal of a small, localized area of diseased lung.
- **Segmental resection** is the removal of lung tissue attached to a bronchiole.
- **Lobectomy** is the removal of a lobe.
- **Pneumonectomy** is the removal of an entire lung.

Tracheotomy is an incision made into the trachea (windpipe) so that a temporary or permanent opening into the windpipe, called a **tracheostomy,** is created (*Figure 8.15*). A tube is placed into the opening to provide an airway. A tracheostomy is used to maintain an airway when there is obstruction or paralysis in the respiratory structures above it.

Mechanical ventilation is a process involving the movement of gases into and out of the lungs via a device programmed to meet the patient's respiratory requirements. A tracheostomy or endotracheal tube must be attached to the mechanical device (**ventilator**). This procedure can augment or replace the patient's own **ventilatory** efforts.

Pulmonary Pharmacology (LO 8.6)

- **Bronchodilators** relax the smooth muscles of the bronchioles. Examples are theophylline, beta2-agonists such as salbutamol and terbutaline, and anticholinergics such as ipratropium bromide.

- **Anti-inflammatory** drugs, such as corticosteroids, are best given by inhalation, but can be used orally or intravenously in acute episodes of asthma or COPD.

- **Mucolytics** are agents that attempt to break up mucus so it can be cleared more effectively from the airways. Examples are guaifenesin (common in over-the-counter cough medications), potassium iodide, and N-acetylcysteine taken through a **nebulizer.**

- **Antibiotics** are used when a bacterial infection is present. Penicillin, erythromycin, cefotaxime, and flucloxacillin are frequently used.

- **Oxygen** is used in hypoxemia and can be given by nasal **cannula** or by mask and intubation. Patients with severe, chronic COPD can be attached to a portable oxygen cylinder.

Word Analysis and Definition

WORD	PRONUNCIATION	ELEMENTS		DEFINITION
bronchodilator	BRONG-koh-die-LAY-tor	S/ R/CF R/	-or *one who does, that which does something* bronch/o- *bronchus* -dilat- *expand, open up*	Agent that increases the diameter of a bronchus
cannula	KAN-you-lah		Latin *reed*	Tube inserted into a blood vessel or cavity as a channel for fluid or gas
immunization	im-you-nih-ZAY-shun	S/ R/	-ation *process* immuniz- *make immune*	Administration of an agent to provide immunity
mucolytic	MYU-koh-LIT-ik	S/ R/CF R/	-ic *pertaining to* muc/o- *mucus* -lyt- *dissolve*	Agent capable of dissolving or liquefying mucus
nebulizer	NEB-you-liz-er	S/ R/	-izer *line of action, affects in a particular way* nebul- *cloud*	Device used to deliver liquid medicine in a fine mist
pneumonectomy	NEW-moh-NECK-toe-me	S/ R/	-ectomy *surgical excision* pneumon- *lung, air*	Surgical removal of a lung
resection resect (verb)	ree-SEK-shun ree-SEKT	S/ P/ R/	-ion *action, condition* re- *back* -sect- *cut off*	Removal of a specific part of an organ or structure
tracheostomy tracheotomy	tray-kee-OST-oh-me tray-kee-OT-oh-me	S/ R/CF S/	-stomy *new opening* trache/o- *trachea* -tomy *surgical incision*	Insertion of a tube into the windpipe to assist breathing Incision made into the trachea to create a tracheostomy
ventilation ventilator	ven-tih-LAY-shun VEN-tih-lay-tor	S/ R/ S/	-ation *a process* ventil- *wind* -ator *person or thing that does something*	Movement of gases into and out of the lungs Device that breathes for the patient

EXERCISES

A. Deconstruct: *Define the elements, and then use any two terms in one sentence each (that is not directly out of the text) to demonstrate that you understand the term's meaning. Fill in the blanks.*   **LO 8.1 and 8.6** *Analyze*

Medical Term	Meaning of Prefix	Meaning of Root/CF	Meaning of Suffix
immunization	1.	2.	3.
nebulizer	4.	5.	6.
mucolytic	7.	8.	9.
bronchodilator	10.	11.	12.

13. _____

_____

14. _____

_____

B. Meet lesson and chapter objectives *by applying the language of pulmonology to answer the following questions correctly.*   **LO 8.2, 8.6, and 8.7** *Apply*

1. Describe the process of *mechanical ventilation.* _____

_____

_____

2. What is the difference between *antibiotic* and *anti-inflammatory* medication? _____

_____

_____

3. A *tracheotomy* creates an opening. What goes in that opening? _____

4. What is the medical term for the *windpipe*? _____

Chapter Review exercises, along with additional practice items, are available in Connect!

The Digestive System

The Essentials of the Language of Gastroenterology

CHAPTER 9

Case Report 9.1

You are . . .

. . . a medical transcriptionist at Fulwood Medical Center.

You are communicating with . . .

. . . one of Fulwood's physicians, Dr. Stewart Walsh, who has dictated this letter to request authorization for a surgical procedure:

Fulwood Medical Center
3333 Medical Parkway, Fulwood, MI 01234
555-247-6100

Center for Bariatric Surgery

Charles Leavenworth, MD
Medical Director
Lombard Insurance Company
One Lombard Place
Haverson, MI 01233

10/06/11
Request for authorization of surgery
Mrs. Martha Jones   Subscriber ID: 056437

Dear Doctor Leavenworth,
Mrs. Jones is a 52-year-old former waitress, recently divorced. She is 5 feet 4 inches tall and weighs 275 pounds. She has type 2 diabetes with frequent episodes of hypoglycemia and also ketoacidosis, requiring three different hospitalizations. She now has diabetic retinopathy and peripheral vasculitis. Complicating this are hypertension (185/110), coronary artery disease, and pulmonary edema. In spite of monthly meetings with our nutritionist, she has gained 25 pounds in the past six months.

To reduce and control her weight, I am proposing to perform a gastric bypass using a laparoscopic approach. We will need to admit her two days prior to surgery to control her blood sugar and cardiovascular problems, and we anticipate that she will remain in the hospital for two days after surgery, barring any complications. She is also very aware of the necessary follow-up to the procedure and the counseling required for a new lifestyle.

We believe not only that this is an essential procedure medically but that it will reduce in the long term the financial burden of her multiple therapies and improve the quality of the patient's life. Enclosed is supportive documentation of her current history and medical problems.

Your company has designated our hospital as a Center of Excellence for bariatric surgery, and I look forward to your prompt agreement with this approach for this patient.

Sincerely,

Stewart Walsh, MD, FACS
Chief of Surgery

Learning Outcomes

As a medical transcriptionist (MT), your job is to accurately transcribe the voice-recorded reports of physicians and any other health care professionals into readable text. To ensure that Mrs. Jones receives the best possible care, you and the health care professionals directly and indirectly involved with her care, need to be able to:

LO 9.1 Use roots, combining forms, suffixes, and prefixes to construct and analyze medical terms related to the digestive system.

LO 9.2 Spell and pronounce correctly medical terms related to the digestive system in order to communicate them with accuracy and precision in any health care setting.

LO 9.3 Define accepted abbreviations related to the digestive system.

LO 9.4 Relate the overall anatomy of the alimentary canal to the actions and functions of digestion.

LO 9.5 Describe the anatomy of the mouth, pharynx, and esophagus; their roles in mastication and swallowing; and their disorders.

LO 9.6 Relate the anatomy of the stomach and small intestine to the digestion that takes place therein and their disorders.

LO 9.7 Explain the anatomy and roles of the liver, gallbladder, and pancreas in digestion and their disorders related to digestion.

LO 9.8 Describe the overall process of digestion and the malabsorption syndromes.

LO 9.9 Relate the anatomy of the large intestine to its functions and disorders.

LO 9.10 Describe the diagnostic and therapeutic procedures and pharmacologic agents used for disorders of the digestive system.

LO 9.11 Apply your knowledge of the medical terms of the digestive system to documentation, medical records, and medical reports.

LO 9.12 Translate the medical terms of the digestive system into everyday language in order to communicate clearly with patients and their families.

In your future career, being able to communicate comfortably, accurately, and effectively with the health professionals involved in the diagnosis and treatment of problems in the **gastroenterological** system is key. You may work directly and/or indirectly with one or more of the following:

- **Gastroenterologists** are medical specialists in the field of gastroenterology.
- **Proctologists** are surgical specialists in diseases of the anus and rectum.
- **Dentists** are qualified practitioners in the anatomy, physiology, and pathology of the oral-facial complex.
- **Periodontists** are specialists in disorders of the tissues surrounding the teeth.
- **Nutritionists** are professionals who prevent and treat illness by promoting healthy eating habits.
- **Dietitians** manage food services systems and promote sound eating habits.

Objectives

There are basic terms and elements of medical terminology that apply throughout the different parts of the digestive system. Understanding these basic terms and elements of the digestive system will enable you to use correct medical terminology to:

9.1.1 Name the health professionals involved in gastroenterology.

9.1.2 List the organs and accessory organs of the digestive system.

9.1.3 Identify the components of the alimentary canal.

9.1.4 Describe the structure and functions of the digestive system.

Lesson 9.1

The Digestive System

Case Report 9.1 (continued)

In Mrs. Jones's case, the **gastric** bypass procedure reduced the size of her stomach from 2 quarts to 2 ounces. The bypass was taken to the mid-ileum (middle part of the small intestine). This resulted in her being able to eat less and to absorb less. She had no complications from the **laparoscopic** procedure and lost 15 pounds in the 2 months that followed.

Alimentary Canal and Accessory Organs (LO 9.4)

Every cell in your body requires a constant supply of nourishment in a form that can be absorbed across its cell membrane. The **digestive system** breaks down the **nutrients** in food into elements that can be transported to the cells via the blood and lymphatics.

The digestive system consists of the **alimentary canal,** or digestive tract, which extends from the mouth to the **anus,** and **accessory organs** connected to the canal to assist in digestion.

Gastroenterology is the study of the digestive system.

The **alimentary canal** *(Figure 9.1)* includes the:

- **Mouth**
- **Pharynx**
- **Esophagus**
- **Stomach**
- **Small intestine**
- **Large intestine**

The **accessory organs** of digestion include the:

- **Teeth**
- **Tongue**
- **Salivary glands**
- **Liver**
- **Gallbladder**
- **Pancreas**

▲ **FIGURE 9.1**
Alimentary Canal.

Word Analysis and Definition

WORD	PRONUNCIATION	ELEMENTS		DEFINITION
alimentary	al-ih-**MEN**-tar-ee	S/ R/	-ary *pertaining to* aliment- *nourishment, food*	Pertaining to the digestive tract
alimentary canal	kah-**NAL**		canal, Latin *a duct or channel*	Digestive tract
anus	**A**-nus		Latin *a ring*	Terminal opening of the digestive tract through which feces are discharged
anal (adj)	**A**-nal	S/ R/	-al *pertaining to* an- *anus*	Pertaining to the anus
bariatric	bar-ee-**AT**-rik	S/ R/	-atric *treatment* bari- *weight*	Treatment of obesity
digestion	die-**JESS**-chun	S/ R/	-ion *action* digest- *to break down food*	Breakdown of food into elements suitable for cell metabolism
digestive (adj)	die-**JEST**-iv	S/	-ive *nature of, quality of*	Pertaining to digestion
esophagus	ee-**SOF**-ah-gus		Greek *gullet*	Tube linking the pharynx and the stomach
gastric (adj)	**GAS**-trik	S/ R/	-ic *pertaining to* gastr- *stomach*	Pertaining to the stomach
gastroenterology	**GAS**-troh-en-ter-**OL**-oh-gee	S/ R/CF R/CF	-logy *study of* gastr/o- *stomach* -enter/o- *intestine*	Medical specialty of the stomach and intestines
gastroenterologist	**GAS**-troh-en-ter-**OL**-oh-jist	S/	-logist *one who studies, specialist*	Medical specialist in gastroenterology
gastrointestinal	**GAS**-troh-in-**TESS**-tin-al	S/ R/CF R/	-al *pertaining to* gastr/o- *stomach* intestin- *gut, intestine*	Pertaining to the stomach and intestines
intestine	in-**TESS**-tin		Latin *intestine, gut*	The digestive tube from stomach to anus
intestinal (adj)	in-**TESS**-tin-al	S/ R/	-al *pertaining to* intestin- *gut, intestine*	Pertaining to the intestines
laparoscopy	lap-ah-**ROS**-koh-pee	S/ R/CF	-scopy *to view, to examine* lapar/o- *abdomen in general*	Examination of contents of abdomen using an endoscope
laparoscope	**LAP**-ah-roh-skope	S/	-scope *instrument for viewing*	Instrument (endoscope) used for viewing abdominal contents
laparoscopic (adj)	**LAP**-ah-roh-**SKOP**-ik	S/	-ic *pertaining to*	Pertaining to laparoscopy
nutrient	**NYU**-tree-ent		Latin *to nourish*	A substance in food required for normal physiologic function
nutritive (adj)	**NYU**-trih-tiv	S/ R/	-ive *nature of, pertaining to* nutrit- *nourishment*	Providing nourishment
nutrition	nyu-**TRISH**-un	S/	-ion *action, condition*	The study of food and liquid requirements for normal function of the human body
nutritionist	nyu-**TRISH**-un-ist	S/	-ist *specialist in*	Certified professional in nutrition science

EXERCISES

A. Review *the Case Report on this, and the chapter opening, spread before answering the questions.*   **LO 9.2, 9.4, 9.10, and 9.11** *Understand*

1. What is the term for the type of surgery being proposed for Mrs. Jones? _____

2. What is the difference between hypoglycemia and hypertension? _____

_____

3. What disease has previously caused Mrs. Jones to be hospitalized? _____

4. What are her complications from the disease in question 3? _____

_____

5. Why does she need to be admitted 2 days prior to her surgery? _____

B. Analyzing *elements can tell you a lot about a medical term. Look closely at the following medical terms, and let the elements be your guide. Review the WAD before you start the exercise. Fill in the blanks.*   **LO 9.1 and 9.4** *Analyze*

gastric   gastroenterology   gastrointestinal   gastroenterologist   gastroscope

1. Based on the root, the term *gastric* pertains to the _____.

2. Analyzing the two combining forms, the term *gastroenterology* pertains to the _____ and the _____.

3. In the term *gastrointestinal*, the root *intestin-* has the same meaning as the combining form _____ in *gastroenterology*.

4. A *gastroscope* would be inserted into the _____ for examination or biopsy.

- Digestion is both mechanical and chemical.
- Water liquefies the food to make it easier to digest and absorb.
- Enzymes break down the food.

Actions and Functions of the Digestive System (LO 9.4)

The actions and functions of your digestive system have these five components:

1. **Propulsion:** The mechanical movement of food from the mouth to the anus *(Figure 9.2).* Normally, this takes 24 to 36 hours.

2. **Digestion:** The breakdown of foods into forms that can be transported to cells and absorbed into these cells. This process has two parts:

    a. **Mechanical digestion** breaks larger pieces of food into smaller ones without altering their chemical composition. **Mastication** (chewing) breaks down the food into smaller particles so that digestive **enzymes** have a larger surface area with which to interact. **Deglutition** (swallowing) moves the **bolus** (mass or lump) of food from the mouth into the esophagus. **Peristalsis** (waves of contraction and relaxation) moves food material through most of the alimentary canal.

    b. **Chemical** digestion breaks down large molecules of food into smaller and simpler chemicals by way of digestive enzymes (made by the salivary glands, stomach, small intestine, and pancreas). The digestive enzymes have three main groups:

    - **Amylases,** which digest carbohydrates
    - **Lipases,** which digest fats
    - **Proteases,** which digest proteins

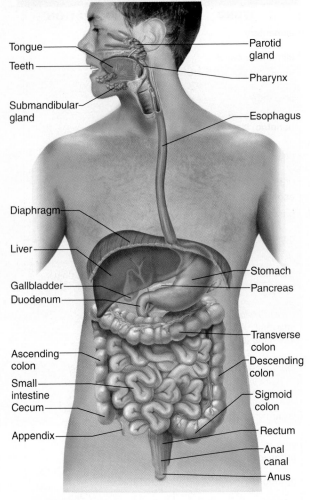

▲ **FIGURE 9.2**
The Digestive System.

3. **Secretion:** The addition of secretions like mucus that lubricate, liquefy, and digest food throughout the digestive tract, while also keeping the tract's lining lubricated.

4. **Absorption:** The movement of nutrient molecules out of the digestive tract, through the epithelial cells lining the tract, and into the blood or lymph for transportation to body cells.

5. **Elimination:** The process by which the body removes undigested food residue.

Word Analysis and Definition

S = Suffix   P = Prefix   R = Root   R/CF = Combining Form

WORD	PRONUNCIATION	ELEMENTS		DEFINITION
amylase	**AM**-ih-laze	S/ R/	-ase *enzyme* amyl- *starch*	One of a group of enzymes that breaks down starch
bolus	**BOH**-lus		Greek *lump*	A single mass of a substance
deglutition	dee-glue-**TISH**-un	S/ R/	-ion *action, condition* deglutit- *to swallow*	The act of swallowing
elimination	ee-lim-ih-**NAY**-shun	S/ R/	-ation *process* elimin- *throw away*	Removal of waste material from the digestive tract
enzyme	**EN**-zime	P/ R/	en- *in* -zyme *fermenting*	Protein that induces changes in other substances
lipase	**LIE**-paze	S/ R/	-ase *enzyme* lip- *fat*	Enzyme that breaks down fat
masticate (verb)	**MAS**-tih-kate	S/ R/	-ate *pertaining to, composed of* mastic- *chew*	To chew
mastication (noun)	mas-tih-**KAY**-shun	S/	-ation *process*	The process of chewing
peristalsis	per-ih-**STAL**-sis	P/ R/	peri- *around* -stalsis *constrict*	Waves of alternate contraction and relaxation of the intestinal wall to move food along the digestive tract
protease	**PRO**-tee-aze	S/ R/CF	-ase *enzyme* prot/e- *protein*	Group of enzymes that breaks down protein

EXERCISES

A. Match *the correct medical term in column 2 to the definition in column 1. The body process, or action, is described for you below. Fill in the blanks.*

   LO 9.4 and 9.8 *Understand*

_____ **1.** swallowing   **A.** mastication

_____ **2.** releasing products of metabolism   **B.** elimination

_____ **3.** chewing   **C.** deglutition

_____ **4.** removal of waste material   **D.** secretion

B. Review *the text to obtain answers to the following questions.*   **LO 9.4 and 9.8** *Understand*

1. What is the mechanical movement of food from mouth to anus called? _____

2. Which organs produce digestive enzymes? _____

3. What lubricates the food in the digestive tract? _____

4. What liquefies the food in the digestive tract? _____

5. What breaks down food in the digestive tract? _____

6. Which body process removes undigested food residue? _____

C. Meet chapter and lesson objectives *by explaining to a fellow student the difference between mechanical and chemical digestion. Be sure to include the appropriate medical terms in your explanation.*   **LO 9.4, 9.8, and 9.11** *Apply*

1. Medical digestion: _____

_____

_____

2. Chemical digestion: _____

_____

_____

3. List here all the medical terms you have included in your explanations: _____

_____

_____

Lesson 9.2

Mouth, Pharynx, and Esophagus

Objectives

When you pop a piece of chicken and some vegetables into your mouth, you start a cascade of digestive tract events that will occur during the next 24 to 36 hours. In this chapter, you will follow the food as it moves through the digestive tract. And in this lesson, you will become familiar with the first stages in the cascade of events, when the food is in the mouth and then swallowed. The information in this lesson will enable you to use correct medical terminology to:

9.2.1 Identify the structures and functions of the teeth, tongue, and salivary glands.

9.2.2 Document the processes and outcomes of mastication and deglutition.

9.2.3 Describe the structures, functions, and disorders of the mouth, pharynx, and esophagus.

The Mouth and Mastication (LO 9.5)

Your **mouth** *(Figure 9.3)* is the gateway to your digestive tract. It's the first site of mechanical digestion, through mastication (chewing), and of chemical digestion, through an **enzyme** in your **saliva.**

The roof of your mouth is called the **palate,** and its anterior two-thirds is the bony **hard palate.** The posterior one-third is the muscular **soft palate.** The skeletal muscle of the soft palate has a projection or flap called the **uvula,** which closes off the **nasopharynx** (upper pharynx) when swallowing.

Your **tongue** moves food around your mouth and helps the cheeks, lips, and gums hold food in place while you chew it. Small, rough, raised areas on the tongue, called **papillae,** contain some 4,000 taste buds that react to the chemical nature of food to give you different taste sensations *(Figure 9.4).* A taste-bud cell lives for 7 to 10 days before it's replaced.

Adult Teeth (LO 9.5)

The average adult has 32 teeth—16 rooted in the upper jaw (maxilla) and 16 in the lower jaw (mandible) *(Figure 9.3).* The bulk of a tooth is composed of

dentine (also spelled *dentin*), a substance like bone but harder, that is covered in **enamel.** The dentine surrounds a central **pulp** cavity, containing blood vessels, nerves, and connective tissue. The blood vessels and nerves reach this cavity from the jaw through tubular root canals.

Salivary Glands (LO 9.5)

Salivary glands secrete saliva. The two **parotid** glands (beside the ears), the two **submandibular** glands (beneath the mandible), the two **sublingual** glands (beneath the tongue) *(Figure 9.5),* and numerous minor salivary glands scattered in the mucosa of the tongue and cheeks secrete more than a quart of saliva daily.

Saliva is 95% water, and its major functions are to begin the digestion of starch and fat and to lubricate food so it's easier to swallow. Imagine you are eating a piece of chicken and some vegetables. By **mastication,** the chicken has been torn and ground into small pieces by your teeth, and its fat has begun to be digested by the lipase in your saliva. The vegetables have also been ground into small pieces, and their starch has begun to be digested by the amylase in your saliva.

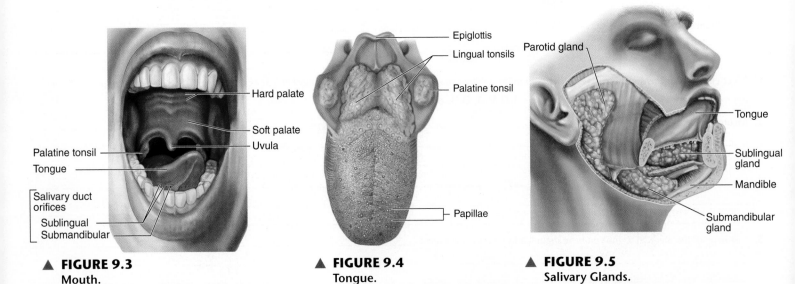

▲ **FIGURE 9.3**
Mouth.

▲ **FIGURE 9.4**
Tongue.

▲ **FIGURE 9.5**
Salivary Glands.

Word Analysis and Definition

WORD	PRONUNCIATION	ELEMENTS		DEFINITION
dentine (*also spelled* **dentin**)	**DEN**-tin	S/ R/	-ine *pertaining to, substance* dent- *tooth*	Dense, ivory-like substance located under the enamel in a tooth
dentist	**DEN**-tist	S/ R/	-ist *specialist* dent- *tooth*	A qualified practitioner in the anatomy, physiology, and pathology of the oral-facial complex
enamel	ee-**NAM**-el		French *enamel*	Hard substance covering a tooth
mastication (noun)	mass-tih-**KAY**-shun	S/ R/	-ation *process* mastic- *chew*	The process of chewing
masticate (verb)	**MASS**-tih-kate	S/	-ate *pertaining to*	To chew
mouth	**MOWTH**		Old English *mouth*	External opening of a cavity or canal
nasopharynx	**NAY**-zoh-**FAIR**-inks	R/CF R/	nas/o- *nose* -pharynx *throat*	Region of the pharynx at the back of the nose and above the soft palate
oral	**OR**-al	S/ R/	-al *pertaining to* or- (os) *mouth*	Pertaining to the mouth
palate	**PAL**-at		Latin *palate*	Roof of the mouth
papilla papillae (pl)	pah-**PILL**-ah pah-**PILL**-ee		Latin *small pimple*	Any small projection
parotid	pah-**ROT**-id	S/ P/ R/	-id *having a particular quality* par- *beside* -ot- *ear*	The parotid gland is the salivary gland beside the ear
pulp	**PULP**		Latin *flesh*	Dental pulp is the connective tissue in the cavity in the center of the tooth
saliva (noun) salivary (adj)	sa-**LIE**-vah **SAL**-ih-var-ee	 S/ R/	Latin *spit* -ary *pertaining to* saliv- *saliva*	Secretion in mouth from salivary glands Pertaining to saliva
sublingual	sub-**LING**-wal	S/ P/ R/	-al *pertaining to* sub- *underneath* -lingu- *tongue*	Underneath the tongue
submandibular	sub-man-**DIB**-you-lar	S/ P/ R/	-ar *pertaining to* sub- *underneath* -mandibul- *mandible*	Underneath the mandible
tongue	**TUNG**		Latin *tongue*	Mobile muscle mass in the mouth; bears the taste buds
uvula	**YOU**-vyu-lah		Latin *grape*	Fleshy projection of the soft palate

EXERCISES

A. Apply *your knowledge of the same elements to various terms, and increase your medical vocabulary. Focus on what is the same and what is different about the following terms. Fill in the chart.*   **LO 9.1, 9.2, and 9.5** *Apply*

Medical Term	Meaning of Prefix	Meaning of Root	Meaning of Suffix	Meaning of Term
submandibular	1.	2.	3.	4.
sublingual	5.	6.	7.	8.
subcutaneous (from Chapter 3)	9.	10.	11.	12.

B. Answer *the following questions based on the above chart.*   **LO 9.1, 9.2, and 9.5** *Analyze*

1. What is similar about every term? _____

2. Which element makes every term different? _____

3. Do all these terms describe size, number, or location? _____

Lesson 9.2 (cont'd)

- **Cleft palate** is a congenital fissure in the median line of the palate. It is often associated with a cleft lip.

- **Glossodynia** is a painful, burning sensation of the tongue. It occurs in postmenopausal women. Its etiology is unknown. There is no successful treatment.

- **Periodontal disease** is thought to be associated with coronary artery disease, but no causal relationship has been established.

Abbreviation

HSV-1   Herpes simplex virus, type 1

Disorders of the Mouth
(LO 9.5)

The human mouth is the entrance to the digestive system, and since so many elements pass through it, the human mouth is prone to tooth disorders and a host of other conditions.

A buildup of **dental plaque** (a collection of oral microorganisms and their products), or **tartar** (calcified deposits at the margin of the teeth along the gums), is a precursor to invasion by dental disease-causing bacteria.

Dental caries, which are tooth decay and cavity formation, are erosions of the tooth surface caused by bacteria *(Figure 9.6)*. If untreated, it can lead to an abscess at the root of the tooth. **Gingivitis** is an infection of the gums. **Periodontal disease** occurs when the gums and the jawbone are involved in a disease process. In **periodontitis,** infection causes the gums to pull away from the teeth, forming pockets that become sources of infection that can spread to underlying bone. Infection of the gums with a purulent or pus-like discharge is called **pyorrhea.**

The term **stomatitis** is used for any infection of the mouth, including:

- **Mouth ulcers,** also called **canker** sores, are erosions of the mucous membrane lining the mouth. **Aphthous** ulcers are the most common and occur in clusters of small ulcers that last for 3 or 4 days. These are usually stress- or illness-related but can also be caused by trauma.

- **Cold sores,** or fever blisters *(Figure 9.7),* are recurrent blisters on the lips, lining of the mouth, and gums due to infection with the virus **herpes simplex type 1 (HSV-1).** These blisters usually clear up spontaneously.

- **Thrush** *(Figure 9.8)* is an infection occurring anywhere in the mouth that is caused by the fungus *Candida albicans.* This fungus is normally found in the mouth, but it can multiply out of control as a result of prolonged antibiotic or steroid treatment, cancer chemotherapy, or diabetes. Newborn babies can acquire oral thrush from the mother's vaginal yeast infection during the birth process. Treatment with antifungal agents is usually successful.

- **Oral cancer** *(Figure 9.9)* occurs most often on the lip, but it can also occur on the tongue. Eighty percent of oral cancers are associated with smoking or chewing tobacco. Metastasis occurs to lymph nodes, bones, lungs, and liver.

Halitosis is the medical term for bad breath, which occurs in association with any of the above mouth disorders.

▲ **FIGURE 9.6**
Dental Caries.

▲ **FIGURE 9.7**
Cold Sores on the inside of the Lower Lip.

▲ **FIGURE 9.8**
Oral Thrush.

— Cancer of the Tongue

▲ **FIGURE 9.9**
Cancer of the Tongue.

Word Analysis and Definition

S = Suffix   P = Prefix   R = Root   R/CF = Combining Form

WORD	PRONUNCIATION		ELEMENTS	DEFINITION
aphthous	AF-thus		Greek *ulcer*	Painful small oral ulcers (canker sores)
canker	KANG-ker		Latin *crab*	Nonmedical term for aphthous ulcer
caries	KARE-eez		Latin *dry rot*	Bacterial destruction of teeth
gingiva gingival (adj)	JIN-jih-vah JIN-jih-val	S/ R/	Latin *gum* -al *pertaining to* gingiv- *gum*	Tissue surrounding the teeth and covering the jaw Pertaining to the gums
gingivitis gingivectomy	jin-jih-VI-tis jin-jih-VEC-toe-me	S/ S/	-itis *inflammation* -ectomy *surgical excision*	Inflammation of the gums Surgical removal of diseased gum tissue
glossodynia	gloss-oh-DIN-ee-ah	S/ R/CF	-dynia *pain* gloss/o- *tongue*	Painful, burning tongue
halitosis	hal-ih-TOE-sis	S/ R/	-osis *condition* halit- *breath*	Bad odor of the breath
periodontal	PER-ee-oh-DON-tal	S/ P/ R/	-al *pertaining to* peri- *around* -odont- *tooth*	Around a tooth
periodontics	PER-ee-oh-DON-tiks	S/	-ics *knowledge*	Branch of dentistry specializing in disorders of tissues around the teeth
periodontist periodontitis	PER-ee-oh-DON-tist PER-ee-oh-don-TIE-tis	S/ S/	-ist *specialist* -itis *inflammation*	Specialist in periodontics Inflammation of tissues around a tooth
plaque	PLAK		French *plate*	Patch of abnormal tissue
pyorrhea	pie-oh-REE-ah	R/ R/CF	-rrhea *flow* py/o- *pus*	Purulent discharge
stomatitis	STOE-mah-TI-tis	S/ R/CF	-itis *inflammation* stomat/i- *oral cavity, mouth*	Inflammation of the mucous membrane in the mouth
tartar	TAR-tar		Latin *crust on wine casks*	Calcified deposit at the gingival margin of the teeth
thrush	THRUSH		Root unknown	Infection with *Candida albicans*

EXERCISES

A. Suffixes: *Find the correct suffix to complete the medical terms, which all appear on this two-page spread. Fill in the blanks.*

LO 9.1 and 9.5 *Remember*

ist   itis   ectomy   rrhea   osis   al   ics

1. inflammation of the gums   gingiv/ _____

2. specialized branch of dentistry   periodont/ _____

3. around a tooth   periodont/ _____

4. bad breath   halit/ _____

5. surgical removal of diseased gum tissue   gingiv/ _____

6. specialist in periodontics   periodont/ _____

7. purulent discharge   pyo/ _____

B. Identify *the following medical terms that have their origin in Greek, Latin, or French.*   **LO 9.2 and 9.5** *Remember*

1. patch of abnormal tissue _____

2. canker sores _____

3. pertaining to the gums _____

4. nonmedical term for a mouth ulcer _____

5. bacterial destruction of teeth _____

C. Terminology challenge: *Recall and review terms from other chapters.*   **LO 9.11** *Remember*

1. In which other body system vocabulary does the medical term *plaque* appear? System: _____

   Define *plaque* in that system: _____

Lesson 9.2 (cont'd)

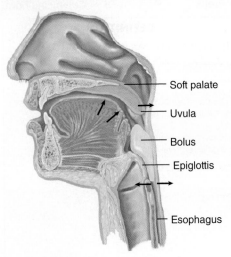

▲ **FIGURE 9.10**
Swallowing.
The bolus of food is
in the oropharynx.

Labels: Soft palate, Uvula, Bolus, Epiglottis, Esophagus

▲ **FIGURE 9.11**
Swallowing.
The bolus of
food is in the
esophagus.

*Labels:* Constriction, Peristaltic wave, Bolus, Relaxation, Shortening

Esophagus (LO 9.5)

The chicken and vegetables that you ingested earlier have now been sliced and ground into small particles by the teeth. These particles are partly digested and lubricated by saliva, and rolled into a bolus between the tongue and the hard palate, the bony roof of the mouth. The bolus is now ready to be swallowed down the oropharynx (upper part of the throat) *(Figure 9.10)* into the **esophagus.**

The bolus enters the esophagus from the lower end of the pharynx. In the esophagus, peristaltic, or wavelike, contractions of the esophageal wall muscles move it downward *(Figure 9.11).* At the lower end of the esophagus, the **cardiac sphincter** relaxes to allow the bolus to enter the stomach.

The **esophagus** *(Figure 9.12)* is a tube 9 to 10 inches long. It pierces the diaphragm at the esophageal **hiatus** to go from the thoracic cavity to the abdominal cavity *(Figure 9.12).*

Disorders of the Esophagus (LO 9.5)

Just like the mouth, the esophagus, too, can be prone to illness. **Esophagitis** is an inflammation of the lining of the esophagus, producing a burning chest pain (**heartburn**) after eating, pain on swallowing, and occasional vomiting of blood (**hematemesis**). The most common cause is **reflux** of the stomach's acid contents into the esophagus, also known as **gastroesophageal reflux disease (GERD).**

Hiatal hernia occurs when a portion of the stomach protrudes through the diaphragm alongside the esophagus at the esophageal hiatus *(Figure 9.13).* Surgical repair—a hiatal **herniorrhaphy**—may be necessary.

Esophageal varices are varicose veins of the esophagus. They are **asymptomatic** until they rupture, causing massive bleeding and hematemesis. They are a complication of cirrhosis of the liver *(see later this chapter).*

Cancer of the esophagus arises from the tube's lining. Symptoms are **dysphagia** (difficulty swallowing), a burning sensation in the chest, and weight loss. Risk factors include cigarettes, alcohol, betel-nut chewing, and esophageal reflux. The cancer metastasizes to the liver, bones, and lungs.

▶ **FIGURE 9.12**
Esophagus.

Labels: Oral cavity, Tongue, Pharynx, Esophagus, Diaphragm, Stomach

▲ **FIGURE 9.13**
Hiatal Hernia.

Labels (Normal): Esophagus, Lower esophageal sphincter, Diaphragm, Flap valve, Stomach, Pylorus, Duodenum

Normal

Labels (Hiatal Hernia): Esophagus, Lower esophageal sphincter, Hiatal Hernia, Diaphragm, Stomach, Pylorus, Duodenum

Hiatal Hernia

Word Analysis and Definition

WORD	PRONUNCIATION	ELEMENTS		DEFINITION
asymptomatic	A-simp-toe-**MAT**-ik	S/ P/ R/	-ic *pertaining to* a- *without* symptomat- *symptom*	Without any symptoms or abnormalities experienced by the patient
symptomatic (with **symptoms**)	simp-toe-**MAT**-ik			Pertaining to the symptoms of a disease
dysphagia	dis-**FAY**-jee-ah	P/ R/	dys- *difficulty* -phagia *swallowing*	Difficulty in swallowing
emesis hematemesis	**EM**-eh-sis he-mah-**TEM**-eh-sis	R/ R/	Greek *to vomit* hemat- *blood* -emesis *to vomit*	Vomit Vomiting of red blood
esophagus esophageal (adj)	ee-**SOF**-ah-gus ee-**SOF**-ah-**JEE**-al	S/ R/	Greek *gullet* -eal *pertaining to* esophag- *esophagus*	Tube linking pharynx to stomach Pertaining to the esophagus
esophagitis	ee-**SOF**-ah-**JI**-tis	S/	-itis *inflammation*	Inflammation of the lining of the esophagus
hernia	**HER**-nee-ah		Latin *rupture*	Protrusion of a structure through the tissue that normally contains it
herniorrhaphy	**HER**-nee-**OR**-ah-fee	S/ R/CF	-rrhaphy *suture* herni/o- *hernia*	Repair of a hernia
hiatus (noun) hiatal (adj)	high-**AY**-tus high-**AY**-tal	S/ R/	Latin *an aperture* -al *pertaining to* hiat- *opening*	An opening through a structure Pertaining to a hiatus
reflux	**REE**-fluks	P/ R/	re- *back* -flux *flow*	Backward flow
sphincter	**SFINK**-ter		Greek *a band*	A band of muscle that encircles an opening; when it contracts, the opening squeezes closed
varix varices (pl) varicose (adj)	**VAIR**-iks **VAIR**-ih-seez **VAIR**-ih-kose	S/ R/	Latin *dilated vein* -ose *full of* varic- *varicosity; dilated, tortuous vein*	Dilated, tortuous vein Characterized by or affected with varices

EXERCISES

A. Knowledge *of elements is your best tool for increasing your medical vocabulary. Each of the following terms has an element in bold. Identify that element and give its meaning. Fill in the chart.* **LO 9.1 and 9.5** *Remember*

Medical Term	Identity of Element (P, R, CF, or S)	Meaning of Element	Meaning of Term
reflux	1.	2.	3.
dysphagia	4.	5.	6.
herniorrhaphy	7.	8.	9.
hematemesis	10.	11.	12.
asymptomatic	13.	14.	15.

B. Apply *the language of gastroenterology and fill in the blanks.* **LO 9.1 and 9.5** *Apply*

1. What is another term for *varicose veins* of the esophagus? _____

2. What is a *bolus*? _____

3. What structure does the esophagus travel through from the *thoracic cavity* to the abdominal cavity? _____

4. What is burning chest pain called? _____

5. What are you vomiting in *hematemesis?* _____

Lesson 9.3

Digestion—Stomach and Small Intestine

Objectives

The bolus of food that you swallowed has now passed down your esophagus and into your stomach. The process of digestion begins in earnest. The stomach continues the mechanical breakdown of the food particles and initiates the chemical digestion of protein and fats. The small intestine is where the greatest amount of food digestion and absorption occurs. The information in this lesson will enable you to use correct medical terminology to:

9.3.1 Define the functions of the stomach and small intestine in digestion.

9.3.2 Explain how food is propelled through the stomach and small intestine.

9.3.3 Describe the process of digestion in the stomach and small intestine.

Abbreviations

HCl	hydrochloric acid
ml	milliliter

Case Report 9.2

You are . . .

. . . a medical interpreter working in Fulwood Medical Center.

You are communicating with . . .

. . . Mr. Xavier Ramirez, a 45-year-old farm worker, who has come to Dr. Susan Lee's primary care clinic. Mr. Ramirez complains of experiencing persistent, burning epigastric pain for several months. He has been a chain-smoker since the age of 14. His pain is eased by antacids but quickly returns. He has been taking aspirin because of joint pain in his fingers while he works. Dr. Lee has decided to refer him to a gastroenterologist for a gastroscopy. Your role is to explain the procedure to Mr. Ramirez and ensure that he keeps his appointments.

Digestion: The Stomach (LO 9.6)

Your stomach's peristaltic contractions mix different boluses of food together and push these contents toward the **pylorus** (the stomach opening that leads to the bowel) *(Figure 9.14)* to produce a mixture of semi-digested food called **chyme.**

The cells of your stomach's lining secrete *(Figure 9.15):*

1. **Mucus,** which lubricates food and protects the stomach lining;

2. **Hydrochloric acid (HCl),** which breaks up the connective tissue of meat and the cell walls of vegetables (think of the chicken-and-vegetables meal you ate earlier);

3. **Pepsin** (an active enzyme), which digests chicken and vegetable proteins;

4. **Intrinsic factor,** which is essential for vitamin B_{12} absorption in the small intestine; and

5. **Gastrin** (a chemical), which stimulates HCl and **pepsinogen** production, and encourages the stomach's peristaltic contractions.

A typical meal like chicken and vegetables takes 3 to 4 hours to exit the stomach as **chyme.** Peristaltic waves squirt 2 to 3 milliliters **(ml)** of this chyme at a time through the **pyloric sphincter** into the **duodenum** (the first part of the small intestine) *(Figure 9.14).*

▲ **FIGURE 9.14**
Stomach.

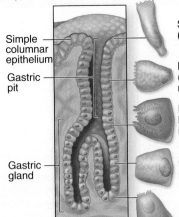

▲ **FIGURE 9.15**
Gastric Cells and Their Secretions.

Word Analysis and Definition

WORD	PRONUNCIATION	ELEMENTS		DEFINITION
chyme	KYME		Greek *juice*	Semifluid, partially digested food passed from the stomach into the duodenum
duodenum	du-oh-**DEE**-num	S/ R/	-um *structure* duoden- *twelve*	The first part of the small intestine; approximately twelve finger-breadths (9 to 10 inches) in length
duodenal (adj)	du-oh-**DEE**-nal	S/	-al *pertaining to*	Pertaining to the duodenum
gastrin	**GAS**-trin	S/ R/	-in *substance, chemical compound* gastr- *stomach*	Hormone secreted in the stomach that stimulates secretion of HCl and increases gastric motility
hydrochloric acid (HCl)	high-droh-**KLOR**-ik **ASS**-id	S/ R/CF R/	-ic *pertaining to* hydr/o- *water* -chlor- *green*	The acid of gastric juice
intrinsic factor	in-**TRIN**-sik **FAK**-tor	S/ R/ R/	-ic *pertaining to* intrins- *on the inside* factor *maker*	Makes the absorption of vitamin B_{12} happen
mucus (noun) mucous (adj) mucin	**MYU**-kus **MYU**-kus **MYU**-sin		Latin *slime*	Sticky secretion of cells in mucous membranes Relating to mucus or the mucosa Protein element of mucus
pepsin pepsinogen	**PEP**-sin pep-**SIN**-oh-jen	S/ R/CF	Greek *to digest* -gen *produce* pepsin/o- *pepsin*	Enzyme produced by the stomach that breaks down protein Converted by HCl in the stomach to pepsin
pylorus	pie-**LOR**-us	S/ R/	-us *pertaining to* pylor- *gate, pylorus*	Exit area of the stomach
pyloric (adj)	pie-**LOR**-ik	S/	-ic *pertaining to*	Pertaining to the pylorus

EXERCISES

A. Review *the Case Report on this spread before answering the questions.*   **LO 9.6, 9.10, and 9.11** *Understand*

1. What are the patient's complaints when he presents to the clinic? _____

2. What is not healthy in the patient's past medical history? _____

3. What do antacids help? _____

4. Why is Mr. Ramirez taking aspirin? _____

5. What is a gastroscopy? _____

B. Grammatical forms *can change with the addition of just one letter. Be aware of the correct spelling of these forms and also how they are used in a sentence. For example, mucus is the noun (person, place, or thing) form of the term, and mucous is the adjective (descriptive) form of the term. Insert the correct grammatical form (noun or adjective) in each of the following sentences. Check your spelling when you are finished.*   **LO 9.6 and 9.11** *Apply*

1. The sticky secretion of the _____ membranes is _____.

2. A sinus infection will produce a lot of _____ in the nasal passages.

3. Some internal organs have a _____ lining or covering.

Demonstrate that you know the difference in the forms of these terms. Create a sentence of patient documentation using any form of one of these terms.

Sentence:

_____

_____

_____

_____

_____

- Difficulty in swallowing is called dysphagia.

GERD   Gastroesophageal reflux disease

NSAID   Nonsteroidal anti-inflammatory drug

Disorders of the Stomach (LO 9.6)

Gastroesophageal reflux disease (GERD) refers to the regurgitation of stomach contents back into the esophagus. The acidity of regurgitated food can irritate and ulcerate the esophageal lining and cause bleeding. Scar tissue can cause an esophageal **stricture** and **dysphagia.**

Vomiting can result from overexpansion or irritation of any part of the digestive tract. The muscles of the diaphragm and abdominal wall forcefully contract and expel the stomach contents upward into the esophagus and mouth.

Gastritis is an inflammation of the stomach lining, producing symptoms of epigastric pain, feeling of fullness, nausea, and occasional bleeding. It can be acute or chronic, and is caused by common medications like aspirin and **NSAIDs,** by radiotherapy and chemotherapy, and by alcohol and smoking. Treatment involves removing the factors causing the gastritis, acid neutralization, and suppression of gastric acid *(see below).*

Peptic ulcers occur in the stomach and duodenum when the mucosal lining breaks down *(Figure 9.16).* Most peptic ulcers are caused by the bacterium *Helicobacter pylori* *(H. pylori),* which produces enzymes that weaken the protective mucus. These ulcers respond to antibiotics. **Dyspepsia** (epigastric pain with bloating and nausea) is the most common symptom.

Gastric ulcers are peptic ulcers that occur in the stomach. If a blood vessel erodes, bleeding may also be present. If untreated, the ulcer can eat into the entire wall, causing a **perforation.**

Gastric cancer can be asymptomatic for a long period and then cause **indigestion, anorexia,** abdominal pain, and weight loss. It affects men twice as often as women. It metastasizes to the lymph nodes, liver, peritoneum, chest, and brain. It is usually treated with surgery and chemotherapy.

Case Report 9.2 (continued)

A **gastroscopy** on Mr. Ramirez reveals a gastric ulcer.

▲ **FIGURE 9.16**
Bleeding Peptic Ulcer.

Stomach

Duodenum

Jejunum

Ileocecal junction

Cecum

Appendix

Ileum

▲ **FIGURE 9.17**
Small Intestine.

Small Intestine (LO 9.6)

The small intestine, called *small* because of its diameter, completes the chemical digestion process. It is responsible for the **absorption** of most of the nutrients. The small intestine extends from the pylorus of the stomach to the beginning of the large intestine, and it has three segments *(Figure 9.17),* as listed below:

1. The **duodenum** is the first 9 to 10 inches of the small intestine. It receives chyme from the stomach, together with pancreatic juices and bile;

2. The **jejunum** makes up about 40% of the small intestine's length. It is the primary region for chemical digestion and nutrient absorption; and

3. The **ileum** makes up about 55% of the small intestine's length. It ends at the **ileocecal** valve, a **sphincter** that controls entry into the large intestine.

Digestion in the Small Intestine (LO 9.6)

After leaving the stomach as chyme, food spends 3 to 5 hours in the small intestine.

Anywhere from 4 to 6 hours after consuming the chicken and vegetables mentioned earlier, the food has passed through the small intestine and is ready to be passed into the large intestine. While in the small intestine, the protein, carbohydrates, and fats have been broken down by enzymes and absorbed into the bloodstream.

WORD	PRONUNCIATION	ELEMENTS		DEFINITION
absorption	ab-**SORP**-shun	S/ R/	-ion *action, condition* absorpt- *to swallow*	Uptake of nutrients and water by cells in the GI tract
anorexia	an-oh-**RECK**-see-ah	S/ P/ R/	-ia *condition* an- *without* -orex- *appetite*	Without an appetite; or an aversion to food
cecum (noun)	**SEE**-kum		Latin *blind*	Blind pouch that is the first part of the large intestine
cecal (adj)	**SEE**-kal	S/ R/	-al *pertaining to* cec- *cecum*	Pertaining to the cecum
dyspepsia	dis-**PEP**-see-ah	S/ P/ R/	-ia *condition* dys- *difficult, bad* -peps- *digestion*	"Upset stomach," epigastric pain, nausea, and gas
gastritis	gas-**TRY**-tis	S/ R/	-itis *inflammation* gastr- *stomach*	Inflammation of the lining of the stomach
gastroesophageal	**GAS**-troh-ee-sof-ah-**JEE**-al	S/ R/CF R/CF	-al *pertaining to* gastr/o- *stomach* -esophag/e- *esophagus*	Pertaining to the stomach and esophagus
gastroscope	**GAS**-troh-skope	S/ R/CF	-scope *instrument for viewing* gastr/o- *stomach*	Endoscope for examining the inside of the stomach
gastroscopy	gas-**TROS**-koh-pee	S/	-scopy *to examine, to view*	Endoscopic examination of the stomach
ileum	**ILL**-ee-um	S/ R/	-um *structure* ile- *ileum*	Third portion of small intestine
ileocecal	**ILL**-ee-oh-**SEE**-cal	S/ R/CF R/	-al *pertaining to* ile/o- *ileum* cec- *cecum*	Pertaining to the junction of the ileum and cecum
indigestion	in-dih-**JESS**-chun	S/ P/ R/	-ion *action, condition* in- *in, not* -digest- *to break down*	Symptoms resulting from difficulty in digesting food
jejunum (noun)	je-**JEW**-num		Latin *empty*	Segment of small intestine between the duodenum and the ileum
jejunal (adj)	je-**JEW**-nal	S/ R/	-al *pertaining to* jejun- *jejunum*	Pertaining to the jejunum
peptic	**PEP**-tik	S/ R/	-ic *pertaining to* pept- *digest*	Relating to the stomach and duodenum
perforation	per-foh-**RAY**-shun	S/ R/	-ion *action, condition* perforat- *bore through*	A hole through the wall of a structure
stricture	**STRICK**-shur		Latin *draw tight*	Narrowing of a tube

EXERCISES

A. Review the Case Report on this spread before answering the questions.   **LO 9.6 and 9.11** *Understand*

1. Mr. Ramirez was diagnosed with a gastric ulcer. What is the difference between a peptic ulcer and a gastric ulcer? _____

_____

2. What type of "scope" did the surgeon use to find the ulcer? _____

3. Name one complication Mr. Ramirez could develop from his gastric ulcer. _____

4. What bacterium causes most peptic ulcers? _____

B. Practice the language of gastroenterology. Review this spread and the WAD before you start the exercise. Use the terms found there to answer the following questions.   **LO 9.6, 9.11, and 9.12** *Apply*

1. Write the three segments of the small intestine in their correct order of location in the intestine.

_____ , _____ , _____

2. A term can often designate more than one area of the gastrointestinal tract (example: *gastrointestinal*).

Find a similar term in the WAD above. _____

The two organs referred to in this term are: _____ and _____

3. Patient education: Explain to your patient the function of a *stricture* in the intestine.

_____

Lesson 9.3 (cont'd) Disorders of the Small Intestine (LO 9.6)

The absorption of nutrients occurs primarily through the small intestine. **Impairment of absorption,** including Crohn disease and lactose intolerance, is covered in *Lesson 9.5* of this chapter.

- **Infections** of the small intestine are common and are caused by a variety of agents.

- **Gastroenteritis,** or inflammation of the stomach and small intestine, can result in acute vomiting and diarrhea. It can be caused by a variety of viruses and bacteria (including, occasionally, the parasite *Giardia lamblia*) and is initiated by contact with contaminated food (food poisoning) and water.

- **Bleeding** from the small intestine is usually caused by a duodenal ulcer.

- **Celiac disease** is an allergy to gluten, which is a protein contained in wheat, rye, barley, and other grains. Celiac disease *(Figure 9.18)* damages the lining of the small intestine and can cause abdominal swelling, gas, pain, weight loss, fatigue, and weakness. Treatment is a strict gluten-free diet.

- The symptoms of **irritable bowel syndrome (IBS)** are chronic abdominal pain, bloating, and either diarrhea or constipation or an alternating pattern of the two. X-rays, scans, and endoscopies of patients with IBS show no abnormality. Treatment is difficult and often unsuccessful.

- An **intussusception** *(Figure 9.19)* occurs when a part of the small intestine slides into a neighboring portion of the small intestine—much like the way that parts of a collapsible telescope slide into each other. Eighty percent of intussusceptions can be cured with an enema; the remaining 20% require surgical intervention.

- **Ileus** is a disruption of the normal peristaltic ability of the small intestine. It can be caused by a bowel obstruction or by intestinal paralysis. Risk factors for **paralytic ileus** include GI surgery, diabetic ketoacidosis *(see Chapter 17),* peritonitis, and medications, such as opiates.

- **Cancer** of the small intestine occurs infrequently compared with tumors in other parts of the GI tract. An **adenocarcinoma** is the most common malignant tumor of the small bowel.

▲ **FIGURE 9.18**
Celiac Disease of the Small Bowel showing atrophy of the villi on the surface of the intestinal lining.

▲ **FIGURE 9.19**
Diagram of intussusception.

Word Analysis and Definition

S = Suffix   P = Prefix   R = Root   R/CF = Combining Form

WORD	PRONUNCIATION	ELEMENTS		DEFINITION
celiac	SEE-lee-ack	S/ R/	-ac *pertaining to* celi- *abdomen*	Relating to the abdominal cavity
celiac disease	SEE-lee-ack diz-EEZ	P/ R/	dis- *apart* -ease *normal function*	Disease caused by a sensitivity to gluten
gastroenteritis	GAS-troh-en-ter-I-tis	S/ R/CF R/	-itis *inflammation* gastr/o- *stomach* -enter- *intestine*	Inflammation of the stomach and intestines
Giardia	jee-AR-dee-ah		Alfred Giard, 1846–1908 French biologist	Parasite that can affect the small intestine
gluten	GLU-ten		Latin *glue*	Insoluble protein found in wheat, barley, and rye
ileus	ILL-ee-us		Greek *intestinal colic*	Dynamic or mechanical obstruction of the small intestine
intussusception	IN-tuss-sus-SEP-shun	S/ P/ R/	-ion *action* intus- *within* -suscept- *to take up*	The slippage of one part of the bowel inside another, causing obstruction

EXERCISES

A. Match *the disorder of the small intestine in column 1 with the statement describing it in column 2.*   **LO 9.6** *Understand*

_____ **1.** ileus

_____ **2.** IBS

_____ **3.** celiac disease

_____ **4.** *Giardia lamblia*

_____ **5.** intussusception

a. Parasite that causes gastroenteritis

b. Part of the small intestine slides into a neighboring part

c. Disruption of the normal peristalsis of the small intestine

d. Treatment is difficult and often unsuccessful

e. Allergy to gluten

B. Use your knowledge *of the small intestine and answer the questions. Rewrite the one incorrect statement on the lines below.*
   LO 9.3 and 9.6 *Remember*

1. The absorption of nutrients occurs primarily through the small intestine.   T   F

2. Gastroenteritis can result in acute vomiting and diarrhea.   T   F

3. Bleeding from the small intestine is usually from an infection.   T   F

4. Chronic abdominal pain, bloating, and either diarrhea or constipation can be signs of IBS.   T   F

5. Risk factors for paralytic ileus include GI surgery, diabetic ketoacidosis, and medicines such as opiates.   T   F

6. Corrected statement:

_____

_____

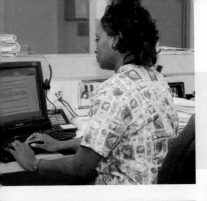

Lesson 9.4

Digestion—Liver, Gallbladder, and Pancreas

Objectives

Your liver and pancreas secrete enzymes that are responsible for the majority of digestion occurring in the small intestine. You will need to be able to use correct medical terminology to:

9.4.1 Describe the digestive functions and common disorders of the liver, gallbladder, bile ducts, and pancreas.

Keynotes

- Only the production of bile relates the liver to digestion.
- Vaccines are available to prevent hepatitis A and B.

Abbreviations

HAV	hepatitis A virus
HBV	hepatitis B virus
HCV	hepatitis C virus

Case Report 9.3

You are . . .

. . . a coder in the Health Information Management department at Fulwood Medical Center.

You are communicating with . . .

. . . Dr. Susan Lee, and you are questioning the documentation of Mrs. Sandra Jacobs's care. Mrs. Jacobs, a 46-year-old mother of four, presented in Dr. Lee's primary care clinic with episodes of cramping pain in her upper abdomen associated with nausea and vomiting. A physical examination reveals an obese white woman with tenderness over her gallbladder. Her BP is 170/90 and she has slight **pedal** edema. A **provisional diagnosis** of gallstones has been made. She has been referred for an ultrasound examination and an appointment has been made to see Dr. Walsh in the surgery department.

The Liver (LO 9.7)

Your **liver** is your largest internal organ. It is a complex structure located under your right ribs just below your diaphragm *(Figure 9.20)*.

As a complex organ, your liver's multiple functions include:

- Manufacturing and excreting **bile;**
- Removing **bilirubin** (a pigment) from the bloodstream;
- Storing excess sugar as **glycogen;** and
- Manufacturing blood proteins, including those needed for clotting *(see Chapter 7).*

Disorders of the Liver (LO 9.7)

Hepatitis is an inflammation of the liver causing **jaundice,** where the skin and sometimes the eyes have a yellowish hue. Viral hepatitis is the most common cause of hepatitis and is related to three major types of virus:

1. **Hepatitis A virus (HAV)** is highly contagious and causes a mild to severe infection. It is transmitted by contaminated food.

2. **Hepatitis B virus (HBV),** or serum hepatitis, is transmitted through contact with blood, semen, vaginal secretions, or saliva, as well as by a needle prick and the sharing of contaminated needles. Vaccines are available to prevent hepatitis A and B.

3. **Hepatitis C virus (HCV)** is the most common blood-borne infection in the United States, occurring mostly through injections given with contaminated syringes and needles. The disease can vary in severity from a mild illness lasting a few weeks to a serious, lifelong condition that can lead to cirrhosis of the liver or liver cancer. More than 3 million Americans are chronically infected with hepatitis C virus. Combination antiviral drugs are used, and new therapeutic agents are being licensed. There is no vaccine yet available.

In addition, **hepatitis D** can occur in association with hepatitis B, making the infection worse. **Hepatitis E** is similar to hepatitis A and occurs mostly in underdeveloped countries.

Chronic hepatitis occurs when the acute hepatitis is not healed after 6 months. It progresses slowly, can last for years, and is difficult to treat.

Cirrhosis of the liver is a chronic irreversible disease, replacing normal liver cells with hard, fibrous scar tissue. Its most common cause is alcoholism. There is no known cure.

Cancer of the liver as a primary cancer usually arises in patients with chronic liver disease, often from HBV infection.

Sternum · 5th rib · Liver

▲ **FIGURE 9.20**
Location of Liver.

S = Suffix   P = Prefix   R = Root   R/CF = Combining Form

WORD	PRONUNCIATION		ELEMENTS	DEFINITION
bile bile acids biliary (adj)	BILE **BILE AH**-sids **BILL**-ee-air-ee	 S/ R/CF	Latin *bile* -ary *pertaining to* bil/i- *bile*	Fluid secreted by the liver into the duodenum Steroids synthesized from cholesterol Pertaining to bile or the biliary tract
bilirubin	bill-ee-**RU**-bin	S/ R/CF	-rubin *rust colored* bil/i- *bile*	Bile pigment formed in the liver from hemoglobin
cirrhosis	sir-**ROE**-sis	S/ R/	-osis *condition* cirrh- *yellow*	Extensive fibrotic liver disease
glycogen	**GLYE**-koh-gen	S/ R/CF	-gen *produce, create* glyc/o- *sugar, glycogen*	The body's principal carbohydrate reserve, stored in the liver and skeletal muscle
hepatic	hep-**AT**-ik	S/ R/	-ic *pertaining to* hepat- *liver*	Pertaining to the liver
hepatitis	hep-ah-**TIE**-tis	S/	-itis *inflammation*	Inflammation of the liver
jaundice	**JAWN**-dis		French *yellow*	Yellow staining of tissues with bile pigments, including bilirubin
liver	**LIV**-er		Old English *liver*	Body's largest organ, located in the right upper quadrant of the abdomen
pedal	**PEED**-al	S/ R/	-al *pertaining to* ped- *foot*	Pertaining to the foot
provisional diagnosis (*also called* **preliminary** diagnosis)	pro-**VIZH**-un-al die-ag-**NO**-sis	S/ R/ P/ R/	-al *pertaining to* provision- *provide* dia- *complete* -gnosis *knowledge of an abnormal condition*	A temporary diagnosis pending further examination or testing The determination of the cause of a disease

EXERCISES

A. Review *the Case Report on this spread before answering the questions.*   **LO 9.7 and 9.11** *Understand*

1. What symptoms did Mrs. Jacobs have when she presented to Dr. Lee's clinic?

_____

2. What does the physical examination reveal? _____

3. Does Mrs. Jacobs have hypertension or hypotension? _____

4. What is pedal edema? _____

5. What is another term for a provisional diagnosis? _____

B. Elements: *Use this exercise as a quick review of the elements in the WAD. Circle the correct choices, and then answer the question.*
   LO 9.1, 9.7, and 9.11 *Remember*

1. In the term *hepatic,* the root means:

   pancreas   stomach   liver

2. The suffix in *cirrhosis* indicates this is:

   a condition   a surgical excision   a structure

3. *Bilirubin* is the color of:

   blood   milk   rust

4. The root in *cirrhosis* indicates a:

   color   size   location

5. Which three terms in the WAD refer to color?

   _____, _____, _____

Gallbladder, Biliary Tract, and Pancreas (LO 9.7)

Gallbladder and Biliary Tract (LO 9.7)

On the underside of your liver is your **gallbladder (GB),** which stores and concentrates the bile produced by the liver. The **cystic duct** from the gallbladder joins with the **hepatic duct** to form the **common bile duct.** This duct system, which moves the bile from the liver to the duodenum, is called the **biliary tract** (*Figure 9.21a and b*).

Disorders of the Gallbladder (LO 9.7)

Gallstones (cholelithiasis) can form in the gallbladder from excess cholesterol, bile salts, and bile pigment (*Figure 9.22*). The stones can vary in size and number. Risk factors are obesity, high-cholesterol diets, multiple pregnancies, and rapid weight loss.

Choledocholithiasis occurs when small stones become impacted in the common bile duct. This can cause biliary colic and jaundice (*see below*).

Cholecystitis is an acute or chronic inflammation of the gallbladder, usually associated with cholelithiasis and obstruction of the cystic duct with a stone.

Jaundice (icterus) is a symptom of many different diseases in the biliary tract and liver. It is a yellow discoloration of the skin and sclera of the eyes caused by deposits of bilirubin just below the skin's outer layers.

Case Report 9.3 (continued)

Mrs. Jacobs presented in the emergency department with the classic gallstone symptoms of severe waves of right upper quadrant pain (biliary colic), nausea, and vomiting.

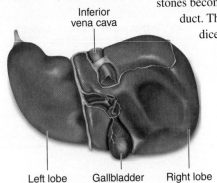

(a)

Inferior vena cava

Left lobe   Gallbladder   Right lobe

The Pancreas (LO 9.7)

Your **pancreas** is a spongy, exocrine gland. **Exocrine** glands secrete fluids. In fact, many of the glands in your body are exocrine glands, including your sweat glands, mammary glands, and other digestive enzyme-releasing glands. The majority of the pancreas secretes digestive juices, but smaller areas of **pancreatic islet cells** secrete the hormones **insulin** and **glucagon** (*see Chapter 12*).

The pancreas produces pancreatic digestive juices that are excreted through the pancreatic duct. This duct joins the common bile duct shortly before it opens into the duodenum (*Figure 9.21b*), which encircles the top or head of the pancreas (*Figure 9.21b*). Pancreatic and bile juices then enter the duodenum.

Other pancreatic cells secrete insulin and glucagon, which go directly into the bloodstream. This part of the pancreas is an **endocrine** (hormone-secreting) gland.

Pancreatic juices contain alkaline electrolytes, which help neutralize the acid chyme as it comes from the stomach, and enzymes, which break down starches, fats, and proteins into simpler elements.

Cystic duct ——— ——— Hepatic duct

Common bile duct ——— ——— Pancreatic duct

Gallbladder ———

Duodenum ———

——— Tail of pancreas

——— Body of pancreas

Jejunum ———

(b)

▲ **FIGURE 9.21**
(a) Underside of liver.
(b) Anatomy of gallbladder, pancreas, and biliary tract.

Disorders of the Pancreas (LO 9.7)

Pancreatitis is an inflammation of the pancreas. The acute disease ranges from a mild, self-limiting episode to an acute life-threatening emergency. In the chronic form, there is a progressive destruction of pancreatic tissue leading to malabsorption and diabetes.

Pancreatic cancer is the fourth leading cause of cancer-related death. Early diagnosis is difficult because the presenting symptoms are very vague. Treatment is surgical resection of the cancer. The prognosis is poor.

Cystic fibrosis (CF) is an inherited disease that becomes apparent in infancy or childhood. With CF, the pancreas, liver, intestines, sweat glands, and lungs all produce abnormally thick mucous secretions. The malabsorption of fat and protein leads to large, bulky, foul-smelling stools. Problems with thick mucous secretions in the lungs lead to chronic lung disease.

◀ **FIGURE 9.22**
Gallstones.
The dime is included to illustrate the relative size of the gallstones.

Word Analysis and Definition

WORD	PRONUNCIATION	ELEMENTS		DEFINITION
cholecystitis	KOH-leh-sis-**TIE**-tis	S/ R/CF R/	-itis *inflammation* chol/e- *bile* -cyst- *bladder*	Inflammation of the gallbladder
cholecystectomy	KOH-leh-sis-**TECK**-toe-me	S/	-ectomy *surgical excision*	Surgical removal of the gallbladder
choledocholithiasis	koh-leh-**DOH**-koh-lih-**THIGH**-ah-sis	S/ R/CF R/	-iasis *condition* choledoch/o- *common bile duct* -lith- *stone*	Presence of a gallstone in the common bile duct
cholelithiasis	KOH-leh-lih-**THIGH**-ah-sis	S/ R/CF R/CF	-iasis *condition* chol/e- *bile* -lith/o- *stone*	Condition of having bile stones (gallstones)
cholelithotomy	KOH-leh-lih-**THOT**-oh-me	S/	-tomy *surgical incision*	Surgical removal of a gallstone(s)
endocrine	**EN**-doh-krin	P/ R/	endo- *within, inside* -crine *secrete*	A gland that produces an internal or hormonal substance and secretes it into the bloodstream
exocrine	**EK**-soh-krin	P/	exo- *outward, outside*	A gland that secretes substances outwardly through excretory ducts
gallstone	**GAWL**-stone	R/ R/	gall- *bitter* -stone *pebble*	Hard mass of cholesterol, calcium, and bilirubin that can be formed in the gallbladder and bile duct
gallbladder	**GAWL**-blad-er		bladder, Old English *receptacle*	Receptacle on the inferior surface of the liver for storing bile
glucagon	**GLU**-kah-gon	R/ R/	gluc- *glucose, sugar* -agon *to fight*	Hormone that mobilizes glucose from body storage
insulin	**IN**-syu-lin	S/ R/	-in *chemical compound* insul- *island*	Pancreatic hormone that suppresses blood glucose levels and transports glucose into cells
pancreas	**PAN**-kree-as		Greek *sweetbread*	Lobulated gland, the head of which is tucked into the curve of the duodenum
pancreatic (adj)	pan-kree-**AT**-ik	S/ R/	-ic *pertaining to* pancreat- *pancreas*	Pertaining to the pancreas
pancreatitis	**PAN**-kree-ah-**TIE**-tis	S/	-itis *inflammation*	Inflammation of the pancreas

EXERCISES

A. Review the *Case Report on this spread before answering the questions.*   **LO 9.1, 9.3, and 9.7** *Understand*

1. What abbreviation could be used in the case report? _____

2. Define "biliary colic." _____
   _____

3. What is the difference between "cholelithiasis" and "choledocholithiasis"? _____
   _____

4. Do both of the terms above involve a stone? _____

5. What type of surgery will Mrs. Jacobs most likely have? _____

B. Roots or combining forms *can remain the same, but the addition of other elements will construct entirely different medical terms. Use this group of elements, in addition to* chol/e, *to form the medical terms that are defined. Some elements you will use more than once; some elements you will not use at all. Fill in the blanks.*   **LO 9.1 and 9.7** *Apply*

The element chol/e *means* _____.

Add these elements to chol/e *to form the medical terms defined below:*

lith   choledoch/o   iasis   chol   ectomy   osis   cyst   otomy   cyst/o   itis

1. condition of gallstones: _____ / _____ / _____

2. surgical removal of gallbladder: _____ / _____ / _____

3. gallstone in the common bile duct: _____ / _____ / _____

4. surgical incision into gallbladder to remove gallstones: _____ / _____ / _____

Lesson 9.5

Absorption and Malabsorption

Objectives

In the previous lessons in this chapter, you learned about the digestive secretions of the different segments of the digestive tract, liver, and pancreas. This information can now be brought together to review the overall process of digestion so that you will be able to use correct medical terminology to:

9.5.1 Explain the chemical digestion and absorption of proteins, carbohydrates, and fats.

9.5.2 Describe disorders of chemical digestion, absorption, and **malabsorption.**

Case Report 9.4

You are . . .

. . . a dietitian working at Fulwood Medical Center.

You are communicating with . . .

. . . Mrs. Jan Stark, a 36-year-old pottery maker, and her husband, Mr. Tom Stark. From her medical record, you see that Mrs. Stark has been referred to you by Dr. Cameron Grabowski, a gastroenterologist.

For the past 10 years, Mrs. Stark has had spasmodic episodes of **diarrhea** and **flatulence** associated with severe headaches and fatigue. During those episodes, her stools were greasy and pale. She has seen several physicians who have recommended low-fat, high-carbohydrate diets, but she has had no relief. Dr. Grabowski has performed an intestinal biopsy through an oral **endoscopy** and diagnosed **celiac disease.** This condition is a sensitivity to the protein **gluten** that is found in wheat, rye, barley, and oats. Dr. Grabowski has asked you to ensure that Mrs. Stark accepts a diet free of gluten-containing foods like breads, cereals, cookies, and beer.

Chemical Digestion, Absorption, and Transport (LO 9.6 and 9.9)

Carbohydrates (LO 9.6 and 9.9)

In your small intestine, carbohydrates like **starches** are broken down into simple sugars—glucose and fructose—which are absorbed by the lining cells and transferred to the capillaries of the **villi** *(Figure 9.23).* The most commonly consumed carbohydrates are bread, soft drinks, cookies, cakes, doughnuts, syrups, jams, potatoes, and rice. From the capillaries of the villi, the simple sugars are carried by the **portal vein** to the liver, where the non-glucose sugars are converted to glucose. Glucose is the major source of energy for all cells.

Glycogen, the storage form of carbohydrate, is found in the liver and skeletal muscle. Glycogen in muscles supplies glucose during high-intensity and endurance exercise.

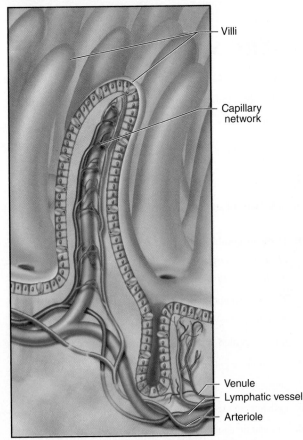

▶ **FIGURE 9.23**
Intestinal Villi.

Word Analysis and Definition

WORD	PRONUNCIATION	ELEMENTS		DEFINITION
celiac disease	SEE-lee-ack diz-EEZ	S/ R/ P/ R/	-ac *pertaining to* celi- *abdomen* dis- *apart* -ease *normal function*	Disease caused by sensitivity to gluten
diarrhea	die-ah-REE-ah	P/ R/	dia- *complete* -rrhea *flow, discharge*	Abnormally frequent and loose stools
endoscopy	en-DOS-koh-pee	P/ S/	endo- *inside, within* -scopy *to examine, view*	The use of an endoscope
endoscope	EN-doh-skope	S/	-scope *instrument for viewing*	Instrument used to examine the interior of a tubular or hollow organ
flatulence	FLAT-you-lents	S/ R/	-ence *forming* flatul- *excessive gas, flatus*	Excessive amount of gas in the stomach and intestines
flatus	FLAY-tus		Latin *blowing*	Gas or air expelled through the anus
glycogen	GLYE-koh-jen	S/ R/CF	-gen *to produce* glyc/o- *sugar/glucose*	The body's principal carbohydrate reserve, stored in the liver and skeletal muscle
malabsorption	mal-ab-SORP-shun	S/ P/ R/	-ion *action, condition* mal- *bad, difficult* -absorpt- *swallow, take in*	Inadequate gastrointestinal absorption of nutrients
portal vein	POR-tal VANE		portal, Latin *gate* vein, Latin *vein*	The vein that carries blood from the intestines to the liver
starch	STARCH		Anglo-Saxon *stiffen*	Complex carbohydrate made of multiple units of glucose attached together
villus villi (pl)	VILL-us VILL-eye		Latin *shaggy hair*	Thin, hairlike projection, particularly of a mucous membrane lining a cavity

EXERCISES

A. Review *the Case Report on this spread before answering the questions.*

LO 9.8, 9.9, and 9.10 *Understand*

1. What is the meaning of the term *spasmodic episodes?* _____

2. What kind of specialist referred Mrs. Stark to the nutritionist?

   _____

3. When Mrs. Stark's condition flares up, what symptoms are present?

   _____

4. What procedure did Dr. Grabowski perform to get a definitive diagnosis for Mrs. Stark?

   _____

5. Why did Mrs. Stark not get any relief from her previous doctor's recommendations for a
   low-fat, high-carbohydrate diet? _____

Study Hint

Endoscope is a generic (general) term that means any instrument *(scope)* used to examine the inside *(endo)* of a tubular or hollow organ. The instrument obtains its specific name from the organ it is used to examine. Thus, an instrument used to view a stomach is a gastroscope specifically, but it is also an endoscope in general.

B. Construct *the correct medical term to match the definitions. Review the WAD before you fill in the blanks.*   **LO 9.1, 9.6, 9.9, and 9.10** *Apply*

1. inadequate gastrointestinal absorption of nutrients

   _____ / _____ / _____
   P   R/CF   S

2. abnormally frequent and loose stools

   _____ / _____ / _____
   P   R/CF   S

3. examination of a hollow structure with a special instrument

   _____ / _____ / _____
   P   R/CF   S

4. excessive amount of gas in stomach and intestines

   _____ / _____ / _____
   P   R/CF   S

5. the instrument used for endoscopy

   _____ / _____ / _____
   P   R/CF   S

Lesson 9.5 (cont'd)

- Proteins are broken down into amino acids.
- Minerals are electrolytes.
- In malnutrition, the body breaks down its own tissues to meet its nutritional and metabolic needs.
- Milk sugar is lactose. The enzyme lactase breaks down lactose into glucose.
- Diarrhea is caused by irritation of the intestinal lining that causes feces to pass through the intestine too quickly for adequate amounts of water to be reabsorbed.

Abbreviations

Ca	calcium
ED	emergency department
K	potassium
Mg	magnesium
Na	sodium

Chemical Digestion, Absorption, and Transport (continued)

Proteins (LO 9.8)

Proteins are only 10 to 20% digested when they arrive in the duodenum and small intestine. Enzymes produced by cells in the small intestine, and the pancreatic enzyme trypsin, break down the remaining proteins into **amino acids.**

The amino acids are carried away in the blood and are transported to cells all over the body to be used as building blocks for new tissue formation.

Lipids (LO 9.8)

Lipids (fats) enter the duodenum and small intestine as large globules. These have to be **emulsified** by the bile salts into smaller droplets so that pancreatic **lipase** (fat-reducing enzymes) can digest them into very small droplets of free **fatty acids** and **monoglycerides.**

These small droplets are taken up by the **lacteals** (lymphatic vessels) inside the villi and then move into the lymphatic system. The droplets now comprise a milky, fatty lymphatic fluid called **chyle,** which eventually reaches the thoracic duct and moves into the bloodstream (see Chapter 7). Chyle is stored in adipose tissue. The fat-soluble vitamins A, D, E, and K are absorbed with the lipids.

Water (LO 9.8)

Water has no caloric value and makes up approximately 60% of your body weight (about 10 gallons). Your small intestine absorbs 92% of your body's water, which is taken into the bloodstream through the capillaries in the villi. Water-soluble vitamins, C and the B complex, are absorbed with water except for B_{12}.

You can survive 6 to 8 weeks without food, but only a few days without water.

Minerals (LO 9.8)

Minerals are absorbed along the whole length of the small intestine. Iron and calcium are absorbed according to the body's needs. The other minerals are absorbed regardless of need, and the kidneys excrete the surplus.

The major minerals are sodium (**Na**), potassium (**K**), calcium (**Ca**), and magnesium (**Mg**).

Disorders of Malabsorption (LO 9.8)

The term **malabsorption syndromes** refers to a group of diseases in which intestinal absorption of nutrients is impaired.

Malnutrition can arise from malabsorption, but can also result from a lack of food, as with famine and poverty. Malnutrition can also result from a loss of appetite in people with cancer or a terminal illness.

Lactose intolerance occurs when the small intestine is not producing enough of the enzyme **lactase** to break down the milk sugar lactose. The result is diarrhea and cramps. Lactase can be taken in pill form before eating dairy products, and milk products can be avoided.

Crohn disease (or **regional enteritis**) is an inflammation of the small intestine, frequently in the ileum and occasionally also in the large intestine. The symptoms are abdominal pain, diarrhea, fatigue, and weight loss. There is no cure.

Celiac disease is an autoimmune disease that damages the villi of the small intestine and interferes with the absorption of nutrients. It is due to an **intolerance** to a protein, **gluten,** found in wheat, barley, and rye products. It affects about 1% of the population in the United States. In addition, there is a nonceliac sensitivity (allergy) to gluten products that affects about 4% of the population.

Constipation occurs when fecal movement through the large intestine is slow and thus too much water is reabsorbed by the large intestine. The feces become hardened. Constipation can be caused by lack of dietary fiber, lack of exercise, and emotional upset.

Gastroenteritis (stomach "flu") is an infection of the stomach and intestine that can be caused by a large number of bacteria and viruses. It causes vomiting, diarrhea, and fever. An outbreak of gastroenteritis can sometimes be traced to contaminated food or water.

Dysentery is a severe form of bacterial gastro-enteritis with blood and mucus in frequent, watery stools.

Malnutrition, malabsorption, and severe forms of diarrhea and vomiting can cause dehydration and an electrolyte imbalance, possibly leading to coma and death.

Word Analysis and Definition

WORD	PRONUNCIATION	ELEMENTS		DEFINITION
amino acid	ah-**ME**-no **ASS**-id	R/CF	amin/o- *nitrogen containing acid*, Latin *sour*	The basic building block for protein
chyle	**KYLE**		Greek *juice*	A milky fluid that results from the digestion and absorption of fats in the small intestine
Crohn disease	**KRONE** diz-**EEZ**		Burrill Crohn, New York gastroenterologist 1884–1983	Narrowing and thickening of terminal small intestine
dysentery	**DISS**-en-tare-ee	P/ R/	dys- *bad, difficult* -entery *condition of the small intestine*	Disease with diarrhea, bowel spasms, fever and dehydration
emulsify	ee-**MUL**-sih-fye	S/ R/	-ify *to become* emuls- *suspend in a liquid*	Break up into very small droplets to suspend in a solution (emulsion)
emulsion (noun)	ee-**MUL**-shun	S/	-ion *condition, action*	The system that contains small droplets suspended in a liquid
gastroenteritis	**GAS**-troh-en-ter-**EYE**-tis	S/ R/ R/CF	-itis *inflammation* -enter- *intestine* gastr/o *stomach*	Inflammation of the stomach and small intestine
lacteal	**LAK**-tee-al	S/ R/CF	-eal *pertaining to* lact- *milk*	A lymphatic vessel carrying chyle away from the intestine
lactose lactase	**LAK**-toes **LAK**-tase	S/ R/	Latin *milk sugar* -ase *enzyme* lact- *milk*	The disaccharide in cows milk Enzyme that breaks down lactose to glucose
lipase	**LIE**-paze	S/ R/	-ase *enzyme* lip- *fat*	Enzyme that breaks down fat
lipid	**LIP**-id		Greek *fat*	General term for all types of fatty compounds; e.g., cholesterol, triglycerides, and fatty acids
mineral	**MIN**-er-al	S/ R/	-al *pertaining to* miner- *mines*	Inorganic compound usually found in the earth's crust

EXERCISES

A. Seek and find *the correct medical terms to fill in the blanks. The answers to the following questions can all be found on the two-page spread open in front of you.* **LO 9.8 and 9.11** *Understand*

1. What proteins break down into: _____

2. Another name for minerals: _____

3. Milky fluid that results from the digestion and absorption of fats: _____

4. Term used to describe all types of fatty compounds: _____

5. Break up into small droplets to suspend in a liquid: _____

B. Continue searching *for the correct answer.* **LO 9.8 and 9.11** *Understand*

1. Lymphatic vessel that carries chyle away from the intestine: _____

2. Inorganic compounds found in the earth's crust: _____

3. Number of calories in an ounce of water: _____

4. Percentage of the body's weight that is water: _____

5. List the four major minerals: _____

Lesson 9.6

The Large Intestine and Elimination

Objectives

Once your small intestine has digested and absorbed the nutrients, the residual materials must be prepared in your large intestine so they can be eliminated from your body. The information in this lesson will enable you to use correct medical terminology to:

9.6.1 Describe the structure and functions of the large intestine.

9.6.2 Outline disorders of the large intestine.

Keynotes

- A sphincter is a ring of smooth muscle that forms a one-way valve.
- Colon: Ascending to transverse to descending to sigmoid to rectum to anus.

Transverse colon —
Hepatic flexure —
Ascending colon (right) —
Ileum —
Ileocecal valve —
Cecum —
Vermiform appendix —
Rectum —
Anal canal —

Splenic flexure
Descending colon (left)
Sigmoid colon
Internal anal sphincter
External anal sphincter

(a)

Cecum —
Appendix —

Descending colon
Sigmoid colon

(b)

◀ **FIGURE 9.24**
Large Intestine.
(a) Surface anatomy.
(b) X-ray of large intestine following barium enema.

Structure and Functions of the Large Intestine (LO 9.9)

Structure of the Large Intestine (LO 9.9)

Your **large intestine** is so named because its diameter is much greater than that of your small intestine. In your abdominal cavity, the large intestine forms a perimeter around the central mass of the small intestine.

At the junction between the small and large intestines, a ring of smooth muscle called the **ileocecal sphincter** forms a one-way valve. This allows chyme to pass into the large intestine and prevents the large intestine's contents from backing into the ileum.

The **cecum** is located at the beginning of the large intestine. It is a pouch in the abdomen's right lower quadrant. A narrow tube with a closed end (the **vermiform appendix**) projects downward from the cecum (*Figure 9.24a and b*). The function of the appendix is not known.

The ascending **colon** begins at the cecum and extends upward to underneath the liver. Here, it makes a sharp turn at the hepatic **flexure** and becomes the transverse colon. At the left side of the abdomen, near the spleen at the splenic flexure, the transverse colon turns downward to form the descending colon. At the pelvic brim, the descending colon forms an S-shaped curve called the **sigmoid** colon. This descends in the pelvis to become the rectum and then the **anal canal.**

The **rectum** has three transverse folds—rectal valves that enable it to retain **feces** while passing gas (flatus).

The anal canal (*Figure 9.25*) is the last 1 to 2 inches of the large intestine, opening to the outside as the **anus.** An internal anal sphincter, composed of smooth muscle from the intestinal wall, and an external anal sphincter, composed of skeletal muscle that can be controlled voluntarily, guard the exit of the anus.

Functions of the Large Intestine (LO 9.9)

Your large intestine has the following key functions:

- **Absorption** of water and electrolytes. The large intestine receives more than 1 liter (1,000 ml) of chyme each day from the small intestine. It reabsorbs water and electrolytes to reduce the volume of chyme to 100 to 150 ml of feces, which are eliminated by **defecation;**

- **Secretion** of mucus that protects the intestinal wall and holds particles of fecal matter together;

- **Digestion** (by the bacteria that inhabit the large intestine) of any food remnants that have escaped the small intestine's digestive enzymes;

- **Peristalsis** happens a few times a day in the large intestine to produce mass movements toward the rectum; and

- **Elimination** of materials that were not digested or absorbed.

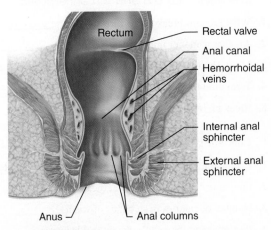

Rectum
Rectal valve
Anal canal
Hemorrhoidal veins
Internal anal sphincter
External anal sphincter
Anus
Anal columns

▲ **FIGURE 9.25**
Anal Canal.

Word Analysis and Definition

S = Suffix   P = Prefix   R = Root   R/CF = Combining Form

WORD	PRONUNCIATION		ELEMENTS	DEFINITION
anus	A-nus		Latin *ring*	Terminal opening of the digestive tract through which feces are discharged
anal (adj)	A-nal	S/	-al *pertaining to*	Pertaining to the anus
		R/CF	an/o- *anus*	
anorectal junction	A-no-**RECK**-tal **JUNK**-shun	R/	-rect- *rectum*	The junction between the anus and rectum
		S/	-ion *condition, action*	
		R/	junct- *joining together*	
appendix	ah-**PEN**-dicks		Latin *appendage*	Small blind projection from the pouch of the cecum
appendicitis	ah-pen-dih-**SIGH**-tis	S/	-itis *inflammation*	Inflammation of the appendix
		R/	appendic- *appendix*	
appendectomy (**Note:** *elimination of "ic" prior to "ec" of* -**ectomy**)	ah-pen-**DEK**-toe-me	S/	-ectomy *surgical excision*	Surgical removal of the appendix
colon	**KOH**-lon		Greek *colon*	The large intestine, extending from the cecum to the rectum
colic (adj)	**KOL**-ik	S/	-ic *pertaining to*	Spasmodic, crampy pains in the abdomen
		R/	col- *colon*	
colitis	koh-**LIE**-tis	S/	-itis *inflammation*	Inflammation of the colon
feces	**FEE**-seez		Latin *dregs*	Undigested, waste material discharged from the bowel
fecal (adj)	**FEE**-kal	S/	-al *pertaining to*	Pertaining to feces
		R/	fec- *feces*	
defecation	def-eh-**KAY**-shun	S/	-ation *process*	Evacuation of feces from rectum and anus
		P/	de- *removal*	
flexure	**FLEK**-shur		Latin *bend*	A bend in a structure
ileum	**ILL**-ee-um		Latin *roll up, twist*	Third portion of the small intestine
ileocecal sphincter	**ILL**-ee-oh-**SEE**-cal **SFINK**-ter	S/	-al *pertaining to*	Band of muscle that encircles the junction of ileum and cecum
		R/CF	ile/o- *ileum*	
		R/	-cec- *cecum*	
			sphincter, Greek *band*	
rectum	**RECK**-tum		Latin *straight*	Terminal part of the colon from the sigmoid to the anal canal
rectal (adj)	**RECK**-tal	S/	-al *pertaining to*	Pertaining to the rectum
		R/	rect- *rectum*	
sigmoid	**SIG**-moyd		Greek *letter "S"*	Sigmoid colon is shaped like an "S"

EXERCISES

A. Apply *the language of the digestive system and answer the following questions.*   **LO 9.2, 9.9, and 9.11** *Apply*

1. What part of the digestive system contains both an internal and external sphincter? _____

2. What body part has no known use or function? _____

3. What is a ring of smooth muscle that forms a one-way valve called? _____

4. How did the "large" intestine get its name? _____

5. Where is the cecum located? _____

6. The *hepatic flexure* is near what major body organ? _____

B. Deconstruct: *Attack a medical term with your analytical skills. Break down these terms into their elements to define the word. Know the meaning of the elements = know the meaning of the term. Fill in the chart.*   **LO 9.1, 9.9, and 9.11** *Analyze*

Medical Term	Meaning of Prefix	Meaning of Root/CF	Meaning of Suffix	Meaning of Term
colitis	1.	2.	3.	4.
defecation	5.	6.	7.	8.
anorectal	9.	10.	11.	12.
ileocecal	13.	14.	15.	16.

Lesson 9.6 (cont'd)

Keynotes

- A proctologist is a surgical specialist in diseases of the anus and rectum.
- Fissures are tears; fistulas are abnormal passages.
- Consuming black licorice, Pepto-Bismol, or blueberries can produce black stools.

Abbreviations

BM	bowel movement
IBS	irritable bowel syndrome

Disorders of the Large Intestine and Anal Canal (LO 9.9)

Disorders of the Large Intestine (LO 9.9)

Appendicitis is the most common cause of acute abdominal pain in the right lower quadrant. If neglected, the inflamed appendix can rupture, leading to **peritonitis**. Appendicitis is treated with a surgical appendectomy, usually performed through laparoscopy.

Diverticulosis is the presence of small pouches (**diverticula**) bulging outward through weak spots in the large intestine's lining *(Figure 9.26)*. The pouches are asymptomatic until they become infected and inflamed, a condition called **diverticulitis.** The most likely cause of **diverticular disease** (diverticulosis and diverticulitis) is a low-fiber diet.

Ulcerative colitis is an extensive inflammation and ulceration of the large intestine's lining. It produces bouts of bloody diarrhea, crampy pain, weight loss, and an electrolyte imbalance.

Irritable bowel syndrome (IBS) is an increasingly common large-bowel disorder presenting with crampy pain, gas, and changes in bowel habits to either constipation or diarrhea. There are no anatomical changes seen in the bowel. The cause is unknown.

Polyps, which vary in size and shape, are masses of tissue arising from the large intestine's wall and protruding into the bowel lumen. Although most polyps are benign, an endoscopic biopsy can determine if they are precancerous or cancerous.

Colon and rectal cancers are the second cause of cancer deaths after lung cancer. The majority of these cancers occur in the rectum and sigmoid colon. They can spread through the bowel wall, extend down the lumen, and metastasize to regional lymph nodes and to liver, lungs, bones, and brain through the bloodstream.

Obstruction of the large bowel can be caused by cancers, large polyps, or diverticulitis.

Proctitis is an inflammation of the rectum's lining, often associated with ulcerative colitis, Crohn disease, or radiation therapy.

Diverticula

▲ **FIGURE 9.26**
Barium Enema Showing Diverticulosis.

Disorders of the Anal Canal (LO 9.9)

Hemorrhoids are dilated veins in the submucosa (connective tissue layer) of the anal canal, often associated with pregnancy, chronic constipation, diarrhea, or aging. They protrude into the anal canal (**internal**) or bulge out along the edge of the anus (**external**) *(Figure 9.27),* producing pain and bright red blood from the anus. A **thrombosed** hemorrhoid, in which blood has clotted, is very painful.

Anal fissures are tears in the anal canal's lining, perhaps from difficult bowel movements (**BMs**). **Anal fistulas** occur following abscesses in the anal glands and are an abnormal passage (fistula) between the anal canal and the skin outside the anus. Surgical procedures—a **fistulectomy** and a **fistulotomy**—are used to treat anal fistulas.

Gastrointestinal (GI) Bleeding (LO 9.6 and 9.9)

GI tract bleeding can have a variety of causes, which are not always easy to recognize. Sometimes, the bleeding can be internal and painless. It can present in different ways, however, to provide a clue as to the site of bleeding:

- **Hematemesis** is the vomiting of bright red blood, which indicates an upper GI source of bleeding (esophagus, stomach, duodenum) that is brisk.
- **Vomiting of "coffee grounds"** occurs when bleeding from an upper GI source has slowed or stopped.
- **Melena,** the passage of black, tarry stools, usually indicates upper GI bleeding.
- **Occult blood** cannot be seen in the stool, but when a chemical fecal occult blood test (**Hemoccult**) is positive, the source of the bleeding can be anywhere in the GI tract.

▲ **FIGURE 9.27**
External Hemorrhoid.

Word Analysis and Definition

S = Suffix   P = Prefix   R = Root   R/CF = Combining Form

WORD	PRONUNCIATION		ELEMENTS	DEFINITION
bowel	BOUGH-el		Latin *sausage*	Another name for intestine
diverticulum	die-ver-**TICK**-you-lum	S/	-um *tissue, structure*	A pouchlike opening or sac from a tubular structure (e.g., intestine)
diverticula (pl)	di-ver-**TICK**-you-lah	R/	diverticul- *byroad*	
diverticulosis	**DIE**-ver-tick-you-**LOW**-sis	S/	-osis *condition*	Presence of a number of small pouches in the wall of the large intestine
diverticulitis	**DIE**-ver-tick-you-**LIE**-tis	S/	-itis *inflammation*	Inflammation of the diverticula
fissure	**FISH**-ur		Latin *slit*	Deep furrow or cleft
fistula	**FIS**-tyu-lah		Latin *pipe, tube*	Abnormal passage
hemorrhoid	**HEM**-oh-royd	S/	-rrhoid *flow*	Dilated rectal vein producing painful anal swelling
hemorrhoids (pl)		R/CF	hem/o- *blood*	
hemorrhoidectomy	**HEM**-oh-royd-**EK**-toh-me	S/	-ectomy *surgical excision*	Surgical removal of hemorrhoids
(**Note:** *This term has two suffixes.*)				
melena	mel-**EN**-ah		Greek *black*	The passage of black, tarry stools
occult blood	oh-**KULT BLUD**		occult, Latin *to hide*	Blood that cannot be seen in the stool but is positive on a fecal occult blood test
Hemoccult test	**HEEM**-o-kult **TEST**			Trade name for a fecal occult blood test
peritoneum	per-ih-toe-**NEE**-um	S/	-um *tissue*	Membrane that lines the abdominal cavity
		R/CF	periton/e- *stretch over*	
peritoneal (adj)	**PER**-ih-toe-**NEE**-al	S/	-al *pertaining to*	Pertaining to the peritoneum
peritonitis	**PER**-ih-toe-**NIE**-tis	S/	-itis *inflammation*	Inflammation of the peritoneum
polyp	**POL**-ip		Latin *foot*	Mass of tissue that projects into the lumen of the bowel
polyposis	pol-ih-**POH**-sis	S/	-osis *condition*	Presence of several polyps
		R/	polyp- *polyp*	
polypectomy	pol-ip-**ECK**-toh-mee	S/	-ectomy *surgical excision*	Excision or removal of a polyp
proctitis	prok-**TIE**-tis	S/	-itis *inflammation*	Inflammation of the lining of the rectum
		R/	proct- *rectum*	
proctologist	prok-**TOL**-oh-jist	S/	-logist *specialist*	A surgical specialist in diseases of the anus and rectum
		R/CF	proct/o- *rectum*	

EXERCISES

A. Suffixes: *This is a two-part exercise. First, insert the correct suffix to complete the term. Then circle the word in the definition that has the same meaning as the suffix. (There are more suffixes than you need.)*   **LO 9.1, 9.4, and 9.9** *Apply*

    osis   ectomy   um   itis   al   ion

1. excision or removal of a polyp   polyp/   _____

2. inflammation of the diverticula   diverticul/   _____

3. membranous structure lining the abdominal cavity   peritone/   _____

4. condition of having multiple polyps   polyp/   _____

5. pertaining to the peritoneum   peritone/   _____

B. Apply *the language of the digestive system and answer the following questions.*   **LO 9.1, 9.2, and 9.9** *Apply*

1. List all the terms on this spread that mean *inflammation of:* _____

2. What is the difference between *diverticulitis* and *diverticulosis?* _____

_____

3. Where else in the body can you have polyps? _____

4. What are dilated veins in the anal canal called? _____

Pyloric sphincter — Pylorus of stomach —

Jejunum — — Duodenum

▲ **FIGURE 9.28**
Barium Meal.

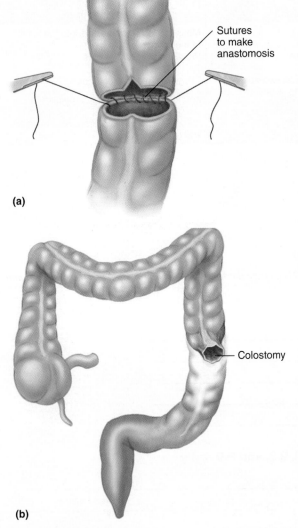

Sutures to make anastomosis

(a)

Colostomy

(b)

▲ **FIGURE 9.29**
Intestinal Resections.
(a) Anastomosis. (b) Ostomy.

Diagnostic and Therapeutic Procedures (LO 9.10)

Procedures for the Biliary System (LO 9.7 and 9.10)

A **cholangiography** requires the intravenous injection of a dye, followed by an x-ray of the biliary system so that the biliary system can be viewed.

A **cholecystectomy** is the surgical removal of the gallbladder.

A **cholelithotomy** is the surgical removal of gallstones.

Diagnostic Procedures for the Digestive Tract (LO 9.10)

Barium swallow involves ingestion of barium sulfate, a contrast material, to show details of the pharynx and esophagus on an x-ray.

Barium meal *(Figure 9.28)* uses barium sulfate to study the distal esophagus, stomach, and duodenum on an x-ray.

Enteroscopy through an oral endoscope is used to visualize and biopsy tumors and ulcers, and to control bleeding from the esophagus, stomach, and duodenum. This procedure is also called **esophagogastroduodenoscopy (EGD).**

Angiography uses dye to highlight blood vessels. It can be used to define the site of a bleed.

Fecal occult blood test (Hemoccult) is used to detect the presence of blood not visible to the naked eye.

Nasogastric aspiration and **lavage** that shows bright red blood indicates active upper GI bleeding. Vomiting of coffee-ground material indicates the bleeding has slowed or stopped.

Upper GI barium x-rays are less accurate than **panendoscopy** at identifying the bleeding lesion.

Barium enema involves the injection of a radiographic contrast material into the large intestine as an enema, and x-ray films are taken.

Endoscopy enables direct visual examination of the intestine with a flexible tube containing light-transmitting glass fibers or a video transmitter. Endoscopy can also be used to perform a biopsy, remove polyps (polypectomy), and coagulate bleeding lesions. **Panendoscopy** examines the esophagus, stomach, and duodenum.

Anoscopy examines the anus and lower rectum with a rigid instrument. **Flexible sigmoidoscopy** examines the rectum and sigmoid colon. **Colonoscopy** examines the whole length of the colon. **Gastroscopy** examines the stomach. **Proctoscopy** examines the anus.

Digital rectal exam (DRE) is performed by the physician, who palpates the rectum and prostate gland with a gloved index finger.

Therapeutic Procedures for the Digestive Tract (LO 9.10)

Excess gastric acid can be neutralized by **antacids,** such as aluminum hydroxide (Maalox) and calcium carbonate (Tums, Rolaids). **Histamine-2 receptor antagonists (H-2 blockers)** block the production of gastric acid. Examples are cimetidine (Tagamet) and ranitidine (Zantac). **Proton pump inhibitors** block the enzyme system in the lining of the stomach that produces gastric acid. Examples are omeprazole (Prilosec) and lansoprazole (Prevacid). **Anti-H. *pylori* therapy** is given with two antibiotics and a proton pump inhibitor.

Intestinal resections are used to surgically remove diseased portions of the intestine. The remaining portions of the intestine can be joined together through an **anastomosis** *(Figure 9.29a)*. If there is insufficient bowel remaining, an **ostomy** *(Figure 9.29b)* can be performed, in which the end of the bowel opens onto the skin at a **stoma** (a surgical, artificial opening). **Ileostomy** and **colostomy** are two common procedures.

Word Analysis and Definition

WORD	PRONUNCIATION	ELEMENTS		DEFINITION
anastomosis anastomoses (pl)	ah-**NAS**-toh-**MOH**-sis ah-**NAS**-toh-**MOH**-seez	S/ R/	-osis *condition* anastom- *provide a mouth*	A surgically made union between two tubular structures
antacid	ant-**ASS**-id	P/ R/	ant- *against* -acid *acid*	Agent that neutralizes acidity
endoscope	**EN**-doh-skope	P/ R/	endo- *within, inside* -scope *instrument for viewing*	Instrument to examine the inside of a hollow or tubular organ
endoscopy	en-**DOS**-koh-pee	R/	-scopy *to examine, to view*	The use of an endoscope
colonoscopy	koh-lon-**OSS**-koh-pee	R/CF	colon/o- *colon*	Examination of the inside of the colon by endoscopy
panendoscopy (**Note:** Two prefixes)	pan-en-**DOS**-koh-pee	P/ P/	pan- *all* -endo- *within, inside*	Examination of the inside of the esophagus, stomach, and upper duodenum using a flexible fiber-optic endoscope
proctoscopy (*also called* **anoscopy**)	prok-**TOSS**-koh-pee	R/CF	proct/o- *anus*	Examination of the inside of the anus by endoscopy
sigmoidoscopy	sig-moi-**DOS**-koh-pee	R/CF	sigmoid/o- *sigmoid colon*	Examination of the sigmoid colon by endoscopy
gastroscopy	gas-**TROSS**-koh-pee	R/CF	gastr/o- *stomach*	Examination of the inside of the stomach by endoscopy
enema	**EN**-eh-mah		Greek *injection*	An injection of fluid into the rectum
ostomy	**OSS**-toe-me	S/ R/	-stomy *new opening* os- *mouth*	Artificial opening into a tubular structure
colostomy	koh-**LOSS**-toe-me	R/CF	col/o- *colon*	Artificial opening from the colon to the outside of the body
ileostomy	ill-ee-**OS**-toe-me	R/CF	ile/o- *ileum*	Artificial opening from the ileum to the outside of the body
proton pump inhibitor	**PRO**-ton **PUMP** in-**HIB**-ih-tor	R/ R/ S/ R/	proton *first* pump *pump* -or *a doer* inhibit- *repress*	Agent in the lining of the stomach that blocks the enzyme system that produces gastric acid.
stoma	**STOW**-mah		Greek *mouth*	Artifical opening

EXERCISES

A. Test yourself *on the elements contained in the WAD. The prefixes and suffixes you will see again in terms in other chapters. Match the element in column 1 with its definition in column 2.*   **LO 9.1, 9.9, and 9.10** *Understand*

_____ **1.** os

_____ **2.** gastro

_____ **3.** endo

_____ **4.** colo

_____ **5.** scope

_____ **6.** procto

_____ **7.** stomy

_____ **8.** ileo

_____ **9.** pan

_____ **10.** osis

A. colon

B. instrument for viewing

C. all

D. mouth

E. condition

F. ileum

G. stomach

H. within

I. new opening

J. anus

B. Cover the WAD *with a piece of paper and spell the following terms correctly. Circle the best answer.*   **LO 9.9 and 9.10** *Remember*

1. procktologist   proctologist   practologist

2. intusception   intussception   intussusception

3. polyp   polip   polypp

4. anastomossis   anastamossis   anastomosis

5. peritineum   peritoneum   peritonium

Additional exercises available in **connect**

Chapter Review exercises, along with additional practice items, are available in Connect!

The Nervous System and Mental Health

The Essentials of the Languages of Neurology and Psychiatry

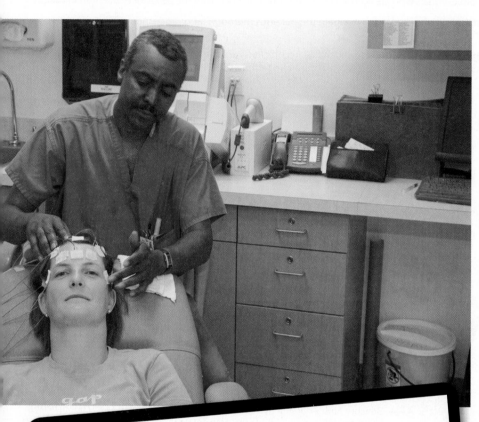

CHAPTER 10

Learning Outcomes

Your roles are to perform electroneurodiagnostic evaluations, communicate with Ms. Gaston and her parents, communicate with other health professionals, and maintain and document Ms. Gaston's history and care. To perform these roles, you must be able to:

LO 10.1 Use roots, combining forms, suffixes, and prefixes to construct and analyze (deconstruct) medical terms related to the nervous system and mental health.

LO 10.2 Spell and pronounce correctly medical terms related to the nervous system and mental health to communicate them with accuracy and precision in any health care setting.

LO 10.3 Define accepted abbreviations related to the nervous system and mental health.

LO 10.4 Relate the structures of the brain, cranial nerves, spinal cord, peripheral nerves, and meninges to their functions.

LO 10.5 Identify the medical terms used in disorders of the brain, cranial nerves, spinal cord, and meninges, and in the management of pain.

LO 10.6 Describe the diagnostic procedures, therapeutic methods, and pharmacologic agents used in treating disorders of the nervous system and mental health.

LO 10.7 Define mental health, the difference between psychiatry and psychology, and the different types of common mental health disorders.

LO 10.8 Apply your knowledge of medical terms relating to the nervous system and mental health to documentation, medical records, and medical reports.

LO 10.9 Translate the medical terms relating to the nervous system and mental health into everyday language in order to communicate clearly with patients and their families.

Case Report 10.1

You are ...

... an **electroneurodiagnostic** technologist working with Gregory Solis, MD, a **neurosurgeon** at Fulwood Medical Center.

You are communicating with ...

... Ms. Roberta Gaston, a 39-year-old woman, who has been referred by Raul Cardenas, MD, a **neurologist,** for evaluation for possible **neurosurgery**. Ms. Gaston has had **epileptic** seizures since the age of 16. She also has daily minor spells in which she stops interacting and blinks rhythmically for about 20 seconds, after which she returns to normal. She is unable to work and is cared for by her parents. Her neurologic examination is normal. Her **electroencephalogram (EEG)** shows diffuse epileptic discharges in the left frontal region. Her CT scan is normal. An MRI shows a 20-mm-diameter mass adjacent to her left ventricle.

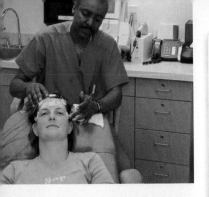

The health professionals involved in the diagnosis and treatment of problems with the neurological system and mental health include the following:

- **Neurologists** are medical doctors who specialize in disorders of the nervous system.

- **Neurosurgeons** are medical doctors who perform surgical procedures on the nervous system.

- **Psychiatrists** are medical doctors who are licensed in the diagnosis and treatment of mental disorders.

- **Anesthesiologists** are medical doctors who are certified to administer anesthetics and can also be responsible for pain management.

- **Psychologists** are professionals who are licensed in the science concerned with the behavior of the human mind.

- **Neuropsychologists** are individuals who evaluate the patient's memory, language, and cognitive functions, and develop appropriate treatment plans.

- **Electroneurodiagnostic technicians** (also called EEG technicians) are professionals who operate specialized equipment that measures the electrical activity of the brain, peripheral nervous system, and spinal cord.

Lesson 10.1

Structure and Functions of the Nervous System

Central nervous system (CNS)
— Brain
— Spinal cord

Peripheral nervous system (PNS)
— Sensory and motor nerves
— Ganglia

Structure of the Nervous System (LO 10.2 and 10.4)

The nervous system *(Figure 10.1)* has two major anatomical subdivisions.

1. The **central nervous system (CNS),** consisting of the brain and spinal cord; and

2. The **peripheral nervous system (PNS),** consisting of all the neurons and nerves outside the central nervous system. It includes 12 pairs of cranial nerves originating from the brain and 31 pairs of spinal nerves originating from the spinal cord.

The peripheral nervous system is further subdivided into:

i. The **sensory division,** in which sensory nerves (**afferent** nerves) carry messages toward the spinal cord and brain from sense organs; and

ii. The **motor division,** in which motor nerves (**efferent** nerves) carry messages away from the brain and spinal cord to muscles and organs.

   a. The **visceral motor division** is called the **autonomic nervous system (ANS).** It carries signals to glands and to cardiac and smooth muscle. It operates at a subconscious level outside your voluntary control, and it has two subdivisions:

   - The **sympathetic division** arouses the body for action by increasing the heart and respiratory rates to increase oxygen supply to the brain and muscles.

   - The **parasympathetic division** calms the body, slowing down the heartbeat but stimulating digestion.

   b. The **somatic motor division** carries signals to the skeletal muscles and is within your voluntary control.

Study Hint

Remember the acronym SAME: Sensory nerves are Afferent (toward the brain). Motor nerves are Efferent (toward the skeleton).

▶ **FIGURE 10.1**
The Nervous System.

S = Suffix   P = Prefix   R = Root   R/CF = Combining Form

WORD	PRONUNCIATION	ELEMENTS		DEFINITION
afferent (Note: *Also called sensory; opposite of efferent*)	AFF-eh-rent		Latin *to bring to*	Moving toward a center; for example, nerve fibers conducting *impulses to the spinal cord and brain*
efferent (Note: *Also called motor; opposite of afferent*)	EFF-eh-rent		Latin *to bring away from*	Moving away from a center; for example, conducting nerve impulses away *from the brain or spinal cord*
electroencephalogram (EEG)	ee-LEK-troh-en-SEF-ah-low-gram	S/ R/CF R/CF	-gram *recording* electr/o- *electricity* -encephal/o- *brain*	Record of the electrical activity of the brain
electroencephalograph	ee-LEK-troh-en-SEF-ah-low-graf	S/	-graph *to write, record*	Device used to record the electrical activity of the brain
electroencephalography	ee-LEK-troh-en-SEF-ah-LOG-rah-fee	S/	-graphy *process of recording*	The process of recording the electrical activity of the brain
electroneurodiagnostic (adj)	ee-LEK-troh-NYUR-oh-die-ag-NOS-tik	S/ R/CF R/CF R/	-ic *pertaining to* electr/o- *electricity* -neur/o- *nerve* -diagnost- *decision*	Pertaining to the use of electricity in the diagnosis of a neurologic disorder
epilepsy	EP-ih-LEP-see		Greek *seizure*	Chronic brain disorder due to paroxysmal excessive neuronal discharges
epileptic (adj) (Note: *An epileptic episode is called a seizure.*)	EP-ih-LEP-tik SEE-zhur	S/ R/	-ic *pertaining to* epilept- *seizure*	Pertaining to or suffering from epilepsy
motor	MOH-tor		Latin *to move*	Structures of the nervous system that send impulses out to cause muscles to contract or glands to secrete
nerve	NERV		Latin *nerve*	A cord of nerve fibers bound together by connective tissue
nervous system	NER-vus SIS-tem	S/ R/	-ous *pertaining to* nerv- *nerve* system, Greek *an organized whole*	The whole, integrated nerve apparatus
neurology	nyu-ROL-oh-jee	S/ R/CF	-logy *study of* neur/o- *nerve*	Medical specialty of disorders of the nervous system
neurologist	nyu-ROL-oh-jist	S/	-logist *one who studies, specialist*	Medical specialist in disorders of the nervous system
neurologic (adj)	NYU-roh-LOJ-ik	S/ R/	-ic *pertaining to* -log- *to study*	Pertaining to the nervous system
neurosurgeon	NYU-roh-SUR-jun	S/ R/	-eon *one who does* -surg- *operate*	One who performs surgery on the nervous system
neurosurgery	NYU-roh-SUR-jer-ee	S/	-ery *process of*	Operating surgically on the nervous system
parasympathetic (Note: *This term contains two prefixes.*)	par-ah-sim-pah-THET-ik	S/ P/ P/ R/	-ic *pertaining to* para- *beside* -sym- *together* -pathet- *suffering*	Division of the autonomic nervous system; has opposite effects to the sympathetic division
sensory	SEN-soh-ree	S/ R/	-ory *having the function of* sens- *feel*	Pertaining to sensation; structures of the nervous system that carry impulses to the brain
somatic	soh-MAT-ik	S/ R/	-ic *pertaining to* somat- *body*	A division of the peripheral nervous system serving the skeletal muscles OR relating to the body in general
sympathetic	sim-pah-THET-ik	S/ P/ R/	-ic *pertaining to* sym- *together* -pathet- *suffering*	Division of the autonomic nervous system operating at an unconscious level
visceral (adj)	VISS-er-al	S/ R/	-al *pertaining to* viscer- *internal organs*	Pertaining to the internal organs
viscus viscera (pl)	VISS-kus VISS-er-ah		Latin *an internal organ*	Any single internal organ

EXERCISE

A. Documentation: *Fill in the following paragraph with the appropriate language of neurology. Review Case Report 10.1 and the WAD before starting this exercise.* **LO 10.2, 10.3, 10.5, and 10.6** *Apply*

electroencephalography   electroneurodiagnostic   epilepsy   electroencephalograph

neurologist   electroencephalogram   neurosurgeon

Roberta Gaston and her parents were sent to this office by her (1) _____.

Dr. Solis has ordered some (2) _____ tests because of her (3) _____.

The particular type of test is an (4) _____, which will produce an EEG on the (device) (5) _____.

After the results of the (6) _____, if Ms. Gaston needs surgery, it will be performed by a(n) (7) _____.

Structure of the Nervous System *(continued)*

▶ **FIGURE 10.2**
Components of the
Nervous System.

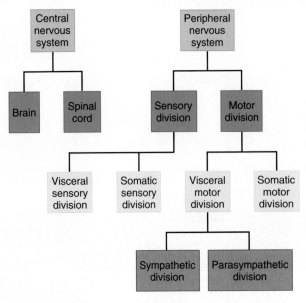

Functions of the Nervous System (LO 10.2 and 10.4)

Optimal communication between your nervous system and all the cells in your body requires that the following five functions are always working smoothly:

1. **Sensory input** to the brain comes from receptors all over your body at both the conscious and subconscious levels. You are conscious of external stimuli that you receive from your body as it interacts with your environment. Inside your body, internal stimuli concerning the amount of oxygen and carbon dioxide in your blood, and other homeostatic variables like your body temperature, are being processed continually at the subconscious level.

2. **Motor output** from your brain stimulates the skeletal muscles to contract, which enables you to move. Your nervous system controls the production of sweat, saliva, and digestive enzymes without active input from you.

3. **Evaluation and integration** occur in your brain and spinal cord to process the **sensory** input, initiate a response, and store the event in memory.

4. **Homeostasis** is maintained by your nervous system taking in internal sensory input and responding to it. For example, the nervous system responds by stimulating the heart to deliver the correct volume of blood to ensure oxygenation of and removal of waste products from cells.

5. **Mental activity** occurs in your brain so that you can think, feel, understand, respond, and remember.

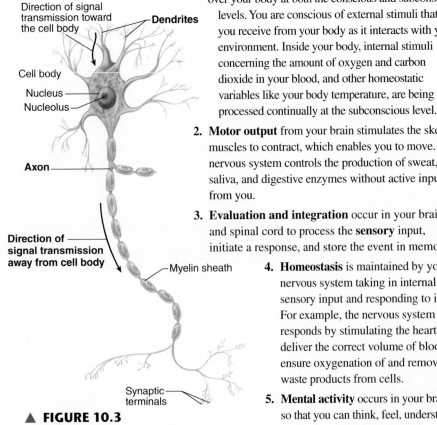

Direction of signal transmission toward the cell body

Dendrites

Cell body

Nucleus

Nucleolus

Axon

Direction of signal transmission away from cell body

Myelin sheath

Synaptic terminals

▲ **FIGURE 10.3**
Neuron.

Cells of the Nervous System
(LO 10.2 and 10.4)

Neurons (nerve cells) receive stimuli and transmit impulses to other neurons or to organ receptors. Each neuron consists of a cell body and two types of processes or extensions, called **axons** and **dendrites** *(Figure 10.3)*.

Dendrites are short, multiple, highly branched extensions of the neuron's cell body. They direct impulses toward the cell body. A single axon, or nerve fiber, arises from the cell body, is covered in a fatty **myelin** sheath, and carries the impulse away from the cell body. Each axon measures a few millimeters to a meter in length.

Bundles of axons appear white in color and create the **white matter** of the brain and spinal cord. Neuron cell bodies, dendrites, and synapses appear gray and create the **gray matter.**

The axon terminates in a network of small branches that ends at a **synapse** (junction) with a dendrite from another neuron, or with a receptor on a muscle cell or gland cell *(Figure 10.4)*. **Neurotransmitters** cross the synapse to stimulate or inhibit another neuron or the cell of a muscle or gland. Examples of neurotransmitters are norepinephrine, serotonin, and **dopamine.**

Groups of cell bodies cluster together to form ganglia, and groups of cell bodies and axons collect together to form nerves.

The trillion neurons in the nervous system are outnumbered 50 to 1 by the supportive **glial** cells **(neuroglia).**

The blood-brain barrier is a physical barrier—composed of glial cells and the capillary blood vessel walls—that prevents foreign substances, toxins, and infections from leaving the bloodstream and affecting the brain cells.

Dendrite

Cell body

Presynaptic neuron

Axon

Direction of signal transmission

Synapses

Dendrite

Synaptic terminals at synapses

Postsynaptic neuron

Axon

Direction of signal transmission

◀ **FIGURE 10.4**
Synapse.

Word Analysis and Definition

WORD	PRONUNCIATION		ELEMENTS	DEFINITION
autonomic	awe-toh-**NOM**-ik	S/ P/ R/	-ic *pertaining to* auto- *self* -nom- *law*	Self-governing visceral motor division of the peripheral nervous system
axon	**ACK**-son		Greek *axis*	Single process of a nerve cell carrying nervous impulses away from the cell body
dendrite	**DEN**-dright		Greek *looking like a tree*	Branched extension of the nerve cell body that receives nervous stimuli
dopamine	**DOH**-pah-meen		Precursor of norepinephrine	Neurotransmitter in some specific small areas of the brain
glia glial (adj) neuroglia	**GLEE**-ah **GLEE**-al nyu-roh-**GLEE**-ah	S/ R/ R/CF	Greek *glue* -al *pertaining to* -glia *glue* neur/o- *nerve*	Connective tissue that holds a structure together Pertaining to glia or neuroglia Connective tissue holding nervous tissue together
myelin	**MY**-eh-lin	S/ R/	-in *substance, chemical compound* myel- *spinal cord*	Material of the sheath around the axon of a nerve
neuron	**NYUR**-on		Greek *nerve*	Technical term for a nerve cell; consists of cell body with its dendrites and axons
neurotransmitter (**Note:** Transmit *is a word itself, so the prefix trans is in the middle of the overall word.*)	**NYUR**-oh-trans-**MIT**-er	S/ R/CF P/ R/	-er *agent* neur/o- *nerve* -trans- *across* -mitt- *send*	Chemical agent that relays messages from one nerve cell to the next
parasympathetic (**Note:** *This term contains two prefixes.*)	par-ah-sim-pah-**THET**-ik	S/ P/ P/ R/	-ic *pertaining to* para- *beside* -sym- *together* -pathet- *suffering*	Division of the autonomic nervous system; has opposite effects to the sympathetic division
sympathetic	sim-pah-**THET**-ik	S/ P/ R/	-ic *pertaining to* sym- *together* -pathet- *suffering*	Division of the autonomic nervous system operating at an unconscious level
synapse	**SIN**-aps	P/ R/	syn- *together* -apse *clasp*	Junction between two nerve cells, or a nerve fiber and its target cell, where electrical impulses are transmitted between the cells

EXERCISE

A. Elements: *Solid knowledge of elements is the key to learning medical terminology. Match each element in column 1 with its correct meaning in column 2.*
LO 10.1 *Understand*

_____ **1.** ic

_____ **2.** sym

_____ **3.** viscer

_____ **4.** auto

_____ **5.** pathet

_____ **6.** para

A. self

B. pertaining to

C. suffering

D. together

E. internal organ

F. beside

B. Deconstruct *the following terms into their elements and give their meanings in your own words.*   **LO 10.1 and 10.4** *Analyze*

1. neurotransmitter _____ / _____ / _____

                      P   R, R/CF   S

   Meaning: _____

2. parasympathetic _____ / _____ / _____

                      P   R, R/CF   S

   Meaning: _____

Lesson 10.2

The Brain and Cranial Nerves

The sensations of smelling the roses, seeing them, and touching them are recognized and interpreted in your brain, as are all sensations. The actions of kneeling down, cutting the rose stem, walking into the house, and placing it in a vase originate in your brain, as do all your voluntary actions. The information in this lesson will enable you to use correct medical terminology to:

10.2.1 Describe the essential structures of the brain and spinal cord.

10.2.2 Identify the major sensory and motor areas of the brain.

10.2.3 Explain how the brain and spinal cord are protected and supported.

Abbreviation

CSF   cerebrospinal fluid

▼ FIGURE 10.5
Brain.
(a) View from the left side.
(b) View from above.

The Brain (LO 10.4)

Your adult brain weighs about 3 pounds. Its size and weight are proportional to your body size, not your intelligence. Your brain is divided into three major regions: the **cerebrum,** the **brain stem,** and the **cerebellum.**

Cerebrum (LO 10.4)

The cerebrum makes up about 80% of your brain. It consists of two **cerebral** hemispheres, which are mirror images of each other. These hemispheres are separated by a deep longitudinal fissure, and at the bottom of this, they are connected by a bridge of nerve fibers (the **corpus callosum**).

On the surface of the cerebrum, numerous ridges, **gyri,** are separated by fissures called **sulci** *(Figure 10.5).* The cerebral hemispheres are covered by a thin layer of gray matter (nerve cells and dendrites) called the cerebral **cortex.** It is folded into the gyri, and sulci, and contains 70% of all the neurons in the nervous system. Below the cerebral cortex is a mass of white matter, in which bundles of myelinated nerve fibers connect the neurons of the cortex to the rest of the nervous system.

Functional Cerebral Regions (LO 10.4)

Each cerebral hemisphere is divided into four lobes:

1. The **frontal lobe,** located behind the forehead, forms the anterior part of the hemisphere. This lobe is responsible for intellect, planning, problem solving, and the voluntary motor control of muscles.

2. The **parietal lobe** is posterior to the frontal lobe. This lobe receives and interprets sensory information, like spoken words.

3. The **temporal lobe** is below the frontal and parietal lobes. This lobe interprets sensory experiences.

4. The **occipital lobe** forms the posterior part of the hemisphere. This lobe interprets visual images and written words.

Deep inside each cerebral hemisphere are spaces called ventricles, which contain watery **cerebrospinal fluid (CSF).** CSF circulates through the ventricles and around the brain and spinal cord. It helps to protect, cushion, and provide nutrition for the brain and spinal cord.

Located beneath the cerebral hemispheres and ventricles are the:

- **Thalamus,** which receives all sensory impulses and channels them to the appropriate region of the cortex for interpretation; and

- **Hypothalamus,** *Figure 10.6* which regulates blood pressure, body temperature, water, and electrolyte balance.

Brainstem and Cerebellum (LO 10.4)

The **brainstem** relays sensory impulses from peripheral nerves to higher brain centers. It also controls vital cardiovascular and respiratory activities.

The **cerebellum,** the most posterior area of the brain, coordinates skeletal muscle activity to maintain the body's posture and balance.

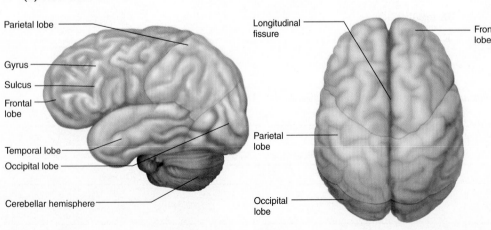

Parietal lobe

Gyrus

Sulcus

Frontal lobe

Temporal lobe

Occipital lobe

Cerebellar hemisphere

(a)

Longitudinal fissure

Frontal lobe

Parietal lobe

Occipital lobe

(b)

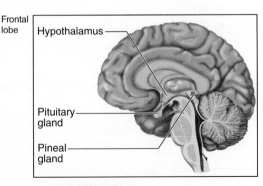

Hypothalamus

Pituitary gland

Pineal gland

▲ FIGURE 10.6
Hypothalamus, Pituitary Gland, and Pineal Gland.

Word Analysis and Definition

WORD	PRONUNCIATION	ELEMENTS		DEFINITION
cerebellum	ser-eh-**BELL**-um	S/ R/	-um *structure* cerebell- *little brain*	The most posterior area of the brain located between the midbrain and the cerebral hemispheres
cerebrospinal (adj) cerebrospinal fluid (CSF)	**SER**-ee-broh-**SPY**-nal	S/ R/CF R/	-al *pertaining to* cerebr/o- *brain* -spin- *spinal cord*	Pertaining to the brain and spinal cord Fluid formed in the ventricles of the brain; surrounds the brain and spinal cord
cerebrum cerebral (adj)	**SER**-ee-brum **SER**-ee-bral	S/ R/	Latin *brain* -al *pertaining to* cerebr- *cerebrum*	Cerebral hemispheres Pertaining to the cerebral hemispheres of the brain
corpus callosum	**KOR**-pus kah-**LOW**-sum	R/ S/ R/	corpus *body* -um *structure* callos- *thickening*	Bridge of nerve fibers connecting the two cerebral hemispheres
frontal lobe	**FRUNT**-al **LOBE**	S/ R/	-al *pertaining to* front- *front of*	Front area of the cerebral hemisphere
gyrus gyri (pl)	**JI**-rus **JI**-ree		Greek *circle*	Rounded elevation on the surface of the cerebral hemispheres
hypothalamus hypothalamic (adj)	high-poh-**THAL**-ah-muss high-poh-thah-**LAM**-ik	P/ S/ S/ R/	hypo- *below* -us *pertaining to* -ic *pertaining to* -thalam- *thalamus*	An endocrine gland in the floor and wall of the third ventricle of the brain Pertaining to the hypothalamus
occipital lobe	ock-**SIP**-it-al **LOBE**	S/ R/	-al *pertaining to* occipit- *back of head*	Posterior area of the cerebral hemisphere
parietal lobe	pah-**RYE**-eh-tal **LOBE**	S/ R/	-al *pertaining to* pariet- *wall*	Area of the brain under the parietal bone
sulcus sulci (pl)	**SUL**-cuss **SUL**-sigh		Latin *furrow, ditch*	Groove on the surface of the cerebral hemispheres that separates gyri
temporal lobe	**TEM**-pore-al **LOBE**	S/ R/	-al *pertaining to* tempor- *time, temple*	Posterior two-thirds of the cerebral hemispheres
thalamus	**THAL**-ah-mus		Greek *inner room*	Mass of gray matter under the ventricle in each cerebral hemisphere

EXERCISES

A. Roots: *The lobes of the brain share the suffix* al, *meaning* pertaining to. *It is the roots that describe their exact location in the brain. Use your knowledge of roots to understand the anatomical location of the lobes. Fill in the blanks.*   **LO 10.1 and 10.4** Understand

1. front/al   root means: _____ ; lobe is located: _____

2. occipit/al   root means: _____ ; lobe is located: _____

3. pariet/al   root means: _____ ; lobe is located: _____

4. tempor/al   root means: _____ ; lobe is located: _____

B. Meet lesson objectives *and use the language of neurology to:*   **LO 10.2, 10.4, and 10.8** Apply

1. Explain the roles of the cerebrospinal fluid. _____

_____

_____

2. Identify the major lobes of the brain. _____

_____

_____

3. Describe the roles of the frontal lobe, brainstem, and cerebellum. _____

_____

_____

_____

Lesson 10.2
(cont'd) Cranial Nerves, Spinal Cord, and Meninges
(LO 10.4)

Cranial Nerves (LO 10.4)

Your brain communicates with the rest of your body through the cranial nerves and spinal cord. The cranial nerves are part of the peripheral nervous system. They originate on the lower or inferior surface of the brain and are identified by names and numbers, the latter written in Roman numerals *(Figure 10.7)*.

The cranial nerves provide sensory and motor functions for your head and neck areas except for the vagus nerve, which supplies your thorax and abdomen.

Oh	(olfactory-I)
once	(optic-II)
one	(oculomotor-III)
takes	(trochlear-IV)
the	(trigeminal-V)
anatomy	(abducens-VI)
final	(facial-VII)
very	(vestibulocochlear-VIII)
good	(glossopharyngeal-IX)
vacations	(vagus-X)
are	(accessory-XI)
heavenly!	(hypoglossal-XII)

▲ **FIGURE 10.7**
Cranial Nerves
This mnemonic device will help you remember the cranial nerves. Use the sentence in column one (read down) to help you remember the correct order and names of the cranial nerves.

Spinal Cord (LO 10.4)

Your spinal cord lies within, and is protected by, the vertebral canal of the spinal column. It has 31 segments, each of which gives rise to a pair of spinal nerves *(Figure 10.8)*. These are the major link between the brain and the peripheral nervous system, and are the pathway for sensory and motor impulses.

Your spinal cord is divided into four regions *(Figure 10.8)*:

1. The **cervical** region is continuous with the brain stem (lower part of the brain). It contains the motor neurons that supply the neck, shoulders, and upper limbs through 8 pairs of cervical spinal nerves (C1–C8);

2. The **thoracic** region contains the motor neurons that supply the thoracic cage, rib movement, vertebral column movement, and postural back muscles through 12 pairs of thoracic spinal nerves (T1–T12);

3. The **lumbar** region supplies the hips and the front of the lower limbs through 5 pairs of lumbar nerves (L1–L5); and

4. The **sacral** region supplies the buttocks, genitalia, and backs of the lower limbs through 5 sacral nerves (S1–S5) and 1 coccygeal nerve, relative to the small bone at the base of the spine.

Meninges
(LO 10.4)

Your brain and spinal cord are protected by the cranium and the vertebrae, cushioned by the CSF, and covered by the **meninges** *(Figure 10.9)*. The meninges have three layers.

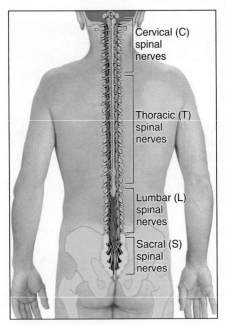

▲ **FIGURE 10.8**
Spinal Cord Regions.

Cervical (C) spinal nerves

Thoracic (T) spinal nerves

Lumbar (L) spinal nerves

Sacral (S) spinal nerves

1. The **dura mater** is the outermost layer of tough connective tissue attached to the cranium's inner surface. Within the vertebral canal the dura mater splits into two sheets, separated by the **epidural space,** into which epidural injections of medication are given to produce **analgesia** during childbirth or for the treatment of low back pain.

2. The **arachnoid mater** is a thin web over the brain and spinal cord. The CSF is contained in the **subarachnoid space** between the arachnoid and pia mater. It is into this space that a needle is introduced to obtain CSF for testing or to place medication in spinal **anesthesia.**

3. The **pia mater** is the innermost layer of the meninges, attached to the surface of the brain and spinal cord. It supplies nerves and blood vessels that nourish the outer cells of the brain and spinal cord.

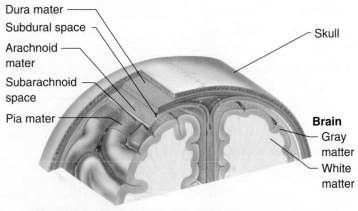

Dura mater
Subdural space
Arachnoid mater
Subarachnoid space
Pia mater

Skull

Brain
Gray matter
White matter

▲ **FIGURE 10.9**
Meninges of Brain.

Word Analysis and Definition

WORD	PRONUNCIATION	ELEMENTS		DEFINITION
analgesia	an-al-**JEE**-zee-ah	S/ P/ R/	-ia *condition* an- *without* -alges- *sensation of pain*	State in which pain is reduced
anesthesia	an-es-**THEE**-zee-ah	S/ P/ R/CF	-ia *condition* an- *without* -esthes- *feeling*	Complete loss of sensation
arachnoid mater	ah-**RACK**-noyd **MAY**-ter	S/ R/ R/	-oid *resembling* arachn- *cobweb, spider* mater *mother*	Weblike middle layer of the three meninges
dura mater (**Note:** *Both terms are stand-alone roots.*)	**DYU**-rah **MAY**-ter	R/ R/	dura *hard* mater *mother*	Hard, fibrous outer layer of the meninges
epidural epidural space	ep-ih-**DYU**-ral	S/ P/ R/	-al *pertaining to* epi- *above* -dur- *dura*	Above the dura Space between the dura mater and the wall of the vertebral canal
meninges meningitis	meh-**NIN**-jeez men-in-**JIE**-tis	 S/ R/	Greek *membrane* -itis *inflammation* mening- *meninges*	Three-layered covering of the brain and spinal cord Inflammation of the meninges
pia mater (stand-alone roots)	**PEE**-ah **MAY**-ter	R/ R/	pia *delicate* mater *mother*	Delicate inner layer of the meninges
subarachnoid space	sub-ah-**RACK**-noyd **SPASE**	S/ P/ R/	-oid *resembling* sub- *under* -arachn -*cobweb, spider*	Space between the pia mater and the arachnoid membrane

EXERCISES

A. Construct the following *medical terms by filling in the missing elements. After you have inserted the correct element, circle the word in the statement that was your clue to the missing element. Fill in the blanks.* **LO 10.1 and 10.4** *Apply*

1. under the arachnoid mater: _____ /arachn/oid

2. inflammation of the meninges: mening/_____

3. weblike middle layer of meninges: _____/_____/oid   mater

4. pertaining to above the dura: _____ /dur/al

5. hard, fibrous outer layer of meninges: _____/_____/_____

B. Continue to use the WAD *and the text on this spread to find your answers.* **LO 10.1, 10.4, and 10.8** *Apply*

1. Which two prefixes in this WAD denote opposite locations?

_____ means _____.

_____ means _____.

2. Which term is a diagnosis? _____/_____/_____

3. CSF is found in the: sub/ _____ /_____ _____.

4. Describe the location of the spinal cord: _____

_____

5. Name the four regions of the spinal cord: _____

_____

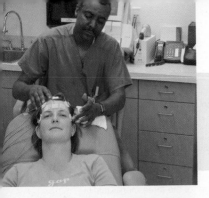

Lesson 10.3

Disorders of the Brain, Cranial Nerves, and Meninges

Objectives

An invaluable benefit of working with patients as a health professional is the opportunity for ongoing learning. By routinely communicating with patients, your education and knowledge of various disorders will continue to be enhanced and reinforced. Information in this lesson will enable you to use correct medical terminology to:

10.3.1 Describe common disorders of the brain, cranial nerves, and meninges.

10.3.2 Communicate about the brain, cranial nerves, and meninges and their disorders with physicians and other health professionals.

Abbreviations

AMS	altered mental state
CVA	cerebrovascular accident
FTD	frontotemporal dementia

Case Report 10.2

You are . . .

. . . a medical assistant working with Dr. Raul Cardenas, a neurologist at Fulwood Medical Center.

You are communicating with . . .

. . . Mr. Lester Rood, a 75-year-old man who was diagnosed with **dementia** a year ago. He lives with his daughter, Judy, and she is with him today.

Patient Interview:

Mr. Rood: "How am I feeling? Scared stiff. Sometimes I don't know where I am. I get so messed up. I can't cook anymore. I forget what I'm doing, can't get things straight. I find myself in the street and don't know how I got there. Judy has to help me shower and remind me to go to the bathroom. And it's only going to get worse. I don't want to be a burden. I used to have 100 people working for me. It's so frustrating, so frightening."

Disorders of the Brain (LO 10.2 and 10.5)

Dementia (LO 10.2 and 10.5)

Your **empathy** allowed Mr. Rood to talk comfortably without interruption. His condition made clear again the specific symptoms of **dementia.** These include an irreversible short-term memory loss, the inability to solve problems, and confusion. Inappropriate behavior, like wandering away, and impaired intellectual function that interferes with normal activities and relationships are also key signs of dementia. Dementia requires a lot of **sympathy** from family and caregivers.

- **Senile dementia** is not a normal part of aging and is not a specific disease. It is a term used for a collection of symptoms that can be caused by a number of disorders affecting the brain.

- **Alzheimer disease** *(Figure 10.10)*—the most common form of dementia—affects 10% of the population over 65, and 50% of the population over 85. Nerve cells in the areas of the brain associated with memory and **cognition** are replaced by abnormal protein clumps and tangles.

- **Vascular dementia**—the second most common form of dementia—can come on gradually when arteries supplying the brain become arteriosclerotic (narrowed or blocked), depriving the brain of oxygen. It can also occur suddenly after a **stroke** *(see later in this chapter).*

- **Frontotemporal dementia (FTD)** is caused by progressive cell degeneration in the brain's frontal and temporal lobes, which control planning and judgment, emotions, speaking and understanding speech, and certain types of movement. It accounts for 10% to 15% of all dementias, but it is more common in those younger than 65.

(a)   (b)

▲ **FIGURE 10.10**
Brain Sections.
(a) MRI scan, normal brain.
(b) MRI scan of Alzheimer disease, showing cerebral atrophy (yellow).

Word Analysis and Definition

WORD	PRONUNCIATION	ELEMENTS		DEFINITION
Alzheimer disease	**AWLZ**-high-mer diz-**EEZ**		Dr. Alois Alzheimer, German physician, 1864–1915	Common form of dementia
cognition	kog-**NIH**-shun		Latin *knowledge*	Process of acquiring knowledge through thinking, learning, and memory
confusion	kon-**FEW**-zhun	S/ R/	-ion *condition, action* confus- *bewildered*	Mental state in which environmental stimuli are not processed appropriately
delirium	de-**LIR**-ee-um	S/ R/	-um *structure* deliri- *disorientation, confusion*	Acute altered state of consciousness with agitation and disorientation
dementia	dee-**MEN**-she-ah	S/ P/ R/	-ia *condition* de- *removal, without* -ment- *mind*	Chronic, progressive, irreversible loss of the mind's cognitive, and intellectual functions
empathy sympathy	**EM**-pah-thee **SIM**-pah-thee	P/ S/ P/ S/	em- *into* -pathy *emotion, disease* sym- *together* -pathy *emotion, disease*	Ability to place yourself into the feelings, emotions, and reactions of another person Appreciation and concern for another person's mental and emotional state
sedative sedation	**SED**-ah-tiv seh-**DAY**-shun	S/ R/ S/	-ive *pertaining to, quality of* sedat- *to calm* -ion *condition, action*	Agent that calms nervous excitement State of being calmed
senile	**SEE**-nile	S/ R/	-ile *pertaining to* sen- *old age*	Characteristic of old age
stroke (same as **cerebrovascular accident, CVA**)	STROHK		Old English *to strike*	Acute clinical event caused by impaired cerebral circulation

EXERCISES

A. Review *the Case Report on this spread before answering the questions.*   **LO 10.2, 10.5, and 10.8** *Understand*

1. What specific symptoms of dementia does Mr. Rood have? _____

_____

2. How long has Mr. Rood had dementia? _____

3. What is "short-term memory"? _____

4. Mr. Rood's short-term memory loss is *irreversible*. What does that mean? _____

_____.

5. What kind of assistance do people with dementia need? _____

_____

6. List some of the key symptoms of dementia. _____

_____

7. Give an example of "inappropriate behavior." _____

_____

B. Identify *the elements in each medical term, and unlock the meaning of the word. Fill in the chart.*   **LO 10.1, 10.5, and 10.8** *Remember*

Medical Term	Meaning of Prefix	Meaning of Root/CF	Meaning of Suffix	Meaning of the Term
dementia	**1.**	**2.**	**3.**	**4.**
sympathy	**5.**	**6.**	**7.**	**8.**
delirium	**9.**	**10.**	**11.**	**12.**
confusion	**13.**	**14.**	**15.**	**16.**
empathy	**17.**	**18.**	**19.**	**20.**
sedation	**21.**	**22.**	**23.**	**24.**

Disorders of the Brain
(continued)

Dementia (continued)
(LO 10.5)

Other conditions causing dementia include reactions to medications, like **sedatives** and antiarthritics; depression in the elderly; and infections, such as AIDS or encephalitis.

Confusion is used to describe people who cannot process information normally. They cannot answer questions appropriately, understand where they are, or remember important facts, like their name and address.

Delirium is an altered mental state **(AMS),** characterized by the sudden onset of disorientation, an inability to think clearly or pay attention. The level of consciousness varies from increased wakefulness to drowsiness. It is not a disease, it is reversible, and it can be part of dementia or a stroke.

Epilepsy (LO 10.5)

Epilepsy is a chronic disorder in which clusters of neurons (nerve cells) discharge their electrical signals in an abnormal rhythm. This disturbed electrical activity (a **seizure** or a **convulsion**) can cause strange sensations and behavior, convulsions, and loss of consciousness. The causes of epilepsy are numerous, from abnormal brain development to brain damage.

The International League Against Epilepsy created the following classification system for seizures:

1. **Partial seizures** occur when the epileptic activity is in one localized area of the brain only, causing, for example, involuntary jerking movements of a single limb.

2. **Generalized seizures** can be categorized into one of the following three types:
   a. **Absence seizures,** previously known as **"petit mal,"** which begin between ages 5 and 10. The child stares vacantly for a few seconds and may be accused of daydreaming.
   b. **Tonic-clonic seizures,** previously called **"grand mal,"** which are dramatic. The person

experiences a **loss of consciousness (LOC),** breathing stops, the eyes roll up, and the jaw is clenched. This "tonic" phase lasts for 30 to 60 seconds. It is followed by the "clonic" phase, in which the whole body shakes with a series of violent, rhythmic jerkings of the limbs. The seizures last for a couple of minutes, and then consciousness returns.
   c. **Febrile seizures,** which are triggered by a fever in infants and toddlers aged 6 months to 5 years. Very few of these children go on to develop epilepsy.

Status epilepticus is considered to be a medical emergency. It is defined as having one continuous seizure or recurrent seizures without regaining consciousness for 30 minutes or more.

Any seizure may be followed by a period of diminished function in the area of the brain surrounding the seizure's main origin. This temporary neurologic deficit is called a **postictal** state.

Tourette syndrome and other **tic** disorders are characterized by episodes of involuntary, rapid, repetitive, fixed movements of individual muscle groups in the face or the limbs. They are associated with meaningless vocal sounds or meaningful words and phrases. The tics may be genetic.

Narcolepsy is a chronic disorder in which patients fall asleep during the day—from a few seconds up to an hour. There is no cure.

Case Report 10.1 (continued from the chapter opening)

For Ms. Roberta Gaston, who was seen in Dr. Solis's neurosurgery clinic, the EEG did not pinpoint an epileptic source. In order to further investigate the source, Dr. Solis inserted deep brain electrodes into the region of the suspicious mass that showed on the MRI. Seizures were recorded arising in the mass itself. Dr. Solis performed a surgical resection of the mass, which was a glioma. Ms. Gaston has been seizure-free since the surgery a year ago.

Case Report 10.1 (continued)

Ms. Gaston suffered from both **absence** and **tonic-clonic** seizures.

Word Analysis and Definition

WORD	PRONUNCIATION	ELEMENTS		DEFINITION
grand mal	**GRAHN** MAL	R/ R/	grand *big* mal *bad*	Previous name for generalized tonic-clonic seizure
narcolepsy	**NAR**-koh-lep-see	S/ R/CF	-lepsy *seizure* narc/o- *stupor*	Involuntary falling asleep
petit mal	peh-**TEE** MAL	R/ R/	petit *small* mal *bad*	Previous name for absence seizures
postictal (adj)	post-**IK**-tal	S/ P/ R/	-al *pertaining to* post- *after* -ict- *seizure*	Transient neurologic deficit after a seizure
ictal (adj)	**IK**-tal	S/	-al *pertaining to*	Pertaining to, or a condition caused by, a stroke or epilepsy
tic	TIK		French *tic*	Sudden, involuntary, repeated contraction of muscles
tonic	**TON**-ik	S/ R/	-ic *pertaining to* ton- *pressure, tension*	State of muscular contraction
tonic-clonic seizure	**TON**-ik-**KLON**-ik **SEE**-zhur	R/ S/ R/	clon- *tumult* -ure *process* seiz- *to grab*	The body alternates between excessive muscular rigidity (tonic) and jerking muscular contractions (clonic)
Tourette syndrome	tur-**ET SIN**-drome		Gilles de la Tourette, French neurologist, 1857–1904	Disorder of multiple motor and vocal tics

EXERCISES

A. Review the Case Report *on this spread before answering the questions.*   **LO 10.2, 10.3, 10.5, and 10.8** *Remember*

1. What were the diagnostic findings of the MRI?

_____

2. Since the EEG did not pinpoint an epileptic source, what additional procedure did Dr. Solis perform?

_____

3. Where did Dr. Solis find the source of the seizures? _____

4. What surgical procedure was then performed? _____

5. What type of seizures did Ms. Gaston have? _____

6. How do you know the surgery was successful for Ms. Gaston? _____

7. What is the postoperative diagnosis for Ms. Gaston? _____

B. Critical thinking: *Employ the language of neurology and answer the following questions. Be prepared to answer aloud in class.*   **LO 10.1, 10.2, 10.5, and 10.8** *Analyze*

1. Use the root in *narcolepsy* in another medical term that also involves "sleep." _____

2. Why is *status epilepticus* considered to be a medical emergency? _____

_____

3. What is a *postictal state?* Describe and define it. _____

4. What triggers a *febrile* seizure? _____

5. What is the difference between an *absence* seizure and a *tonic-clonic* seizure? _____

_____

Disorders of the Brain (continued)

Cerebrovascular Accidents (CVAs) or Strokes (LO 10.3 and 10.5)

A stroke (also known as a cerebrovascular accident or CVA) occurs when the blood supply to a part of the brain is suddenly interrupted, depriving the brain cells of oxygen. Some cells die; others are badly damaged. With timely treatment, the damaged cells can be saved. There are two types of stroke:

1. **Ischemic strokes** account for 90% of all strokes and are caused by:
   a. **Atherosclerosis:** Plaque in the wall of a cerebral artery *(Figure 10.11a);* or
   b. **Embolism:** A blood clot in a cerebral artery originating from elsewhere in the body *(Figure 10.11b).*

   Treatment of ischemic strokes is by thrombolysis together with clot busters like **tissue plasminogen activator (tPA).** This must occur within 3½ hours of the stroke, using supportive measures followed by rehabilitation.

2. **Hemorrhagic strokes (intracranial hemorrhage)** occur when a blood vessel in the brain bursts or when a cerebral **aneurysm** ruptures.

   Cerebral arteriography can determine the site of bleeding in hemorrhagic stroke. A surgical procedure can be performed to stop the bleed or clip off the aneurysm.

Transient Ischemic Attack (TIA) (LO 10.3 and 10.5)

Transient ischemic attacks **(TIAs)** are small, short-term strokes with symptoms lasting for less than 24 hours. If neurologic symptoms persist for more than 24 hours, the condition is a full-blown stroke with brain cell damage and death.

The most frequent cause of TIAs is a small embolus that occludes (blocks) a small artery in the brain. Often, the embolus arises from a clot in the atrium in atrial fibrillation or from an atherosclerotic plaque in a carotid artery. Treatment is directed at the underlying cause. A **carotid endarterectomy** may be necessary if a carotid artery is significantly blocked with plaque.

Atherosclerosis   Residual lumen of artery

(a)

Embolus

(b)

◀ **FIGURE 10.11**
Causes of Ischemic Strokes.
(a) Atherosclerosis in a cerebral artery, leaving a small, residual lumen.
(b) Embolus blocking an artery. Healthy tissue is on the left (pink) and blood-starved tissue is on the right (blue).

Other Brain Disorders (LO 10.3 and 10.5)

Parkinson disease is caused by the degeneration of neurons in the basal ganglia that produce a neurotransmitter called dopamine. Motor symptoms of abnormal movements, **tremor** of the hands, rigidity, a shuffling gait, and weak voice appear, and gradually become more and more severe. There is no cure.

Creutzfeld-Jakob disease (CJD) produces a rapid deterioration of mental function, with difficulty in muscle movement coordination. Some cases are linked to the consumption of beef from cattle with mad cow disease (**bovine spongiform encephalopathy, BSE**).

Syncope (fainting or passing out) is a temporary loss of consciousness and posture. It is usually due to hypotension and the associated deficient oxygen supply (hypoxia) to the brain.

Migraine produces an intense throbbing, pulsating pain in one area of the head, often with nausea and vomiting. It can be preceded by an aura, visual disturbances like flashing lights, or temporary loss of vision. Prevention is difficult.

Encephalitis, an inflammation of the parenchyma (tissue) of the brain, is often caused by a virus such as HIV, West Nile virus, herpes simplex, or childhood measles, mumps, chickenpox, and rubella.

Brain abscess is usually a direct spread of infection from sinusitis, otitis media (middle ear infection), or mastoiditis (an infection in the skull bone behind the ear). It can also result from blood-borne pathogens arising from lung or dental infections.

Brain tumors are often secondary tumors that have metastasized from cancers in the lung, breast, skin, or kidney. Primary brain tumors arise from any of the glial cells and are called gliomas. In Case Report 10.1, Ms. Gaston has a glioma.

Autism spectrum disorder (ASD) is a range of complex developmental disorders characterized by communication difficulties, impaired social interactions, and rigid or repetitive patterns of behavior. It is estimated that more than 1% of children aged eight will have an ASD, and it is four times as likely to occur in males than females. It occurs in all ethnic and socioeconomic groups. Twenty to 30% of children with an ASD develop epilepsy before reaching adulthood. Treatment is with highly structured educational and behavioral interventions. Medications can be used to treat autism-related symptoms, such as depression and seizures.

Word Analysis and Definition

WORD	PRONUNCIATION	ELEMENTS		DEFINITION
aneurysm	**AN**-yur-izm		Greek *dilation*	Small, circumscribed dilation of an artery or cardiac chamber
arteriography	ar-teer-ee-**OG**-rah-fee	S/ R/CF	-graphy *recording* arteri/o- *artery*	X-ray visualization of an artery after injection of contrast material
autism	**AWE**-tizm		Greek *self*	A disorder with severely abnormal social and communication skills
autistic	awe-**TIS**-tik	S/ R/	-tic *pertaining to* autis- *autism*	Pertaining to autism
bovine spongiform encephalopathy (BSE)	**BO**-vine **SPON**-jee-form en-sef-ah-**LOP**-ah-thee	S/ R/ S/ R/CF S/ R/CF	-ine *pertaining to* bov- *cattle* -form *appearance of* spong/i- *sponge* -pathy *disease* encephal/o- *head*	Disease of cattle ("mad cow disease") that can be transmitted to humans, causing Creutzfeldt-Jakob disease
carotid endarterectomy	kah-**ROT**-id **END**-ar-ter-**EK**-toe-me	S/ P/ R/	carotid, Greek *large neck artery* -ectomy *surgical excision* end- *inside* -arter- *artery*	Surgical removal of diseased lining from the carotid artery to leave a smooth lining and restore blood flow
Creutzfeldt-Jakob disease (CJD)	**KROITS**-felt **YAK**-op **DIZ**-eez		Hans Creutzfeldt, 1885–1964, and Alfons Jakob, 1884–1931, German psychiatrists	Progressive, incurable, neurologic disease caused by infectious prions
encephalitis	en-**SEF**-ah-**LIE**-tis	S/ R/	-itis *inflammation* encephal- *brain*	Inflammation of brain cells and tissues
migraine	**MY**-grain	P/ R/	mi- *derived from hemi, half* -graine *head pain*	Paroxysmal severe headache confined to one side of the head
Parkinson disease	**PAR**-kin-son diz-**EEZ**		James Parkinson, British physician, 1755–1824	Disease of muscular rigidity, tremors, and a mask-like facial expression
prion	**PREE**-on		Latin *protein*	Small, infectious protein particle
syncope	**SIN**-koh-pee		Greek *cutting short*	Temporary loss of consciousness and postural tone due to diminished cerebral blood flow
tremor	**TREM**-or		Latin *to shake*	Small, shaking, involuntary, repetitive movements of hands, extremities, neck, or jaw

EXERCISES

A. Diagnosis: *Patient documentation is given to you below. Circle the correct language of neurology for the diagnosis.*   **LO 10.5 and 10.8**
Understand

1. Patient is experiencing shaking, involuntary movements of her extremities.

   Diagnosis: *syncope   prion   tremor*

2. Radiologic studies show a small, circumscribed dilation of the cerebral artery.

   Diagnosis: *Parkinson disease   aneurysm   migraine*

3. The patient's paroxysmal headache is confined to the left temporal region.

   Diagnosis: *syncope   tremor   migraine*

4. Tests and studies have confirmed inflammation of the brain cells and tissues to make this diagnosis.

   Diagnosis: *meningitis   fasciitis   encephalitis*

5. This patient has experienced loss of consciousness due to diminished cerebral blood flow.

   Diagnosis: *syncope   tremor   migraine*

B. Continue working *with the text and the WAD to answer the following questions.*   **LO 10.5 and 10.8** *Understand*

1. What is another medical term for *intracranial hemorrhage?* _____

2. *Hemorrhage* (noun) and *hemorrhagic* (adjective) both signify the presence of _____.

3. What are the probable causes of a stroke? _____

   _____

4. What is an abbreviation used for stroke? _____

Traumatic Brain Injury (TBI) (LO 10.3 and 10.5)

Traumatic brain injury (TBI) results from any one of many types of injuries to the head, from a bad fall on a hard surface to a car accident to war injuries. Every year, physicians treat over 1 million patients who have experienced TBI; as many as 10% of these have long-term damage affecting their normal **activities of daily living (ADLs).**

Imagine driving your car along the highway at 50 miles per hour. Suddenly, you are hit head-on by another driver. Your brain goes from 50 miles per hour to zero—instantly. Your soft brain is propelled forward and squished against the front of your hard skull **(coup).** Next, you rebound backward, and your brain slams against the back of your skull **(contrecoup).** Your brain now has at least one bruise or **contusion,** if not worse damage.

A mild head injury **(concussion)** may leave you feeling dazed, confused, or unable to recall the event that caused your concussion. Repeated concussions, like those experienced by famous boxer Muhammad Ali, have a cumulative effect, leading to a reduced mental ability and reaction time, and/or trauma-induced Parkinson's disease.

A severe injury may include torn blood vessels that bleed into the brain. The brain may also tear, or swell within the hard, inflexible skull, cutting off important signals and connections.

Shaken baby syndrome (SBS) is a type of TBI produced when a baby is violently shaken. A baby has weak neck muscles and a heavy head. Shaking makes the brain bounce back and forth in the skull, leading to severe brain damage.

Posttraumatic stress disorder is discussed later in this chapter, in Lesson 10.5 Mental Health.

Disorders of the Meninges (LO 10.5)

Meningitis is an inflammation of the membranes (meninges) covering the brain and spinal cord. Viral meningitis—the most common form—can occur at any age. Bacterial meningitis predominantly affects the very young or very old. **Meningococcal** meningitis is contagious, transmitted through a simple cough or sneeze. It is most commonly passed among people who live in close quarters—such as students in college dormitories. Vaccines are available to prevent most types of meningitis.

A **subdural hematoma** is bleeding into the subdural space below the dura mater, which is frequently associated with closed-head injuries and bleeding from broken veins caused by violent head rotations.

An **epidural hematoma** is a pooling of blood in the epidural space between the skull and the dura mater, often associated with a fractured skull and bleeding from an artery within the meninges.

▲ **FIGURE 10.12**
Bell Palsy of Left Side of Face.

Disorders of the Cranial Nerves (LO 10.5)

Bell palsy is a facial nerve (vii) disorder characterized by a sudden weakness or paralysis of muscles on one side of the face. The inability to smile or whistle, the uncontrollable drooping of the mouth and drooling of saliva, and an inability to close the eye *(Figure 10.12)* are common symptoms. The use of steroids in the early stages can prevent the paralysis from becoming permanent.

Trigeminal neuralgia (TN), **tic douloureux,** is an extremely painful chronic disorder of the trigeminal (v) cranial nerve caused by nerve injury or compression of the nerve by a blood vessel. The facial pain can be constant or sporadic and is very intense. The anticonvulsant carbamazepine (Tegretol) is the first-line treatment, and opiates can be prescribed for pain. The evidence for a good result from surgical treatment is poor.

An **acoustic neuroma** is a benign, slow-growing tumor on the vestibulocochlear (viii) nerve that causes hearing loss, tinnitus, and dizziness. Treatment is with surgery and/or radiation.

Pain Management (LO 10.5)

It's estimated that more than 6 million Americans are affected by the acute or chronic pain of **fibromyalgia,** 5 million are disabled by back pain, and 40 million suffer from recurrent headaches. Interventional procedures (such as nerve blocks or trigger point injections) can target the tissue or the organ causing pain, and physical medicine and rehabilitation **(physiatry)** can use physical techniques such as heat, electrotherapy, therapeutic exercises, and biofeedback techniques. Pain management practitioners include anesthesiologists, physiatrists, physiotherapists, occupational therapists, and chiropractors.

Medications prescribed based on the severity of the pain include:

- **Analgesics** (such as acetaminophen) and nonsteroidal anti-inflammatory drugs (NSAIDs) for mild pain;

- **Opiates** (codeine, hydrocodone, and oxycodone) in combination with analgesics for moderate pain; and

- Higher doses of opiates for severe pain. These are often used on their own, and include **morphine** and fentanyl.

Word Analysis and Definition

S = Suffix   P = Prefix   R = Root   R/CF = Combining Form

WORD	PRONUNCIATION	ELEMENTS		DEFINITION
acoustic	ah-**KYU**-stik		Greek *hearing*	Pertaining to hearing
analgesia	an-al-**JEE**-zee-ah	S/ P/ R/	-ia *condition* an- *without* -alges- *sensation of pain*	State in which pain is reduced
analgesic (adj)	an-al-**JEE**-zik	S/	-ic *pertaining to*	Substance that produces analgesia
Bell palsy	BELL **PAWL**-zee		Charles Bell, Scottish -surgeon, 1774–1842	Paresis, or paralysis, of one side of the face
concussion	kon-**KUSH**-un	S/ R/	-ion *action, condition* concuss- *shake or jar violently*	Mild brain injury
contrecoup	**KON**-treh-koo		French *counterblow*	Injury to the brain at a point directly opposite the point of contact
contusion	kon-**TOO**-zhun	S/ R/	-ion *action, condition* contus- *bruise*	Hemorrhage into a tissue (bruising), including the brain
coup	KOO		French *a blow*	Injury to the brain directly under the skull at the point of contact
fibromyalgia	fie-broh-my-**AL**-jee-ah	S/ R/CF R/	-algia *pain* fibr/o- *fiber* -my- *muscle*	Pain in the muscle fibers
meningococcal	meh-nin-goh-**KOK**-al	S/ R/CF R/	-al *pertaining to* mening/o- *meninges* -cocc- *round bacterium*	Pertaining to the meningococcus bacterium
neuroma	nyu-**ROH**-mah	S/ R/	-oma *tumor* neur- *nerve*	Any tumor arising from cells in the nervous system
subdural space	sub-**DYU**-ral SPASE	S/ P/ R/	-al *pertaining to* sub- *below* -dur- *dura, hard*	Space between the arachnoid and dura mater layers of the meninges
trauma traumatic	**TRAW**-mah traw-**MAT**-ik	S/ R/	Greek *wound* -tic *pertaining to* trauma- *injury*	A physical or mental injury Pertaining to or caused by trauma
trigeminal	try-**GEM**-in-al	S/ P/ R/	-al *pertaining to* tri- *three* -gemin- *double*	Fifth (v) cranial nerve with three branches supplying the face
neuralgia	nyu-**RAL**-jee-ah	S/ R/	-algia *pain* neur- *nerve*	Trigeminal neuralgia; painful facial muscles supplied by the trigeminal nerve
tic douloureux	TIK duh-luh-**RUE**		douloureux French *painful tic*	Synonym for trigeminal neuralgia

EXERCISES

A. Insert medical terms *found in this spread to fill in the answer blanks.*   **LO 10.5 and 10.8** *Understand*

1. These related neurological injuries occur very often in motor vehicle accidents: _____

2. Medicine given to reduce pain is an _____.

3. Hemorrhaging into surrounding brain tissue produces a _____.

4. _____ is a mild brain injury that occurs often in sports.

5. Pain in the muscle fibers is termed _____.

B. Terminology challenge: *Use the language of neurology to describe the difference between a* subdural hematoma *and an* epidural hematoma.
   LO 10.5 and 10.8 *Analyze*

1. _____

_____

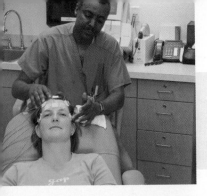

Lesson 10.4

Disorders of the Spinal Cord and Peripheral Nerves

Objectives

Many disorders of the nervous system can affect the spinal cord and the peripheral nerves without affecting the brain. In this lesson, the information will enable you to use correct medical terminology to:

10.4.1 Discuss disorders of the spinal cord and peripheral nerves.

10.4.2 Communicate about the nervous system and its disorders with patients and other health professionals.

10.4.3 Name common congenital disorders of the nervous system.

▲ FIGURE 10.13
Multiple Sclerosis of the Spinal Cord.
Areas of demyelination are arrowed and shown in red.

Abbreviations

MS	multiple sclerosis
PNS	peripheral nervous system
VEP	visual evoked potential

Case Report 10.3

You are . . .

. . . Tanisha Colis, an electroneurodiagnostic technologist working for Raul Cardenas, MD, a neurologist at Fulwood Medical Center.

You are communicating with . . .

. . . Mrs. Suzanne Kalish, a 42-year-old social worker employed by the medical center. Mrs. Kalish has recently had an exacerbation of her symptoms due to multiple sclerosis (MS). She is going to have a visual evoked potential **(VEP)** test, followed by an MRI of her brain and spinal cord.

Patient Interview:

Tanisha: "Good morning, Mrs. Kalish. I'm Tanisha Colis, the technologist who'll be performing your visual evoked potential test. How are you feeling?"

Mrs. Kalish: "I've been doing OK for the last 4 or 5 years. Then, a few weeks ago, I started dragging my right foot like a wounded witch. I've got to hang onto the walls to stay vertical. I'm tired out, can't come to work. It's a struggle to walk the few yards just to pick up the mail."

Tanisha: "The MRI you are going to have today will give us a lot of information about what's going on."

Mrs. Kalish: "My mind is going 'wheelchair, wheelchair, wheelchair.' Especially since in the last couple of days the vision in my right eye has gotten all blurred."

Tanisha: "That's the reason you are having the visual evoked potential test."

Mrs. Kalish: "I hate this disease. If I had cancer, I've got a chance. I'd fight it to the end, whatever that would be. Nobody's ever beat MS. You can only lose. It can be kind and leave you for a while, but it's never far away."

Tanisha: "Let me help you up, and we'll go get this test done."

Mrs. Kalish: "I can manage, thank you."

Disorders of the Myelin Sheath of Nerve Fibers
(LO 10.5)

When the myelin sheath surrounding nerve fibers is damaged, nerves do not conduct impulses normally. In newborns, many of their nerves have immature myelin sheaths, which is why some of their movements are jerky and uncoordinated.

Demyelination, the destruction of an area of the myelin sheath, can occur in the PNS and be caused by inflammation, vitamin B_{12} deficiency, poisons, and some medications.

Multiple sclerosis (MS), a chronic, progressive disorder, is the most common condition in which demyelination of nerve fibers in the brain, spinal cord, and optic nerves can occur *(Figure 10.13).* **Intermittent** myelin damage and scarring slow nerve impulses. This leads to muscle weakness, pain, abnormal sensations **(paresthesias),** numbness, and vision loss. Because different nerve fibers are affected at different times, MS symptoms often worsen **(exacerbations)** or show partial or complete reduction **(remissions).** Suzanne Kalish is now in an exacerbation.

Word Analysis and Definition

S = Suffix   P = Prefix   R = Root   R/CF = Combining Form

WORD	PRONUNCIATION	ELEMENTS		DEFINITION
demyelination	dee-**MY**-eh-lin-A-shun	S/ P/ R/	-ation *process* de- *without* -myelin- *myelin*	Process of losing the myelin sheath of a nerve fiber
exacerbation (contrast remission)	ek-zas-er-**BAY**-shun	S/ R/	-ation *process* exacerbat- *increase, aggravate*	Period when there is an increase in the severity of a disease
intermittent	IN-ter-**MIT**-ent	S/ P/ R/	-ent *end result* inter- *between* -mitt- *send*	Alternately ceasing and beginning again
modify	**MOD**-ih-fie		Latin *to limit*	Change the form or qualities of something; here, the pathology of MS
paresthesia paresthesias (pl) (**Note:** the "a" following the "r" in *para* is dropped for ease of pronunciation.)	par-es-**THEE**-ze-ah	S/ P/ R/	-ia *condition* par(a)- *abnormal* -esthes- *sensation*	Abnormal sensation; e.g., tingling, burning, pricking
remission (contrast exacerbation)	ree-**MISH**-un	S/ P/ R/	-ion *condition, action* re- *back* -miss- *send*	Period when there is a lessening or absence of the symptoms of a disease
sclerosis	skleh-**ROH**-sis	S/ R/CF	-sis *abnormal condition* scler/o- *hardness*	Thickening and hardening of a tissue; in the nervous system, hardening of nervous tissue by fibrous and glial connective tissue

EXERCISES

A. Review *the Case Report on this spread before answering the questions.*   **LO 10.2, 10.5, and 10.8** *Understand*

1. What symptoms made Mrs. Kalish come to see Dr. Cardenas? _____

2. Is the change in her symptoms sudden? _____

3. What diagnostic test is Mrs. Kalish having? _____

4. What type of comments from the patient make her sound depressed about her condition? _____

5. What does it mean if a disease is *chronic* and *progressive?* _____

6. Can this disease be cured? _____

B. Test yourself *on the elements and terms in the above WAD box. Practice pronouncing the terms before you start the exercise. Circle the best answer.*   **LO 10.1 and 10.5** *Analyze*

1. The term *intermittent* contains:

   prefix, root, and suffix   prefix and root   combining form and suffix

2. *Remission* is the opposite of:

   intermittent   exacerbation   demyelination

3. *To modify* something is to:

   dispose of it   change it   renew it

4. In the term *demyelination* the prefix means:

   without   in front of   half

5. If a disease is *exacerbated,* it:

   is more severe   has not changed   is less severe

   Have you pronounced each word correctly?

Lesson 10.4
(cont'd)

Keynote

- Approximately half a million people in the United States have spinal cord injuries (SCIs). There are approximately 8,000 new injuries each year, of which 82% involve males between the ages of 16 and 30.

Abbreviations

SCI	spinal cord injury
PPS	Postpolio syndrome
ALS	Amyotrophic lateral sclerosis
POLIO	Poliomyelitis

▼ **FIGURE 10.14**
Spinal Cord Injuries.
(a) Severed spinal cord from fracture-dislocation of vertebra.
(b) Compressed spinal cord with vertebral fracture.

Severed spinal cord

(a) Fracture-dislocation of vertebra

(b) Fractured vertebra

Disorders of the Myelin Sheath of Nerve Fibers *(continued)* (LO 10.5)

MS, most common in women, has an average age of onset between 18 and 35 years. Its cause is unknown, but it is thought to be an autoimmune disease. There is no known cure for MS, but currently there are 10 medications that help to slow the disease's progress. For people with relapsing MS, like Mrs. Kalish, high doses of corticosteroids are used to treat severe exacerbations, and three oral and four injectable medications are available for less severe exacerbations. Other drugs are in the research pipeline. Rehabilitation programs that focus on function are also of value.

Disorders of the Spinal Cord (LO 10.5)

Trauma (LO 10.5)

The spinal cord can be injured in three ways:

1. **Severed,** by a fractured vertebra *(Figure 10.14a);*
2. **Contused,** as in a sudden, violent jolt to the spine; and
3. **Compressed,** by a dislocated vertebra, bleeding, or swelling *(Figure 10.14b).*

Because of its anatomy—with nerve fibers and tracts going up and down, to and from the brain—a spinal cord injury results in a loss of function below the injury site. For example, if the cord is injured in the thoracic region, the arms function normally but the legs can be **paralyzed.** Both muscle control and sensation are lost. **Paresis** is partial paralysis.

If the spinal cord is severed, the loss of function is permanent. Contusions can cause temporary loss, lasting days, weeks, or months.

Compression of the cord can also occur from a tumor in the cord or spine or from a **herniated disc.** The intervertebral disc *(see Lesson 4.2 of Chapter 4)* can move out of place (herniate, slip) or break open (rupture) from injury or strain. This causes pressure on the spinal nerves leading to pain, numbness, and/or weakness. Cancer or osteoporosis can cause a vertebra to collapse and also compress the cord.

Other Disorders of the Spinal Cord (LO 10.5)

Acute transverse myelitis is a localized spinal cord disorder that blocks the transmission of impulses up and down the spinal cord.

Subacute combined degeneration of the spinal cord is due to a deficiency of vitamin B_{12}. The spinal cord's sensory nerve fibers degenerate, producing weakness, clumsiness, tingling, and a sensory loss as to the position of the limbs. Treatment involves vitamin B_{12} injections.

In **syringomyelia,** fluid-filled cavities form in the spinal cord and compress nerves that detect pain and temperature. There is no specific cure.

Poliomyelitis (POLIO) is an acute infectious disease, occurring mostly in children, due to the poliovirus. The virus destroys motor neurons. It is preventable by vaccination and has almost been eradicated worldwide.

Postpolio syndrome (PPS) is when people develop tired, painful, and weak muscles many years after recovery from polio.

Amyotrophic lateral sclerosis (ALS), or "Lou Gehrig's disease," occurs when motor nerves in the spinal cord progressively deteriorate. There is no cure.

Disorders of Peripheral Nerves (LO 10.5)

Peripheral neuropathy is used here as any disorder affecting one or more peripheral nerves. **Mononeuropathy** is damage to a single peripheral nerve. Examples are:

- **Carpal tunnel syndrome,** in which the median nerve at the wrist is compressed between the wrist bones and a strong overlying ligament.
- **Ulnar nerve palsy,** which results from nerve damage as the forearm's ulnar nerve crosses close to the surface over the humerus at the back of the elbow.
- **Peroneal nerve palsy,** which arises from nerve damage as the peroneal or lower leg bone nerve passes close to the surface near the back of the knee. Compression of this nerve occurs in people who are bedridden or strapped in a wheelchair.

Polyneuropathy is damage to, and the simultaneous malfunction of, many motor and/or sensory peripheral nerves throughout the body. There are many causes of peripheral polyneuropathy; diabetes is a common cause. Symptoms include numbness, pain, tingling sensations, and weakness. Treatment is aimed at the underlying problem and pain reduction.

Herpes zoster, or **shingles,** is an infection of peripheral nerves arising from a reactivation of the dormant childhood chickenpox (varicella) virus.

Word Analysis and Definition

S = Suffix   P = Prefix   R = Root   R/CF = Combining Form

WORD	PRONUNCIATION	ELEMENTS		DEFINITION
amyotrophic	a-my-oh-**TROH**-fik	S/ P/ R/CF R/	-ic *pertaining to* a- *without* -my/o- *muscle* -troph- *nourishment, development*	Pertaining to muscular atrophy
compression	kom-**PRESH**-un	S/ P/ R/	-ion *action, condition* com- *together* -press- *squeeze*	Squeeze together to increase density and/or decrease a dimension of a structure
herniation	her-nee-**AY**-shun	S/ R/	-ation *process* herni- *rupture*	Protrusion of an anatomical structure from its normal location
hernia (noun) herniate (verb)	**HER**-nee-ah **HER**-nee-ate	S/	-ate *composed of*	Protrusion of a structure through the tissue that normally contains it
myelitis	**MY**-eh-**LIE**-tis	S/ R/	-itis *inflammation* myel- *spinal cord*	Inflammation of the spinal cord
neuropathy	nyu-**ROP**-ah-thee	S/ R/CF	-pathy *disease* neur/o- *nerve*	Any disorder of the nervous system
mononeuropathy polyneuropathy	**MON**-oh-nyu-**ROP**-ah-thee **POL**-ee-nyu-**ROP**-ah-thee	P/ P/	mono- *one* poly- *many*	Disorder affecting a single nerve Disorder affecting many nerves
paralyze (verb)	**PAR**-ah-lyze	P/ R/	para- *beside, abnormal* -lyze *destroy*	To make incapable of movement
paralysis (noun) paralytic (adj)	pah-**RAL**-ih-sis par-ah-**LYT**-ik	R/ S/ R/	-lysis *destruction* -ic *pertaining to* -lyt- *destroy*	Loss of voluntary movement Suffering from paralysis
paresis hemiparesis	par-**EE**-sis **HEM**-ee-pah-**REE**-sis	P/ R/	Greek *weakness* hemi- *half* -paresis *weakness*	Partial paralysis (weakness) Weakness of one side of the body
poliomyelitis (Note: abbreviated as polio) postpolio syndrome (PPS)	**POE**-lee-oh-**MY**-eh-lie-tis post-**POE**-lee-oh **SIN**-drome	S/ R/ R/ P/ R/ P/ R/	-itis *inflammation* polio- *gray matter* -myel- *spinal cord* post- *after* -polio *gray matter* syn- *together* -drome *running*	Inflammation of the gray matter of the spinal cord, leading to paralysis of the limbs and muscles of respiration Progressive muscle weakness in a person previously affected by polio
syringomyelia	sih-**RING**-oh-my-**EE**-lee-ah	S R/CF R/	-ia *condition* syring/o- *tube, pipe* -myel- *spinal cord*	Abnormal longitudinal cavities in the spinal cord that cause paresthesias and muscle weakness
trauma traumatic	**TRAW**-mah traw-**MAT**-ik	S/ R/	Greek *wound* -tic *pertaining to* trauma- *injury*	A physical or mental injury Pertaining to or caused by trauma

EXERCISES

A. Use the language *of neurology to demonstrate your knowledge of the spinal cord.* **LO 10.5 and 10.8** *Apply*

1. Name the three ways the spinal cord can be injured: _____

2. Where does loss of function occur in a spinal cord injury? _____

3. What is lost in paralysis? _____

4. What is partial paralysis called? _____

5. What can cause compression of the spinal cord? _____

B. Identify the element, *and give its meaning. Complete the exercise by listing a medical term that contains this element. Review the WAD box above before you start the exercise. Fill in the chart.* **LO 10.1 and 10.5** *Remember*

Element	Element Identity (P, R, CF, or S)	Meaning of Element	Medical Term Containing This Element
myo	1.	2.	3.
herni	4.	5.	6.
pathy	7.	8.	9.
troph	10.	11.	12.

Lesson 10.4 (cont'd)

Congenital Anomalies of the Nervous System (LO 10.5)

Keynote

- Classification of CP by number of limbs impaired:
  - Quadriplegia: All four limbs are affected.
  - Paraplegia: Both lower extremities are affected.
  - Hemiplegia: The arm and leg of one side of the body are affected.
  - Monoplegia: Only one limb is affected, usually an arm.

Some of the most devastating congenital neurologic abnormalities develop in the first 8 to 10 weeks of pregnancy, when the nervous system is in its early stages of formation. These malformations can be detected using ultrasonography and amniocentesis *(see Chapter 15)*. Many of these can be prevented by the mother taking 4 mg/day of folic acid before conception and during early pregnancy.

A **teratogen** is an agent that can cause **anomalies** of an embryo or fetus *(see Chapter 15)*. It can be a chemical, a virus, or radiation. Some teratogens found in the workplace include textile dyes, photographic chemicals, semiconductor materials, and the metals lead, mercury, and cadmium.

Anencephaly is the absence of the cerebral hemispheres and is incompatible with life. **Microcephaly,** decreased head size, is associated with small cerebral hemispheres and moderate to severe motor and mental retardation.

Hydrocephalus *(Figure 10.15)* is ventricular enlargement in the cerebral hemispheres with excessive CSF; it is usually due to a blockage that prevents the CSF from exiting the ventricles to circulate around the spinal cord. Treatment involves placing a tube (shunt) into the ventricle to divert the excess fluid into the abdominal cavity or a neck vein.

Spina bifida (neural tube defect) occurs mostly in the lumbar and sacral regions. It is variable in its presentation and symptoms. **Spina bifida occulta** has a small partial defect in the vertebral arch. The spinal cord or meninges do not protrude. Often the only sign is a tuft of hair on the skin overlying the defect.

In **spina bifida cystica** there is no vertebral arch formed. The spinal cord and meninges protrude through the opening and may or may not be covered with a thin layer of skin *(Figure 10.16a and b)*. Protrusion of only the meninges is called a **meningocele.** Protrusion of the meninges and spinal cord is called a **meningomyelocele** (myelomeningomyelocele). The lower limbs may be paralyzed.

Fetal alcohol syndrome (FAS) can occur when a pregnant woman drinks alcohol. A child born with FAS has a small head, narrow eyes, and a flat face and nose. Intellect and growth are impaired. FAS is the third most common cause of mental retardation in newborns.

▲ **FIGURE 10.15**
Infant with Hydrocephalus.

Cerebral Palsy (LO 10.5)

Cerebral palsy (CP) is the term used to describe the motor impairment resulting from brain damage in an infant or young child. It is not hereditary. In congenital CP, the cause is often unknown but can be a brain malformation or maternal use of cocaine. CP developed at birth or in the neonatal period is usually related to an incident causing hypoxia of the brain.

Cerebral palsy causes delay in the development of normal milestones in infancy and childhood. The affected limbs can be **spastic** (muscles are tight and resistant to stretch) and may show **athetoid** movements, where the limbs involuntarily writhe and constantly move. A poor sense of balance and coordination may also be present, leading to **ataxia.**

A rehabilitation program focused on function is the key component in treatment of cerebral palsy.

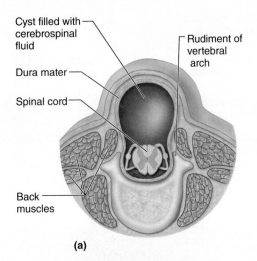

Cyst filled with cerebrospinal fluid

Dura mater

Spinal cord

Rudiment of vertebral arch

Back muscles

(a)

(b)

▲ **FIGURE 10.16**
Spina Bifida Cystica.
(a) Cross section of a spinal meningocele.
(b) Child with spina bifida cystica.

Word Analysis and Definition

WORD	PRONUNCIATION	ELEMENTS		DEFINITION
anencephaly	AN-en-SEF-ah-lee	S/ P/ R/	-aly condition an- without -enceph- brain	Born without cerebral hemispheres
microcephaly	MY-kroh-SEF-ah-lee	P/ R/	micro- small -ceph- head	An abnormally small head
ataxia	a-TAK-see-ah	S/ P/ R/	-ia condition a- without -tax- coordination	Inability to coordinate muscle activity, leading to jerky movements
ataxic (adj)	a-TAK-sik	S/	-ic pertaining to	Pertaining to or suffering from ataxia
athetosis	ath-eh-TOE-sis	S/ R/	-osis condition athet- without position, uncontrolled	Slow, writhing involuntary movements
athetoid (adj)	ATH-eh-toyd	S/	-oid resembling	Resembling or suffering from athetosis
hemiplegia	hem-ee-PLEE-jee-ah	S/ P/ R/	-ia condition hemi- half -pleg- paralysis	Paralysis of one side of the body
hemiplegic (adj) hemiparesis	hem-ee-PLEE-jik HEM-ee-pah-REE-sis	S/ R/	-ic pertaining to -paresis weakness	Pertaining to or suffering from hemiplegia Weakness of one side of the body
meningocele	meh-NIN-goh-seal	S/ R/CF	-cele hernia mening/o- meninges	Protrusion of the meninges from the spinal cord or brain through a defect in the vertebral column or cranium
meningomyelocele	meh-nin-goh-MY-el-oh-seal	S/ R/CF	-cele hernia -myel/o- spinal cord	Protrusion of the spinal cord and meninges through a defect in the vertebral arch of one or more vertebrae
monoplegia	MON-oh-PLEE-jee-ah	S/ P/ R/	-ia condition mono- one -pleg- paralysis	Paralysis of one limb
monoplegic (adj)	MON-oh-PLEE-jik	S/	-ic pertaining to	Pertaining to or suffering from monoplegia
palsy	PAWL-zee		Latin paralysis	Paralysis or paresis from brain damage
paraplegia	par-ah-PLEE-jee-ah	S/ P/ R/	-ia condition para- abnormal -pleg- paralysis	Paralysis of both lower extremities
paraplegic (adj)	par-ah-PLEE-jik	S/	-ic pertaining to	Pertaining to or suffering from paraplegia
quadriplegia	kwad-rih-PLEE-jee-ah	S/ P/ R/	-ia condition quadri- four -pleg- paralysis	Paralysis of all four limbs
quadriplegic (adj)	kwad-rih-PLEE-jik	S/	-ic pertaining to	Pertaining to or suffering from quadriplegia
spina bifida	SPY-nah BIH-fih-dah	R/CF P/ R/	spin/a spine bi- two -fida split	Failure of one or more vertebral arches to close during fetal development
spina bifida cystica	SIS-tik-ah	S/ R/	-ica pertaining to cyst- cyst	Meninges and spinal cord protruding through the absent vertebral arch and having the appearance of a cyst
spina bifida occulta	OH-kul-tah	R/CF	occult/a hidden	The deformity of the vertebral arch is not apparent from the surface
teratogen	TER-ah-toe-gen	S/ R/CF	-gen create, produce terat/o- monster, malformed fetus	Agent that produces fetal deformities

EXERCISE

A. Search and find *the correct term for the element you are given. Circle the best answer.*   **LO 10.1 and 10.5** *Understand*

1. Find the term with the prefix meaning *without:*

   hydrocephalus   anencephaly   bifida

2. Find the term with the suffix meaning *hernia:*

   meningocele   cystica   teratogen

3. Find the term with the root meaning *hidden:*

   spina bifida   spina bifida cystica   spina bifida occulta

4. Find the term with the root meaning *coordination:*

   monoplegia   athetosis   ataxia

Lesson 10.4 (cont'd) Diagnostic Procedures in Neurology (LO 10.2 and 10.6)

Abbreviations

CT scan	Computed tomography
EEG	Electroencephalography
LP	Lumbar puncture
MRI	Magnetic resonance imaging
PET scan	Positron emission tomography

- **Lumbar puncture (LP or spinal tap)** enables laboratory examination of the CSF to be made and helps diagnose meningitis, damage to the spinal cord, and brain hemorrhage.

- **Electroencephalography (EEG)** records the brain's electrical activity to help identify epilepsy, sleep disturbances, degenerative brain disease, and brain damage *(Figure 10.17)*.

- **Computed tomography (CT scan)** generates images of slices of the brain to detect tumors, tissue damage, and birth defects.

- **Magnetic resonance imaging (MRI)** produces highly detailed anatomical images of most neurologic disorders *(Figure 10.18)*.

- **Cerebral angiography** involves an injection of radiopaque dye into the blood vessels of the neck and brain to detect partial or complete blockages of blood vessels and aneurysms.

- **Color Doppler ultrasonography** uses high-frequency sound (ultrasound) waves to evaluate the rates of blood flow through arteries of the neck or base of the brain.

- **Positron emission tomography (PET scan)** involves attaching radioactive molecules to glucose to look at brain function *(Figure 10.19)*.

- **Evoked responses** are a procedure in which stimuli for vision, sound, and touch are used to activate areas of the brain, and their responses are measured with EEG or PET scans. They are used to give information about how a specific area of the brain is functioning.

- **Electromyography** involves placing small needles into a muscle to record its electrical activity at rest and during contraction.

- **Nerve conduction studies** measure the speed at which sensory and motor nerves conduct impulses to focus on the function of peripheral nerves.

Alpha (α)
Beta (β)
Theta (θ)
Delta (δ)

1 second

▲ **FIGURE 10.17**
Four Classes of Brain Waves on EEG.

(a)   (b)

▲ **FIGURE 10.18**
MRI Scans of Brain Sections.
(a) Colored MRI scan of a Section of Normal Brain.
(b) Colored MRI Scan of Brain Section showing Cerebral Atrophy (in yellow) in a Patient with Alzheimer Disease.

Primary motor cortex

▲ **FIGURE 10.19**
PET Scan of the Brain Showing the Motor Cortex.

Word Analysis and Definition

WORD	PRONUNCIATION	ELEMENTS		DEFINITION
angiography	an-jee-**OG**-rah-fee	S/ R/CF	-graphy *process of recording* angi/o- *blood vessel*	X-ray visualization of blood vessels after injection of contrast material
electromyography	ee-**LEK**-troh-my-**OG**-rah-fee	S/ R/CF R/CF	-graphy *process of recording* electr/o- *electricity* -my/o- *muscle*	Recording of electrical activity in muscle
neuromuscular	**NYUR**-oh-**MUSS**-kyu-lar	S/ R/CF R/	-ar *pertaining to* neur/o- *nerve* -muscul- *muscle*	Pertaining to both nerves and muscles
ultrasonography	**UL**-trah-son-**NOG**-rah-fee	S/ P/ R/CF	-graphy *process of recording* ultra- *beyond* -son/o- *sound*	Imaging using ultrasound that detects direction, velocity, and turbulence of blood flow

EXERCISES

A. Demonstrate *your knowledge of the use of diagnostic procedures in neurology.*   **LO 10.2, 10.6, and 10.8** *Understand*

1. Which procedures can be considered *invasive* procedures? _____

_____

2. What makes a procedure invasive? _____

_____

3. Which procedures involve injections of dye or radioactive material? _____

_____

4. Which procedures involve sound waves? _____

_____

5. Which procedures measure electrical activity? _____

_____

B. Deconstruct *each medical term into its elements and give its meaning. Every word does not have a prefix and suffix, and some words have more than one of the same element.*   **LO 10.1, 10.6, and 10.8** *Analyze*

1. angiography _____/_____/_____

                P   R, R/CF   S

   Meaning: _____

2. ultrasonography _____/_____/_____

                P   R, R/CF   S

   Meaning: _____

3. neuromuscular _____/_____/_____

                P   R, R/CF   S

   Meaning: _____

4. electromyography _____/_____/_____

                P   R, R/CF   S

   Meaning: _____

Lesson 10.5
Mental Health

Objectives

To be an effective member of the mental health team that will be responsible for Mr. Costello's care, you will need to be able to:

10.5.1 Define mental health, and differentiate between psychiatry and psychology.

10.5.2 Discuss psychosis and schizophrenia.

10.5.3 Review common mood disorders.

10.5.4 Describe the major types of anxiety disorders.

10.5.5 Identify personality disorders.

10.5.6 Explain the effects of common psychoactive drugs.

Keynotes

- A specialist in **psychiatry** is a physician called a **psychiatrist,** who is licensed to prescribe medications.

- A specialist in **psychology** is a **psychologist,** who is not licensed to prescribe medications.

- **Insanity** is a legal term for a severe mental illness that impairs a defendant's ability to understand the **moral** wrong of the act he/she committed. It is not a medical diagnosis.

◀ **FIGURE 10.20**
Homeless Schizophrenic Man on the Street.

Case Report 10.4

You are . . .

. . . a **psychiatric technician** employed in the Psychiatric Department of Fulwood Medical Center. Your patient has been referred from the Emergency Department, where he was seen earlier this morning.

Your patient is . . .

. . . Mr. Dante Costello, a 21-year-old homeless man, brought in by the police after he was found sitting immobile in the middle of a main street (**catatonia**).

Mr. Costello's explanation is "the voices told me to do it." He has heard voices (**hallucinations**) telling him to do things for the past year. The voices often comment on his behavior. He has isolated himself from other people because "they are not who they say they are, and they are trying to get me" (**delusions**). He is taking no drugs or medications, and he denies any **suicidal** or homicidal intent.

Mr. Costello is dirty and disheveled, with poor hygiene. He can give no home or family address. His **affect** is **congruent,** though expressionless. His speech is slow, and his thoughts are disorganized and confused.

The most probable diagnosis is **schizophrenia.** He needs to be admitted to the hospital because he is a danger to himself and other people.

Mental Health Definitions
(LO 10.7 and 10.8)

- **Mental health** is defined by the World Health Organization (**WHO**) as "a state of wellbeing in which the individual realizes his or her own abilities, can cope with the normal stresses of life, can work productively and fruitfully, and is able to make a contribution to the community."

- **Psychology** is the scientific study of behavior—talking, reading, sleeping, interacting with others—and mental processes—thinking, feeling, remembering, and dreaming.

- **Psychiatry** is the medical specialty concerned with the origin, diagnosis, prevention, and treatment of mental, emotional, and behavioral disorders.

- **Mental health disorders** are of different types and will be considered in this chapter under the headings Psychosis and Schizophrenia, Mood Disorders, Anxiety Disorders, Personality Disorders, and Substance Abuse and Chemical Dependence.

Psychosis and Schizophrenia
(LO 10.7)

Psychosis is an abnormal mental state in which the individual has a loss of contact with reality. People suffering from psychosis are described as **psychotic.**

Schizophrenia is a form of psychosis in which the individual loses contact with reality. People with schizophrenia do *not* have a "split personality," but their perceptions are separated from reality, their words are separated from their meanings, and their behaviors are separated from their thought processes. They perceive things without stimulation (**hallucinations**). They suffer from mistaken beliefs that are contrary to facts (**delusions**). The delusions can be **paranoid,** with pervasive distrust and suspicion of others. Their speech is disorganized and can be incoherent, and they may refuse or be unable to speak (**mute**) *(Figure 10.20)*. In the Case Report above, Mr. Costello showed all of these symptoms.

Word Analysis and Definition

WORD	PRONUNCIATION		ELEMENTS	DEFINITION
affect	AFF-ekt		Latin *state of mind*	External display of feelings, emotions, and thoughts
congruent	KON-gru-ent	S/ P/ R/	-ent *end result* con- *with* -gru- *to move*	Coinciding or agreeing with
delusion	dee-LOO-zhun	S/ R/	-ion *condition* delus- *deceive*	Fixed, unyielding false belief despite strong evidence to the contrary
hallucination	hah-loo-sih-NAY-shun	S/ R/	-ation *condition* hallucin- *imagination*	Perception of an object or event when there is no such thing present
mute	MYUT		Latin *silent*	Unable or unwilling to speak
paranoia	par-ah-NOY-ah	P/ R/	para- *abnormal* -noia *to think*	Presence of persecutory delusions
paranoid	PAR-ah-noyd	S/	-oid *resembling*	Having persecutory delusions
psychiatry	sigh-KIGH-ah-tree	S/ R/	iatry- *treatment* psych- *mind*	Diagnosis and treatment of mental disorders
psychiatrist	sigh-KIGH-ah-trist	S/	-iatrist *one who treats*	Licensed medical specialist in psychiatry
psychology	sigh-KOL-oh-jee	S/ R/CF	-logy *study of* psych/o- *mind*	Science concerned with the behavior of the human mind
psychologist	sigh-KOL-oh-jist	S/	-logist *one who treats*	Licensed specialist in psychology
psychosis	sigh-KOH-sis	S/ R/	-osis *condition* psych- *mind*	Disorder with loss of contact with reality
psychotic	sigh-KOT-ik	S/ R/CF	-tic *pertaining to* psych/o- *mind*	Affected by psychosis
schizophrenia	skitz-oh-FREE-nee-ah	S/ R/CF R/	-ia *condition* schiz/o- *to split* -phren- *mind*	Disorder of perception and behavior with loss of reality
schizophrenic	skitz-oh-FREN-ik	S/	-ic *pertaining to*	Suffering from schizophrenia
suicide	SOO-ih-side	R/CF R/CF	su/i- *self* -cid/e *kill*	The act of killing oneself
suicidal	SOO-ih-SIGH-dal	S/	-al *pertaining to*	Wanting to kill oneself

EXERCISE

A. Define *the following terms in your own words:*   **LO 10.1, 10.7, and 10.9** *Understand*

1. psychologist _____

   _____

2. psychiatrist _____

   _____

3. psychosis _____

   _____

4. hallucination _____

   _____

5. delusion _____

   _____

Lesson 10.5 Mood Disorders
(cont'd) (LO 10.3 and 10.7)

▲ **FIGURE 10.21**
Depressed Woman at a Window.

Major depression, also called **unipolar disorder** *(Figure 10.21),* occurs when a person is deeply sad, despairing, and hopeless for at least two weeks; sees nothing but sorrow and despair in the future; and may not want to live anymore. Moderate exercise has been shown to reduce the symptoms of depression by 47%, and medication will ease the symptoms *(see later).* **Electroconvulsive therapy (ECT)** is used in severe depression that has not responded to other treatment.

- **Bipolar disorder,** which used to be called **manic-depressive disorder,** is the alternation of major episodes of depression with periods of excessive overexcitement, impulsive behavior, **insomnia,** and lack of fatigue, called **mania.** Untreated mixed (manic and depressive) episodes usually last around four to five months.

- **Dysphoric mania** combines the frenetic energy of mania with dark thoughts and paranoid delusions. It may be the cause of some mass shootings.

- **Seasonal affective disorder (SAD)** has episodes of depression that occur in the fall and winter months. It appears to be related to a lack of sunshine causing increased melatonin production by the pineal gland *(see Chapter 12).* It can be helped by **phototherapy** with bright white fluorescent lights and by antidepressant medications.

▲ **FIGURE 10.22**
The remains of an American Humvee, one of four that were disabled by massive IEDs, lies on a dirt road on August 4, 2007, in Hawr Rajab, Iraq.

Anxiety Disorders
(LO 10.2, 10.3, and 10.7)

Anxiety disorders are the most common category of mental disorder found in the United States. They are characterized by an unreasonable anxiety and fear so intense and persistent that it disrupts the person's life. There are five categories of anxiety disorders:

1. **Generalized anxiety disorder (GAD)** consists of uncontrollable anxiety not focused on one situation or event that has lasted for six months or more. People with the disorder develop physical fear reactions, including palpitations, insomnia, difficulty concentrating, and irritability.

2. **Posttraumatic stress disorder (PTSD)** affects about 7.7 million American adults. It arises after significant trauma, such as a life-threatening incident, loss of a loved one, abuse, torture or combat in war, or a high level of stress in daily life *(Figure 10.22).* Symptoms include flashbacks of the traumatic event, nightmares, intense physical reactions to reminders of the event, feeling emotionally numb, irritability, outbursts of anger, and difficulty concentrating. Alcohol and drug abuse are common. Treatment is with **cognitive behavioral therapy (CBT),** in which the traumatic experiences are relived and worked through; **cognitive processing therapy (CPT),** in which the thoughts and beliefs generated by the trauma are explored and reframed; and antidepressants.

3. **Panic disorder** is characterized by sudden, brief attacks of intense fear that cause physical symptoms, occur often for no reason, and peak in 10 minutes or less. Treatment is with CBT and medication with benzodiazepines or selective serotonin reuptake inhibitors **(SSRI)** *(see later in this lesson).*

4. **Phobias** differ from panic attacks in that a *specific* situation or event brings on the strong fear response. There are two categories of phobias:
   - **Situational phobias** involve a fear of specific situations. Examples are **acrophobia** (fear of heights), **agoraphobia** (fear of crowded places), and **claustrophobia** (fear of confined spaces).
   - **Social phobias** involve a fear of being embarrassed in social situations. The most common are fear of public speaking and fear of eating in public.

5. In **obsessive-compulsive disorder (OCD),** most patients have both **obsessions** and **compulsions.** Obsessions are recurrent thoughts, fears, doubts, images, or impulses. Compulsions are recurrent, irresistible impulses to perform actions such as counting, hand washing, checking, and systematically arranging things. Treatment is with CBT and/or an SSRI.

Psychosomatic disorder is a real physical illness in which anxiety and stress play a causative role. Examples are tension headaches and low back pain. Treatment is with **biofeedback** and relaxation techniques *(Figure 10.23).*

A person called a **hypochondriac** has **hypochondriasis** and interprets some minor symptom such as a cough or a bruise as a sign of serious disease, and cannot believe normal physical examinations and reassurances.

▲ **FIGURE 10.23**
Person Undergoing Biofeedback.

Abbreviations

CBT	cognitive behavioral therapy
CPT	cognitive processing therapy
GAD	generalized anxiety disorder
ECT	Electroconvulsive therapy
OCD	obsessive-compulsive disorder
PTSD	posttraumatic stress disorder
SAD	seasonal affective disorder
SSRI	selective serotonin reuptake inhibitor

Word Analysis and Definition

S = Suffix   P = Prefix   R = Root   R/CF = Combining Form

WORD	PRONUNCIATION	ELEMENTS		DEFINITION
acrophobia	ak-roh-**FOH**-be-ah	S/ R/CF	-phobia *fear* acr/o- *peak, highest point*	Pathologic fear of heights
agoraphobia	ah-gor-ah-**FOH**-be-ah	S/ R/CF	-phobia *fear* agor/a- *marketplace*	Pathologic fear of being trapped in a public place
anxiety	ang-**ZI**-eh-tee		Greek *distress, anxiety*	Distress caused by fear
biofeedback (Note: This term has no prefix or suffix.)	bi-oh-**FEED**-back	R/CF R/ R/	bi/o- *life* -feed- *to give food, nourish* -back *back, return*	Training techniques to achieve voluntary control of responses to stimuli
bipolar disorder	bi-**POH**-lar dis-**OR**-der	S/ P/ R/	-ar *pertaining to* bi- *two* -pol- *pole*	A mood disorder with alternating episodes of depression and mania
claustrophobia	klaw-stroh-**FOH**-be-ah	S/ R/CF	-phobia *fear* claustr/o- *confined space*	Pathologic fear of being trapped in a confined space
cognitive	**KOG**-nih-tiv	S/ R/	-ive *quality of* cognit- *thinking*	Pertaining to the mental activities of thinking and learning
cognitive behavioral therapy (CBT) (Note: Behavioral has two suffixes to make the word flow.)	**KOG**-nih-tiv be-**HAYV**-yur-al **THAIR**-ah-pee	S/ R/ S/ S/ R/ R/	-ive *quality of* cognit- *thinking* -al *pertaining to* -ior- *pertaining to* behav- *mental activity* therapy *medical treatment*	Psychotherapy that emphasizes thoughts and attitudes in one's behavior
cognitive processing therapy (CPT)	**KOG**-nih-tiv **PROS**-es-ing **THAIR**-ah-pee	S/ R/ S/ P/ R/	-ive *quality of* cognit- *thinking* -ing *doing* pro- *before* -cess- *going forward*	Psychotherapy to build skills to deal with effects of trauma in other areas of life
compulsion	kom-**PULL**-shun	S/ R/	-ion *action, condition* compuls- *drive, compel*	Uncontrollable impulses to perform an act repetitively
compulsive (adj)	kom-**PULL**-siv	S/	-ive *nature of, quality of*	Possessing uncontrollable impulses to perform an act repetitively
depression	de-**PRESH**-un	S/ R/	-ion *condition, process* depress- *press down*	Mental disorder with feelings of deep sadness and despair
electroconvulsive therapy	ee-**LEK**-troh-kon-**VUL**-siv **THAIR**-ah-pee	S/ R/CF P/ R/	-ive *quality of* electr/o- *electricity* -con- *with* -vuls- *tear, pull*	Passage of electric current through the brain to produce convulsions and treat persistent depression, mania, and other disorders
hypochondriac	high-poh-**KON**-dree-ack	S/ P/ R/	-iac *pertaining to* hypo- *below* -chondr- *cartilage*	A person who exaggerates the significance of symptoms
hypochondriasis	**HIGH**-poh-kon-**DRY**-ah-sis	S/	-iasis *condition, state of*	Belief that a minor symptom indicates a severe disease
insomnia	in-**SOM**-nee-ah	S/ P/ R/	-ia *condition* in- *not* -somn- *sleep*	Inability to sleep
mania	**MAY**-nee-ah		Greek *frenzy*	Mood disorder with hyperactivity, irritability, and rapid speech
manic	**MAN**-ik	S/ R/	-ic *pertaining to* man- *mania*	Pertaining to or characterized by mania
manic-depressive disorder	**MAN**-ik-de-**PRESS**-iv dis-**OR**-der	S/ R/	-ive *quality of* depress- *press down*	An outdated name for bipolar disorder
obsession	ob-**SESH**-un	S/ R/	-ion *action, Condition* obsess- *besieged by thoughts*	Persistent, recurrent, uncontrollable thoughts or impulses
obsessive (adj)	ob-**SES**-iv	S/	-ive *nature of, quality of*	Possessing persistent, recurrent, uncontrollable thoughts or impulses
phobia	**FOH**-be-ah		Greek *fear*	Pathologic fear or dread
posttraumatic	post-traw-**MAT**-ik	S/ P/ R/	-ic *pertaining to* post- *after* -traumat- *wound*	Occurring after and caused by trauma
psychosomatic	sigh-koh-soh-**MAT**-ik	S/ R/CF R/	-tic *pertaining to* psych/o- *mind* -soma- *body*	Pertaining to disorders of the body usually resulting from disturbances of the mind
unipolar disorder	you-nih-**POLE**-ar dis-**OR**-der	S/ P/ R/	-ar *pertaining to* uni- *one* -pol- *pole (at the pole of depression)*	Depression

EXERCISES

A. Demonstrate *your knowledge of medical terminology for mental health. Fill in the blanks.*   **LO 10.2, 10.3, and 10.7** *Apply*

1. What symptom do patients with unipolar disorder exhibit? _____ and _____

2. Name three different phobias and define them:

   a. _____

   b. _____

   c. _____

3. What characterizes anxiety disorders? _____

4. What is *bipolar disorder?* _____

Personality Disorders
(LO 10.3 and 10.7)

Personality is defined as an individual's unique and stable patterns of thoughts, feelings, and behaviors. When these patterns become rigid and inflexible in response to different situations, they can cause impairment of the individual's ability to deal with other people (i.e., to function socially).

- **Borderline personality disorder (BPD)** is a frequent diagnosis in people who are impulsive, unstable in mood, and manipulative. They can be exciting, charming, and friendly one moment and angry, irritable, and sarcastic the next. Their identity is fragile and insecure, their self-worth low. They can be promiscuous and self-destructive; for example, with **self-mutilation (self-injury)** *(Figure 10.24)* or suicide. People with **narcissistic personality disorder** have an exaggerated sense of self-importance and seek constant attention.

- **Antisocial personality disorder,** used interchangeably with the terms **sociopath** and **psychopath,** describes people who lie, cheat, steal, and have no sense of responsibility and no anxiety or guilt about their behavior. Psychopaths have these characteristics but tend to be more violent and anger easily.

- **Schizoid** and **paranoid personality disorders** describe people who are absorbed with themselves, untrusting, and fearful of closeness with others.

- Treatment for personality disorders is not successful.

▲ **FIGURE 10.24**
Self-Mutilated Arm.

▲ **FIGURE 10.25**
Dissociative Identity Disorder (Multiple Personality Disorder).

Dissociative Disorders
(LO 10.3 and 10.7)

Dissociative disorders involve a disassociation (splitting apart) of past experiences from present memory or consciousness. The development of distinctly separate personalities is called **dissociative identity disorder (DID).** It was formerly called **multiple personality disorder (MPD).** Two or more distinct personalities, each with its own memories and behaviors, inhabit the same person at the same time *(Figure 10.25).* The basic origin of all these disorders is the need to escape, usually from extreme trauma, and most often from sexual, emotional, or physical abuse in childhood. Treatment is with psychotherapy.

Impulse Control Disorders
(LO 10.3 and 10.7)

Impulse control disorders involve an inability to resist an impulse to perform an action that is harmful to the individual or to others. These disorders include:

- **Kleptomania,** which is characterized by stealing—not for gain but to satisfy an irresistible urge to steal. Behavior therapy can help, and SSRIs appear to be of value.
- **Trichotillomania (TTM),** which is characterized by the repeated urge to pull out one's own scalp, beard, pubic, and other body hair.
- **Pyromania,** which is repeated fire setting with no motive other than a fascination with fire and fire engines. Some pyromaniacs end up as volunteer firefighters.

Treatment with behavior therapy is sometimes successful.

Substance Abuse and Chemical Dependence
(LO 10.3 and 10.7)

Substance abuse involves a person's continued use of psychoactive drugs, including alcohol and illicit drugs, despite having significant problems or distress related to their use. This continued use can lead to a **dependence** syndrome, which includes the strong need to take the drug, persistence in its use despite harmful consequences to the user and others, daily priority given to drug use, and increased **tolerance.** Tolerance is the process by which the body continually adapts to a substance and requires increasingly larger amounts to achieve the original effects.

- **Addiction** includes dependence syndrome, but it refers to not only psychoactive drugs but also such entities as exercise addiction, food addiction, computer addiction, and gambling. The patterns of behavior and habits of use associated with an addiction are characterized by immediate gratification coupled with the long-term harmful effects, which include changes in the structure and function of the brain.

- **Abused substances** include tobacco, alcohol, marijuana, cocaine, heroin, methamphetamines, Ecstasy, LSD, and PCP. In addition, prescription drug abuse is increasing dramatically. The three classes of prescription drugs being abused are:
  1. **Opioids,** which include oxycodone (Oxycontin), hydrocodone (Vicodin), meperidine (Demerol), hydromorphone (Dilaudid), and fentanyl (Duragesic and others).
  2. **CNS depressants** such as the benzodiazepines Xanax and Valium.
  3. **CNS stimulants** such as Adderall and Ritalin.

Abuse of prescription drugs now ranks second to marijuana among illicit drug users, and the number of fatal poisonings from prescription opioid analgesics outnumbers total deaths from heroin and cocaine.

Abbreviations

BPD	borderline personality disorder
DID	dissociative identity disorder
MPD	multiple personality disorder
TTM	trichotillomania

Word Analysis and Definition

S = Suffix   P = Prefix   R = Root   R/CF = Combining Form

WORD	PRONUNCIATION		ELEMENTS	DEFINITION
addict	ADD-ikt	P/	ad- *toward*	Person with a psychologic or physical depen-dence on a substance or practice
addiction	ah-DIK-shun	R/	-dict *surrender*	Habitual psychologic and physiologic depen-dence on a substance or practice
		S/	-ion *condition, action*	
antisocial personality disorder	AN-tee-SOH-shal per-son-AL-ih-tee dis-OR-der	S/	-al *pertaining to*	Disorder of people who lie, cheat, steal, and have no guilt about their behavior
		P/	anti- *against*	
		R/	-soci- *partner, ally, community*	
		S/	-ity *condition, state*	
		S/	-al- *pertaining to*	
		R/	person- *person*	
dissociative identity disorder	di-SO-see-ah-tiv eye-DEN-tih-tee dis-OR-der	S/	-ative *quality of*	Mental disorder in which part of an individual's personality is separated from the rest, leading to multiple personalities
		P/	dis- *apart, away from*	
		R/	-soci- *partner, ally, community*	
kleptomania	klep-toe-MAY-nee-ah	S/	-mania *frenzy*	Uncontrollable need to steal
		R/CF	klept/o- *to steal*	
narcissism	NAR-sih-sizm		Greek mythical character, Narcissus, who was in love with his own reflection in water	Self-love; person interprets everything purely in relation to himself or herself
narcissistic (adj)	NAR-sih-SIS-tik	S/	-ism *a process*	Relating everything to oneself
		S/	-istic *pertaining to*	
		R/	narciss- *selflove*	
pathologic gambling	path-oh-LOJ-ik GAM-bling	S/	-ic *pertaining to*	Morbid, constant, uncontrollable, destructive gambling
		R/CF	path/o- *disease*	
		R/	-log- *study of*	
psychopath	SIGH-koh-path	S/	-path *disease*	Person with antisocial personality disorder
		R/CF	psych/o- *mind*	
pyromania	pie-roh-MAY-nee-ah	S/	-mania *frenzy*	Morbid impulse to set fires
		R/CF	pyr/o- *fire*	
schizoid	SKITZ-oyd	S/	-oid *resemble*	Withdrawn, socially isolated
		R/	schiz- *split*	
self-mutilation	self-myu-tih-LAY-shun	S/	-ation *process*	Injury or disfigurement made to one's own body
		R/	self- *own individual*	
		R/	-mutil- *to maim*	
sociopath	SO-see-oh-path	S/	-path *disease*	Person with antisocial personality disorder
		R/CF	soci/o- *partner, ally, community*	

EXERCISES

A. In your own words, *describe the behaviors of a:*   **LO 10.2, 10.7, and 10.8** *Understand*

1. sociopath _____

_____

2. kleptomaniac _____

_____

3. pyromaniac _____

_____

▼ **TABLE 10.1**

PSYCHOACTIVE DRUGS (LO 10.6 AND 10.7)

Type/Mode of Action	Name	Common Effects	Effects of Abuse
Stimulants ("uppers") Speed up activity in the CNS	Caffeine	Wakefulness, shorter reaction time, alertness	Restlessness, insomnia, heartbeat irregularities
	Nicotine	Varies from alertness to calmness, appetite for carbohydrates decreases	Heart disease; high blood pressure; vasoconstriction; bronchitis; emphysema; lung, throat, mouth cancer
	Amphetamines	Wakefulness, alertness, increased metabolism, decreased appetite	Nervousness, high blood pressure, delusions, psychosis, convulsions, death
	Cocaine	**Euphoria,** high energy, illusions of power	Excitability, paranoia, anxiety, panic, depression, heart failure, death
Depressants ("downers") Slow down activity in the CNS	Alcohol	1–2 drinks—reduced inhibitions and anxiety Many drinks—slow reaction time, poor coordination and memory	Blackouts, mental and neurologic impairment, psychosis, cirrhosis of liver, death
	Barbiturates and **tranquilizers**	Reduced anxiety and tension, sedation	Impaired motor and sensory functions, amnesia, loss of consciousness, death
Narcotics Mimic the actions of natural **endorphins**	Codeine, opium, morphine, heroin	Euphoria, pleasure, relief of pain	High tolerance of pain, nausea, vomiting, constipation, convulsions, coma, death
Psychedelics Disrupt normal thought processes	Marijuana	Relaxation, euphoria, increased appetite, pain relief	Sensory distortion, hallucinations, paranoia, throat and lung damage
	LSD, mescaline, MDMA (Ecstasy)	Exhilaration, euphoria, hallucinations, insightful experiences	Panic, extreme delusions, bad trips, paranoia, psychosis
Antidepressants Affect the neurotransmitters serotonin, norepinephrine, and dopamine	Selective serotonin reuptake inhibitors (SSRIs)—Prozac, Paxil, Zoloft	Enhanced mental clarity, improved sleep, diminished depression	Anxiety, decreased sex drive, insomnia, restlessness, fatigue, headaches
	Serotonin and norepinphrine reuptake inhibitors (SNRIs)—Effexor XR, Pristiq, Cymbalta	Diminished depression, pain relief	Raised blood pressure, liver and kidney failure, fatal outcome with overdose
	Tricyclic antidepressants (TCAs)—amitriptyline, Tofranil	Effective relief of depression but numerous side effects	Decreased sex drive and outcomes, difficulty urinating, sedation, weight gain, dry mouth, fatal outcome with overdose
Anxiolytics (anti-anxiety) Affect inhibitory neurotransmitters and their synaptic receptors	Benzodiazepines—Librium, Valium, Xanax	Relief of anxiety and panic disorder in the short term with rapid action	Habit forming, addiction tendencies, drowsiness, dizziness, worsen the effects of alcohol
	Selective serotonin reuptake inhibitors (SSRIs) (see above)	Used because they are not addictive	Fatigue, nausea, depression, insomnia
	Azaspirones—BuSpar	Effective in mild to moderate anxiety—takes 2–4 weeks to have effect; not addictive	Overdose leads to unconsciousness
	Beta blockers—Inderal, Tenormin (see Chapter 6)	Greatly reduce certain anxiety symptoms, such as shaking, palpitations, and sweating	Nausea, diarrhea, bronchospasm, bradycardia, insomnia, erectile dysfunction
Antiepileptic drugs (AEDs) (anticonvulsants) Do not cure epilepsy, but suppress seizures while medications are in the body	Broad-spectrum AEDs—Depakote, Lamictal, Topamax, Keppra	Effective for a wide range of all types of seizures	Weight gain, tremor, hair loss, osteoporosis, low blood count, memory problems
	Narrow-spectrum AEDs—phenobarbital, Dilantin, Tegretol, Lyrica	Effective for specific types of seizures	GI upset, weight gain, blurred vision, low blood counts, fatigue

Word Analysis and Definition

S = Suffix   P = Prefix   R = Root   R/CF = Combining Form

WORD	PRONUNCIATION	ELEMENTS		DEFINITION
antiepileptic	AN-tih-epi-LEP-tik	S/ P/ R/	-ic *pertaining to* anti- *against* -epilept- *seizure*	An agent to suppress seizures
anxiolytic	ANG-zee-oh-LIT-ik	S/ R/CF	-lytic *soluble* anxi/o *anxiety*	An agent that reduces the symptoms of anxiety
dependence	dee-PEN-dense		Latin *to hang from*	State of needing someone or something
depressant	dee-PRESS-ant	S/ R/	-ant *agent* depress- *press down*	Substance that diminishes activity, sensation, or tone
antidepressant	AN-tih-dee-PRESS-ant	P/	anti- *against*	An agent to suppress the symptoms of depression
endorphin	en-DOR-fin	P/ R/	end- *within* -orphin *morphine*	Natural substance in the brain that has the same effect as opium
euphoria	yoo-FOR-ee-ah	S/ P/ R/	-ia *condition* eu- *normal* -phor- *bear, carry*	Exaggerated feeling of well-being
narcotic	nar-KOT-ik	S/ R/CF	-tic *pertaining to* narc/o- *sleep, stupor*	Drug derived from opium or a synthetic drug with similar effects
psychedelic	sigh-keh-DEL-ik	S/ R/ R/	-ic *pertaining to* psyche- *mind, soul* -del- *manifest, visible*	Agent that intensifies sensory perception
psychoactive	sigh-koh-AK-tiv	S/ R/CF R/	-ive *quality of, nature of* psych/o- *mind, soul* -act- *performance*	Able to alter mood, behavior, and/or cognition
stimulant	STIM-you-lant	S/ R/	-ant *agent* stimul- *excite*	Agent that excites or strengthens functional activity
tolerance	TOL-er-ans	S/ R/	-ance *condition, state of* toler- *endure*	The capacity to become accustomed to a stimulus or drug
tranquilizer	TRANG-kwih-lie-zer	S/ R/	-izer *affect in a particular way* tranquil- *calm*	Agent that calms without sedating or depressing

EXERCISES

A. Deconstruct *each medical term into its basic elements to better understand the meaning of the term:*   **LO 10.1, 10.6, and 10.7** *Analyze*

1. psychoactive _____/_____/_____
                          P   R, R/CF   S

   Meaning: _____

2. psychedelic _____/_____/_____
                          P   R, R/CF   S

   Meaning: _____

3. euphoria _____/_____/_____
                          P   R, R/CF   S

   Meaning: _____

4. antidepressant _____/_____/_____
                          P   R, R/CF   S

   Meaning: _____

5. tranquilizer _____/_____/_____
                          P   R, R/CF   S

   Meaning: _____

Chapter Review exercises, along with additional practice items, are available in Connect!

CHAPTER 11

Special Senses of the Eye and Ear

The Essentials of the Languages of Ophthalmology and Otology

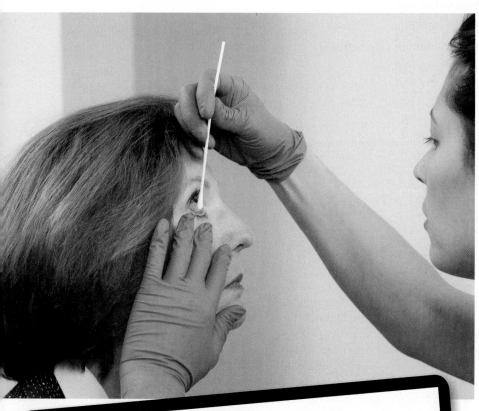

Learning Outcomes

In order to make correct decisions in situations like Mrs. Hughes' case, to communicate with Dr. Chun about the patient, to participate in patient education, and to document the patient's care, you need to be able to:

LO 11.1 Use roots, combining forms, suffixes, and prefixes to construct and analyze (deconstruct) medical terms related to the eye and ear.

LO 11.2 Spell and pronounce correctly medical terms related to the eye and ear in order to communicate them with accuracy and precision in any health care setting.

LO 11.3 Define accepted abbreviations related to the eye and ear.

LO 11.4 Relate the position and anatomy of the accessory structures and extrinsic muscles of the eye to their functions, disorders, and treatments.

LO 11.5 Relate the anatomy of the eyeball and retina to vision and refraction and their disorders and treatments.

LO 11.6 Describe the three chambers of the ear, their roles in hearing and balance, and their disorders and treatments.

LO 11.7 Apply your knowledge of medical terms relating to the eye and ear to documentation, medical records, and medical reports.

LO 11.8 Translate the medical terms relating to the eye and ear into everyday language in order to communicate clearly with patients and their families.

NOTE: The sense of smell is discussed as an integral part of the respiratory system; the sense of taste, as an integral part of the digestive system; and the sense of touch, as an integral part of the nervous system.

Case Report 11.1

You are . . .

. . . an **ophthalmic** technician (OT) working in the office of **ophthalmologist** Angela Chun, MD, a member of the Fulwood Medical Group.

You are communicating with . . .

. . . Mrs. Jenny Hughes, a 30-year-old computer software consultant. She walked into the office with painful, red, swollen eyelids and a sticky, purulent discharge from both eyes. The administrative medical assistant did not hold her in the reception area but brought her directly to you. Mrs. Hughes complains of headache and **photophobia**, and says her eyelids were stuck together when she woke up this morning. She tells you that a couple of days earlier, she had gone into a small business office to install software at the firm's 10 workstations. One of the employees was absent with **pink eye**. Mrs. Hughes wants to know if she could have contracted the disease from that employee's keyboard, and how to prevent her husband and two children from getting it. In your hand, you have a pen and clipboard with the office Notice of Privacy Practices and sign-in sheet for her to sign. How do you proceed?

Objectives

*Mrs. Jenny Hughes' "pink eye" involved her **conjunctiva** and eyelids—two of the **periorbital** accessory structures of the eye, located around the **orbit** and in front of the eyeball. All the accessory structures support and protect the exposed front surface of the eyes.*

The information in this lesson will enable you to use correct medical terminology to:

11.1.1 Describe the accessory structures of the eye.

11.1.2 Link the anatomy of each of the accessory structures to its functions.

11.1.3 Discuss disorders of the accessory structures.

11.1.4 Explain the effects of disorders of the extrinsic muscles on the eye.

Lesson 11.1

Accessory Structures of the Eye (LO 11.2 and 11.4)

A beam of light travels to the eye at 186,000 miles per second, or 671 million miles per hour. Before it can reach the eyeball it passes through external accessory structures, which have important functions that support and protect the exposed front surface of the eye.

The **eyebrows** *(Figure 11.1)* keep sweat from running into the eyes and function in nonverbal -communication to show how you're feeling in response to certain stimuli.

The **eyelids** protect the eyes from foreign objects. They blink to move tears across the eyes' surface and sweep debris away. They close in sleep to keep out visual stimuli. They are covered in the body's thinnest layer of skin.

The **eyelashes** are strong hairs that help keep debris out of the eyes. They arise from hair follicles with their sebaceous glands on the edge of the lids.

The **conjunctiva** is a transparent mucous membrane that lines the inside of both eyelids. It moves freely over the eyeball and covers the front of the eye but not the central portion (the **cornea**). In the conjunctiva, numerous goblet cells secrete a thin film of mucin (a complex protein) that keeps the eyeball moist. It has numerous small blood vessels and is richly supplied with nerve endings that make it very sensitive to pain.

The **lacrimal apparatus** *(Figure 11.2)* consists of the **lacrimal (tear) gland** located in the superolateral corner of the orbit. This gland secretes tears, and short ducts carry the tears to the conjunctiva's surface. After washing across the conjunctiva, the tears leave the eye at its medial corner by draining into the **lacrimal sac.** They then flow into the **nasolacrimal duct,** which carries the tears into the nose, from where they are swallowed.

The functions of tears are to:

- **Clean and lubricate** the surface of the eyes;
- **Deliver** nutrients and oxygen to the conjunctiva; and
- **Prevent infection** through bactericidal (bacteria-killing) enzymes.

Eyelashes   Eyebrow   Pupil   Upper ey   Lower ey   Conjunctiva

▲ **FIGURE 11.1**
External Anatomy of the Eye.

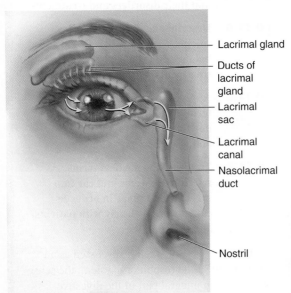

- Lacrimal gland
- Ducts of lacrimal gland
- Lacrimal sac
- Lacrimal canal
- Nasolacrimal duct
- Nostril

▲ **FIGURE 11.2**
Lacrimal Apparatus.

Word Analysis and Definition

WORD	PRONUNCIATION		ELEMENTS	DEFINITION
conjunctiva conjunctival (adj) conjunctivitis "pink eye"	kon-junk-**TIE**-vah kon-junk-**TIE**-val kon-junk-tih-**VI**-tis	 S/ R/ S/	Latin *inner lining of eyelids* -al *pertaining to* conjunctiv- *conjunctiva* -itis *inflammation* Lay term for conjunctivitis	Inner lining of eyelids Pertaining to the conjunctiva Inflammation of the conjunctiva Conjunctivitis
cornea corneal (adj)	**KOR**-nee-ah **KOR**-nee-al	 S/ R/	Latin *web, tunic* -al *pertaining to* corne- *cornea*	The central, transparent part of the outer coat of the eye covering the iris and pupil
lacrimal nasolacrimal duct	**LAK**-rim-al **NAY**-zoh-**LAK**-rim-al DUKT	S/ R/ R/CF R/	-al *pertaining to* lacrim- *tear* nas/o- *nose* duct *to lead*	Pertaining to tears and the tear apparatus Passage from the lacrimal sac to the nose
ophthalmology ophthalmologist ophthalmic (adj)	off-thal-**MALL**-oh-jee off-thal-**MALL**-oh-jist off-**THAL**-mik	S/ R/CF S/ S/ R/	-logy *study of* ophthalm/o- *eye* -logist *one who studies, specialist* -ic *pertaining to* ophthalm- *eye*	Diagnosis and treatment of diseases of the eye Medical specialist in ophthalmology Pertaining to the eye
orbit orbital (adj) periorbital	**OR**-bit **OR**-bit-al per-ee-**OR**-bit-al	 S/ R/ P/	Latin *circle* -al *pertaining to* orbit- *orbit* peri- *around*	The bony socket that holds the eyeball Pertaining to the orbit Pertaining to tissues around the orbit
photophobia photophobic (adj)	foh-toe-**FOH**-bee-ah foh-toe-**FOH**-bik	S/ R/CF R/ S/	-ia *condition* phot/o- *light* -phob- *fear* -ic *pertaining to*	Abnormal sensitivity to light due to pain in the eyes Pertaining to or suffering from photophobia

EXERCISES

A. Build *your medical vocabulary. Many of the prefixes and suffixes you see in this chapter you will meet in later chapters and use to build your knowledge of additional medical terms. Fill in the chart.*   **LO 11.1 and 11.4** *Apply*

Medical Term	Prefix	Meaning of Prefix	Root(s)/CF(s)	Meaning of R/CF	Suffix	Meaning of Suffix
nasolacrimal	1.	2.	3.	4.	5.	6.
conjunctivitis	7.	8.	9.	10.	11.	12.
periorbital	13.	14.	15.	16.	17.	18.
ophthalmologist	19.	20.	21.	22.	23.	24.
photophobia	25.	26.	27.	28.	29.	30.

B. Continue *working with the terms in the WAD.*   **LO 11.1 and 11.4** *Apply*

1. Take the term *ophthalmologist,* add two different suffixes to the same root/combining form, and construct two new medical terms:

_____ / _____ means _____
    R/CF   S

_____ / _____ means _____
    R/CF   S

Lesson 11.1
(cont'd)
Disorders of the Accessory Glands
(LO 11.4)

The accessory glands of the eyes can be affected by a number of different disorders, most of which cause noticeable discomfort.

Conjunctivitis *(Figure 11.3)*, an inflammation of the conjunctiva, is more commonly viral than bacterial; it can also be caused by irritants like chlorine, soaps, fumes, and smoke.

Eyelid edema, a generalized swelling of the eyelids, is often produced by an allergic reaction *(see Chapter 8)* from cosmetics, pollen in the air, or insect stings and bites.

A **stye** or **hordeolum** is an infection of an eyelash follicle that produces an abscess *(Figure 11.4)*, with localized pain, swelling, redness, and pus at the edge of the eyelid.

Blepharitis occurs when multiple eyelash follicles become infected. The eyelid's margin shows persistent redness and crusting and may become ulcerated *(Figure 11.5)*.

Ptosis, in which the upper eyelid is constantly drooped over the eye, is due to **paresis** of the muscle that raises the upper lid *(Figure 11.6)*. The term **blepharoptosis** defines the sagging of the eyelids from excess skin. The plastic surgery procedure of **blepharoplasty** is used to repair the eyelid.

Dry eye disease (dysfunctional tear syndrome) is due to decreased tear production by the lacrimal glands. It leads to ocular discomfort and potential damage to the conjunctiva and cornea. Some cases are due to **Sjogren's syndrome,** in which the lacrimal glands are affected by autoimmune processes. Dry eye is more common in females and the elderly, and in people who wear contact lenses.

▲ **FIGURE 11.3**
Conjunctivitis.

Stye

▲ **FIGURE 11.4**
Stye Showing Pus-Filled Cyst.

Abbreviation

q4h — Every four hours.

Case Report 11.1 (continued)

Mrs. Hughes' pink eye is called acute **contagious** conjunctivitis *(Figure 11.3)*. It responds well to **antibiotic** eyedrops. Her hands were **contaminated** from the keyboard of the employee who had left work and gone home with pink eye. She transmitted the infection to her eye by touching or rubbing it. Your documentation of Mrs. Hughes' office visit could read:

Progress Note: 04/10/14

Mrs. Jenny Hughes was brought directly into the clinical area at 1030 hrs with what appeared to be conjunctivitis, "pink eye." Both eyelids were red and swollen with a **purulent discharge.** She complained of headache and photophobia. Dr. Chun prescribed three drops q4h of Neosporin eyedrops and sent a swab of the discharge to the laboratory. I instructed and watched Mrs. Hughes wash her hands and use an alcohol-based hand gel. I then had her sign in and sign our Notice of Privacy Practices. I instructed her in the use of the eyedrops and emphasized home care and hand care measures to prevent the infection from spreading to her family. She was given a return appointment in 1 week and told to call the office if the eyedrops do not help.

—Daphne Butras, OT, 1055 hrs.

Study Hint

Note that the term *ptosis* is a stand-alone term and has a meaning in its own right. It can also function as a suffix specifically relating to the eyelids when it is added to the combining form *blephar/o.*

▲ **FIGURE 11.5**
Blepharitis of the Lower Lid.

▲ **FIGURE 11.6**
Ptosis of Right Eyelid.

Word Analysis and Definition

WORD	PRONUNCIATION		ELEMENTS	DEFINITION
antibiotic	AN-tih-bye-OT-ik	S/ P/ R/	-tic *pertaining to* anti- *against* -bio- *life*	A substance that has the capacity to inhibit the growth of or destroy bacteria and other microorganisms
blepharitis	blef-ah-RYE-tis	S/ R/	-itis *inflammation* blephar- *eyelid*	Inflammation of the eyelid
blepharoptosis	BLEF-ah-ROP-toe-sis	S/ R/CF	-ptosis *drooping* blephar/o- *eyelid*	Drooping of the upper eyelid
blepharoplasty	BLEF-ah-roh-plas-tee	S/	-plasty *surgical repair*	Surgical repair of the eyelid
conjunctivitis		S/ R/	-itis *inflammation* conjunctiv- *conjunctiva*	Inflammation of the conjunctiva
contagious	kon-TAY-jus		Latin *touch closely*	Infection can be transmitted from person to person or from a person to a surface to a person
contaminate (verb)	kon-TAM-in-ate	S/ P/ R/	-ate *composed of, pertaining to* con- *together* -tamin- *touch*	To cause the presence of an infectious agent to be on any surface
contamination (noun)	KON-tam-ih-NAY-shun	S/	-ation *process*	The presence of an infectious agent on any surface
hordeolum (*also called* stye)	hor-DEE-oh-lum		Latin *stye in the eye*	Abscess in an eyelash follicle
paresis	par-EE-sis		Greek *paralysis*	Partial paralysis
ptosis (Notes: *When a word begins with two consonants, the first is silent.* Ptosis *can also be used as a suffix.*)	TOE-sis		Greek *drooping*	Drooping down of the upper eyelid or an organ
purulent	PURE-you-lent	S/ R/	-ulent *abounding in* pur- *pus*	Showing or containing a lot of pus

EXERCISES

A. Review *the Case Report on this spread before answering the questions.*   **LO 11.2, 11.4, and 11.7** *Remember*

1. What are the symptoms Mrs. Hughes was experiencing?_____

2. Explain each of the terms in Mrs. Hughes' diagnosis. _____

   _____

3. What was the source of contamination for Mrs. Hughes? _____

4. What is the correct medical term for *pink eye?* _____

5. How can she prevent her family from getting this infection from her? _____

   _____

B. The chapter objectives *can be met by inserting the correct medical terminology in the following patient documentation. Use only the terms contained in the WAD box above. Remember to proofread your work for correct spelling! Fill in the blanks.*   **LO 11.2, 11.4, and 11.7** *Understand*

1. The patient's drooping left eyelid has been diagnosed as _____, and the surgical procedure
   _____ will correct this condition.

2. The patient has been advised to wipe down all household surfaces with a disinfectant to reduce the chance of further
   _____ in the household.

3. The _____ on the patient's right eyelid has a _____ drainage.

4. Mrs. Hughes' eye infection will be helped by the prescribed _____.

C. Terminology challenge: *Apply your knowledge of the language of ophthalmology and answer the following question.*   **LO 11.1** *Apply*

1. Which element in the WAD that functions as a suffix is also a medical term in its own right? _____.

Case Report 11.2

You are . . .

. . . an ophthalmic technician employed by Angela Chun, MD, an ophthalmologist at Fulwood Medical Center.

You are communicating with . . .

. . . Mrs. Jenny Hughes, the mother of Sam Hughes, a 2½-year-old boy, who has been referred by his pediatrician to Dr. Chun.

Mrs. Hughes states that for the past couple of months, Sam's right eye has turned in. The only visual difficulty she has noticed is that he sometimes misses a Cheerio when he tries to grab it.

You are responsible for documenting Sam's diagnostic and therapeutic procedures and explaining their significance to his mother.

Extrinsic Muscles of the Eye (LO 11.2 and 11.4)

Humans have two eyes positioned on the face, one on either side of the nose facing forward, which work closely together. This eye configuration gives us very good three-dimensional perception (**stereopsis**) and hand-eye coordination. Stereopsis depends on an accurate alignment of the two eyes.

Six coordinated **extrinsic** eye muscles in each eye—attached to the inner wall of the orbit and outer surface of the eyeball—keep the eyes properly aligned, and move the eyes in all directions.

When there is a muscle imbalance in one eye, the alignment breaks down and **strabismus** *(Figure 11.7).* also known as a "cross-eyed" condition, results. It can be cured by vision therapy or surgery.

Esotropia is a condition where the eye is turned in toward the nose. In congenital or infantile esotropia, both eyes look in toward the nose—the right eye looks to the left and the left eye looks to the right *(Figure 11.8).* Children with this condition require surgery.

Accomodative esotropia is an inward eye turn, usually noticed around age 2 in 1 to 2% of children. Sam Hughes had an accommodative esotropia in one eye. Wearing glasses and perhaps a patch over the stronger eye will help to correct Sam's problem.

Exotropia, an outward eye turn, is noticed in children around ages 2 to 4. It will often respond to vision therapy, which includes eye exercises and glasses, from an **optometrist.** Eye muscle surgery can establish good **ocular** alignment.

▲ **FIGURE 11.7**
Strabismus.

Amblyopia, or "lazy eye," occurs in children when vision in one eye has not developed as well as vision in the other. Instead, it occurs because the eye and the brain won't cooperate for the affected eye. Amblyopia is treated with a patch over the stronger eye in order to develop the vision in the weaker eye.

Nystagmus is a term to describe fast, uncontrollable movements of the eye that may be side to side (horizontal nystagmus), up and down (vertical nystagmus), or **rotary** (rotary nystagmus). The condition can be congenital or acquired from head injury, inner ear disorders *(see the next section of this chapter),* stroke, or drugs, such as excess alcohol, sedatives, or anti-epilepsy drugs *(see Chapter 10).* There is no cure, but some cases improve spontaneously.

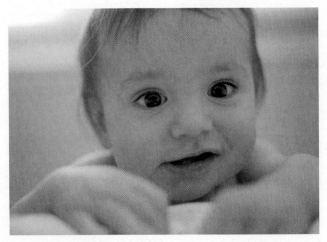

▲ **FIGURE 11.8**
Congenital Esotropia (both eyes are affected).

Word Analysis and Definition

S = Suffix   P = Prefix   R = Root   R/CF = Combining Form

WORD	PRONUNCIATION	ELEMENTS		DEFINITION
accommodation (noun)	ah-kom-oh-**DAY**-shun	S/ P/ R/	-ion *action* ac- *toward* -commodat- *adjust*	The act of adjusting something to make it fit the needs; in this case the lens of the eye adjusts itself
accommodate (verb)	ah-**KOM**-oh-date	S/ S/	-ate *pertaining to, composed of*	To adapt to meet a need
accommodative (adj)	ah-kom-oh-**DAY**-tiv		-ive *pertaining to*	Pertaining to accommodation
amblyopia	am-blee-**OH**-pee-ah	R/ S/	ambly- *dull* -opia *sight*	Failure or incomplete development of the pathways of vision to the brain
esotropia	es-oh-**TROH**-pee-ah	S/ P/ R/	-ia *condition* eso- *inward* -trop- *turn*	Turning the eye inward toward the nose
exotropia	ek-soh-**TROH**-pee-ah	P/	exo- *outward*	Turning the eye outward away from the nose
extrinsic	eks-**TRIN**-sik		Latin *on the outer side*	Any muscle located entirely on the outside of the structure under consideration; e.g., the eye
intrinsic	in-**TRIN**-sik		Latin *on the inner side*	Any muscle located entirely within (inside) the structure under consideration; e.g., the eye
nystagmus	nis-**TAG**-muss		Greek *nodding*	Fast, uncontrollable movements of the eyeballs
ocular	**OCK**-you-lar	S/ R/	-ar *pertaining to* ocul- *eye*	Pertaining to the eye
optometrist	op-**TOM**-eh-trist	S/ R/CF	-metrist *skilled in measurement* opt/o- *vision*	Someone skilled in the measurement of vision but who cannot treat eye diseases or prescribe medication
optometry	op-**TOM**-eh-tree	S/	-metry *process of measuring*	The profession of the measurement of vision
rotary	**ROW**-tah-ree		Latin *to revolve*	Circular movement
stereopsis	ster-ee-**OP**-sis	S/ R/	-opsis *vision* stere- *three-dimensional*	Three-dimensional vision
strabismus	strah-**BIZ**-mus	S/ R/	-ismus *take action* strab- *squint*	Turning of an eye away from its normal position

EXERCISES

A. Review *the Case Report on this spread before answering the questions.*   **LO 11.2 and 11.4** *Remember*

1. What did Mrs. Hughes notice about Sam's right eye? _____

2. Other than #1 above, what other visual difficulty has Mrs. Hughes noticed that Sam has? _____
_____

3. Who referred Sam to the ophthalmologist? _____

4. What is the name of the specialty department where Dr. Chun sees her patients? _____

5. What is Sam's diagnosis? _____

6. How can this condition be corrected in Sam's case? _____

B. Deconstruct *the following medical terms into their elements. Complete the chart. Notice in this exercise that not every medical term needs a prefix and/or a suffix but every medical term does contain one or more roots and/or combining forms.*   **LO 11.1 and 11.4** *Analyze*

Medical Term	Prefix	Root(s)/ Combining Form(s)	Suffix	Meaning of Term
exotropia	1.	2.	3.	4.
optometrist	5.	6.	7.	8.
esotropia	9.	10.	11.	12.
amblyopia	13.	14.	15.	16.
stereopsis	17.	18.	19.	20.
ocular	21.	22.	23.	24.

Lesson 11.2

The Eyeball and Seeing

Objectives

Although your eyeball may appear to be solid, it's actually a hollow sphere that measures around 1 inch in diameter. Knowledge of its terminology, structure, and function allows you to understand how we see and what major problems and disorders can arise with the eye. In this lesson, the information will enable you to use correct medical terminology to:

11.2.1 Identify the principal structures of the eyeball and their functions.

11.2.2 Explain the role of the cornea and the problems that can occur in that structure.

11.2.3 Describe the structures and functions of the lens and its associated structures.

11.2.4 Link the different components of the retina to their functions.

11.2.5 Discuss disorders of the eyeball.

Keynotes

- The cornea protects the eye and, by changing shape, provides about 60% of the eye's focusing power.
- The iris controls the amount of light entering the eye.
- The lens changes its shape to focus rays of light on the retina.
- Medical shorthand for a quick, normal eye examination can be PERRLA: Pupils Equal, Round, Reactive to Light and Accommodation.

The Eyeball (Globe)

(LO 11.5)

The functions of the eyeball are to continuously:

1. **Adjust** the amount of light it lets in to reach the retina;

2. **Focus** on near and distant objects; and

3. **Produce** images of those objects and instantly transmit them to the brain.

As shown earlier in this chapter, the front of the eyeball is covered by the conjunctiva. This thin layer of tissue lines the inside of the eyelids and curves over the eyeball to meet the **sclera** *(Figure 11.9).* the tough, white outer layer of the eye.

At the center of the front of the eye is the **cornea,** a transparent, dome-shaped membrane. The cornea has no blood supply and obtains its nutrients from tears and from fluid in the anterior chamber behind it.

When light rays strike the eye, they pass through the cornea. Because of its dome curvature, those rays striking the edge of the cornea are bent toward its center. The light rays then go through the **pupil,** the black opening in the center of the colored area (the **iris)** in the front of the eye.

The iris controls the amount of light entering the eye. For example, when you're in the dark outside at night the iris opens **(dilates)** to allow more light into the eye. When you're in bright sunlight or in a well-lit room, the iris closes **(constricts)** to allow less light into the eye.

After traveling through the pupil, the light rays pass through the transparent **lens.** This lens can become thicker and thinner, enabling it to bend light rays and focus them on the **retina** at the back of the eye. Accommodation is the process of changing focus, and **refraction** is the process of bending light rays.

The lens does not contain blood vessels **(avascular)** or nerves, and with increasing age, it loses its elasticity. Because of this reduced elasticity, when you reach your forties, your eyes may have difficulty focusing on near objects, a condition called **presbyopia.**

▲ **FIGURE 11.9**
Anatomy of the Eyeball.

Word Analysis and Definition

WORD	PRONUNCIATION	ELEMENTS		DEFINITION
avascular	a-**VAS**-cue-lar	S/ P/ R/	-ar *pertaining to* a- *without* -vascul- *blood vessel*	Without a blood supply
constrict (verb)	kon-**STRIKT**	P/ R/	con- *with, together* -strict *narrow*	Become or make narrow
constriction (noun)	kon-**STRIK**-shun	S/	-ion *action, condition*	A narrowed portion of a structure
dilate (verb) dilation (noun)	**DIE**-late die-**LAY**-shun	S/ R/	Latin *dilate* -ion *action, condition* dilat- *dilate*	To perform or undergo dilation Stretching or enlarging an opening or a structure
iris	**EYE**-ris		Greek *diaphragm of the eye*	Colored portion of the eye with the pupil in its center
lens	**LENZ**		Latin *lentil shape*	Transparent refractive structure behind the iris
presbyopia	prez-bee-**OH**-pee-ah	S/ R/	-opia *sight* presby- *old man*	Difficulty in nearsighted vision occurring in middle and old age
pupil	**PYU**-pill		Latin *pupil*	The opening in the center of the iris that allows light to reach the lens
pupillary (adj) (Note: Change to ll.)	**PYU**-pill-ah-ree	S/ R/	-ary *pertaining to* pupill- *pupil*	Pertaining to the pupil
refract (verb) refraction (noun)	ree-**FRAKT** ree-**FRAKT**-shun	S/ R/	Latin *break up* -ion *condition* refract- *bend*	Bend or change direction of a ray of light The bending of light
retina retinal (adj)	**RET**-ih-nah **RET**-ih-nal	S/ R/	Latin *net* -al *pertaining to* retin- *retina*	Light-sensitive innermost layer of the eyeball Pertaining to the retina
sclera	**SKLAIR**-ah		Greek *hard*	Fibrous outer covering of the eyeball and the white of the eye
scleral (adj)	**SKLAIR**-al	S/ R/	-al *pertaining to* scler- *hardness, white of eye*	Pertaining to the sclera
scleritis	sklair-**RI**-tis	S/	-itis *inflammation*	Inflammation of the sclera

EXERCISES

A. Define the statements in column 1 using the language of ophthalmology in colum 2. These medical terms all relate to the vision process. Fill in the blanks.   **LO 11.5** *Remember*

_____ **1.** colored portion of the eye   **A.** lens

_____ **2.** bend a ray of light   **B.** retina

_____ **3.** opening in the iris   **C.** avascular

_____ **4.** transparent, refractive structure   **D.** pupil

_____ **5.** difficulty in nearsighted vision   **E.** refract

_____ **6.** innermost layer of the eyeball   **F.** iris

_____ **7.** fibrous, outer covering of the eye   **G.** presbyopia

_____ **8.** without a blood supply   **H.** sclera

B. The WAD contains 3 pairs of noun/verb terms. Choose one pair and write a brief sentence for each term that is NOT a definition.   **LO 11.2, 11.5, and 11.7** *Apply*

1. _____

_____

2. _____

_____

Lesson 11.2 The Eyeball (Globe) (continued)
(cont'd)

The Retina (LO 11.2 and 11.5)

The retina is the size of a postage stamp and has ten layers of cells. Located at the back of the eye *(Figure 11.10a),* it's the final destination for light rays. The retina has 130 million **rods** *(Figure 11.10b),* which perceive only light, not color, and function mostly in dim lighting. The retina has 6.5 million light- and color-activated **cones** *(Figure 11.10b),* which have precise **visual acuity** (sharpness). Different cones respond to red, blue, and green light. The perception of color is based on the intensity of various color mixtures from the three cone types.

Some people have a hereditary lack of response by one or more of the three cone types and show color blindness. The most common form of this is red-green color blindness. Here, red-green colors and related shades cannot be distinguished from each other.

The rods and cones convert the light rays' energy into electrical impulses. The **optic nerve**—a bundle of more than a million nerve fibers—transmits these impulses to the visual cortex at the back of the brain. The area where the optic nerve leaves the retina is called the **optic disc.** Because it has no rods and cones, the optic disc cannot form images; as a result, it's called the "blind spot."

Just lateral to the optic disc at the back of the retina is a circular, yellowish region called the **macula lutea** *(Figure 11.10a).* In the center of the macula is a small pit called the **fovea centralis,** which has 4,000 tiny cones but no rods. Each cone has its own nerve fiber, and this gives the fovea area the sharpest vision. As you read this text, the words are precisely focused on your fovea centralis.

Behind the light-sensitive **photoreceptor** layer of the retina is a vascular layer called the **choroid.** This layer, together with the iris and its muscle, is called the **uvea.**

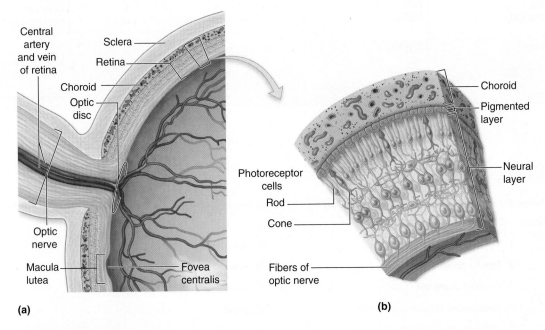

(a)

(b)

▲ **FIGURE 11.10**
Structure of the Retina.
(a) Retina. (b) Rods and cones.

Word Analysis and Definition

WORD	PRONUNCIATION	ELEMENTS		DEFINITION
choroid	KOR-oid		Greek *membrane*	Region of the retina and uvea
fovea centralis	FOH-vee-ah sen-TRAH-lis	S/ R/	fovea Latin *a pit* -is *pertaining to* central- *center*	Small pit in the center of the macula that has the highest visual acuity
macula lutea	MACK-you-lah LOO-tee-ah		macula Latin *small spot* lutea Latin *yellow*	Yellowish spot on the back of the retina; contains the fovea
optic optical (adj)	OP-tik OP-tih-kal	S/ R/	Greek *eye* -al *pertaining to* optic- *eye*	Pertaining to the eye or vision Pertaining to the eye or vision
photoreceptor	foh-toe-ree-SEP-tor	S/ R/CF R/	-or *that which does something* phot/o- *light* -recept- *receive*	A photoreceptor cell receives light and converts it into electrical impulses
uvea uveitis	YOU-vee-ah you-vee-EYE-tis	S/ R/	Latin *vascular layer* -itis *inflammation* uve- *uvea*	Middle coat of the eyeball; includes the iris, ciliary body, and choroid Inflammation of the uvea
visual acuity	VIH-zhoo-wal ah-KYU-ih-tee		acuity Latin *sharpen*	Sharpness and clearness of vision

EXERCISES

A. The language of ophthalmology *will be your answers in this exercise. Review the WAD before you begin the exercise. Circle the best answer.*

LO 11.1 and 11.5 *Understand*

1. Sharpness and clearness of vision is called:

   a. optical

   b. acuity

   c. vascular

   d. sclera

   e. choroid

2. Because it has no rods and cones, the optic disc cannot form images and thus is called the:

   a. fovea

   b. blind spot

   c. uvea

   d. visual cortex

   e. optic nerve

3. The term *photoreceptor* has:

   a. two combining forms and a suffix

   b. a prefix, a root, and a suffix

   c. a combining form, a root, and a suffix

   d. two roots and a suffix

   e. a suffix and a root

4. The area of sharpest vision is the:

   a. cornea

   b. rods

   c. macula lutea

   d. fovea centralis

   e. cones

B. Meet chapter *and lesson objectives and apply the language of ophthalmology to answer the questions.* **LO 11.2 and 11.5** *Apply*

1. Where is the choroid located? _____

2. What does the term *vascular* mean in *vascular layer*? _____

3. What is the opposite of *vascular*? _____

4. What is the final destination of light rays in the eye? _____

5. What is the pit called that is in the center of the macula? _____

Lesson **11.2** **Refraction** (LO 11.5)

(cont'd) The optic nerves leave each orbit through the optic **foramen.** Light travels at 186,000 miles per second, and even when it hits the eye, this speed remains the same. Light rays that hit the center of the cornea pass straight through the eye, while rays that hit away from the center then bend toward the center. These light rays then hit the lens and bend again, and in normal vision, the image is focused sharply on the retina *(Figure 11.11).*

Farsighted people are said to have **hyperopia** *(Figure 11.12).* Because the eyeball is shortened, objects close to the eye are focused behind the retina and vision is blurred. **Convex** lenses help to correct the problem.

Nearsighted people are said to have **myopia** *(Figure 11.13).* Because the eyeball is elongated, faraway objects are focused in front of the retina. Vision is blurred. **Concave** lenses help to correct the problem.

In **presbyopia,** a condition mentioned earlier in this chapter, the lens loses its flexibility, making it difficult to focus for near vision. This usually occurs when you reach your forties. Convex bifocal or transitional lenses help to correct this problem.

In **astigmatism,** unequal curvatures of the cornea cause unequal focusing and blurred images. This problem can be corrected with cylindrical lenses, which refract light more in one plane than in another.

A surgical procedure, **radial keratotomy,** is used to treat myopia. Radial cuts, like the spokes of a wheel, flatten the cornea so it can refract the light rays to focus on the retina.

Laser surgery can also change the shape of the cornea. It can flatten it to correct myopia, or it can alter the cornea's outer edges to correct hyperopia.

Laser-assisted in situ keratomileusis (LASIK) is used to treat myopia, hyperopia, and astigmatism. LASIK involves a computer-controlled laser that uses a cold beam of ultraviolet light, which alters the shape of the cornea by vaporizing the tissue.

▲ **FIGURE 11.11**
Normal Vision.

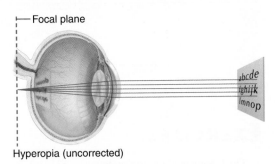

Hyperopia (uncorrected)

▲ **FIGURE 11.12**
Hyperopia (Farsightedness).

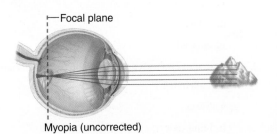

Myopia (uncorrected)

▲ **FIGURE 11.13**
Myopia (Nearsightedness).

Abbreviation

LASIK   laser-assisted in situ keratomileusis

Word Analysis and Definition

WORD	PRONUNCIATION	ELEMENTS		DEFINITION
astigmatism	ah-**STIG**-maht-izm	S/ P/ R/	-ism *process* a- *without* -stigmat- *focus*	Inability to focus light rays that enter the eye in different planes
concave convex	kon-**KAVE** kon-**VEKS**		Latin concavus *arched* Latin convexus *vaulted*	Having a hollowed surface A surface that is evenly curved outward
foramen foramina (pl)	fo-**RAY**-men fo-**RAM**-ih-nah		Latin *hole*	An opening through a structure
hyperopia	high-per-**OH**-pee-ah	P/ S/	hyper- *beyond* -opia *sight*	Able to see distant objects but unable to see close objects
in situ	IN **SIGH**-tyu		Latin *in its original place*	In the correct place
keratomileusis	ker-ah-**TOE**-mill-oo-sis	R/CF R/	kerat/o- *cornea* -mileusis *lathe*	Cuts and shapes the cornea
keratotomy	ker-ah-**TOT**-oh-mee	S/ R/CF	-tomy *surgical incision* kerat/o- *cornea*	Incision in the cornea
myopia (Note: *One "op" is removed to allow the term to flow.*)	my-**OH**-pee-ah	R/ S/	myop- *to blink* -opia *sight*	Able to see close objects but unable to see distant objects
radial (adj)	**RAY**-dee-al	S/ R/	-al *pertaining to* radi- *radius*	Diverging in all directions from any given center

EXERCISES

A. Construct *the correct medical term to match the meaning given in column 1. Write each element in the correct column to form the complete term. Fill in the chart.*   **LO 11.1 and 11.5** *Apply*

Meaning of Medical Term	Prefix	Root(s)/Combining Form(s)	Suffix
inability to focus light rays	1.	2.	3.
able to see distant objects but not close ones	4.	5.	6.
able to see close objects but not distant ones	7.	8.	9.

B. Terminology challenge: *Use the information from this and previous spreads to answer the challenge questions.*   **LO 11.2 and 11.5** *Understand*

1. What other medical term ending in *opia* means difficulty in nearsighted vision that occurs in middle and old age? _____

2. What is the medical term for "nearsightedness"? _____

3. What eye conditions can laser surgery correct? _____

4. What is a medical term describing the condition that is opposite to the term in question 2? _____

C. Meet lesson objectives *and use the language of ophthalmology to answer the following questions.*   **LO 11.2 and 11.5** *Understand*

1. Name two procedures that correct myopia: _____ and _____

2. How does LASIK surgery alter the shape of the cornea? _____

3. What corrects astigmatism? _____

4. Why is myopia known as *nearsightedness?* _____

5. What helps to correct *hyperopia?* _____

Lesson 11.3

Disorders of the Eye and Ophthalmic Procedures

Objectives

Many eye disorders can threaten a patient's vision, but if detected early, the majority of these conditions can be cured or treated to slow or prevent the progression of vision loss. Routine eye exams are important for early detection and prevention, and are recommended at different times throughout life. The information in this lesson will enable you to use correct medical terminology to:

11.3.1 Discuss common disorders of the eye and their effects on vision.

11.3.2 Describe common ophthalmic procedures performed in the doctor's office.

Disorders of the Anterior Eyeball (LO 11.5)

Conjunctivitis is the infectious, contagious, "blood-shot eyes"-causing condition that Mrs. Jenny Hughes had in the opening Case Report of this chapter. It can be caused by viruses and bacteria, and by organisms that cause sexually transmitted diseases (STDs) *(Chapter 15)*. Four other types of conjunctivitis are:

- **Allergic conjunctivitis,** which can be part of seasonal hay fever or produced by year-round allergens like animal dander and dust mites *(Chapter 8)*;

- **Irritant conjunctivitis,** which can be caused by air **pollutants** (smoke and fumes), chemicals like chlorine, and some ingredients found in soaps and cosmetics; and

- **Neonatal conjunctivitis (ophthalmia neonatorum),** which is specific to babies and can be caused by a blocked tear duct, by the antibiotic eye drops given routinely at birth, or by sexually transmitted bacteria from an infected mother's birth canal.

  - **Keratoconjunctivitis** is a combined inflammation of the cornea and conjunctiva. It can be viral, bacterial, or allergic in origin.

    Corneal abrasions are caused by foreign bodies, by direct trauma (like being poked by a fingernail), or by ill-fitting contact lenses. An abrasion can grow into an ulcer. This ulcer or lesion can be stained with drops of the dye **fluorescein** to make it more easily visible on examination *(Figure 11.14)*. If the cornea is scarred by trauma or infection and vision is impaired, a corneal transplant or graft **(keratoplasty)** from a deceased donor can be performed.

    Scleritis is an inflammation of the sclera (the white outer covering of the eyeball) that can affect one or both eyes.

    Glaucoma results if fluid from inside the eyeball cannot escape from the eye into the bloodstream. The fluid continues to be produced and pressure builds up inside the eye. This pressure interferes with the blood supply to the retina, causing retinal cells to die and

damage to the optic nerve fibers. Glaucoma is a major cause of blindness *(Figure 11.15)*, and it's treated with a lifelong use of eye drops, which help to prevent the condition from worsening.

A **cataract** is a cloudy or opaque area in the lens *(Figure 11.16)*. It is caused by aging and may be associated with diabetes and cigarette smoke. Symptoms include blurred vision and **photosensitivity.** A cataract may also be discovered during a routine eye exam. It is another major cause of blindness.

Congenital (present at birth) cataracts occur in less than 0.5% of newborns and can be unilateral (present in one eye) or bilateral (present in both eyes). They are treated in the same way as any other cataract.

When a cataract interferes with a patient's vision *(Figure 11.17)*, the lens needs to be removed and replaced with an artificial **intraocular** lens, which becomes a permanent part of the eye. The lens is removed by **phacoemulsification,** a process in which the lens is fragmented with an ultrasonic handpiece and aspirated from the eye.

Ulcer

▲ **FIGURE 11.14**
Fluorescein-Stained Corneal Ulcer.

▲ **FIGURE 11.15**
Vision with Glaucoma.

Cataract

▲ **FIGURE 11.16**
Cataract.

▲ **FIGURE 11.17**
Vision with Cataract.

Word Analysis and Definition

S = Suffix   P = Prefix   R = Root   R/CF = Combining Form

WORD	PRONUNCIATION	ELEMENTS		DEFINITION
cataract	KAT-ah-ract		Latin *to break down*	Complete or partial opacity of the lens
fluorescein	flor-ESS-ee-in	P/ R/	fluo- *fluorine* -rescein *resin*	Dye that produces a vivid green color under a blue light to diagnose corneal abrasions and foreign bodies
glaucoma	glau-KOH-mah	S/ R/	-oma *mass, tumor* glauc- *lens opacity*	Loss of vision due to increased intraocular pressure
intraocular	in-trah-OCK-you-lar	S/ P/ R/	-ar *pertaining to* intra- *inside* -ocul- *eye*	Pertaining to the inside of the eye
keratoplasty	KER-ah-toh-PLAS-tee	S/ R/	-plasty *repair* kerat/o *cornea*	Corneal transplant or graft
keratoconjunctivitis	KER-ah-toh-con-junk-tih-VI-tis	S/ R/	-itis *inflammation* -conjunctiv- *conjunctiva*	Combined inflammation of the cornea and conjunctiva
ophthalmia neonatorum	off-THAL-me-ah ne-oh-nay-TOR-um	S/ R/ S/ P/ R/	-ia *condition* ophthalm- *eye* -orum *function of* neo- *new* -nat- *born*	Conjunctivitis of the newborn
phacoemulsification	FAKE-oh-ee-MUL sih-fih-KAY-shun	S/ P/ R/	-ation *process* phaco- *lens* -emulsific- *to milk out*	Technique used to fragment the lens into very tiny pieces and suck them out of the eye
photosensitivity photosensitive (adj)	FOH-toe-sen-sih-TIV-ih-tee foh-toe-SEN-sih-tiv	S/ R/CF R/	-ity *condition* phot/o- *light* -sensitiv- *feeling*	When light produces pain in the eye
pollution	poh-LOO-shun		Latin *to defile*	Condition that is unclean, impure, and a danger to health
pollutant	poh-LOO-tant	S/ R/	-ant *pertaining to* pollut- *unclean*	Substance that makes an environment unclean or impure

EXERCISES

A. Review *the medical terms contained on the two pages open in front of you. Use these terms to complete the following sentences. You may use a term only one time. Fill in the blanks.*   **LO 11.2 and 11.5** Apply

1. _____ can be the cause of bloodshot eyes.

2. Dust mites and pollen are _____ .

3. Scratching your eye with a tree branch can produce a(n) _____ .

4. _____ produces increased intraocular pressure.

5. When light causes pain in the eye, this is termed _____ .

B. Use critical thinking *and the language of ophthalmology to answer the following questions.*   **LO 11.2 and 11.5** Understand

1. What is a "foreign body"? _____

2. Name two other kinds of foreign bodies that could get into your eye: _____ and _____

3. What type of safety equipment prevents foreign bodies from getting into your eyes? _____

4. What occupations are at greater risk for getting foreign bodies in their eyes? _____

5. Which of the terms in the WAD is a major cause of blindness? _____

6. What is the correct medical term for "conjunctivitis of the newborn"? _____

C. Deconstruct *the following medical terms into their elements and give their meanings.*   **LO 11.1 and 11.5** Analyze

1. photosensitivity _____/_____/_____

              P   R, R/CF   S

    Meaning: _____

2. intraocular _____/_____/_____

              P   R, R/CF   S

    Meaning: _____

Lesson **11.3**
(cont'd)

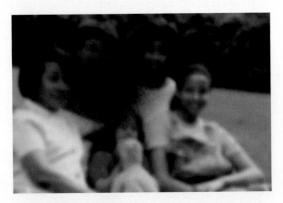

▲ **FIGURE 11.18**
Vision with Macular Degeneration.

Macular degeneration

▲ **FIGURE 11.19**
Ophthalmoscopic View of Macular Degeneration.

Hemorrhage

▲ **FIGURE 11.20**
Ophthalmoscopic View of Diabetic Retinopathy Showing Areas of Hemorrhage.

Disorders of the Retina (LO 11.5)

An impaired retina affects your ability to see in the same way that an injured leg affects your ability to walk. In either case, your level of functioning in normal, daily life is limited.

Macular Degeneration (LO 11.5)

Degeneration of the central macula results in a loss of visual acuity or sharpness, with a dark blurry area of vision loss in the center of the visual field *(Figure 11.18)*. Photoreceptor cell loss and bleeding with capillary proliferation and scar formation *(Figure 11.19)* also occur. Macular degeneration can progress to blindness. Most cases occur in people over 55. Although there is currently no known cure, laser **photocoagulation** may be used to destroy abnormal capillaries, which slows the pace of vision loss.

Retinal Detachment (LO 11.5)

In retinal detachment, the retina may separate partially or completely from its underlying choroid layer, creating a retinal tear or hole. This detachment—visible on an **ophthalmoscopic** exam—can happen suddenly, without pain, but is considered a surgical emergency. The patient sees a dark shadow invading his or her peripheral vision. **Laser surgery** is used to treat the small lesions and to "weld" the retina back into place.

Diabetic Retinopathy (LO 11.5)

Some 50% of diabetics have **retinopathy.** Patients may experience hemorrhages (bleeding), which can lead to the destruction of the photoreceptor cells (rods and cones) and visual difficulties.

An ophthalmoscopic examination shows the disease *(Figure 11.20)*, and fluorescein **angiography** with pictures taken as the dye passes through the retina reveals more details.

Laser photocoagulation is often effective in controlling the lesions, but once vision is lost from an area of the retina, it usually doesn't return *(Figure 11.21)*.

Cancer of the Eye (LO 11.5)

Tumors of the skin of the eyelids include the **squamous cell** and basal cell carcinomas and melanoma described in Chapter 3.

Retinoblastoma is the most common cancer in children and is diagnosed most frequently around 18 months of age. Of those children affected, 20% have the cancer in both eyes. This condition can be hereditary. With early detection and aggressive chemotherapy and laser surgery treatment, 90% of these cases can be cured.

In adults, the most common eye cancers are metastases to the eye from lung cancer in men and breast cancer in women.

▲ **FIGURE 11.21**
Vision with Diabetic Retinopathy.

Word Analysis and Definition

S = Suffix   P = Prefix   R = Root   R/CF = Combining Form

WORD	PRONUNCIATION	ELEMENTS		DEFINITION
angiography	an-jee-OG-rah-fee	S/ R/CF	-graphy *process of recording* angi/o- *blood vessel*	X-ray visualization of vessels after injection of contrast material
angiogram	AN-jee-oh-gram	S/	-gram *a record*	X-ray images obtained after injection of radiopaque material into blood vessels
laser surgery	LAY-zer SUR-jer-ee	S/ R/	Light Amplification by Simulated Emission of Radiation -ery *process of* surg- *operate*	Use of a concentrated, intense narrow beam of electromagnetic radiation for surgery
ophthalmoscope	off-THAL-moh-skope	S/ R/CF	-scope *instrument for viewing* ophthalm/o- *eye*	Instrument for viewing the retina
ophthalmoscopy	OFF-thal-MOS-koh-pee	S/	-scopy *to view, examine*	The process of viewing the retina
ophthalmoscopic (adj)	OFF-thal-moh-SCOP-ik	S/	-ic *pertaining to*	Pertaining to the use of an ophthalmoscope
photocoagulation	foh-toe-koh-ag-you-LAY-shun	S/ R/CF R/	-ation *process* phot/o- *light* -coagul- *clotting*	Using light (laser beam) to form a clot
retinoblastoma	RET-in-oh-blas-TOE-mah	S/ R/CF R/	-oma *tumor, mass* retin/o- *retina* -blast- *immature cell*	Malignant neoplasm of primitive retinal cells
retinopathy	ret-ih-NOP-ah-thee	S/	-pathy *disease*	Degenerative disease of the retina

EXERCISES

A. Elements *help build your knowledge of the language of ophthalmology. One element in each of the following medical terms is bolded. Identify the type of element (P, R/CF, S) in column 2, and then write the meaning of the element in column 3. Fill in the chart.* **LO 11.1 and 11.5** *Understand*

Medical Term	P, R/CF, S	Meaning of Element
retino**blast**oma	1.	2.
ophthalmo**scope**	3.	4.
angio**graphy**	5.	6.
ophthalmoscopy	7.	8.
photo**coagul**ation	9.	10.
retino**pathy**	11.	12.
angiogram	13.	14.
ophthalmoscop**ic**	15.	16.

B. Apply *the terms in Exercise A to the questions in Exercise B.* **LO 11.2 and 11.5** *Apply*

1. List all the terms from the above chart that are medical procedures: _____

2. List all the terms from the above chart that are diagnoses: _____

3. Which term is an adjective? _____

4. Which term is an instrument used in a procedure? _____

5. Which term is a malignant neoplasm of retinal cells? _____

6. Which term contains an element meaning *light*? _____

Lesson 11.3 (cont'd) Ophthalmic Diagnostic Procedures (LO 11.2 and 11.5)

A number of procedures, which are detailed in the following paragraphs, can be used to effectively examine the eye for various purposes.

Arteriole
Venule
Fovea centralis
Macula lutea
Optic disc

▲ **FIGURE 11.22**
Anatomy of the Fundus.

Examination of the Retina (LO 11.5)

A **fundoscopy** examines the retina with an ophthalmoscope to identify the optic disc (*Figure 11.22*), where the optic nerve leaves the back of the eye. The optic disc has no receptor cells and, as mentioned earlier in this chapter, it produces a "blind spot" in the visual field of each eye. In the middle of the optic disc, a retinal artery enters to supply the intraocular structures, and a retinal vein leaves the eye.

Color Vision (LO 11.5)

The **Ishihara color system** is used to test color vision. In the example in *Figure 11.23*, people with red-green color blindness would not be able to see the number 16 among the colored dots.

▲ **FIGURE 11.23**
Test for Color Blindness. Reproduced with permission from *Ishihara's Tests for Color Deficiency*, published by Kanehara Trading Inc., Tokyo, Japan. Tests for color deficiency cannot be conducted with this figure. For accurate testing, the original plates should be used.

▶ **FIGURE 11.24**
Visual Acuity Tests. (a) Snellen letter chart for distant vision. (b) Jaeger reading card for near vision.

Distance Vision (LO 11.5)

The **Snellen letter chart** is used to test distance vision (*Figure 11.24a*). The results are recorded as a fraction. For example, when the chart is viewed from 20 feet, line 8 is the smallest line a person with standard vision can read. This is recorded as 20/20. If the patient using her or his left eye misses two letters on line 8, this is documented as **OS** 20/20–2. The right eye is documented as **OD**, the left eye as **OS,** and the use of both eyes is noted as **OU.**

Near Vision (LO 11.5)

Near vision is measured using handheld charts or **Jaeger reading cards** with printed paragraphs of different sizes of print (*Figure 11.24b*).

Visual Fields (LO 11.5)

Visual fields are tested in the following way: Sit 2 feet in front of your patient, and instruct the patient to cover one eye. Next, cover your own opposite eye. Now, bring a pencil into the horizontal and vertical fields to compare the patient's **peripheral vision** with your own.

Intraocular Pressure (LO 11.5)

Intraocular pressure is measured with a **tonometer,** which determines the eyeball's resistance to indentation or tension. Increased intraocular pressure indicates glaucoma.

Abbreviations

OD	right eye
OS	left eye
OU	both eyes

(a)

V = .50 D.

The fourteenth of August was the day fixed upon for the sailing of the brig Pilgrim, on her voyage from Boston round Cape Horn, to the western coast of North America. As she was to get under way early in the afternoon, I made my appearance on board at twelve o'clock in full sea-rig, and with my chest, containing an outfit for a two or three years voyage, which I had undertaken from a determination to cure, if possible, by an entire change of life, and by a long absence from books and study, a weakness of the eyes which had obliged me to give up my pursuits, and which no medical aid seemed likely to cure. The change from the tight dress coat, silk cap and kid gloves of an undergraduate at Cambridge, to the

V = .75 D.

loose duck trousers, checked shirt and tarpaulin hat of a sailor, though somewhat of a transformation, was soon made, and I supposed that I should pass very well for a Jack tar. But it is impossible to deceive the practiced eye in these matters; and while I supposed myself to be looking as salt as Neptune himself, I was, no doubt, known for a landsman by every one on board, as soon as I hove in sight. A sailor has a peculiar cut to his clothes, and a way of wear-

V = 1. D.

ing them which a green hand can never get. The trousers, tight around the hips, and thence hanging long and loose around the feet, a superabundance of checked shirt, a low-crowned, well-varnished black hat, worn on the back of the head, with half a fathom of black ribbon hanging over the left eye, and a peculiar tie to the black silk neckerchief, with sundry other *details*, are signs the want of which betray the beginner at once.

V = 1.25 D.

Beside the points in my dress which were out of the way, doubtless my complexion and hands would distinguish me from the regular *salt*, who, with a sun-browned cheek, wide step and rolling gait, swings his bronzed and toughened hands athwartships half open, as though just to ready to grasp a rope. "With all my imperfections

V = 1.50 D.

on my head," I joined the crew, and we hauled out into the stream and came to anchor for the night. The next day we were employed in preparation for sea, reeving and studding-sail gear, crossing royal yards, putting on chafing gear, and taking on board our powder. On the

(b)

WORD	PRONUNCIATION		ELEMENTS	DEFINITION
fundus	FUN-dus		Latin *bottom*	Part farthest from the opening of a hollow organ
fundoscopy	fun-DOS-koh-pee	S/	-scopy *to examine*	Examination of the fundus (retina) of the eye
		R/CF	fund/o- *fundus*	
fundoscopic (adj)	fun-doh-SKOP-ik	S/	-ic *pertaining to*	Pertaining to fundoscopy
Ishihara color system	ish-ee-HAR-ah		Shinobu Ishihara, Japanese ophthalmologist, 1879–1963	Test for color vision defects
Jaeger reading cards	YA-ger		Eduard Jaeger, Austrian ophthalmologist, 1818–1884	Type of different sizes for testing near vision
peripheral	peh-RIF-er-al	S/	-al *pertaining to*	Pertaining to the periphery or external boundary
		R/	peripher- *external boundary*	
peripheral vision	peh-RIF-er-al VIZH-un	S/	-ion *action, condition*	Ability to see objects as they come into the outer edges of
		R/	vis- *sight*	the visual field
Snellen letter chart	SNEL-en		Hermann Snellen, Dutch ophthalmologist, 1834–1908	Test for acuity of distant vision
tonometer	toe-NOM-eh-ter	S/	-meter *measure*	Instrument for determining intraocular pressure
		R/CF	ton/o- *pressure, tension*	
tonometry	toe-NOM-eh-tree	S/	-metry *process of measuring*	The measurement of intraocular pressure

EXERCISES

A. Communication is key. *The OT in Dr. Chun's office needs to be familiar with all the WAD terms in order to communicate with Dr. Chun and her patients. Show your understanding of the language of ophthalmology by circling the correct answer.* **LO 11.2 and 11.5** *Understand*

1. Which of these instrument(s) can be found in the Eye Clinic?

    a. tonometer

    b. cystoscope

    c. ophthalmoscope

    d. a and b

    e. a and c

2. Which is used to test color vision?

    a. Snellen

    b. Jaeger

    c. Ishihara system

    d. visual fields

    e. otoscope

3. The abbreviation *OD* means:

    a. right eye

    b. both eyes

    c. left eye

    d. does not pertain to the eye

    e. normal eye

4. A test for near vision is:

    a. Snellen chart

    b. ophthalmoscope

    c. Jaeger cards

    d. Ishihara

    e. visual fields

B. Continue using *the language of ophthalmology to answer the following questions.* **LO 11.2, 11.5, and 11.8** *Apply*

1. Explain to your patient the phrase *intraocular pressure.* _____

_____

2. What is the instrument that is used to measure intraocular pressure? _____

3. The instrument named in question #2 above measures the eyeball's resistance to what?

_____

4. What does increased ocular pressure indicate is present? _____

Lesson 11.3 Ophthalmic Pharmacology (LO 11.4 and 11.5)

(cont'd)

- **Fluorescein** eye drops are used extensively as a tool for the diagnosis of corneal abrasions, corneal ulcers, and herpetic corneal infections.

- **Ocular local (topical) anesthetics** are used in the initial assessment of minor trauma and for removal of conjunctival and corneal foreign bodies. The most commonly used agent is **lidocaine** hydrochloride.

- **Injected ocular anesthetics** are used in ocular surgery, most commonly in cataract removal. The injections can be given subconjunctivally, or through the lower lid, or into the space between the conjunctiva and the lens. Lidocaine or **tetracaine** are most frequently used.

- **Hydrocortisone** (corticosteroid) drops and eye ointment are used following surgery and for allergic and inflammatory conditions, but not for infections.

- **Bacterial conjunctivitis** (a form of "pink eye") is often treated empirically without a culture using drops or ointments containing such antibiotics as trimethoprim, polymyxin, and bacitracin.

- **Ophthalmia neonatorum,** which is caused by acquiring gonorrhea or chlamydia infection during passage down the birth canal of an infected mother, is prevented by routinely giving 0.5% erythromycin eye drops to all newborns within two hours of birth. Untreated, the infections can cause blindness.

- **Dry eye syndrome** and irritable eyes can be treated with more than 20 over-the-counter (OTC) drops or ointments.

- **Herpetic keratoconjunctivitis** requires **acyclovir** in eye ointment or drops.

- **Mydriatics,** agents to dilate the pupils of the eye, are used to examine the interior of the eye, to determine refractive error in children, and to treat amblyopia. Atropine and homatropine are mydriatics. The opiate class drugs—heroin, codeine, morphine, and methadone—contract (**miosis**) the pupils.

- Anesthetics used prior to cataract surgery can be injected by the **intracameral** route. After the surgery, antibiotics can be given by the same route to prevent **endophthalmitis.**

- **Glaucoma** treatment can start with **prostaglandin** eye drops, which increase the outflow of the aqueous humor fluid in the eye to reduce the pressure. Medications such as beta blockers or alpha-adrenergic agonists reduce the production of fluid in the eye. If eye drops are insufficient to bring down the intraocular pressure, an oral medication such as a **carbonic anhydrase inhibitor** can be added. If medication is insufficient, surgery involving laser treatment or surgery to the eye can help reduce the pressure. The surgery does not reverse vision loss.

- Medications to treat diabetic retinopathy that are in clinical practice and in clinical trials are given by **intravitreal** injection. They include the synthetic corticosteroid **triamcinalone** and monoclonal antibodies such as Avastin and Lucentis, but these medications have not achieved as robust an effect as focal laser treatment.

- Surgical therapeutic interventions have been described previously with each disorder of the different elements of the eye.

Word Analysis and Definition

WORD	PRONUNCIATION		ELEMENTS	DEFINITION
endophthalmitis	EN-dof-thal-MY-tis	S/ P/ R/	-itis *inflammation* end- *inside* -ophthalm- *eye*	Inflammation of tissues inside the eye
fluorescein	flor-ESS-ee-in	P/ R/	fluo- *fluorine* -rescein *resin*	Dye that produces a vivid green color under blue light to diagnose corneal abrasions and foreign bodies in the eye
graft	GRAFT		French *transplant*	The transplanted tissue or the act of transplantation of tissue
intracameral	in-trah-CAM-er-al	S/ P/ R/	-al *pertaining to* intra- *inside* -camer- *chamber*	Introduction of an anesthetic agent into the anterior chamber of the eye during surgery
intravitreal	in-trah-VIT-ree-al	S/ P/ R/	-eal *pertaining to* intra- *inside* -vitr- *glass*	Injection of various agents into the vitreous body of the eye to treat retinal disorders
miosis miotic	my-OH-sis my-OT-ik	 S/ R/	Greek *a lessening* -ic *pertaining to* miot- *a lessening*	Contraction of the pupil An agent that contracts the pupil
mydriasis mydriatic	mih-DRY-ah-sis mih-dree-AT-ik	 S/ R/	Greek *to dilate* -ic *pertaining to* mydriat- *dilate*	Dilation of the pupil An agent that dilates the pupil
prostaglandin	PROSS-tah-GLAN-din	S/ R/ R/	-in *chemical* prosta- *prostate* -gland- *gland*	Hormone present in many tissues; first isolated in the prostate gland
transplant transplantation	TRANZ-plant TRANZ-plan-TAY-shun	P/ R/ S/	trans- *across* -plant *plant* -ation *process*	Tissue or organ used, or the act of transferring tissue from one person to another The process of moving tissue from one person or place to another

EXERCISES

A. Translate *the following sentences into everyday language so that your patients can understand their significance.*   **LO 11.2, 11.5, and 11.8** *Apply*

1. Ophthalmia neonatorum is caused by acquiring gonorrhea or chlamydia infection during the passage down the vagina of an infected mother in childbirth, and can be prevented by giving erythromycin eye drops within 2 hours of birth. Translation: _____

_____

_____

2. Treatment of glaucoma can start with the use of eye drops, which reduce the outflow of the fluid aqueous humor from the eye to reduce the pressure in the eye. Translation: _____

_____

_____

B. List *three terms that have a prefix showing location*   **LO 11.1**

1. _____

2. _____

3. _____

The Ear and Hearing

The Language of Otology

Case Report 11.3

You are . . .

. . . a medical assistant working for primary care physician Susan Lee, MD, of the Fulwood Medical Group.

You are communicating with . . .

. . . Mrs. Carmen Cardenas, who has brought in her 3-year-old son, Eddie. She tells you that Eddie has had a cold for a couple of days. Early this morning, he woke up screaming, felt hot, and was tugging his ears. She gave him **acetaminophen** with some orange juice, and he threw up. She also tells you this is the third similar episode in the past year, and, since the last time, she is concerned that he is not hearing normally. You see a worried mother and a restless toddler with a green nasal discharge. His oral temperature taken with an electronic digital thermometer is 102.4°F, and his pulse is 100. You tell Mrs. Cardenas that Dr. Lee will be in to see Eddie as soon as possible.

Lesson 11.4

The Ear and Hearing

Objectives

In order to understand and to address Eddie Cardenas' condition, you must be able to use correct medical terminology to:

11.4.1 Recognize the structures and functions of the three regions of the ear.

11.4.2 Explain how sound waves progress through the ear, are transferred to the brain, and are recognized as sounds.

11.4.3 Identify common diseases of the ear that interfere with the process of hearing.

11.4.4 Relate the appropriate structures of the ear to disorders of equilibrium and balance.

11.4.5 Recognize health professionals involved in the diagnosis and treatment of problems of the ear.

Your ear has three major sections (*Figure 11.25*):

1. The external ear
2. The middle ear
3. The inner ear

In your future career, being able to communicate comfortably, accurately, and effectively with the health professionals involved in the diagnosis and treatment of problems of the ear is key. You may work directly and/or indirectly with one or more of the following:

- **Otologists** are medical specialists in diseases of the ear.

- **Otorhinolaryngologists** are medical specialists in diseases of the ear, nose, and throat.

- **Audiologists** are specialists in the evaluation of hearing function.

Case Report 11.3 (continued)

Clinical Note. 05/10/14
Examination by Dr. Lee showed that Eddie has a **bilateral acute otitis media (BOM)** with an upper respiratory infection **(URI).** Dr. Lee is also concerned that Eddie has a **chronic** otitis media with **effusion (OME)** that is causing a hearing loss. She prescribed Amoxicillin 250 mg **q.i.d.** with acetaminophen 160 **mg p.r.n.** for 10 days, when she will see Eddie again. If, after the acute infection subsides, there remains an effusion with hearing loss, Dr. Lee may need to refer Eddie to an **otologist.** I explained this to Mrs. Cardenas.

—Luis Guittierez, CMA 1115 hrs.

Abbreviations

BOM	bilateral otitis media
mg	milligram
OME	otitis media with effusion
p.r.n.	when necessary
q.i.d.	four times each day
URI	upper respiratory infection

▲ **FIGURE 11.25**
Anatomical Regions of the Ear.

Word Analysis and Definition

S = Suffix   **P = Prefix**   R = Root   R/CF = Combining Form

WORD	PRONUNCIATION	ELEMENTS		DEFINITION
acetaminophen	ah-seat-ah-**MIN**-oh-fen		Generic drug name	Medication that is an analgesic and antipyretic
acute	ah-**KYUT**		Latin *sharp*	Disease of sudden onset
audiology	aw-dee-**OL**-oh-jee	S/ R/CF	-logy *study of* audi/o *hearing*	Study of hearing disorders.
audiologist	aw-dee-**OL**-oh-jist	S/	-logist *one who studies*	Specialist in the evaluation of hearing function
bilateral	by-**LAT**-er-al	S/ P/ R/	-al *pertaining to* bi- *two* -later- *side*	On two sides; e.g., in both ears
chronic	**KRON**-ik		Greek *time*	A persistent, long-term disease
effusion	eh-**FYU**-shun		Latin *pouring out*	Collection of fluid that has escaped from blood vessels into a cavity or tissues
otitis media	oh-**TIE**-tis **ME**-dee-ah	S/ R/ R/	-itis *inflammation* ot- *ear* Latin *middle*	Inflammation of the middle ear
otologist	oh-**TOL**-oh-jist	S/ R/CF	-logist *specialist* ot/o- *ear*	Medical specialist in diseases of the ear
otology otorhinolaryngologist	oh-**TOL**-oh-jee oh-toe-rye-no-lah-rin-**GOL**-oh-jist	S/ R/CF R/CF	-logy *study of* -rhin/o- *nose* -laryng/o- *larynx*	Diagnosis and treatment of disorders of the ear Ear, nose, and throat medical specialist

EXERCISES

A. Review *the Case Report and Case Report (continued) before you answer the following questions.*   **LO 11.2, 11.6, and 11.7** *Remember*

1. What symptoms did Eddie have this morning? _____

2. Is this condition a recurring one for Eddie? _____

3. What two factors in the Case Report indicate that Eddie has an infection? _____

_____

4. What is Mrs. Cardenas's big concern about Eddie now? _____

5. What is Eddie's diagnosis after examination by Dr. Lee? _____

6. Eddie has both "acute" and "chronic" conditions. What is the difference? _____

_____

7. How often does Eddie take the antibiotic? _____

B. Deconstruct *these medical terms into their basic elements. Complete the chart, and fill in the blanks.*   **LO 11.1 and 11.6** *Analyze*

Medical Term	Prefix	Root(s)/ Combining Form(s)	Suffix	Meaning of Term
otology	1.	2.	3.	4.
otitis media	5.	6.	7.	8.
otologist	9.	10.	11.	12.
otorhinolaryngologist	13.	14.	15.	16.

Lesson 11.4

(cont'd)

Keynotes

- The external auditory canal is the only skin-lined cul-de-sac in the body.
- Cerumen combines with dead skin cells to form earwax.

External Ear (LO 11.6)

The external ear comprises several structures that keep it functioning effectively.

The **auricle** or **pinna** is a wing-shaped structure that directs sound waves into the ear canal through the external **auditory meatus.** The external auditory canal ends at the very delicate **tympanic** membrane, otherwise known as the eardrum *(Figure 11.26)*. When using an otoscope to examine the tympanic membrane, the pinna should be pulled up and out to straighten the external auditory canal.

The meatus and canal are lined with skin that contains many modified sweat glands called **ceruminous** glands, which secrete **cerumen.**

If a foreign body, like a small bead, gets into the auditory canal, or if cerumen becomes **impacted** in the canal, the result can be hearing loss.

Disorders of the External Ear (LO 11.6)

Some disorders of the external ear include infections and earwax buildup.

Otitis externa *(Figure 11.27)* is a bacterial or fungal infection of the external auditory canal lining. An **otoscopic** exam shows a painful, red, swollen ear canal, sometimes with a purulent drainage. Treatment entails thorough cleansing of the ear canal, applying a hydrocortisone **topical** solution with 2% acetic acid, and using antibiotic drops. Occasionally, a wick is used to help the topical medications penetrate down the canal.

Swimmer's ear is a form of otitis externa resulting from swimming, particularly if the water is polluted.

Excessive earwax can be removed in your physician's office by ear **irrigation** or with a **curette,** a small metal ring at the end of a handle.

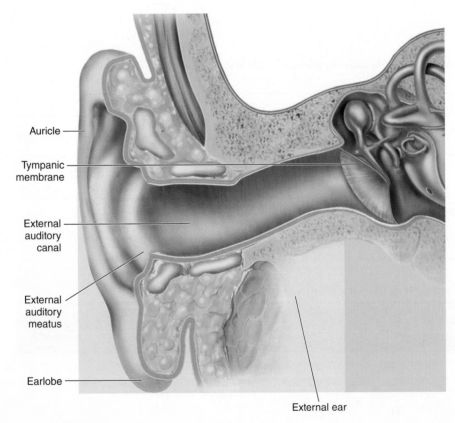

Auricle

Tympanic membrane

External auditory canal

External auditory meatus

Earlobe

External ear

▲ **FIGURE 11.26**
External Ear.

External auditory canal

▲ **FIGURE 11.27**
Otoscopic View of Otitis Externa.

Word Analysis and Definition

WORD	PRONUNCIATION	ELEMENTS		DEFINITION
auditory (adj)	AW-dih-tor-ee		Latin *hearing*	Relating to hearing or the organs of hearing
auricle (Note: *same as* pinna)	AW-ri-kul		Latin *ear*	The shell-like external ear
cerumen ceruminous (adj)	seh-**ROO**-men seh-**ROO**-mih-nus	S/ R/	Latin *wax* -ous *pertaining to* cerumin- *cerumen*	Waxy secretion of glands of the external ear Pertaining to cerumen
curette curettage (**Note:** *The final "e" of* curette *is dropped because the suffix* -age *begins with a vowel)*	kyu-**RET** kyu-reh-**TAHZH**	S/ R/ S/	-ette *little* cur- *cleanse, cure* -age *pertaining to*	Scoop-shaped instrument for scraping or removal of new growths (or earwax) The use of a curette
impacted	im-**PAK**-ted		Latin *driven in*	Immovably wedged, as with earwax blocking the external canal
irrigation	ih-rih-**GAY**-shun	S/ R/	-ation *process* irrig- *to water*	Use of water; e.g., to remove wax from the external ear canal
meatus meatal (adj)	me-**AY**-tus me-**AY**-tal		Latin *go through*	Passage or channel; also the external opening of a passage
otoscope otoscopy otoscopic (adj)	**OH**-toe-skope oh-**TOS**-koh-pee oh-toe-**SKOP**-ik	S/ R/CF S/ S/	-scope *instrument for viewing* ot/o- *ear* -scopy *to examine* -ic *pertaining to*	Instrument for examining the ear Examination of the ear Pertaining to examination with an otoscope
pinna pinnae (pl)	**PIN**-ah **PIN**-ee		Latin *wing*	Another name for auricle
topical	**TOP**-ih-kal	S/ R/	-al *pertaining to* topic- *local*	Medication applied to the skin to obtain a local effect
tympanic	tim-**PAN**-ik	S/ R/	-ic *pertaining to* tympan- *eardrum*	Pertaining to the tympanic membrane (eardrum) or tympanic cavity

EXERCISES

A. Test *your knowledge of the language of otology by matching correct answers. Every part of the body has its own specialized vocabulary. Fill in the blanks.*   **LO 11.6** *Understand*

_____ **1.** pertaining to the eardrum

_____ **2.** external opening of a passage

_____ **3.** instrument for examining the ear

_____ **4.** procedure for removing ear wax

_____ **5.** scoop-shaped instrument

_____ **6.** shell-like external ear

A. meatus

B. curette

C. curettage

D. auricle

E. tympanic

F. otoscope

B. Meet *lesson and chapter objectives using the language of otology to answer the questions.*   **LO 11.2, 11.6, and 11.7** *Apply*

1. Name the structures in the external ear: _____

2. Explain the keynote: "The external auditory canal is the only skin-lined cul-de-sac in the body." _____

_____

3. What is another name for the auricle? _____

4. Describe the difference between an otoscope and a curette _____

_____

_____

Lesson 11.4 Middle Ear (LO 11.2 and 11.6)

(cont'd) The middle ear has the following four components *(Figure 11.28).*

Keynote

- The three ossicles amplify sound so that soft sounds can be heard. The stapes is the smallest bone in the body.

1. The **tympanic membrane** (eardrum) rests at the inner end of the external auditory canal. It vibrates freely as sound waves hit it. It has a good nerve supply and is very sensitive to pain. When examined through the otoscope, it is transparent and reflects light *(Figure 11.29).*

2. The **tympanic cavity** is immediately behind the tympanic membrane. It is filled with air that enters through the eustachian tube, and the cavity is continuous with the **mastoid** air cells in the bone behind it. The cavity contains small bones called **ossicles.**

3. The three **ossicles**—the **malleus, incus,** and **stapes**—work to amplify sounds and are attached to the tympanic cavity wall by tiny ligaments. The malleus is attached to the tympanic membrane and vibrates with the membrane when sound waves hit it. The malleus is also attached to the incus, which vibrates, too, and passes the vibrations onto the stapes. The stapes is attached to the oval window, an opening that transmits the vibrations to the inner ear.

4. The **eustachian (auditory) tube** connects the middle ear with the **nasopharynx** (throat), into which it opens near the pharyngeal **tonsils (adenoids)** *(Figure 11.30).* In children under 5 years of age, this tube is not fully developed. It is short and horizontal, and valve-like flaps in the throat that protect it are not yet developed.

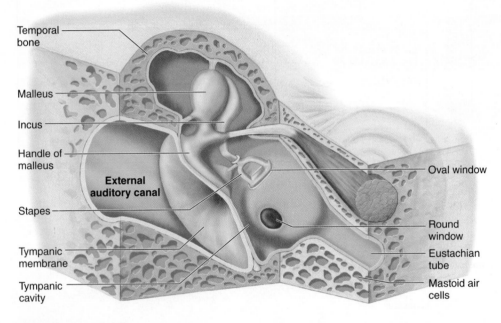

▲ FIGURE 11.28
Middle Ear.

▲ FIGURE 11.29
Otoscopic View of Normal Tympanic Membrane.

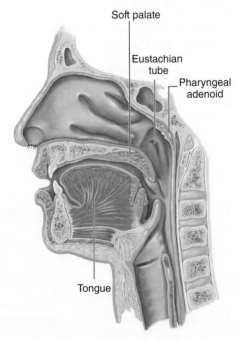

▲ FIGURE 11.30
Nasopharynx (Throat).

Word Analysis and Definition

WORD	PRONUNCIATION	ELEMENTS		DEFINITION
adenoid	ADD-eh-noyd	S/ R/	-oid *resembling* aden- *gland*	Single mass of lymphoid tissue in the midline at the back of the throat
eustachian tube *(Note: same as auditory tube)*	you-**STAY**-shun TYUB		Bartolomeo Eustachio, Italian anatomist, 1524–1574	Tube that connects the middle ear to the nasopharynx
incus	**IN**-cuss		Latin *anvil*	Middle one of the three ossicles in the middle ear; shaped like an anvil
malleus	**MAL**-ee-us		Latin *hammer*	Outer (lateral) one of the three ossicles in the middle ear; shaped like a hammer
mastoid	**MASS**-toyd	S/ R/	-oid *resembling* mast- *breast*	Small bony protrusion immediately behind the ear
nasopharynx nasopharyngeal (adj)	**NAY**-zoh-fair-inks **NAY**-zoh-fair-**RIN**-jee-al	R/CF R/ S/ R/	nas/o- *nose* -pharynx *throat* -eal *pertaining to* -pharyng- *pharynx*	Region of the pharynx at the back of the nose and above the soft palate Pertaining to the nasopharynx
ossicle	**OSS**-ih-kel	S/ R/CF	-cle *small* oss/i- *bone*	A small bone, particularly relating to the three bones in the middle ear
stapes	**STAY**-peez		Latin *stirrup*	Inner (medial) one of the three ossicles of the middle ear; shaped like a stirrup

EXERCISES

A. Review *the terms in the WAD box before you start this exercise. Pay special attention to the spelling. Circle the best choice.*   **LO 11.1 and 11.6**
Remember

1. In the term *mastoid,* the suffix means:

condition   resembling   inflammation

2. The element *mast* means:

throat   breast   ear

3. The element *pharynx* means:

throat   nose   tongue

4. The term *nasopharynx* is composed of:

prefix + suffix   root + root   combining form + root

5. Shaped like a hammer:

malleus   malleolus   maleus

B. Employ *the language of otology and fill in the blanks.*   **LO 11.2, 11.6, and 11.7** *Understand*

1. Meet a lesson objective by describing the four componenets of the middle ear.

_____

_____

_____

_____

2. The femur is the largest bone in the body, which is the smallest? _____

3. Write a synonym for *eustachian tube.* _____

4. What is the medical term for *eardrum?* _____

5. The pharyngeal tonsils are the _____ .

6. What is the medical term for *throat?* _____

Lesson 11.4
(cont'd)

Abbreviations

AOM	acute otitis media
PE tube	pressure-equalization tube
URI	upper respiratory infection

Disorders of the Middle Ear (LO 11.6)

The middle ear can be susceptible to the disorders outlined below.

- **Acute otitis media (AOM)** is the presence of pus in the middle ear with ear pain, fever, and redness of the tympanic membrane. AOM occurs most often in the first 2 to 4 years of age. If the infection is viral, it will go away on its own; if it's bacterial, oral antibiotics may be necessary.

- **Chronic otitis media** occurs when the acute infection subsides but the eustachian tube is blocked. The fluid in the middle ear caused by the infection cannot drain, and it gradually becomes stickier. This is called **chronic otitis media with effusion (OME)** and produces hearing loss because the sticky fluid prevents the ossicles from vibrating. You can see the fluid through the otoscope *(Figure 11.31)*. Dr. Lee was concerned that this had happened to Eddie in his previous ear infection.

- If the sticky fluid persists, a **myringotomy** can be performed, and a small, hollow plastic tube may have to be inserted through the tympanic membrane to allow the effusion to drain. These ear tubes have several names: **tympanostomy** tubes, **pressure-equalization tubes,** and, most commonly, **PE tubes** *(Figure 11.32)*. The tubes are inserted under general anesthesia as outpatient surgery. They remain in the ear for 6 to 18 months before they drop out on their own.

- A **perforated** tympanic membrane *(Figure 11.33)* can occur in acute otitis media **(AOM)** and chronic otitis media when pus in the middle ear cannot escape down the eustachian tube. The pus builds up pressure and punctures the eardrum. Most perforations will heal spontaneously in a month, leaving a small scar. Other perforation causes include a Q-tip puncture, an open-handed slap to the ear, or induced pressure as in scuba diving.

- **Cholesteatoma** is a complication of chronic otitis media with fluid or effusion (OME). Chronically inflamed middle ear cells multiply and collect into a tumor. They damage the ossicles and can spread to the inner ear. Surgical removal is required.

- **Otosclerosis** is a middle-ear disease that usually affects people between 18 and 35 years. It can impair one ear or both and produces a gradual hearing loss for low and soft sounds. Its etiology is unknown. Spongy bone forms around the junction of the oval window and stapes, preventing the stapes from conducting sound vibrations to the inner ear. The only treatment is to replace the stapes with a metal or plastic **prosthesis.**

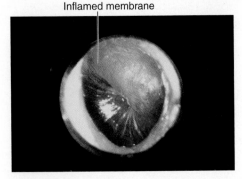

Inflamed membrane

▲ **FIGURE 11.31**
Otoscopic View of Acute Otitis Media.

PE tube

▲ **FIGURE 11.32**
Otoscopic View of PE Tube in Tympanic Membrane.

Perforation

▲ **FIGURE 11.33**
Otoscopic View of Chronic Otitis Media with Perforation.

Word Analysis and Definition

S = Suffix   P = Prefix   R = Root   R/CF = Combining Form

WORD	PRONUNCIATION	ELEMENTS		DEFINITION
cholesteatoma	koh-less-tee-ah-**TOE**-mah	S/ R/CF R/	-oma *tumor, mass* chol/e- *bile* -steat- *fat*	Yellow, waxy tumor arising in the middle ear
coryza (Note: *same as acute rhinitis*)	koh-**RYE**-zah		Greek *catarrh*	Viral inflammation of the mucous membrane of the nose
myringotomy	mir-in-**GOT**-oh-me	S/ R/CF	-tomy *surgical incision* myring/o- *tympanic membrane*	Incision in the tympanic membrane
otosclerosis	oh-toe-sklair-**OH**-sis	S/ R/CF R/CF	-sis *abnormal condition* ot/o- *ear* -scler/o- *hard*	Hardening at the junction of the stapes and oval window that causes loss of hearing
perforated perforation	**PER**-foh-ray-ted per-foh-**RAY**-shun	S/ R/	Latin *to bore through* -ion *action* perforat- *bore through*	Punctured with one or more holes A hole through the wall of a structure
prosthesis	**PROS**-thee-sis		Greek *addition*	Manufactured substitute for a missing or diseased part of the body
tympanostomy	tim-pan-**OS**-toe-me	S/ R/CF	-stomy *new opening* tympan/o- *eardrum*	Surgically created new opening in the tympanic membrane to allow fluid to drain from the middle ear

EXERCISES

A. Review *the Case Report on this spread before answering the questions.*   **LO 11.2, 11.3, 11.6, and 11.7** *Remember*

1. What other terms in the Case Report can be used interchangeably with the word *cold?* _____

2. What is the difference between a *UTI* and a *URI?* _____
_____

3. How did the infection move from Eddie's throat into his middle ear? _____

4. What is the difference between *AOM* and *OME?* _____
_____

5. What is the medical term for the fluid in Eddie's ear? _____

B. Precision in communication *is very important because some terms can look very similar but have very different meanings. Define the following terms, then answer the challenge questions.*   **LO 11.2, 11.6, 11.7, and 11.8** *Remember*

1. transfusion _____

2. infusion _____

3. effusion _____

4. In what other location in the body can you have *effusion?* _____

5. What body system does this represent? _____

C. Match *the correct element in column 1 to the correct meaning in column 2 below.*   **LO 11.1 and 11.6** *Understand*

_____ 1. tympan/o   **A.** tumor, mass

_____ 2. myring/o   **B.** fat

_____ 3. oma   **C.** eardrum

_____ 4. steat   **D.** bile

_____ 5. chol/e   **E.** tympanic membrane

Lesson 11.4 Inner Ear for Hearing (LO 11.6)

(cont'd)

The inner ear is a **labyrinth** of complex, intricate passage systems. The passages in the **cochlea**, a part of the labyrinth *(Figure 11.34)*, contain receptors that convert vibrations into electrical nerve impulses so the brain can interpret them as different sounds.

Sound waves cause the tympanic membrane and the ossicles to vibrate *(Figure 11.35)*. The stapes moves the oval window's membrane to create pressure waves in the fluid inside the inner ear's cochlea. These pressure waves make the **basilar** membranes in the cochlea vibrate. Hair cells attached to the membrane convert this motion into nerve impulses, which travel via the cochlear nerve to the brain. The excess pressure waves in the cochlea escape to the middle ear through the round window *(Figure 11.35)*.

Today, the most common cause of hearing loss is damage to the fine hairs in the cochlea by repeated loud noises—from the work-related use of jackhammers or leaf blowers to the leisure-related exposure to amplified music at concerts, personal listening devices, and motorcycles. This is a **sensorineural hearing loss.**

Hearing aids are becoming more sophisticated and smaller, but they do not help people with cochlear damage. **Cochlear implants** are used to bypass the damaged hair cells and directly stimulate cochlear nerve endings.

A **conductive hearing loss** occurs when sound is not conducted efficiently through the external auditory canal to the tympanic membrane and the ossicles. Causes of this include:

- A middle-ear pathology, like acute otitis media, otitis media with effusion, or a perforated eardrum;

- An infected external auditory canal; or

- The presence of a foreign body in the external canal.

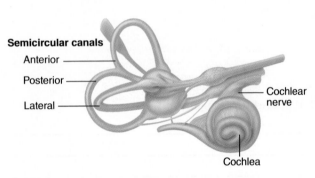

Semicircular canals
Anterior
Posterior
Lateral
Cochlear nerve
Cochlea

Superior view

▲ **FIGURE 11.34**
Labyrinth of Inner Ear.

Hearing Test Procedures (LO 11.6)

Hearing tests are available to accurately measure just how much, and at what frequencies, a patient is able to hear. Some hearing test procedures are described below.

- **Whispered speech testing:** Ask the patient to cover one ear. Stand 2 feet away from the uncovered ear, whisper words, and ask the patient to repeat them. If the patient cannot repeat the words, say the words more loudly. This is a simple, but unmeasured, screening method.

- **Weber test:** Place a vibrating tuning fork in the middle of the patient's forehead and ask whether the tone is louder in one ear or equal on both sides. This determines on which side a hearing loss is located.

- **Rinne test:** Place a high-frequency tuning fork against the patient's mastoid bone and ask the patient to tell you when the sound is no longer heard. Then, quickly place the tuning fork 1 to 2 cm from the auditory canal on the same side and ask the patient whether he can hear the tuning fork. With normal hearing, air conduction should be greater than bone, and the patient should hear the fork next to the pinna when he can no longer hear it when held against the mastoid. The reverse indicates a conductive hearing loss.

- **Audiometer:** After proper training, you may use an audiometer to test for hearing loss. The audiometer is an electronic device that generates sounds in different frequencies and intensities and can print out the patient's responses.

In recording the results of hearing testing, **AD** is shorthand for the right ear, **AS** for the left ear, and **AU** for both ears.

Auditory ossicles
Malleus   Stapes
Incus
Cochlea
Oval window
Cochlear nerve
External auditory canal
Vestibular membrane
Basilar membrane
Tympanic membrane
Round window   Auditory (eustachian) tube

◀ **FIGURE 11.35**
Model of the Hearing Process.

Word Analysis and Definition

WORD	PRONUNCIATION	ELEMENTS		DEFINITION
audiometer	aw-dee-**OM**-eh-ter	S/ R/CF	-meter *measure* audi/o- *hearing*	Instrument to measure hearing
audiometric (adj)	**AW**-dee-oh-**MET**-rik	S/	-metric *pertaining to measurement*	Pertaining to the measurement of hearing
basilar	**BAS**-ih-lar	S/ R/	-ar *pertaining to* basil- *base, support*	Pertaining to the base of a structure
cochlea cochlear (adj)	**KOK**-lee-ah **KOK**-lee-ar		Latin *snail shell*	An intricate combination of passages; used to describe the inner ear
conductive hearing loss	kon-**DUK**-tiv		Latin *to lead*	Hearing loss in the outer ear or middle ear
implant	im-**PLANT**		Latin *to plant*	To insert material into tissues; or the material inserted into tissues
labyrinth labyrinthitis	**LAB**-ih-rinth **LAB**-ih-rin-**THI**-tis	S/ R/	Greek *labyrinth* -itis *inflammation* labyrinth -*inner ear*	The inner ear Inflammation of the inner ear
Rinne test	**RIN**-eh TEST		Friedrich Rinne, German otologist, 1819–1868	Test for conductive hearing loss
sensorineural hearing loss	**SEN**-sor-ih-**NYUR**-al	S/ R/CF R/	-al *pertaining to* sensor/i- *sensory* -neur- *nerve*	Hearing loss of the inner ear or the auditory nerve
Weber test	**VA**-ber TEST		Ernst Weber, German physiologist, 1794–1878	Test for sensorineural hearing loss

EXERCISES

A. Match *the meaning of the element in column 1 with the correct element in column 2. Fill in the blanks.*   **LO 11.1 and 11.6** *Understand*

_____ **1.** hearing

_____ **2.** nerve

_____ **3.** pertaining to

_____ **4.** measure

_____ **5.** inner ear

_____ **6.** sensory

A. meter

B. al

C. sensor/i

D. audi/o

E. neur

F. labyrinth

B. Review *the WAD to find the answers to the questions below.*   **LO 11.2, 11.6, and 11.7** *Remember*

1. What are the two eponyms in the WAD? _____ and _____

2. What is the most common cause today of hearing loss? _____

3. What is a *perforated* eardrum? _____

C. Meet lesson *and chapter objectives by using the correct medical language for your answers to the following questions.*   **LO 11.2, 11.6, and 11.7** *Apply*

1. Describe the difference between *conductive hearing loss* and *sensorineural hearing loss.* _____

_____

_____

2. What is the difference between a *transplant* and an *implant?* _____

_____

_____

_____

▲ FIGURE 11.36
Vestibule of the Inner Ear.

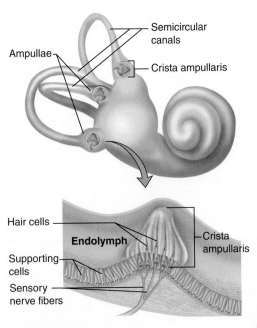

▲ FIGURE 11.37
Semicircular Canals.

Abbreviation

BPPV   benign paroxysmal positional vertigo

Case Report 11.4

You are . . .

. . . Sonia Ramos, a medical assistant working with Sylvia Thompson, MD, an otorhinolaryngologist at Fulwood Medical Center.

You are communicating with . . .

. . . Mr. Ernesto Santiago, a 44-year-old man who was referred to Dr. Thompson. Mr. Santiago complains of recurrent attacks of nausea, vomiting, a sense of spinning or whirling, and ringing in his ears. The attacks last about 24 hours and are getting more frequent. He has been having trouble hearing quiet speech on his left side. Your role is to document his examination, diagnosis, and care, and to act as translator between Mr. Santiago and Dr. Thompson.

Inner Ear for Equilibrium and Balance

(LO 11.6)

The inner ear contains the organs in your body responsible for maintaining the true sense of balance. The **vestibule** and the three semicircular canals *(Figures 11.36 and 11.37)* in the inner ear maintain an individual's balance. These are the true organs of balance. Inside the fluid-filled vestibule are two raised, flat areas covered with hair cells and a jelly-like material. This gelatinous material contains calcium and protein crystals called **otoliths.** The position of the head alters the amount of pressure this gelatinous mass applies to the hair cells. The hair cells respond to horizontal and vertical changes and send impulses to the brain relating how the head is tilted.

Each of the three fluid-filled semicircular canals has a dilated end called an **ampulla.** The ampulla contains a mound of hair cells set in a gelatinous material that together are called the **crista ampullaris** *(Figure 11.37)*. This detects rotational movements of the head that distort the hair cells and lead to stimulation of connected nerve cells. The nerve impulses travel through the vestibular nerve to the brain. From the brain, nerve impulses travel to the muscles to maintain **equilibrium** and balance.

The sensation of spinning or whirling that Mr. Santiago experiences is called **vertigo,** often described by patients as dizziness. The ringing in his ears is called **tinnitus.** Both sensations arise in the inner ear. Tinnitus can also sound like hissing, buzzing, roaring, or clicking and may be associated with difficulty hearing, sleeping, or working. Treatment includes hearing aids, sound-masking devices, and learning ways to cope with the problem.

Benign paroxysmal positional vertigo (BPPV) is another type of intermittent vertigo caused by fragments of the otoliths in the vestibule migrating into the semicircular canals. The otolith fragments brush against the hair cells, sending conflicting signals to the brain. This produces vertigo.

Acute labyrinthitis is an acute viral infection of the labyrinth producing extreme vertigo, nausea, and vomiting. It usually lasts 1 to 2 weeks.

Case Report 11.4 (continued)

The recurrent attacks that Mr. Santiago suffered are called **Ménière disease.** The disease involves the destruction of inner-ear hair cells, but the etiology is unknown and there is no cure. Dr. Thompson prescribed medication to control Mr. Santiago's nausea and vomiting.

Word Analysis and Definition

WORD	PRONUNCIATION		ELEMENTS	DEFINITION
ampulla	am-**PULL**-ah		Latin *two-handled bottle*	Dilated portion of a canal or duct
crista ampullaris	**KRIS**-tah am-**PULL**-air-is	R/ S/ R/	crista *crest* -aris *pertaining to* ampull- *bottle-shaped*	Mound of hair cells and gelatinous material in the ampulla of a semicircular canal
equilibrium	ee-kwi-**LIB**-ree-um	P/ R/	equi- *equal* -librium *balance*	Being evenly balanced
Ménière disease	men-**YEAR** diz-**EEZ**		Prosper Ménière, French physician, 1799–1862	Disorder of the inner ear with acute attacks of tinnitus, vertigo, and hearing loss
otolith	**OH**-toe-lith	R/CF R/	ot/o- *ear* -lith *stone*	A calcium particle in the vestibule of the inner ear
paroxysmal	par-ock-**SIZ**-mal	S/ R/	-al *pertaining to* paroxysm- *sudden, sharp attack*	Occurring in sharp, spasmodic episodes
tinnitus	**TIN**-ih-tus		Latin *jingle*	Persistent ringing, whistling, clicking, or booming noise in the ears
vertigo	**VER**-tih-go		Latin *dizziness*	Sensation of spinning or whirling
vestibule vestibular (adj)	**VES**-tih-byul ves-**TIB**-you-lar	S/ R/	Latin *entrance chamber* -ar *pertaining to* vestibul- *vestibule*	Space at the entrance to a canal Pertaining to the vestibule

EXERCISES

A. Review *Case Report 11.4 and the Case Report (continued) before answering the questions.*   **LO 11.2, 11.6, and 11.8** *Remember*

1. What are Mr. Santiago's chief complaints? _____

2. What is a *recurrent* attack? _____

3. What shows Mr. Santiago's condition is getting worse? _____

4. Which side of his body is most affected with hearing loss? _____

5. What is Mr. Santiago's final diagnosis? _____

6. What does *its etiology is unknown* mean? _____

7. If there is no cure for this disease, what is the treatment plan? _____

B. Terminology challenge: *Analyze the following challenge questions and employ medical language for your answers.*   **LO 11.2, 11.3, and 11.6** *Analyze*

1. What other body system has terminology using the element *lith?* _____

2. Can you give an example of a term in this body system? _____

3. How can vertigo affect your equilibrium? _____

4. Define each medical term represented by the abbreviation *BPPV.*

   B _____

   P _____

   P _____

   V _____

C. Use the language *of otology for your answers to the following questions.*   **LO 11.2, 11.6, and 11.7** *Apply*

1. Where are the organs located that are responsible for maintaining the body's true sense of balance? _____

   _____

2. Name the specific organs in your answer for question 1 above. _____

   _____

3. What travels from the brain to the muscles to help the body maintain equilibrium and balance? _____

   _____

Chapter Review exercises, along with additional practice items, are available in Connect!

CHAPTER 12

The Endocrine System

The Essentials of the Language of Endocrinology

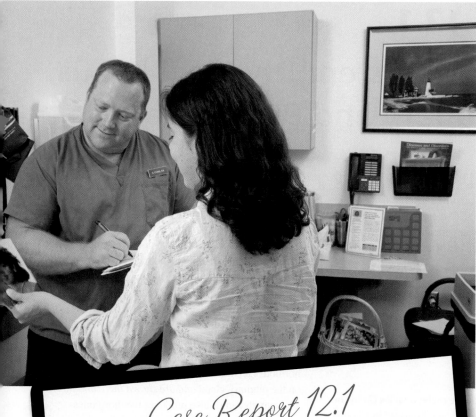

Case Report 12.1

You are . . .

. . . a registered nurse working with endocrinologist Sabina Khalid, MD, in the Endocrinology Clinic at Fulwood Medical Center.

You are communicating with . . .

. . . Mrs. Gina Tacher, a 33-year-old schoolteacher. She complains of coarsening of her facial features and enlargement of the bones of her hands. Over the past 10 years, Mrs. Tacher's nose and jaw have increased in size and her voice has become husky. She has brought photos of herself at ages 9 and 16. She has no other health problems.

Learning Outcomes

The **endocrine** system is a communication system. The **hormones** produced by this system are blood-borne messengers secreted by endocrine glands; they circulate in the bloodstream, gaining access to all other body cells. They are distributed anywhere the blood travels, but only affect the target cells that have receptors for them. These hormones alter the metabolism of the target cells. The information in this chapter will enable you to:

LO 12.1 Use roots, combining forms, suffixes, and prefixes to construct and analyze (deconstruct) medical terms related to the endocrine system.

LO 12.2 Spell and pronounce correctly medical terms related to the endocrine system in order to communicate them with accuracy and precision in any health care setting.

LO 12.3 Define accepted abbreviations related to the endocrine system.

LO 12.4 Identify the anatomical positions of the hypothalamus, pituitary, and pineal glands; the functions of the hormones they secrete; and their disorders and treatments.

LO 12.5 Describe the hormones secreted by the thyroid, parathyroid, and thymus glands; their functions; and their disorders and treatments.

LO 12.6 Compare the hormones secreted by the adrenal cortex and medulla, their functions, and their disorders and treatments.

LO 12.7 Relate the hormones secreted by the endocrine cells of the pancreas to the different types of diabetes mellitus and their symptoms, signs, and treatments.

LO 12.8 Apply your knowledge of medical terms relating to the endocrine system to documentation, medical records, and medical reports.

LO 12.9 Translate the medical terms relating to the endocrine system into everyday language in order to communicate clearly with patients and their families.

The health professionals involved in the diagnosis and treatment of problems with the endocrine system include:

- **Endocrinologists,** who are medical specialists concerned with the production and effects of hormones.
- **Endocrine physician assistants,** who work with endocrinologists to provide care and education to endocrine and diabetes patients.
- **Endocrine nurse practitioners,** who are registered nurses with specialized training in endocrinology.
- **Certified diabetic educators,** who are certified to possess specialized knowledge in diabetes self-management education and monitoring.

Lesson 12.1

Endocrine System, Hypothalamus, and Pituitary and Pineal Glands

The Endocrine System (LO 12.4)

The endocrine system comprises several major organs *(Figures 12.1 and 12.2).* These organs, with their respective names and numbers in parentheses below, work together to ensure that this system operates smoothly:

- **Pituitary gland (1)** and the nearby **hypothalamus (1).**
- **Pineal gland (1).**
- **Thyroid gland (1).**
- **Parathyroid glands (4).**
- **Thymus gland (1).**
- **Adrenal glands (2).**
- **Pancreas (1).**
- **Gonads: testes (2) in the male; ovaries (2) in the female** (The male gonads are discussed in *Chapter 14* and the female in *Chapter 15.*)

In addition, endocrine cells found in tissues throughout the body secrete particular hormones. For example:

- **Cells in the upper GI tract** secrete hormones that include gastrin, which stimulates gastric secretions.
- **Cells in the kidney** secrete erythropoietin, which stimulates erythrocyte (red blood cell) production.
- **Fat cells** secrete leptin, which helps suppress appetite. Lack of leptin can lead to overeating and obesity.
- **Cells in tissues throughout the body** secrete **prostaglandins,** which act locally to dilate blood vessels, relax airways, stimulate uterine contractions in menstrual cramps or labor, and lower acid secretion in the stomach. When tissues are injured, prostaglandins promote an inflammatory response.

Hypothalamus (LO 12.2 and 12.4)

The hypothalamus, which is the size of an almond, is the part of the brain located just above the pituitary gland. It connects the brain to the endocrine system through blood vessels between the hypothalamus and the pituitary gland, thus enabling hypothalamic hormones to control pituitary hormone secretion. The hypothalamus secretes a total of eight hormones: four are releasing hormones that stimulate the secretion of hormones by the anterior lobe of the pituitary gland; two are inhibitory hormones that inhibit the secretion of anterior lobe pituitary gland hormones. These releasing and inhibitory hormones are named and described in the next section on the pituitary gland *and are shown there in italics.* The hypothalamus also produces two hormones—vasopressin and oxytocin—that travel directly to the posterior lobe of the pituitary, where they are stored. These two hormones are also described in the next section.

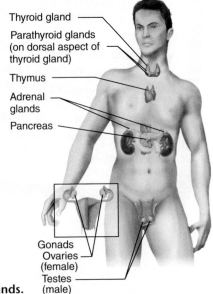

Thyroid gland
Parathyroid glands (on dorsal aspect of thyroid gland)
Thymus
Adrenal glands
Pancreas

Gonads
Ovaries (female)
Testes (male)

▶ **FIGURE 12.2**
Major Endocrine Glands.

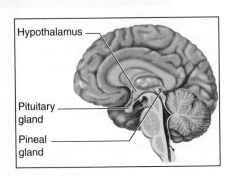

Hypothalamus

Pituitary gland

Pineal gland

▲ **FIGURE 12.1**
Hypothalamus, Pituitary Gland, and Pineal Gland.

WORD	PRONUNCIATION	ELEMENTS		DEFINITION
antidiuretic (**Note:** *Two prefixes*)	**AN**-tih-die-you-**RET**-ik	S/ P/ P/ R/	-ic *pertaining to* anti- *against* -di- *complete* -uret- *urination*	An agent that decreases urine production
endocrine	**EN**-doh-krin	P/ R/CF	endo- *within* -crine *secrete*	A gland that produces an internal or hormonal secretion
endocrinology (**Note:** *The "e" in crine changes to "o" for better flow.*)	**EN**-doh-krih-**NOL**-oh-jee	S/	-logy *study of*	Medical specialty concerned with the production and effects of hormones
endocrinologist	**EN**-doh-krih-**NOL**-oh-jist	S/	-logist *one who studies, specialist*	A medical specialist in endocrinology
hormone	**HOR**-mohn		Greek *to set in motion*	Chemical formed in one tissue or organ and carried by the bloodstream to stimulate or inhibit a function of another tissue or organ
hormonal (adj)	hor-**MOHN**-al	S/ R/	-al *pertaining to* hormon- *hormone*	Pertaining to hormones
hypothalamus	high-poh-**THAL**-ah-muss	S/ P/	-us *pertaining to* hypo- *below*	An endocrine gland in the floor and wall of the third ventricle of the brain
hypothalamic (adj)	high-poh-thal-**AM**-ik	S/ R/	-ic *pertaining to* -thalam- *thalamus*	Pertaining to the hypothalamus
melatonin	mel-ah-**TONE**-in	S/ R/ R/	-in *substance* mela- *black* -ton- *tension, pressure*	Hormone formed by the pineal gland
oxytocin	**OCK**-see-**TOE**-sin	S/ R/ R/	-in *substance* oxy- *oxygen* -toc- *labor and childbirth*	Pituitary hormone that stimulates the uterus to contract
pineal	**PIN**-ee-al		Latin *like a pine cone*	Pertaining to the pineal gland
pituitary	pih-**TYU**-ih-tary	S/ R/	-ary *pertaining to* pituit- *pituitary*	Pertaining to the pituitary gland
prostaglandin	**PROS**-tah-**GLAN**-din	S/ R/ R/	-in *chemical* prosta- *prostate* -gland- *gland*	Hormone present in many tissues, but first isolated from the prostate gland
serotonin	ser-oh-**TOE**-nin	S/ R/CF R/	-in *substance* ser/o- *serum* -ton- *tension, pressure*	Neurotransmitter in central and peripheral nervous systems

EXERCISES

A. Review *the Case Report on the previous spread before answering the questions.* **LO 12.2, 12.4, and 12.8** *Understand*

1. What are Mrs. Tacher's chief complaints? _____

2. What has been happening to Mrs. Tacher's facial features over the past ten years? _____

3. What change has there been in Mrs. Tacher's voice? _____

4. Why was it important for Mrs. Tacher to bring the photos with her? _____

5. Does Mrs. Tacher have any other health problems? _____

B. Elements *remain your best tool for understanding medical terms. The elements are listed in column 1. Identify the type of element in column 2, its meaning in column 3, and an example of a term containing that element in column 4. Fill in the chart.* **LO 12.1** *Remember*

Element	Type of Element (P, R, CF, or S)	Meaning of Element	Medical Term Containing This Element
anti	1.	2.	3.
di	4.	5.	6.
endo	7.	8.	9.
hypo	10.	11.	12.
logist	13.	14.	15.
mela	16.	17.	18.

The Endocrine System (continued)

Pineal Gland
(LO 12.2 and 12.4)

The pineal gland is located on the roof of the brain's third ventricle, posterior to the hypothalamus. It secretes the feel-good hormone **serotonin** by day, and at night, converts it to **melatonin,** which helps to regulate sleep and wake cycles. This gland reaches its maximum size in childhood and may regulate puberty's timing.

Case Report 12.1 (continued)

Dr. Khalid's examination of Mrs. Tacher shows a protruding mandible and an enlarged, deeply grooved tongue. Her feet and hands are enlarged, her ribs are thickened, and her heart is enlarged. X-rays show a thickened skull and enlarged nasal sinuses. Blood tests display high growth hormone levels. CT and MRI scans show a tumor in the pituitary gland, and as a result, Mrs. Tacher is scheduled for surgery to remove the tumor.

Pituitary Gland
(LO 12.2, 12.3, and 12.4)

Each hormone plays its part in maintaining the body's homeostasis, but the pituitary gland and hypothalamus work together and often influence hormone production in the other endocrine glands. The pituitary gland is suspended from the hypothalamus, and it has two components:

- A large anterior lobe; and
- A small posterior lobe.

There are six **anterior-lobe hormones,** which are listed here with their functions:

1. **Follicle-stimulating hormone (FSH)** stimulates target cells in the ovaries to develop eggs, as well as sperm production in the testes.

2. **Luteinizing hormone (LH)** stimulates ovulation. It also encourages a corpus luteum (a yellow tissue mass) to form in the ovary *(see Chapter 15)* to secrete estrogen and progesterone. In the male, LH stimulates testosterone production *(see Chapter 14). Both FSH and LH production are stimulated by the **gonadotropin-releasing hormone (GnRH)** of the hypothalamus.*

3. **Thyroid-stimulating hormone (TSH),** or **thyrotropin,** stimulates the growth of the thyroid gland and the production of the chief thyroid hormone, thyroxine. *TSH production is stimulated by the **thyrotropin-releasing hormone (TRH)** of the hypothalamus.*

4. **Adrenocorticotropic hormone (ACTH),** or **corticotropin,** stimulates the adrenal glands to produce hormones called **corticosteroids,** including **hydrocortisone (cortisol)** and **cortisone.** *ACTH production is stimulated by the **cortico-releasing hormone (CRH)** of the hypothalamus.*

5. **Prolactin (PRL)** encourages the mammary glands to produce milk after pregnancy. In the male, it sensitizes the testes to LH, which enhances testosterone production. *Prolactin production is stimulated by the **thyrotropin-releasing hormone (TRH)** of the hypothalamus.*

6. **Growth hormone (GH),** or **somatotrophin,** stimulates cells to enlarge and divide. The body produces at least a thousand times more GH than any other pituitary hormone. *This production of growth hormone is stimulated by the **growth hormone-releasing hormone (GHRH)** of the hypothalamus.*

An **overproduction of growth hormone** in children produces gigantism. In adults, this overproduction produces **acromegaly,** the condition that Mrs. Tacher has. An **underproduction of growth hormone,** present at birth, leads to dwarfism.

Tropic hormones are hormones that stimulate other endocrine glands to produce their hormones. FSH and LH are called **gonadotropins** because they stimulate **gonadal** (reproductive organ) functions.

In addition to the six anterior-lobe hormones, there are the **posterior-lobe hormones.** These hormones are produced in the hypothalamus and stored and released in the pituitary posterior lobe *(Figure 12.3).* The two types of posterior-lobe hormones and their functions are:

1. **Oxytocin (OT)** in childbirth stimulates uterine contractions, and in lactation, it forces milk to flow down ducts to the nipple. In both sexes, its production increases during social interaction and sexual intercourse to help give the feelings of satisfaction and emotional bonding.

2. **Antidiuretic hormone (ADH),** also called **vasopressin,** reduces the volume of urine produced by the kidneys.

Diabetes insipidus (DI) (not diabetes mellitus) results from a decreased production of ADH. Symptoms of DI are excessive urine production leading to excessive thirst.

Nuclei of hypothalamus
Paraventricular nucleus
Supraoptic nucleus

Optic chiasm

Third ventricle of brain
Floor of hypothalamus

Anterior lobe

Posterior lobe

Oxytocin
Antidiuretic hormone

▲ **FIGURE 12.3**
Hormones of the Posterior Lobe of the Pituitary Gland.

Word Analysis and Definition

S = Suffix   P = Prefix   R = Root   R/CF = Combining Form

WORD	PRONUNCIATION	ELEMENTS		DEFINITION
acromegaly	ak-roe-**MEG**-ah-lee	S/ R/CF	-megaly *enlargement* acr/o- *peak, highest point*	Enlargement of head, face, hands, and feet due to excess growth hormone after growth plates have closed
adrenocorticotropic	ah-**DREE**-noh-**KOR**-tih-koh-**TROH**-pik	S/ R/CF R/CF	-tropic *a turning, change* adren/o- *adrenal gland* -cortic/o- *from the cortex*	Hormone of the anterior pituitary that stimulates the cortex of the adrenal gland to produce its own hormones
corticosteroid	**KOR**-tih-koh-**STAIR**-oyd	S/ R/CF	-steroid *steroid* cortic/o- *from the cortex*	A hormone produced by the adrenal cortex
corticotropin	**KOR**-tih-koh-**TROH**-pin	S/ R/CF	-tropin *stimulation* cortic/o- *from the cortex, cortex*	Pituitary hormone that stimulates the cortex of the adrenal gland to secrete cortisone
cortisone	**KOR**-tih-sohn	S/ R/	-one *hormone* cortis- *from the cortex*	A corticosteroid produced in small amounts by the adrenal cortex
diabetes insipidus (DI)	dye-ah-**BEE**-teez in-**SIP**-ih-dus	 S/ P/ R/	diabetes, Greek *siphon* -us *pertaining to* in- *not* -sipid- *flavor*	Excretion of large amounts of dilute urine as a result of inadequate antidiuretic hormone production
gonadotropin	**GO**-nad-oh-**TROH**-pin	S/ R/CF	-tropin *stimulation* gonad/o- *testis, ovary*	Any hormone that stimulates gonadal function
gonad	**GO**-nad		gonad, Latin *seed*	An organ that produces sex cells; a testis or an ovary
hydrocortisone (also called **cortisol**)	high-droh-**KOR**-tih-sohn	S/ R/CF R/	-one *hormone* hydr/o- *water* -cortis- *from the cortex*	Potent glucocorticoid with antiinflammatory properties
prolactin	pro-**LAK**-tin	S/ P/ R/	-in *substance* pro- *before* -lact- *milk*	Pituitary hormone that stimulates the production of milk
somatotrophin (also called **growth hormone, GH**)	**SO**-mah-toh-**TROH**-fin	S/ R/CF	-trophin *stimulation* somat/o- *the body*	Hormone of the anterior pituitary that stimulates the growth of body tissues
thyrotropin	thigh-roe-**TROH**-pin	S/ R/CF	-tropin *stimulation* thyr/o- *thyroid*	Hormone from the anterior pituitary gland that stimulates function of the thyroid gland

EXERCISES

A. Review *the Case Report on this spread before answering the questions.*   **LO 12.2, 12.4, and 12.8** *Understand*

1. What does Dr. Khalid learn from his physical examination of Mrs. Tacher? _____

2. List below one of the diagnostic tests Mrs. Tacher had, and the results of that test.

_____

3. Which test(s) pinpointed the source of Mrs. Tacher's problems? _____

4. What is the next step in her treatment plan? _____

B. Abbreviations *will be your answers in this matching exercise. Match the correct abbreviation to its description.*

   LO 12.1, 12.3, and 12.4 *Understand*

_____ **1.** stimulates ovulation   **A.** LH

_____ **2.** stimulates production of corticosteroids   **B.** ADH

_____ **3.** stimulates uterine contractions   **C.** ACTH

_____ **4.** stimulates ovaries to develop eggs   **D.** TSH

_____ **5.** reduces volume of urine   **E.** OT

_____ **6.** stimulates production of thyroxin   **F.** FSH

Lesson 12.2
Thyroid, Parathyroid, and Thymus Glands

Objectives

In order to understand what is happening to Ms. Norma Leary in the Case Report, to be able to help her, and to communicate about her situation with her parents and her physician, it's necessary to learn the correct medical terminology provided in this lesson to:

12.2.1 Describe the location and anatomy of the thyroid gland.

12.2.2 Explain how the three thyroid hormones are produced and secreted.

12.2.3 Specify the functions of the thyroid hormones.

12.2.4 Discuss common disorders of the thyroid gland.

12.2.5 Locate the positions of the parathyroid and thymus glands.

12.2.6 Name the hormones produced by the parathyroid and thymus glands and state their functions.

Case Report 12.2

You are . . .

. . . an EMT working in the Emergency Department at Fulwood Medical Center at 0200 hours in the morning.

You are communicating with . . .

. . . the parents of Ms. Norma Leary, a 22-year-old college student who is living with her parents for the summer. Ms. Leary is **emaciated**, extremely agitated, and at times disoriented and confused. Her parents tell you that in the past 3 or 4 days she has been coughing and not feeling well. In the past 12 hours, she has become feverish and been complaining of a left-sided chest pain. Upon questioning, the parents reveal that prior to this acute illness, Ms. Leary had lost about 20 pounds in weight, although she was eating voraciously. Her **VS** are T 105.2, P 180 and irregular, R 24, BP 160/85.

You call for Dr. Hilinski, an emergency physician, STAT. On his initial examination, he believes that the patient is in thyroid storm, which is a medical emergency. There are no immediate laboratory tests that can confirm this diagnosis.

Thyroid Gland (LO 12.5)

Shaped like a bow tie and measuring about 2 inches wide, the **thyroid** gland lies just beneath the skin of the neck and below the thyroid cartilage ("Adam's apple"). Two lobes extend up on either side of the trachea (or windpipe) and are joined by an isthmus *(Figure 12.4)*.

Cells in the thyroid gland secrete the two thyroid hormones **T3** and **T4.** The latter is known as **thyroxine.** The term **thyroid hormone** refers to T3 and T4 collectively, and it performs the following functions:

- **Stimulates** almost every tissue in the body to produce proteins;
- **Increases** the amount of oxygen that cells use; and
- **Controls** the speed of the body's chemical functions, known as the **metabolic rate.**

The thyroid also produces the hormone **calcitonin,** which promotes calcium deposition and bone formation.

Abbreviations

PTH	parathyroid hormone
T3	triiodothyronine
T4	tetraiodothyronine (thyroxine)
VS	vital signs: measurement of temperature (T), pulse (P), respiration (R), and blood pressure (BP)

▲ **FIGURE 12.4**
Anatomy of the Thyroid Gland.

Labels: Thyroid cartilage; Thyroid gland; Isthmus; Trachea

Parathyroid Glands (LO 12.5)

Most people have four **parathyroid** glands, and these are partially embedded in the posterior surface of the thyroid gland. The parathyroid glands secrete **parathyroid hormone (PTH).** PTH stimulates bone resorption to bring calcium back into the blood, and calcitonin takes calcium from the blood to stimulate bone deposition *(see Chapter 4).*

Thymus Gland (LO 12.5)

The **thymus** gland is located in the mediastinum *(Figure 12.5).* This gland is large in children and over time, it decreases in size until it is mostly fibrous tissue in the elderly. It secretes a group of hormones that stimulate the production of T lymphocytes (see *Chapter 7*).

▶ **FIGURE 12.5**
Position of the Thymus Gland.

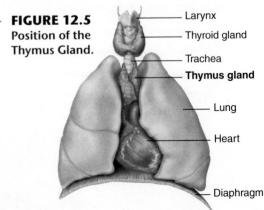

Labels: Larynx; Thyroid gland; Trachea; **Thymus gland**; Lung; Heart; Diaphragm

Word Analysis and Definition

WORD	PRONUNCIATION	ELEMENTS		DEFINITION
calcitonin	kal-sih-**TONE**-in	S/ R/CF R/	-in *substance* calc/i- *calcium* -ton- *tension, pressure*	Hormone produced by the thyroid gland that moves calcium from blood to bones
emaciation	ee-may-see-**AY**-shun	S/ R/CF	-ation *process* emac/i- *make thin*	Abnormal thinness
emaciated (adj)	ee-may-see-**AY**-ted	S/	-ated *pertaining to a condition*	Pertaining to or suffering from emaciation
parathyroid	par-ah-**THIGH**-royd	S/ P/ R/	-oid *resembling* para- *adjacent, beside* -thyr- *thyroid*	Endocrine glands embedded in the back of the thyroid gland
thymus	**THIGH**-mus		Greek *sweetbread*	Endocrine gland located in the mediastinum
thyroid	**THIGH**-royd		Greek *an oblong shield*	Endocrine gland in the neck; or a cartilage of the larynx
thyroxine	thigh-**ROCK**-sin	S/ R/ R/	-ine *pertaining to* thyr- *thyroid gland* -ox- *oxygen*	Thyroid hormone T4, tetraiodothyronine

EXERCISES

A. Review *the Case Report on this spread before answering the questions.*   **LO 12.2, 12.3, 12.5, and 12.8** *Understand*

1. What are the outward signs Ms. Leary presents with in the ED? _____

2. What were her symptoms 4 days ago? _____

3. What additional symptoms has she developed in the last 12 hours? _____

4. Name one vital sign that shows Ms. Leary is now a medical emergency: _____

5. What does Dr. Hilinski believe is Ms. Leary's diagnosis? _____

B. Critical thinking: *Apply your knowledge of the language of endocrinology and answer these additional questions about the Case Report.*
   LO 12.2, 12.3, 12.5, and 12.8 *Apply*

1. Why was Dr. Hilinski called to the ED STAT? _____

2. What information about Ms. Leary's weight is surprising, based on her eating pattern? _____
   _____

3. Will Dr. Hilinski order diagnostic tests for Ms. Leary? _____

C. Meet lesson *and chapter objectives and use the language of endocrinology to answer the following questions.*   **LO 12.2 and 12.8** *Apply*

1. What is the *speed of the body's chemical functions* known as? _____

2. What is *bone resorption?* _____
   _____
   _____

3. What is the role of calcitonin in bone deposition? _____
   _____
   _____

4. The processes in questions 2 and 3 are *antagonistic.* What does that mean? _____
   _____
   _____

Lesson 12.2 (cont'd)

Disorders of the Thyroid and Parathyroid Glands

▲ **FIGURE 12.6**
Hyperthyroidism May Cause the Eyes to Protrude (Exophthalmos).

Hyperthyroidism (Thyrotoxicosis) (LO 12.5)

The symptoms of **hyperthyroidism** (excessive thyroid hormone production) are those of an increased body metabolism. These include tachycardia (rapid heart rate), hypertension, sweating, shakiness, anxiety, weight loss despite increased appetite, and diarrhea.

Graves disease is an autoimmune disorder *(see Chapter 7)* in which an antibody stimulates the thyroid to produce and secrete excessive amounts of thyroid hormone into the blood. It presents with **exophthalmos** (bulging of the eyes) *(Figure 12.6),* a **goiter** (an enlarged thyroid gland) *(Figure 12.7),* and a non-pitting, waxy edema of the lower leg.

Hypothyroidism (LO 12.2 and 12.5)

Hypothyroidism is the opposite of hyperthyroidism and results from an inadequate production of thyroid hormone. This decreases the body's metabolism. Primary hypothyroidism affects 10% of older women. Symptoms develop gradually and include hair loss; dry, scaly skin; a puffy face and eyes; slow, hoarse speech; weight gain; constipation; and a high sensitivity to cold temperatures. No specific cause has been found.

Severe hypothyroidism is called **myxedema.** In developing countries, a common cause of this is a lack of **iodine** in the diet. In the United States, iodine is added to table salt to prevent hypothyroidism. Iodine is also found in dairy products and seafood.

Thyroiditis is an inflammation of the thyroid gland. It presents most commonly as **Hashimoto thyroiditis,** an autoimmune disease with lymphocytic infiltration of the gland. Hypothyroidism results, necessitating lifelong thyroid hormone replacement therapy.

Cretinism *(Figure 12.8)* is a congenital form of thyroid deficiency that severely retards mental and physical growth. If diagnosed and treated early with thyroid hormones, the patient can achieve significant improvement.

Thyroid cancer usually presents as a symptomless nodule in the thyroid gland. It can metastasize (spread) to cervical and mediastinal lymph nodes, and to the liver, lungs, and bones. A total **thyroidectomy** with local lymph node dissection is the first step in treating thyroid cancer.

Disorders of the Parathyroid Glands (LO 12.5)

Hypoparathyroidism is a deficiency of parathyroid hormone (PTH) that lowers levels of blood calcium. Most symptoms of this are neuromuscular (in nerve and muscle tissue), ranging from tingling in the fingers, to muscle cramps, to the painful muscle spasms of **tetany** (not **tetanus,** which is caused by a toxin acting on the central nervous system).

Hyperparathyroidism is an excess of PTH and is more common than hypoparathyroidism. It is usually caused by one of the four glands enlarging and working out of pituitary control. It leads to calcium depletion in bones (making bones brittle), high blood calcium levels, and kidney stones.

Case Report 12.2 (continued)

Thyroid storm is the condition Ms. Norma Leary presented with in the Emergency Department. It is the most extreme state of **hyperthyroidism,** with severely exaggerated effects of the thyroid hormones causing **hyperpyrexia,** tachycardia, agitation, and delirium. The weight loss prior to her illness becoming acute was part of her undiagnosed hyperthyroidism.

▲ **FIGURE 12.7**
Elderly Woman with Hypothyroidism and Goiter.

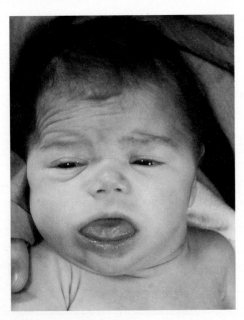

▶ **FIGURE 12.8**
Infant with Cretinism.

Word Analysis and Definition

WORD	PRONUNCIATION		ELEMENTS	DEFINITION
cretin cretinism	**KREH**-tin **KREH**-tin-izm	S/ R/	French *cretin* -ism *condition, process* cretin- *cretin*	Severe congenital hypothyroidism Condition of severe congenital hypothyroidism
exophthalmos	ek-sof-**THAL**-mos	P/ R/	ex- *out* -ophthalmos *eye*	Protrusion of the eyeball
goiter	**GOY**-ter		Latin *throat*	Benign enlargement of the thyroid gland
Graves disease	**GRAVZ** diz-**EEZ**		Robert Graves, Irish physician, 1796–1853	Hyperthyroidism with toxic goiter
Hashimoto disease	hah-shee-**MOH**-toe diz-**EEZ**		Hakaru Hashimoto, Japanese surgeon, 1881–1934	Autoimmune disease of the thyroid gland
hyperparathyroidism (**Note:** *Two suffixes and two prefixes*)	**HIGH**-per-par-ah-**THIGH**-royd-izm	S/ S/ P/ P/ R/	-ism *condition* -oid- *resembling* hyper- *excessive* -para- *adjacent* -thyr- *thyroid*	Excessive levels of parathyroid hormone
hypoparathyroidism	**HIGH**-poh-par-ah-**THIGH**-royd-izm	P/	hypo- *deficient, below*	Deficient levels of parathyroid hormone
hyperpyrexia	**HIGH**-per-pie-**REK**-see-ah	S/ P/ R/	-ia *condition* hyper- *excessive* -pyrex- *fever*	Extremely high body temperature or fever
hyperthyroidism (**Note:** *Two suffixes*) (*Also called* thyrotoxicosis.)	high-per-**THIGH**-royd-izm	S/ S/ P/ R/	-ism *condition* -oid- *resembling* hyper- *excessive* -thyr- *thyroid*	Excessive production of thyroid hormones
hypothyroidism (**Note:** *Two suffixes*)	high-poh-**THIGH**-royd-izm	S/ S/ P/ R/	-ism *condition* -oid- *resembling* hypo- *deficient, below* -thyr- *thyroid*	Deficient production of thyroid hormones
iodine	**EYE**-oh-dine or **EYE**-oh-deen	S/ R/	-ine *pertaining to* iod- *violet*	Chemical element, the lack of which causes thyroid disease
myxedema	miks-eh-**DEE**-muh	P/ R/	myx- *mucus* -edema *swelling*	Nonpitting, waxy edema of the skin in hypothyroidism
tetany	**TET**-ah-nee		Greek *convulsive tension*	Severe muscle twitches, cramps, and spasms
thyroidectomy	thigh-roy-**DEK**-toe-me	S/ S/ R/	-ectomy *surgical excision* -oid- *resembling* thyr- *thyroid*	Surgical removal of the thyroid gland
thyroiditis	thigh-roy-**DIE**-tis	S/	-itis *inflammation*	Inflammation of the thyroid gland
thyrotoxicosis (*also called* hyperthyroidism)	**THIGH**-roe-toks-ih-**KOH**-sis	S/ R/CF R/CF	-sis *condition* thyr/o- *thyroid* -toxic/o- *poison*	Disorder produced by excessive thyroid hormone production

EXERCISES

A. Review *the Case Report on this spread before answering the questions.* **LO 12.2, 12.5, and 12.8** *Understand*

1. What is the most extreme state of hyperthyroidism called? _____

2. What is the difference between hyperthyroidism and hyperpyrexia? _____
   _____

3. What three terms in the Case Report (continued) signify body processes that have speeded up or are in an excessive state?
   _____, _____, and _____.

4. What condition did Ms. Leary have that had been undiagnosed until it reached an acute state? _____

B. Meet lesson objectives *and apply the language of endocrinology to answer the following questions.* **LO 12.2, 12.5, and 12.8** *Apply*

1. Describe the difference between *tetany* and *tetanus*. _____
   _____

2. List some of the common disorders of the thyroid gland. _____

Lesson 12.3

Adrenal Glands and Hormones

Objectives

Your adrenal glands produce several key hormones that help to maintain homeostasis. The information in this lesson will enable you to use correct medical terminology to:

12.3.1 Locate the adrenal glands.

12.3.2 Differentiate between the adrenal cortex and the medulla.

12.3.3 Identify the functions of the hormones produced by the cortex and medulla.

12.3.4 Detail how the body adapts to stress.

12.3.5 Explain common disorders of the adrenal glands.

Adrenal Glands
(LO 12.6)

An **adrenal (suprarenal)** gland is anchored like a cap on the upper pole of each kidney *(Figure 12.10 inset)*. The outer layer of the gland—the adrenal cortex *(Figure 12.10)*—synthesizes more than 25 **steroid** hormones known collectively as **adrenocortical** hormones, or corticosteroids. These hormones include:

1. **Glucocorticoids,** mainly **hydrocortisone (cortisol),** which help regulate blood glucose levels, particularly in response to stress. They also have an anti-inflammatory effect, and are often found in dermatologic lotions and ointments;

2. **Mineralocorticoids,** mostly **aldosterone,** which promote sodium retention and potassium excretion by the kidneys; and

3. **Sex steroids,** which include a weak androgen that is converted to testosterone *(see Chapter 14)* and estrogen *(see Chapter 15).*

The inner layer of the adrenal gland, the adrenal medulla *(Figure 12.10),* also secretes hormones. These hormones are called **catecholamines,** and principally include **epinephrine (adrenaline)** and **norepinephrine (noradrenaline).** These hormones prepare the body for physical activity and are responsible for the "flight or fight" response.

Disorders of the Adrenal Glands (LO 12.6)

Adrenocortical hypofunction, most commonly seen as **Addison disease,** is caused by the **idiopathic** atrophy (wasting away) of the adrenal cortex. Symptoms are weakness, fatigue, increased susceptibility to infection, and diminished resistance to stress. This disorder is treated with hormone replacement therapy, which John F. Kennedy received until he died.

Adrenocortical hyperfunction most commonly appears as **Cushing syndrome.** Excess production of the steroid hormones produces "moon" **facies** (facial features and expressions), muscle wasting and weakness, kidney stones, and reduced resistance to infection. Most cases are due to a pituitary tumor secreting

▲ **FIGURE 12.9**
John F. Kennedy.

Case Report 12.3

John Fitzgerald Kennedy (JFK) (1917–1963) was elected president of the United States of America in 1960 at the age of 43 *(Figure 12.9).* He had health problems from the age of 13, when he was first diagnosed as having colitis. At age 27, he had lower back pain that necessitated lower back surgery. He was then diagnosed as having adrenal gland insufficiency (Addison disease) with osteoporosis of his lumbar spine. This required lower back surgery on three more occasions. JFK received adrenal hormone replacement therapy for the rest of his life, together with pain medication for his lower back pain, until his assassination in Dallas, Texas, in 1963. In medical retrospect, instead of colitis, JFK probably had celiac disease *(see Chapter 9),* which has strong associations with Addison disease.

too much ACTH, causing the adrenal glands to produce an excess of steroids. Sometimes, Cushing syndrome can be produced by the administration of excess steroid medications.

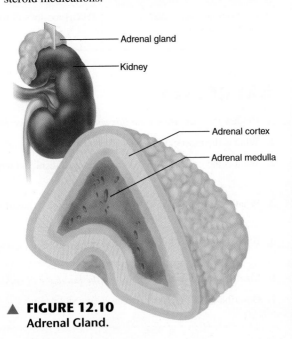

— Adrenal gland

— Kidney

— Adrenal cortex

— Adrenal medulla

▲ **FIGURE 12.10**
Adrenal Gland.

Word Analysis and Definition

S = Suffix   P = Prefix   R = Root   R/CF = Combining Form

WORD	PRONUNCIATION	ELEMENTS		DEFINITION
Addison disease	**ADD**-ih-son diz-**EEZ**		Thomas Addison, English physician, 1793–1860	An autoimmune disease leading to decreased production of adrenocortical steroids
adrenal (*same as* **suprarenal**)	ah-**DREE**-nal	S/ P/ R/ P/	-al *pertaining to* ad- *to, toward* -ren- *kidney* supra- *above*	Endocrine gland on the upper pole of each kidney
adrenaline (*also called* **epinephrine**)	ah-**DREN**-ah-lin ep-ih-**NEF**-rin	S/ P/ R/	-ine *pertaining to* epi- *above* -nephr- *kidney*	Main catecholamine produced by the adrenal medulla
adrenocortical	ah-dree-noh-**KOR**-tih-kal	S/ R/CF R/	-al *pertaining to* adren/o- *adrenal* -cortic- *cortex*	Pertaining to the cortex of the adrenal gland
aldosterone	al-**DOS**-ter-own	S/ R/CF R/	-one *hormone* ald/o- *organic compound* -ster- *steroid*	Mineralocorticoid hormone of the adrenal cortex
catecholamine	kat-eh-**COAL**-ah-meen	S/ R/	-amine *nitrogen-containing substance* catechol- *tyrosine containing*	Major elements produced by the adrenal cortex in the stress response; include epinephrine and norepinephrine
Cushing syndrome	**KUSH**-ing **SIN**-drohm		Harvey Cushing, U.S. neurosurgeon, 1869–1939	Hypersecretion of cortisol (hydrocortisone) by the adrenal gland
facies	**FASH**-eez		Latin *appearance*	Facial features and expressions
glucocorticoid	glu-co-**KOR**-tih-koyd	S/ R/ R/CF	-oid *resembling* -cortic- *cortisone* gluc/o- *glucose*	Hormone of the adrenal cortex that helps regulate glucose metabolism
hydrocortisone (*also called* **cortisol**)	high-droh-**KOR**-tih-sohn	S/ R/CF R/	-one *hormone* hydr/o- *water* -cortis- *cortisone*	Potent glucocorticoid with anti-inflammatory properties
idiopathic	id-ih-oh-**PATH**-ik	S/ R/CF R/	-ic *pertaining to* idi/o- *unknown* -path- *disease*	Pertaining to a disease of unknown etiology
mineralocorticoid	**MIN**-er-al-oh-**KOR**-tih-koyd	S/ R/CF R/	-oid *resemble* mineral/o- *inorganic material* -cortic- *cortex*	Hormone of the adrenal cortex that influences sodium and potassium metabolism
norepinephrine (**Note:** *Two prefixes: also called* **noradrenaline**)	**NOR**-ep-ih-**NEFF**-rin	S/ P/ P/ R/	-ine *pertaining to* nor- *normal* -epi- *above* -nephr- *kidney*	Catecholamine hormone of the adrenal gland that is a parasympathetic neurotransmitter
steroid	**STER**-oyd	S/ R/	-oid *resembling* ster- *solid*	Large family of chemical substances found in many drugs, hormones, and body components

EXERCISE

A. Review *the Case Report on this spread before answering the questions.*   **LO 12.2, 12.6, and 12.8** *Understand*

1. What is *colitis* and what body system does it affect?

   Definition _____

   Body system _____

2. *Adrenal gland insufficiency* is also known as _____ .

3. What lumbar spine problem did John F. Kennedy also have? _____

4. What two conditions did John F. Kennedy treat with medications?

   _____ and _____

5. What other disease has a *strong association* with Addison disease? _____

6. What does *strong association with* mean in this case? _____

Lesson 12.4

The Pancreas

Objectives

The pancreas measures approximately 6 inches in length, rests across the back of the abdomen, and has many important functions, including the secretion of digestive juices and the production of hormones. The information provided in this lesson will enable the learner to use correct medical terminology to:

12.4.1 Distinguish between the different cells of the pancreas and their secretions.

12.4.2 Identify the functions of the hormones produced by the pancreas.

12.4.3 Explain common disorders of the pancreatic hormones.

Keynotes

- Glucagon is not the only hormone that raises blood glucose; epinephrine, hydrocortisone, and growth hormone do as well.

- Insulin is the only hormone that lowers blood glucose.

Case Report 12.4

You are . . .

. . . a certified medical assistant working with Susan Lee, MD, in her Primary Care Clinic at Fulwood Medical Center.

You are communicating with . . .

. . . Mrs. Martha Jones, who is here for her monthly checkup. She is a 53-year-old type 2 diabetic on insulin. Mrs. Jones has diabetic retinopathy and diabetic neuropathy of her feet. Bariatric surgery has enabled her to reduce her weight from 275 to 156 pounds. The time is 0930 hrs. She is complaining of having a cold and cough for the past few days. Now, she is feeling drowsy and nauseous and has a dry mouth. As you talk with her, you notice that her speech is slurred. She cannot remember if she gave herself her morning insulin. Examination of her lungs reveals rales (wet, crackly lung noises) at her right base.

Her VS: T 97.8, P 120, R 20, BP 100/50. You perform her blood **glucose** measurement. The reading is 600 milligrams per deciliter (mg/dL). A recommended value 2 hours after breakfast is < 145 mg/dL.

The Pancreas (LO 12.2 and 12.7)

The location and structure of the pancreas are further detailed in *Chapter 9*. Most of your pancreas is an **exocrine** gland (external secretion gland) that secretes digestive juices through a duct *(Figure 12.11a)*. Scattered throughout the pancreas are clusters of endocrine cells grouped around blood vessels. These clusters are called **pancreatic islets (islets of Langerhans).** Within the islets are three distinct cell types *(Figure 12.11b)*:

1. **Alpha cells:** Secrete the hormone **glucagon** in response to low blood **glucose.** Glucagon's actions are:

   a. In the liver, to stimulate **gluconeogenesis, glycogenolysis,** and the release of glucose into the bloodstream; and

   b. In adipose tissue, to stimulate fat catabolism and the release of free fatty acids.

2. **Beta cells:** Secrete **insulin** in response to a high blood glucose level. Insulin has the opposite effects to those of glucagon, and its actions are:

   a. In muscle and fat cells, to enable them to absorb glucose, and to store glycogen and fat; and

   b. In the liver, to stimulate the conversion of glucose to glycogen.

3. **Delta cells:** Secrete **somatostatin,** which acts within the pancreas to prevent the secretion of glucagon and insulin.

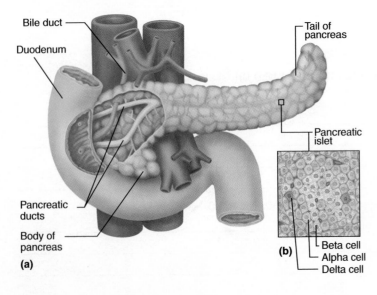

Bile duct
Duodenum
Pancreatic ducts
Body of pancreas
(a)

Tail of pancreas
Pancreatic islet
Beta cell
Alpha cell
Delta cell
(b)

◀ **FIGURE 12.11**
Pancreas.
(a) Anatomy of the pancreas. (b) Alpha, beta, and delta cells.

Word Analysis and Definition

S = Suffix   P = Prefix   R = Root   R/CF = Combining Form

WORD	PRONUNCIATION	ELEMENTS		DEFINITION
exocrine	EK-soh-krin	P/ R/CF	exo- *outward* -crine *secrete*	A gland that secretes outwardly through excretory ducts
glucagon	GLU-kah-gon	S/ R/	-agon *to fight* gluc- *sugar, glucose*	Pancreatic hormone that supports blood glucose levels
gluconeogenesis	GLU-koh-nee-oh-JEN-eh-sis	S/ P/ R/CF	-genesis *creation* -neo- *new* gluc/o- *sugar, glucose*	Formation of glucose from noncarbohydrate sources
glucose	GLU-kose	S/ R/	-ose *full of* gluc- *sugar, glucose*	The final product of carbohydrate digestion and the main sugar in the blood
glycogenolysis	GLYE-koh-jen-oh-LYE-sis	S/ R/CF R/CF	-lysis *separate, dissolve* glyc/o- *glycogen* -gen/o- *create*	Conversion of glycogen to glucose
insulin	IN-syu-lin	S/ R/	-in *a substance* insul- *an island*	Hormone produced by the islet cells of the pancreas
islets of Langerhans	EYE-lets of LAHNG-er-hahnz		Paul Langerhans, German anatomist, 1847–1888	Areas of pancreatic cells that produce insulin and glucagon
somatostatin	SOH-mah-toh-STAT-in	S/ R/CF	-statin *inhibit* somat/o- *body*	Hormone that inhibits release of growth hormone and insulin

EXERCISES

A. Review *the Case Report on this spread before answering the questions.*   **LO 12.2, 12.7, and 12.8** *Understand*

1. What body system is affected by diabetic retinopathy? _____

2. What type of surgery has Mrs. Jones had to help reduce her weight? _____

3. What are her complaints that caused her to see Dr. Lee? _____
_____

4. Explain what *rales* are and how you detect them. _____
_____

5. In which body system would you have the term *neuropathy?* _____

6. What symptoms is Mrs. Jones experiencing now? _____
_____
_____

7. What outward signs does the CMA notice in Mrs. Jones? _____

8. Why is it important for Mrs. Jones to go for monthly checkups? _____
_____
_____

9. Is Mrs. Jones' blood glucose measurement too high or too low? _____

10. Which other specialists might Mrs. Jones have to consult for her other conditions? _____ and _____

B. Build the correct medical term *that matches the definition. Insert each missing element on the line, and label what type of element it is under the line.* *Then answer question 5.*   **LO 12.1, 12.2, and 12.7** *Apply*

1. Conversion of glycogen to glucose: _____ / _____ /lysis

2. Main sugar in the blood: _____ / _____ /ose

3. Hormone that inhibits release of GH and insulin: _____ / _____ /statin

4. The formation of glucose from noncarbohydrate sources: gluco/_____ /genesis

5. What is unusual about the elements in the term in question 4 above? _____

Diabetes Mellitus (DM)
(LO 12.7)

Diabetes mellitus is a condition characterized by hyperglycemia, resulting from an impairment of insulin secretion and/or insulin action. Diabetes affects the body's ability to make use of the energy found in food, disrupting the normal process of carbohydrate, fat, and protein metabolism. It is the world's most prevalent metabolic disease and the leading cause of blindness, renal failure, and gangrene of the lower extremities. There is a spectrum of types of diabetes, the main ones being:

1. **Type 1 diabetes,** also called **insulin-dependent diabetes mellitus (IDDM),** accounts for 10 to 15% of all cases of DM. It is the predominant type of DM found in patients under the age of 30. When symptoms become apparent, 90% of the pancreatic insulin-producing cells have already been destroyed by **autoantibodies** (antibodies that attack the patient's own system).

2. **Type 2 diabetes,** also called **non-insulin-dependent diabetes mellitus (NIDDM),** accounts for 85 to 90% of all DM cases. Nearly 18 million people in the United States have been diagnosed with type 2 DM. Not only is there an impairment of insulin response, but there is also a decreased glucose uptake by tissues due to insulin resistance. In addition to contributing to type 2 DM, insulin resistance leads to other common disorders like hypertension, hyperlipidemia, and coronary artery disease.

3. **Latent autoimmune diabetes in adults (LADA or Type 1.5)** accounts for roughly 10% of people with diabetes. It occurs in adults who have the same autoantibodies as Type 1 diabetics, but there is no need for insulin treatment in the first 6 months after diagnosis. It is a more slowly progressing variation of Type 1 diabetes.

4. **Gestational diabetes** occurs in about 5% of pregnancies. While most cases of gestational diabetes resolve after the pregnancy, a woman who has this complication of pregnancy has a 30% chance of developing type 2 DM within 10 years.

5. **Mature-onset diabetes of the young (MODY)** is a selection of genetically linked forms of diabetes usually found in thin people under 55 years of age. Many forms of MODY will respond to small doses of insulin or to sulfonylurea drugs.

Hypoglycemia (LO 12.7)

Hypoglycemia is present when blood glucose is below 70 mg/dL. Because brain metabolism depends primarily on glucose, the brain is the first organ affected by hypoglycemia. This disorder presents clinically as an impaired mental efficiency, followed by shakiness, anxiety, confusion, tremor, seizures, and, if untreated, loss of consciousness. Symptomatic hypoglycemia is sometimes called **insulin shock.** Low blood glucose can be raised to normal in minutes by taking 10 to 20 g carbohydrate (3 to 4 ounces), such as orange, apple, or grape juice, or a sugar-containing soft drink.

Hyperglycemia (LO 12.7)

In **hyperglycemia,** the classic symptoms are **polyuria** (excessive urination), **polydipsia** (excessive thirst), and **polyphagia** (excessive hunger), with unexplained weight loss.

Symptomatic hyperglycemia is how type 1 DM usually presents. Type 2 DM can be symptomatic or asymptomatic, and is often found during a routine health exam.

Because of high glucose levels, hyperglycemia damages capillary endothelial cells in the retina, renal glomerulus *(see Chapter 13),* and neurons and Schwann cells in peripheral nerves *(see Chapter 10).* Of all diabetics, 85% develop some degree of **diabetic retinopathy;** 30% develop diabetic **nephropathy,** which can progress to end-stage renal disease *(see Chapter 13).* Diabetic **neuropathy** causes sensory defects with numbness, tingling, and **paresthesias** (abnormal skin sensations) in the feet and/or hands.

In larger blood vessels, hyperglycemia contributes to endothelial cell-lining damage and atherosclerosis. Coronary artery disease and peripheral vascular disease with claudication *(see Chapter 6)* are complications. Hyperglycemia is the most common cause of foot ulcers and gangrene of the lower extremity, sometimes requiring **amputation.** The risk of infection is increased by the cellular hyperglycemia and the circulatory deficits.

The complications of hyperglycemia can be kept at bay by stringent control of blood glucose levels.

Word Analysis and Definition

WORD	PRONUNCIATION	ELEMENTS		DEFINITION
amputation	am-pyu-**TAY**-shun	S/ R/	-ation *a process* amput- *to prune, lop off*	Process of removing a limb, part of a limb, a breast, or other projecting part
autoantibody (**Note:** *Two prefixes*)	awe-toe-**AN**-tee-bod-ee	P/ P/ R/	auto- *self, same* -anti- *against* -body *body*	Antibody produced in response to an antigen from the host's own tissue
coma comatose (adj)	**KOH**-mah **KOH**-mah-toes	 S/ R/	Greek *deep sleep* -ose *full of* comat- *coma*	State of deep unconsciousness In a state of coma
diabetes mellitus diabetic (adj)	dye-ah-**BEE**-teez **MEL**-ih-tus dye-ah-**BET**-ik	 S/ R/	diabetes, Greek *a siphon* mellitus, Latin *sweetened with honey* -ic *pertaining to* diabet- *diabetes*	Metabolic syndrome caused by absolute or relative insulin deficiency and/or ineffectiveness Pertaining to or suffering from diabetes
hyperglycemia hyperglycemic (adj)	**HIGH**-per-gly-**SEE**-me-ah **HIGH**-per-gly-**SEE**-mik	S/ P/ R/ S/	-emia *a blood condition* hyper- *above* -glyc- *glucose* -emic *pertaining to a blood condition*	High level of glucose (sugar) in the blood Pertaining to or having hyperglycemia
hypoglycemia hypoglycemic (adj)	**HIGH**-poh-gly-**SEE**-me-ah **HIGH**-poh-gly-SEE-mik	S/ P/ R/ S/	-emia *a blood condition* hypo- *below, deficient* -glyc- *glucose* -emic *pertaining to a blood condition*	Low level of glucose (sugar) in the blood Pertaining to or suffering from low blood sugar
nephropathy	neh-**FROP**-ah-thee	S/ R/CF	-pathy *disease* nephr/o- *kidney*	Any disease of the kidney
neuropathy	nyu-**ROP**-ah-thee	S/ R/	-pathy *disease* neur/o- *nerve*	Any disease of the nervous system
paresthesia paresthesias (pl)	par-es-**THEE**-ze-ah	S/ P/ R/	-ia *condition* par- *abnormal* -esthes- *sensation*	An abnormal sensation; e.g., tingling, burning, pricking
polydipsia	pol-ee-**DIP**-see-ah	S/ P/ R/	-ia *condition* poly- *many, excessive* -dips- *thirst*	Excessive thirst
polyphagia	pol-ee-**FAY**-jee-ah	S/ P/ R/	-ia *condition* poly- *many, excessive* -phag- *eat*	Excessive eating
polyuria	pol-ee-**YOU**-ree-ah	S/ P/ R/	-ia *condition* poly- *many, excessive* -ur- *urine*	Excessive production of urine
retinopathy	ret-ih-**NOP**-ah-thee	S/ R/CF	-pathy *disease* retin/o- *retina of the eye*	Degenerative disease of the retina

EXERCISES

A. Diabetes *is the world's most prevalent metabolic disease. Many patients have diabetes as a concurrent condition with other health problems, which always makes it a consideration in treatment and the prescribing of medications. Test your knowledge of this disease by answering the following questions. Circle the correct choice.*   **LO 12.2 and 12.7** *Understand*

1. Diabetes is the leading cause of:

   blindness   renal failure   gangrene   all of these   none of these

2. The first organ affected by hypoglycemia is the:

   kidney   heart   pancreas   brain   liver

3. Impairment of insulin response and decreased insulin effectiveness is termed insulin:

   production   resistance   autoantibodies   control   conversion

4. Most cases of gestational diabetes resolve after:

   medication   treatment   testing   pregnancy   surgery

B. Apply *your knowledge of the endocrine system and the correct medical terminology to answer the following questions.*   **LO 12.2, 12.7, and 12.8** *Apply*

1. What are the three classic symptoms of diabetes? _____, _____, and _____

2. Hyperglycemia can result in _____.

3. What is the correct medical term for abnormal skin sensations? _____

Diabetes Mellitus (continued) (LO 12.7)

Diabetic ketoacidosis (DKA) is a state of marked hyperglycemia with dehydration, **metabolic acidosis** (abnormal increase in blood acidity), and **ketone** formation. This is seen mostly in type 1 DM and usually results from a lapse in insulin treatment, an acute infection, or a trauma that makes the usual insulin treatment inadequate.

DKA presents with polyuria, vomiting, and lethargy and can progress to coma. The ketone **acetone** can be smelled on the breath. DKA is a medical emergency. There is a 2% to 5% mortality rate from circulatory collapse if the DKA is not promptly controlled.

Diabetic coma is a severe medical emergency, caused by hyperglycemia.

Insulin shock is another severe medical emergency, caused by hypoglycemia.

A blood glucose test will differentiate hypoglycemia from hyperglycemia.

Treatment of Diabetes Mellitus (LO 12.7)

The basic principle of diabetes treatment is to avoid hyperglycemia and hypoglycemia. The areas of treatment are as follows:

- **Diet and exercise** to achieve weight reduction of 2 pounds per week in overweight type 2 DM patients is essential.

- **Patient education** is necessary so that the patient understands the disease process, can recognize the indications for seeking immediate medical care, and will follow a foot care regimen.

- **Plasma glucose monitoring** is an essential skill that all diabetics must learn. Patients on insulin must learn to adjust their insulin doses. Home glucose analyzers use a drop of blood obtained from the fingertip or forearm by a spring-powered lancet. The frequency of testing varies individually.

  - **Assessment of the patient** should be performed on routine physician visits for symptoms or signs of complications.

  - **Periodic laboratory evaluation** includes **BUN** and serum creatinine (kidney function), lipid profile, ECG, and an annual complete ophthalmologic evaluation.

Glycosylated hemoglobin (Hb A1c) is used to monitor plasma glucose control during the preceding 1 to 3 months.

Oral antidiabetic drugs are used for type 2 DM but not type 1 DM. There are numerous drugs available, and they produce their effect in four main ways:

- Stimulate the beta cells of the pancreas to produce more insulin. **Sulfonylureas** are an example; the oldest one, chlorpropamide (Diabinese), has been available for 50 years. The second-generation sulfonylureas include glipizide (Glucotrol) and glyburide (Micronase). **Meglitinides**—repaglinide (Prandin)—act in the same way.

- Decrease glucose production by the liver. **Biguanides**—metformin (Glucophage)—act in this way.

- Block the breakdown of starches in the intestine. **Alpha-glucosidase inhibitors**—acarbose (Precose)—act in this way.

- Increase insulin production and decrease glucose production. **DPP-4 inhibitors**—sitagliptin (Januvia)—are an example of this type.

Combinations of these different-acting drugs are often used.

Injectable insulin preparations are used in type 1 DM and sometimes in type 2 DM. They are classified by their speed of action. *(see Table below)*

The injectable insulins are supplied in vials, cartridges, and prefilled pens.

For some patients requiring frequent doses of insulin, continuous subcutaneous insulin infusion is given by an implanted battery-powered, programmable pump *(Figure 12.12)*. This pump provides continuous insulin through a small needle in the abdominal wall.

Pump

Canula cover

◀ **FIGURE 12.12**
Photograph of Insulin Pump—with Cannula Inserted in the Subcutaneous Tissue of the Abdominal Wall.

Word Analysis and Definition

S = Suffix   P = Prefix   R = Root   R/CF = Combining Form

WORD	PRONUNCIATION	ELEMENTS		DEFINITION
acetone	ASS-eh-tone		Latin *vinegar*	Ketone that is found in blood, urine, and breath when diabetes mellitus is out of control
ketoacidosis	KEY-toe-ass-ih-DOE-sis	S/ R/CF R/	-osis *condition* ket/o- *ketone* -acid- *acid*	Excessive ketones in the blood, making it acidic
ketone ketosis	KEY-tone key-TOE-sis	S/ R/	Greek *acetone* -osis *condition* ket- *ketone*	Chemical formed in uncontrolled diabetes or in starvation Excessive production of ketones
lethargy lethargic (adj)	LETH-ar-jee le-THAR-jik		Greek *drowsiness*	Abnormal drowsiness in depth or length of time
metabolic acidosis	met-ah-BOL-ik ass-ih-DOE-sis	S/ R/ S/ R/	-ic *pertaining to* metabol- *change* -osis *condition* acid- *acid*	Decreased pH in blood and body tissues as a result of an upset in metabolism
saline	SAY-leen		Latin *salt*	Salt solution, usually sodium chloride

PHARMACOLOGY: CLASSES OF INSULIN LO 12.7

Insulin Type	Onset of Action*	Peak of Action*	Duration of Action*	Examples
Rapid acting	15 min	30–60 min	3–5 hr	Humalog, NovoLog
Regular acting	30–60 min	100–120 min	5–8 hr	Humulin R, Novolin R
Intermediate acting (NPH)	1–3 hr	7–8 hr	18–24 hr	Humulin N, Novolin N
Long acting	4–8 hr	minimal peak effects	16–24 hr	Lantus, Levemir
Premixed	30 min	2–4 hrs	14–24 hrs	Humulin 70/30, Novolin 70/30

*min = minutes; hr = hours.

EXERCISES

A. Case Report (*continued*): *Read aloud the Case Report on the opposite page. Read it a second time, and highlight or underline the medical terms. Answer the following questions based on this Case Report.*   **LO 12.2, 12.3, 12.7, and 12.8** *Apply*

1. "Diabetic ketoacidosis is a state of marked hyperglycemia with dehydration." Explain this in layperson's language. _____
_____
_____

2. Mrs. Jones' pneumonia is in her right lower lobe. How many lobes are in the right lung? _____

3. Define pneumonia: _____
_____

4. Name an abbreviation that could have been used in this Case Report: _____, which stands for _____
_____

5. What chemical is contained in a *saline* solution? _____

6. Name three possible causes of DKA: _____, _____, and _____

7. If DKA is not promptly controlled, _____ and _____ can result, which can cause death.

B. Terminology challenge *on the Case Report and Case Report (continued). Challenge yourself to use all the correct medical terminology in your answers.*   **LO 12.2, 12.7, and 12.9** *Apply*

1. What was the probable cause of Mrs. Jones' coma? _____

2. What diagnostic tests did Mrs. Jones have? _____

3. Why did Mrs. Jones have an *infusion* and not a *transfusion?* _____

4. Diabetic coma is caused by _____. Conversely, insulin shock is caused by _____.

5. What is the chemical produced in uncontrolled diabetes or starvation? _____

6. Define *metabolic acidosis.* _____
_____
_____

7. Which specific ketone can be smelled on the breath? _____

Additional exercises available in

Chapter Review exercises, along with additional practice items, are available in Connect!

The Urinary System

The Essentials of the Language of Urology

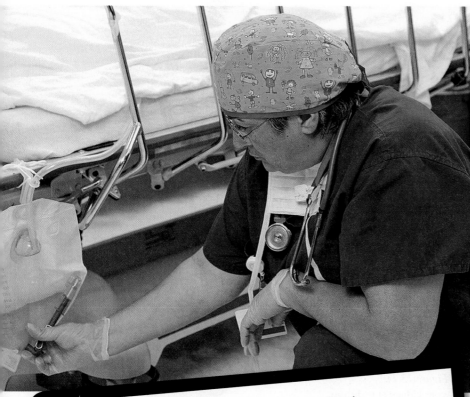

CHAPTER 13

Learning Outcomes

In order to understand and to assess Mr. Hughes' situation, define and recognize the areas of concern, communicate with Dr. Johnson and the patient, and document the patient's progress, you need to be able to:

LO 13.1 Use roots, combining forms, suffixes, and prefixes to construct and analyze (deconstruct) medical terms related to the urinary system.

LO 13.2 Spell and pronounce correctly medical terms related to the urinary system in order to communicate them with accuracy and precision in any health care setting.

LO 13.3 Define accepted abbreviations related to the urinary system.

LO 13.4 Relate the structure of the kidneys and ureters to their functions and disorders.

LO 13.5 Relate the structure of the urinary bladder and urethra and associated organs to their functions and disorders.

LO 13.6 Describe the diagnostic and therapeutic procedures and the pharmacologic agents used for disorders of the urinary system.

LO 13.7 Apply your knowledge of medical terms relating to the urinary system to documentation, medical records, and medical reports.

LO 13.8 Translate the medical terms relating to the urinary system into everyday language in order to communicate clearly with patients and their families.

Case Report 13.1

You are . . .

. . . a surgical physician assistant working with **urologist** Phillip Johnson, MD, at Fulwood Medical Center.

You are communicating with . . .

. . . Mr. Nelson Hughes, a 58-year-old school principal. You are making your afternoon hospital visits to Dr. Johnson's patients. Earlier today, you assisted at Mr. Hughes' surgery. A laparoscopic radical nephrectomy (kidney removal) for a **TNM** Stage II **renal** cell carcinoma (cancer) with no evidence of local invasion or lymph node involvement (metastasis) was performed. Your job is to assess Mr. Hughes' postoperative state and determine whether postoperative complications exist.

Abbreviation

TNM   tumor, node, metastasis
(tumor staging method)

In your future career, being able to communicate comfortably, accurately, and effectively with the health professionals involved in the diagnosis and treatment of problems with the urologic system is key. You may work directly and/or indirectly with one or more of the following:

- **Urologists** are specialists in the diagnosis and treatment of diseases of the urinary system.

- **Nephrologists** are specialists in the diagnosis and treatment of diseases of the kidney.

- **Urologic nurses** and **nurse practitioners** are registered nurses with advanced academic and clinical experience in urology.

Lesson 13.1

Urinary System, Kidneys, and Ureters

Objectives

Your body's metabolism continually produces metabolic waste products. If these wastes are not eliminated, they will poison your body. Your **urinary** *system carries the major burden of excreting these wastes, and within this system, the kidney is the organ that does the actual eliminating. So, the kidney is a vital organ to understand, and it brings with it a whole new set of terminology.*

In this lesson, the information will enable you to use correct medical terminology to:

13.1.1 Name and locate the organs of the urinary system.

13.1.2 Identify the structures and functions of the kidneys and ureters.

13.1.3 Describe disorders of the kidneys and ureters.

Keynotes

• The kidney removes waste products from the blood by a process of **filtration.**

• Each renal cortex contains about 1 million **nephrons,** the functional filtration unit of the kidney.

• The filtrate from the kidney's filtration process is urine. It consists of excess water, electrolytes, and urea.

Urinary System
(LO 13.4, and 13.5)

Your **urinary system** *(Figure 13.1)* consists of **six organs:**

• Two **kidneys**

• Two **ureters**

• A single **urinary bladder**

• A single **urethra**

The process of removing metabolic wastes is called excretion, and it's essential in maintaining your body's homeostasis *(see Chapter 2).* Metabolic wastes include carbon dioxide, excess water and electrolytes, **nitrogenous** compounds including **ammonia** (from the breakdown of proteins), and **urea.** If these wastes are not eliminated, they will poison the entire body.

The Kidneys (LO 13.4)

Each of your kidneys is a bean-shaped organ about the size of your clenched fist. One kidney is located on each side of the vertebral column and lies against the deep muscles of your back *(Figure 13.1).*

Waste-laden blood enters your kidney at its **hilum** (an opening for nerves and vessels) *(Figure 13.2)* through the **renal** artery. Excess water, urea, and other waste products are **filtered** from the blood by the more than 1 million **nephrons** in each kidney's cortex. The renal artery *(Figure 13.2)* divides into smaller and smaller arterioles, each of which then enters a nephron and divides into a network of capillaries known as a **glomerulus** *(Figure 13.3),* which is encased in **Bowman's capsule.** Because the blood is under pressure and the capillaries are permeable, much of the fluid from the blood filters through the capillary walls into the surrounding renal tubules, including the loop of Henle. The tubules join to form the collecting duct, and collecting ducts join to form **calyces,** which join to form the **ureter** *(Figure 13.2).* The ureters carry the **filtrate,** now called **urine,** from the kidneys to the urinary **bladder.**

The **excretion functions of the kidneys** are to:

• **Filter** blood to eliminate wastes;

• **Regulate** blood volume and pressure by eliminating or conserving water; and

• **Maintain homeostasis** by controlling the amounts of water and electrolytes that are eliminated.

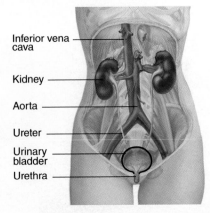

▲ **FIGURE 13.1**
Urinary System.

▲ **FIGURE 13.2**
Section of kidney.

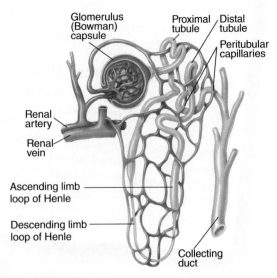

▲ **FIGURE 13.3**
Nephron.

Word Analysis and Definition

WORD	PRONUNCIATION	ELEMENTS		DEFINITION
ammonia	ah-**MOAN**-ih-ah	S/ R/	-ia *condition* ammon- *ammonia*	Toxic breakdown product of amino acids (proteins)
bladder	**BLAD**-er		Old English *bladder*	Hollow sac that holds fluid; e.g., urine or bile
calyx calyces (pl) calices (syn)	**KAY**-licks **KAY**-lih-seez		Greek *cup of a flower*	Funnel-shaped structure
filter (noun or verb)	**FIL**-ter		Latin *strain through material*	Porous substance used to separate liquids and gases from particulate matter; or to subject a substance to the action of a filter
filtrate	**FIL**-trate	S/ R/	-ate *composed of, pertaining to* filtr- *strain through*	Liquid that has passed through a filter
filtration	fil-**TRAY**-shun	S/	-ation *process*	Process of passing liquid through a filter
glomerulus	glo-**MER**-you-lus		Latin *small ball of yarn*	Network of capillaries in a nephron
hilum hila (pl)	**HIGH**-lum **HIGH**-lah		Latin *small bit*	The opening where the nerves and blood vessels enter and leave an organ
kidney	**KID**-nee		Old English *kidney*	Organ of excretion
nephron	**NEF**-ron		Greek *kidney*	Filtration unit of the kidney; comprised of glomerulus and renal tubule
nephrology	neh-**FROL**-oh-jee	S/ R/CF	-logy *study of* nephr/o- *kidney*	Medical specialty of diseases of the kidney
nephrologist	neh-**FROL**-oh-jist	S/	-logist *one who studies, specialist*	Medical specialist in disorders of the kidney
nitrogenous (adj)	ni-**TRO**-jen-us	S/ R/CF R/	-ous *pertaining to* nitr/o- *nitrogen* -gen- *create*	Containing or generating nitrogen
renal (adj)	**REE**-nal	S/ R/	-al *pertaining to* ren- *kidney*	Pertaining to the kidney
urea	you-**REE**-ah		Greek *urine*	End product of nitrogen metabolism
ureter	you-**REE**-ter		Greek *urinary canal*	Tube that connects each kidney to the urinary bladder
ureteral (adj)	you-ree-**TER**-al	S/ R/	-al *pertaining to* ureter- *ureter*	Pertaining to a ureter
urine	**YUR**-in		Latin *urine*	Fluid and dissolved substances excreted by the kidney
urinary (adj)	**YUR**-in-ary	S/ R/	-ary *pertaining to* urin- *urine*	Pertaining to urine
urinate (verb) urination	**YUR**-in-ate yur-ih-**NAY**-shun	S/ S/	-ate *composed of, pertaining to* -ation *process*	To pass urine Process of passing urine
urology	yur-**ROL**-oh-jee	S/ R/CF	-logy *study of* ur/o- *urinary system*	Medical specialty that studies the urinary system
urologist urological (adj)	yur-**ROL**-oh-jist yur-roh-**LOJ**-ik-al	S/ S/	-logist *one who studies, specialist* -ical *pertaining to*	Specialist in urology Pertaining to urology

EXERCISE

A. Construct *the following terms by inserting the correct elements. After you insert an element, write the identity (P, R, CF, or S) of the element below the line. Review the terms in the WAD box first. Fill in the blanks.*   **LO 13.1 and 13.4** *Apply*

1. specialist in the urinary system: _____ / _____ / _____

2. containing or generating nitrogen: _____ / _____ / _____

3. pertaining to the ureter: _____ / _____ / _____

4. study of diseases of the kidney: _____ / _____ / _____

5. pertaining to the kidney: _____ / _____ / _____

6. liquid that has passed through a filter: _____ / _____ / _____

Lesson 13.1
(cont'd)

Disorders of the Kidneys (LO 13.4)

Renal cell carcinoma, the most common form of kidney cancer, occurs twice as often in men as in women. The cancer develops in the lining cells of the renal tubules, which is why Mr. Hughes had hematuria. Radical **nephrectomy** is the most common treatment for renal cell carcinoma.

Wilms tumor, or **nephroblastoma,** is a malignant childhood kidney tumor, usually occurring between the ages of 3 and 8. It is treated effectively with a combination of surgery and chemotherapy.

Renal adenomas (benign kidney tumors) are usually asymptomatic (produce no symptoms), are discovered by chance, and are not life threatening.

Hematuria (blood in the urine) can be caused by lesions or stones anywhere in the urinary system. These lesions may result from trauma, infections, and congenital diseases like sickle cell anemia. In microscopic hematuria, the urine is not red, and red blood cells can be seen only under a microscope or identified by a urine dipstick.

Acute glomerulonephritis is an inflammation of the kidney's filtration unit (the nephron). It damages the glomerular capillaries and allows protein and red blood cells to leak into the urine. It can develop rapidly after a strep throat infection, especially in children.

Chronic glomerulonephritis can occur with no history of kidney disease and present as kidney failure. It also occurs in **diabetic nephropathy** and can be associated with autoimmune diseases like lupus erythematosus (a disease of the connective tissues).

Nephrotic syndrome is caused by different disorders that damage the kidneys, causing large amounts of protein to leak into the urine, so the level of protein in the blood drops. The most obvious symptom is fluid retention, with edema of the ankles and legs. This is treated with **diuretics,** by restricting salt in the diet, and by reducing fluid intake. Minimal change disease *(Table 13.1)* is the most common cause in children. Membranous nephropathy *(Table 13.1)* is the most common cause in adults.

Case Report 13.1 (continued)

Mr. Nelson Hughes had been well until a few months before his surgery, when he noticed a vague, aching pain in the left side of his abdomen. One week prior to his surgery, he suddenly passed bright red urine. A urinalysis showed red blood cells **(hematuria)** and a physical examination revealed an enlarged left kidney. **Intravenous pyelogram (IVP)** *(Figure 13.4)* and other imaging tests showed a tumor 3 inches in diameter in the center of his left kidney. His bone scan was normal, indicating no metastases to the bones.

Kidney

Ureter

Urinary bladder

▲ **FIGURE 13.4**
Colored Intravenous Pyelogram (IVP).

▼ **TABLE 13.1**

TYPES OF NEPHROTIC SYNDROME (LO 13.4)

Disease (as Seen on Biopsy)	Description
Minimal change disease	Most common in children; responds to steroids
Focal segmental glomerulosclerosis (FSGS)	Cause unknown; little response to treatment
Membranous nephropathy	Cause unknown; may respond to immunosuppressive treatment
Diabetes	Occurs if blood sugar has been poorly controlled

Word Analysis and Definition

WORD	PRONUNCIATION	ELEMENTS		DEFINITION
diuretic (adj) (**Note:** *The "a" is dropped from dia to enable the word to flow.*)	die-you-**RET**-ik	S/ P/ R/	-etic *pertaining to* di(a)- *complete* -ur- *urine*	Agent that increases urine output
diuresis (noun)	die-you-**REE**-sis	S/	-esis *condition*	Excretion of large volume of urine
glomerulonephritis	glo-**MER**-you-low-nef-**RYE**-tis	S/ R/CF R/	-itis *inflammation* glomerul/o- *glomerulus* -nephr- *kidney*	Infection of the glomeruli of the kidney
hematuria	he-mah-**TYU**-ree-ah	S/ R/	-uria *urine* hemat- *blood*	Blood in the urine
nephrectomy	neh-**FREK**-toe-me	S/ R/	-ectomy *surgical excision* nephr- *kidney*	Surgical removal of a kidney
nephroblastoma (Wilms tumor) Wilms tumor	**NEF**-roh-blas-**TOE**-mah WILMZ **TOO**-mor	S/ R/CF R/	-oma *tumor, mass* nephr/o- *kidney* -blast- *immature cell* Max Wilms, German surgeon, 1867–1918	Cancerous kidney tumor of childhood
nephropathy	neh-**FROP**-ah-thee	S/ R/CF	-pathy *disease* nephr/o- *kidney*	Any disease of the kidney
nephrotic syndrome nephrosis (*same as* nephrotic syndrome)	neh-**FROT**-ik **SIN**-drohm neh-**FROH**-sis	S/ R/CF S/ R/	-tic *pertaining to* nephr/o- *kidney* -osis *condition* nephr- *kidney*	Glomerular disease with marked loss of protein
pyelogram	**PIE**-el-oh-gram	S/ R/CF	-gram *record, recording* pyel/o- *renal pelvis*	X-ray image of renal pelvis and ureters using contrast media

EXERCISES

A. Review *the Case Report on this spread before answering the questions.*   **LO 13.2, 13.3, 13.4, and 13.7** *Understand*

1. What are Mr. Hughes' chief complaints? _____

2. What does the doctor find on physical examination of Mr. Hughes? _____

   _____

3. Define the two medical terms in the abbreviation *IVP.* _____

   _____

4. What does a "normal bone scan" mean for Mr. Hughes? _____

   _____

B. Unscramble *the terms at the right to match them with their definitions. Check the correct spelling in the WAD box. Fill in the blanks.*
   LO 13.2 and 13.4 *Understand*

1. infection of the glomeruli of the kidney: eeopilrnrtohisugml   _____

2. also known as Wilms tumor: hbsaelmoanprto   _____

3. any disease of the kidney: teopyahnprh   _____

4. excretion of large volume of urine: iessudri   _____

5. X-ray image of renal pelvis and ureters: lrgeyoapm   _____

6. blood in the urine: arameithu   _____

Lesson 13.1 Disorders of the Kidneys (continued) (LO 13.4)

(cont'd)

Keynotes

- Acute interstitial nephritis causes 15% of all cases of acute renal failure.
- Acute renal failure is usually reversible.
- Chronic renal failure has no cure.

Abbreviations

ARF	acute renal failure
CAPD	continuous ambulatory peritoneal dialysis
CKD	chronic kidney disease
CRF	chronic renal failure
ESRD	end-stage renal disease
NSAID	nonsteroidal anti-inflammatory drug
PKD	polycystic kidney disease
UTI	urinary tract infection

Interstitial nephritis is an inflammation (often acute and temporary) of the kidney tissue between the renal tubules. It can be an allergic reaction to or a side effect of drugs like penicillin or ampicillin, **NSAIDs,** and diuretics.

Pyelonephritis is an infection of the renal parenchyma, calyces, and pelvis. This usually occurs as part of a total urinary tract infection **(UTI),** beginning in the urinary bladder *(see the next lesson in this chapter).* It has a high mortality rate in the elderly and in people with a compromised immune system.

Polycystic kidney disease (PKD) is an inherited disease. Large fluid-filled cysts grow within the kidneys and press against the kidney tissue. Eventually, the kidneys cannot function effectively.

Acute renal failure (ARF) makes the kidneys suddenly stop filtering waste products from the blood. Initially, **oliguria** and then **anuria** are associated with confusion, seizures, and coma.

The causes of acute renal failure include: severe burns; trauma; septicemia; toxins like mercury and excess alcohol; excessive amounts of drugs like aspirin and ibuprofen; and antibiotics like streptomycin and gentamycin.

When caring for a patient who has ARF, the goal is to treat the underlying disease. **Dialysis** may be necessary while the kidneys are healing.

Chronic renal failure (CRF), or **chronic kidney disease (CKD),** is a gradual loss of renal function. Symptoms and signs may not appear until the kidney's level of functioning is less than 25% of normal. The causes of chronic renal failure are diabetes, hypertension, kidney disease (including chronic glomerulonephritis, nephrotic syndrome), and lead poisoning.

Uremia is the complex of symptoms resulting from excess nitrogenous waste products in the blood, as seen in renal failure.

End-stage renal disease (ESRD) means the kidneys are functioning at less than 10% of their normal capacity. At this point, life cannot be maintained, and either dialysis or a kidney transplant is needed.

Dialysis is an artificial method of removing waste materials and excess fluid from the blood. It is not a cure but can prolong life. There are several types of kidney dialysis:

- **Hemodialysis** *(Figure 13.5)* filters the blood through an artificial kidney machine **(dialyzer).** Most patients require 12 hours of hemodialysis a week, usually in three sessions.

- **Peritoneal dialysis** uses a dialysis solution that is infused into and drained out of your abdominal cavity through a small, flexible, **implanted** catheter. The dialysis solution extracts wastes and excess fluid from the network of capillaries in the peritoneal lining of the abdominal cavity.

- **Continuous ambulatory peritoneal dialysis (CAPD)** is performed by the patient at home through an implanted abdominal catheter *(Figure 13.6),* usually four times a day, 7 days a week.

- **Continuous cycling peritoneal dialysis** uses a machine to automatically infuse dialysis solution into and out of the abdominal cavity during sleep.

Kidney transplant provides a better quality of life than dialysis—if a suitable donor can be found. The donor has to match the recipient's blood type, cell surface proteins, and antibodies. A **sibling** or a blood relative can often qualify as a donor. If not, tissue banks across the country can search for a kidney from an accident victim or a donor who has died.

▲ FIGURE 13.5
Hemodialysis.

▲ FIGURE 13.6
Continuous Ambulatory Peritoneal Dialysis.

Word Analysis and Definition

WORD	PRONUNCIATION	ELEMENTS		DEFINITION
anuria	an-**YOU**-ree-ah	S/ P/ R/	-ia *condition* an- *a lack of, no* -ur- *urine*	Absence of urine production
dialysis	die-**AL**-ih-sis	P/ S/	dia- *complete* -lysis *destruction*	An artificial method of filtration to remove excess waste materials and water from the body
hemodialysis	**HE**-moh-die-**AL**-ih-sis	R/CF	hem/o- *blood*	An artificial method of filtration to remove excess waste materials and water directly from the blood
nephritis	neh-**FRY**-tis	S/ R/	-itis *inflammation* nephr- *kidney*	Inflammation of the kidney
oliguria	ol-ih-**GYUR**-ee-ah	S/ R/ R/	-ia *condition* olig- *scanty* -ur- *urine*	Scanty production of urine
polycystic	pol-ee-**SIS**-tik	S/ P/ R/	-ic *pertaining to* poly- *many* -cyst- *sac, bladder, cyst*	Composed of many cysts
pyelonephritis	**PIE**-eh-loh-neh-**FRY**-tis	S/ R/CF R/	-itis *inflammation* pyel/o- *renal pelvis* -nephr- *kidney*	Inflammation of the kidney and renal pelvis
sibling	**SIB**-ling	S/ R/	-ling *small* sib- *relative*	Brother or sister
transplant	**TRANZ**-plant	P/ R/	trans- *across* -plant *insert, plant*	The act of transferring tissue from one person to another
uremia	you-**REE**-me-ah	S/ R/	-emia *a blood condition* ur- *urine*	The complex of symptoms arising from renal failure

EXERCISES

A. Build your knowledge *of the elements contained in the language of urology. First slash the term into elements. A specific element in each term is bolded. Write the identity (P, R, CF, or S) of the bolded element under it, and write the meaning of that element on the line next to the term.*
LO 13.1 and 13.4 *Apply*

1. **hemo**dialysis   _____

2. **poly**cystic   _____

3. **an**uria   _____

4. ur**emia**   _____

5. **olig**uria   _____

6. **pyelo**nephritis   _____

Remember: Every element at the beginning of a medical term is not necessarily a prefix!

7. Give an example from this exercise: _____

B. Meet chapter and lesson objectives *and use the language of urology for your answers.*   **LO 13.2, 13.3, and 13.4** *Understand*

1. What is the difference between ARF and CRF?

   ARF _____

   CRF _____

2. Which specific kidney disease is inherited? _____

3. Which type of RF has no cure? _____

4. Which diagnosis has a high mortality rate in the elderly? _____

▲ FIGURE 13.7
Urinalysis Dipstick Being
Compared Against Color
Chart on Container.

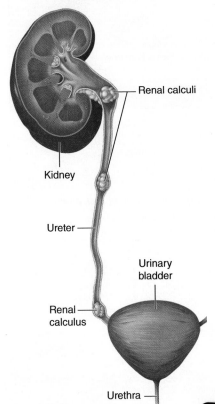

Renal calculi

Kidney

Ureter

Urinary
bladder

Renal
calculus

Urethra

▲ FIGURE 13.8
Renal Calculi.
Calculi can become
lodged at sites along the
urinary tract.

Abbreviations

ESWL	extracorporeal shock wave lithotripsy
IV	intravenous
KUB	X-ray of abdomen to show Kidneys, Ureters, and Bladder

Case Report 13.2

Clinical Note   **Emergency Department, Fulwood Medical Center**
9/12/14

Mr. Justin Leandro, a 37-year-old construction worker, presented at 1520 hrs. He complained of a sudden onset of excruciating pain in his right abdomen and back an hour previously, while at work. The pain is spasmodic and radiates down into his **groin**.

He has vomited once, and keeps having the urge to urinate. He has no previous medical history of significance.

VS: T 99.4°F, P 92, R 20, BP 130/86.

Patient's abdomen is slightly distended, with tenderness in the right upper and lower quadrants and **flank**. A **dipstick** (Figure 13.7) test showed blood in his urine.

Provisional diagnosis by Mark Eagle, MD: stone in the right ureter.

An IV line was started, and 2 mg of morphine sulfate was given by IV push at 1540 hrs. He is going to X-ray STAT for KUB and IVP.

—Andrea Facundo, EMT-P, 1555 hrs.

The Ureters (LO 13.4, and 13.7)

Each ureter is a muscular tube, about 10 inches long and ¼ inch wide. The ureters carry urine from the renal pelvis to the urinary bladder. Each ureter lies on the posterior abdominal wall. This is why Mr. Leandro had pain in his back.

The ureters pass obliquely through the bladder's muscle wall. As pressure builds in the filling bladder, the muscle wall compresses the ureters and prevents urine from being forced back up the ureters to the kidneys (**reflux).**

In addition to gravity, muscular **peristaltic** waves, originating in the renal pelvis, squeeze urine down the ureters and squirt it into the bladder. The peristaltic waves are intermittent (come and go), which is why Mr. Leandro's pain was spasmodic.

Kidney and Ureteral Stones (Nephrolithiasis)
(LO 13.4, and 13.7)

Stones (**calculi**) begin in the pelvis of the kidney as a tiny grain of undissolved material, usually the minerals uric acid or calcium oxalate (Figure 13.8). When the urine flows out of the kidney, this grain of material is left behind. Over time, more material is deposited and a stone is formed. Most stones enter one of the ureters while they are still small enough to pass down the ureter into the bladder and out of the body in urine.

Case Report 13.2 (continued)

Mr. Leandro's KUB (X-ray of **k**idney, **u**reter, and **b**ladder) showed a suspicious lesion halfway down his right ureter. IVP confirmed that this was a stone (renal **calculus**) blocking the ureter and showed the pelvis of the right kidney to be slightly dilated.

Mr. Leandro's stone was large enough to be lodged in the ureter, blocking the flow of urine, with the backflow pressure leading to **hydronephrosis** of the kidney.

Mr. Leandro was kept in the hospital overnight with IV pain medication but did not pass the stone. **Extracorporeal shock wave lithotripsy (ESWL)** was successful in crumbling the stone. He urinated through a strainer so that the stone fragments could be recovered and chemically analyzed.

Word Analysis and Definition

S = Suffix   P = Prefix   R = Root   R/CF = Combining Form

WORD	PRONUNCIATION	ELEMENTS		DEFINITION
calculus calculi (pl)	KAL-kyu-lus KAL-kyu-lie		Latin *pebble*	Small stone
dipstick	DIP-stik			A strip of plastic or paper bearing squares of reagent that change color to indicate presence of chemicals
extracorporeal	EKS-tra-kor-**POH**-ree-al	S/ P/ R/	-eal *pertaining to* extra- *outside* -corpor- *body*	Outside the body
flank	FLANK		Latin *broad*	Side of the body between the pelvis and the ribs
groin	GROYN		Old English *groin*	Crease where the thigh joins the abdomen
hydronephrosis	HIGH-droh-neh-**FRO**-sis	S/ R/CF R/CF	-osis *condition* hydr/o- *water* -nephr/o- *kidney*	Dilation of the pelvis and calyces of a kidney
hydronephrotic (adj)	HIGH-droh-neh-**FROT**-ik	S/	-tic *pertaining to*	Pertaining to or suffering from the dilation of the pelvis and calyces of the kidney
lithotripsy	**LITH**-oh-trip-see	S/ R/CF	-tripsy *crushing* lith/o- *stone*	Crushing stones by sound waves
lithotripter	**LITH**-oh-trip-ter	S/	-tripter *crusher*	Instrument that generates sound waves
nephrolithiasis	NEF-roe-lih-**THIGH**-ah-sis	S/ R/CF R/	-iasis *condition, state of* nephr/o- *kidney* -lith- *stone*	Presence of a kidney stone
peristalsis	per-ih-**STAL**-sis	P/ R/	peri- *around* -stalsis *constrict*	Waves of alternate contraction and relaxation of the muscle wall of a tube

EXERCISES

A. Review *the Case Report on this spread before answering the questions.*   **LO 13.2, 13.3, 13.4, and 13.7** *Understand*

1. Where in the Case Report can abbreviations be substituted for medical terms? _____

2. Where is Mr. Leandro's stone lodged, and what is it blocking? _____

3. What are his diagnoses? _____

4. What procedure will he have as part of his treatment plan? _____

5. What is the medical term for *blood in the urine?* _____

6. Why was Mr. Leandro given morphine? _____

7. What is the medical term for a kidney stone? _____

8. What diagnostic tests were ordered for Mr. Leandro? _____

9. What is *urinary reflux?* _____

B. Match *the element in column 1 with the correct meaning in column 2.*   **LO 13.1 and 13.4** *Understand*

_____ **1.** extra	**A.** body	
_____ **2.** lith	**B.** crushing	
_____ **3.** corpor	**C.** water	
_____ **4.** tripsy	**D.** stone	
_____ **5.** hydro	**E.** outside	

Lesson 13.2

Urinary Bladder and Urethra

Objectives

*The urinary bladder is a temporary storage place for urine before it is **voided** through the **urethra**. A moderately full bladder contains about 500 mL (1 pint) of urine. The maximum capacity of the bladder is around 750 to 800 mL (1½ pints). **Urination**, or emptying of the bladder, is also called **micturition**. The information in this lesson will enable you to use correct medical terminology to:*

13.2.1 Describe the structure and functions of the urinary bladder.

13.2.2 Contrast the differences in structure of the male and female urethras and the incidence of urinary tract infections in the two sexes.

13.2.3 Discuss common disorders of the bladder and urethra.

Case Report 13.3

You are ...

... a medical assistant working in the office of Dr. Susan Lee, a primary care physician, at Fulwood Medical Center.

You are communicating with ...

... Mrs. Caroline Dobson, a 32-year-old housewife. You have asked her the reason for her visit to the office today.

   Mrs. Dobson: "Since yesterday afternoon, I've had a lot of pain low down in my belly and in my lower back. I keep having to go to the bathroom every hour or so to pee. It's often difficult to start, and it burns as it comes out. I've had this problem twice before when I was pregnant with my two kids, so I've started drinking cranberry juice. I've been shivering since I woke up this morning, and the last urine I passed was pink. Was that due to the cranberry juice?"

The Urinary Bladder and Urethra (LO 13.5)

Urinary Bladder (LO 13.5)

The urinary bladder is a hollow, muscular organ on the floor of the pelvic cavity, posterior to the pubic symphysis *(Figure 13.9)*.

Urethra (LO 13.5)

The urethra, a thin-walled tube, transports urine from the floor of the bladder to the outside. The base of the bladder's muscular wall is thickened to form the **internal urethral sphincter.** As the urethra passes through the skeletal muscles of the pelvic floor, the **external urethral sphincter** provides voluntary control of urination.

   In the male *(Figure 13.9a)*, the urethra is 7 to 8 inches long and passes through the penis. In the female *(Figure 13.9b)*, the urethra is only about 1½ inches long, and it opens to the outside just above the vagina.

   In both the male and female, the opening of the urethra to the outside is called the **external urinary meatus.**

Micturition (LO 13.5)

When the bladder contains about 200 mL or 7 fluid ounces (just less than a cup) of urine, stretch receptors in its wall trigger the **micturition reflex.** Parasympathetic nerves stimulate the bladder's muscle wall to contract and the internal sphincter to relax, and the need to urinate feels urgent. However, voluntary control of the external sphincter can keep that sphincter contracted and can hold urine in the bladder until urination is initiated voluntarily. Involuntary micturition during sleep in older children or adults is called **enuresis.**

Ureter
Ureteral openings
Internal urethral sphincter
Prostate gland
Prostatic urethra
Pelvic floor
External urethral sphincter
Spongy (penile) urethra
Penis
External urinary meatus

(a)

Ureter
Ureteral openings
Internal urethral sphincter
External urethral sphincter
External urinary meatus

(b)

▲ **FIGURE 13.9**
Urinary Bladder.
(a) Male anatomy. (b) Female anatomy.

Word Analysis and Definition

S = Suffix   P = Prefix   R = Root   R/CF = Combining Form

WORD	PRONUNCIATION	ELEMENTS		DEFINITION
enuresis	en-you-**REE**-sis	S/ R/	-esis *condition* enur- *urinate* in	Involuntary bedwetting
meatus	me-**AY**-tus		Latin *a passage*	The external opening of a passage
micturition (noun) micturate (verb)	mik-choo-**RISH**-un **MIK**-choo-rate	S/ R/ S/	-ition *process* mictur- *pass urine* -ate *pertaining to*	Act of passing urine Pass urine
reflex	**REE**-fleks		Latin *to bend back*	An involuntary response to a stimulus
sphincter	**SFINK**-ter		Greek *a band*	A band of muscle that encircles an opening; when it contracts, the opening squeezes closed
urethra (**Note:** *One "e" = one tube.*) urethral	you-**REE**-thra	S/ R/	Greek *passage for urine* -al *pertaining to* urethr- *urethra*	Tube that carries urine from bladder to outside Pertaining to the urethra
void (verb)	**VOYD**		Latin *to empty*	To evacuate urine or feces
voluntary involuntary	**VOL**-un-tare-ee in-**VOL**-un-tare-ee	P/	Latin *voluntary* in- *not*	Acting in obedience to the will Independent of or contrary to the will

EXERCISES

A. Reread *the Case Report on the opposite page and review all the terms and elements in the WAD box above. Fill in the blanks.*
   LO 13.2, 13.5, and 13.7 *Understand*

1. List all of Mrs. Dobson's symptoms:

   _____

   _____

   _____

   _____

2. Has Mrs. Dobson ever had this condition before?

   _____

3. If Dr. Lee feels that Mrs. Dobson might need a referral to a specialist, what kind of specialist would she recommend?

   _____

4. According to the terms in the WAD, what symptom does Mrs. Dobson not have?

   _____

5. What substance may be in Mrs. Dobson's urine, as indicated by the urine's pink color? _____

B. Apply your knowledge *of the language of urology to answer the following questions relating to chapter and lesson objectives.*
   LO 13.2, 13.5, and 13.7 *Apply*

1. Describe the location, structure, and function of the urinary bladder: _____

   _____

   _____

2. What is the function of a sphincter? _____

3. Voiding and micturition can both be used to mean which body function? _____

   _____

4. What is the function of a meatus? _____

   _____

Lesson 13.2

(cont'd)

Disorders of the Urinary Bladder and Urethra

(LO 13.2, 13.5, and 13.8)

Keynotes

- Ten million doctor visits each year are for UTIs.
- Incontinence is not a way of life. It can be helped.
- Cigarette smoking contributes to more than 50% of bladder cancers.

Abbreviation

UTI   urinary tract infection

Urinary Tract Infection (UTI) (LO 13.5)

A urinary tract infection occurs when bacteria invade and multiply in the urinary tract. The bacteria's point of entry is through the urethra. Because the female urethra is shorter than that of the male and opens to the surface near the anus *(Figure 13.10)*. bacteria from the GI tract, like *E. coli*, can more easily invade the female urethra. This is why women are more prone to UTIs than men. Once UTIs have occurred, they often recur.

Case Report 13.3 *(continued)*

Mrs. Dobson described many of the symptoms of cystitis. She had **suprapubic** and lower back pain. She had increased frequency of micturition with **dysuria** (difficulty with and pain or burning on urination). Her pink urine is probably hematuria.

An infection of the urethra is called **urethritis; cystitis** is an infection of the urinary bladder. If cystitis is untreated, infection can spread up the ureters to the renal pelvis, causing **pyelitis.** The infection can then travel to the renal cortex and nephrons, causing pyelonephritis.

Pyelonephritis, an inflammation of the renal parenchyma, calyces, and pelvis, is commonly caused by bacterial infection that has spread up the urinary tract, often in association with structural abnormalities in the urinary tract, kidney stones, prostate disease, or **vesicoureteral reflux.** 70- to 80% of the infections are caused by *E. coli* and require aggressive, appropriate antibiotic therapy.

The diagnosis of a UTI can be made through a urinalysis. A culture of the infection-causing organism and testing of its sensitivity to different antibiotics allows the appropriate antibiotic therapy to be prescribed. Cranberry juice can make the urine more acidic and resistant to infection.

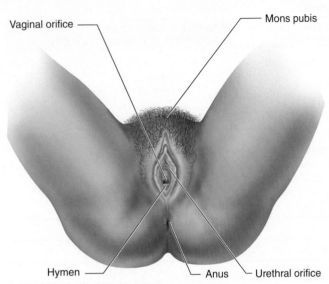

Vaginal orifice — Mons pubis

Hymen — — Anus — Urethral orifice

▲ **FIGURE 13.10**
Female External Genitalia.

Urinary Incontinence (LO 13.5)

Urinary incontinence is a loss of bladder control, which results in wet clothes and bedding. About 12 million adults in America have this condition. Urinary incontinence is most common in women over the age of 50, and it's also seen frequently in elderly men. However, aging alone is not a cause of urinary incontinence.

- **Stress incontinence** is the loss of urine when pressure is exerted on the bladder by coughing, laughing, exercising, or lifting.
- **Urge incontinence** is a sudden, intense urge to urinate followed by an involuntary loss of urine.
- **Overflow incontinence** is the frequent or constant dribbling of urine. It can occur with a damaged bladder; blocked urethra; nerve damage from diabetes, multiple sclerosis, or spinal cord injury; and in men with prostate gland hypertrophy.
- **Functional incontinence** occurs in older adults when a physical or mental impairment prevents them from getting to the toilet in time.
- **Mixed incontinence** is when there are more than one type of incontinence producing symptoms.
- **Total incontinence** is the continuous leakage of urine day and night.

Urinary Retention (LO 13.5)

Urinary retention is the abnormal, involuntary holding of urine in the bladder. **Acute retention** can be caused by an obstruction in the urinary system, like an enlarged prostate in the male. Neurologic problems, like multiple sclerosis, can also be responsible. **Chronic retention** can be caused by an untreated obstruction in the urinary tract, like an enlarged prostate gland.

Bladder Cancer (LO 13.5)

Bladder cancer is more common in men than in women. In fact, it's the fourth most common cancer in men and the eighth most common in women.

Word Analysis and Definition

S = Suffix   P = Prefix   R = Root   R/CF = Combining Form

WORD	PRONUNCIATION	ELEMENTS		DEFINITION
cystitis	sis-**TIE**-tis	S/ R/	-itis *inflammation* cyst- *bladder*	Inflammation of the urinary bladder
dysuria	dis-**YOU**-ree-ah	S/ P/ R/	-ia *condition* dys- *bad, difficult* -ur- *urine*	Difficulty or pain with urination
incontinence	in-**KON**-tin-ence	S/ P/ R/	-ence *state of* in- *not* -contin- *hold together*	Inability to prevent discharge of urine or feces
incontinent	in-**KON**-tin-ent	S/	-ent *pertaining to*	Denoting incontinence
pyelitis	pie-eh-**LYE**-tis	S/ R/	-itis *inflammation* pyel- *renal pelvis*	Inflammation of the renal pelvis
pyelonephritis	**PIE**-eh-loe-neh-**FRIE**-tis	S/ R/ R/CF	-itis *inflammation* nephr- *kidney* pyel/o *pelvis*	inflammation of the kidney and renal pelvis
retention	ree-**TEN**-shun		Latin *hold back*	Holding back in the body what should normally be discharged (e.g., urine)
suprapubic	**SOO**-prah-**PYU**-bik	S/ P/ R/	-ic *pertaining to* supra- *above* -pub- *pubis*	Above the symphysis pubis
urethritis	you-ree-**THRI**-tis	S/ R/	-itis *inflammation* urethr- *urethra*	Inflammation of the urethra
vesicoureteral reflux	**VEE**-sik-oh-you-**REE**-ter-al **REE**-flucks	S/ R/CF R/ P/ R/	-al *pertaining to* vesic/o- *bladder* -ureter- *ureter* re- *back* -flux *flow*	Backward flow of urine from the bladder into the ureter.

EXERCISES

A. Review *the Case Report on this spread before answering the questions.*   **LO 13.2, 13.5, and 13.7** *Understand*

1. Mrs. Dobson was diagnosed with dysuria and hematuria. Explain to Mrs. Dobson, in language she can understand, the difference in the medical terms.

   Dysuria _____

   Hematuria _____

2. Describe on the body the location of *suprapubic* pain. _____

3. What is the diagnosis for Mrs. Dobson? _____

4. Define the diagnosis in question 3 above. _____

B. Deconstruct *the language of urology found in the WAD above. Knowledge of elements is your best key to understanding the meaning of a term. Slash the terms in column 1 into elements, and fill in the chart. Then fill in the blanks.*   **LO 13.1 and 13.2** *Analyze*

Medical Term	Meaning of Root/CF	Meaning of Suffix	Meaning of Term
pyelitis	**1.**	**2.**	**3.**
urethritis	**4.**	**5.**	**6.**
cystitis	**7.**	**8.**	**9.**

10. How are the terms in the chart the same? _____

    _____

11. How are they different? _____

    _____

12. What, then, is *pyelonephritis?* _____

    _____

Lesson 13.2

(cont'd)

Methods of Urine Collection

- Random urine collection is taken with no precautions regarding contamination. It is often used for collecting drug testing samples.

- Early morning urine collection is used to determine the ability of the kidneys to concentrate urine following overnight dehydration.

- Clean-catch, midstream urine specimen is collected after the external urethral meatus is cleaned. The first part of the urine is passed, and the sterile collecting vessel is introduced into the urinary stream to collect the last part.

- Twenty-four-hour urine collection is used to determine the amount of protein being excreted and to estimate the kidneys' filtration ability.

- Suprapubic transabdominal needle aspiration of the bladder is used in newborns and small infants to obtain a pure sample of urine.

- Catheterization of the bladder can be used as a last resort to obtain a urine specimen. A soft plastic or rubber tube (catheter) is inserted through the urethra into the bladder to drain and collect urine.

Diagnostic Procedures
(LO 13.6)

Urinalysis (LO 13.3, and 13.6)

A **dipstick** (a plastic strip bearing paper squares of reagent) is the most cost-effective method of screening urine *(Figure 13.11)*. After the stick is dipped into the urine specimen, the color change in each segment of the dipstick is compared to a color chart on the container. Dipsticks can screen for pH, specific gravity, protein, blood, glucose, ketones, bilirubin, **nitrite,** and leukocyte esterase *(see below)*.

A **routine urinalysis (UA)** in the lab can include the following tests:

- **Visual observation** examines color and clarity. Normal, healthy urine is pale yellow or amber in color and clear. Cloudiness indicates excess cells or cellular material. Red and cloudy indicates red blood cells.

- **Odor** of normal urine has a slight "nutty" scent. Infected urine has a foul odor. **Ketosis** gives urine a fruity odor.

- **pH** measures how acidic or alkaline urine is.

- **Specific gravity (SG)** measures how dilute or concentrated the urine is.

- **Protein** is not normally detected in urine; its presence (**proteinuria**) indicates infection or urinary tract disease.

- **Glucose** in the urine (**glycosuria**) is a spillover of sugar into the urine when the nephrons are damaged or diseased, or blood sugar is high in uncontrolled diabetes.

- **Ketones** are present in the urine in diabetic **ketoacidosis** *(see Chapter 12)* or in starvation.

- **Leukocyte esterase** indicates the presence of white blood cells in the urine, which can point to a UTI.

- **Urine culture** from a clean-catch specimen *(see box)* is the definitive test for a UTI.

A **microscopic urinalysis** is performed on the solids deposited by centrifuging a specimen of urine. It can reveal:

- **Red blood cells (RBCs), white blood cells (WBCs),** and renal tubular epithelial cells stuck together to form **casts,** WBCs stuck together to form casts, and bacteria.

Other Diagnostic Procedures
(LO 13.3, and 13.6)

Other diagnostic procedures used to test for urinary bladder and urethra infections include:

- **KUB.** An x-ray of the abdomen shows the kidneys, ureters, and bladder.

- **Intravenous pyelogram (IVP).** A contrast material containing iodine is injected intravenously, and its progress through the urinary tract is recorded on a series of x-ray images.

- **Retrograde pyelogram.** Contrast material is injected through a urinary catheter into the ureters and kidneys to locate stones and other obstructions.

- **Voiding cystourethrogram (VCUG).** Contrast material is inserted into the bladder through a catheter and x-rays are taken as the patient voids.

- **CT scan.** X-ray images show cross-sectional views of the kidneys and bladder.

- **MRI.** Magnetic fields are used to generate cross-sectional images of the urinary tract.

- **Ultrasound imaging.** High-frequency sound waves and a computer generate noninvasive images of the kidneys.

- **Renal angiogram.** X-rays with contrast material are used to assess blood flow to the kidneys.

- **Cystoscopy.** A pencil-thin, flexible, tube-like optical instrument is inserted through the urethra into the bladder to examine the bladder's lining and to take a biopsy if needed *(Figure 13.12)*.

Abbreviations

IVP	Intravenous pyelogram
RBC	red blood cell
SG	specific gravity
UA	urinalysis
VCUG	voiding cystourethrogram
WBC	white blood cell

▲ **FIGURE 13.11**
Urinalysis Dipstick Being Compared Against Color Chart on Container.

▲ **FIGURE 13.12**
Cystoscopy.

Word Analysis and Definition

WORD	PRONUNCIATION	ELEMENTS		DEFINITION
cast	KAST		Latin pure	A cylindrical mold formed by materials in kidney tubules
cystoscope	SIS-toh-skope	S/	-scope instrument for viewing	An endoscope inserted to view the inside of the bladder
		R/CF	cyst/o- bladder	
cystoscopy	sis-TOS-koh-pee	S/	-scopy to examine	The process of using a cystoscope
cystourethrogram	sis-toh-you-REETH-roe-gram	S/	-gram a record	X-ray image during voiding to show structure and function of bladder and urethra
		R/CF	cyst/o- bladder	
		R/CF	-urethr/o- urethra	
glycosuria (Note: The "s" is added to make the word flow.)	GLYE-koh-SYU-ree-ah	S/	-ia condition	Presence of glucose in urine
		R/CF	glyc/o- glucose	
		R/	-ur- urinary system	
ketone	KEY-tone		Greek acetone	Chemical formed in uncontrolled diabetes or in starvation
ketosis	key-TOE-sis	S/	-sis abnormal condition	Excess production of ketones
		R/CF	ket/o- ketones	
ketoacidosis	KEY-toe-as-ih-DOE-sis	R/CF	-acid/o- acid, low pH	Excessive production of ketones, making the blood acid
nitrite	NI-trite		Greek niter, saltpeter	Chemical formed in urine by E. coli and other microorganisms
proteinuria	pro-tee-NYU-ree-ah	S/	-ia condition	Presence of protein in urine
		R/	protein- protein	
		R/	-uri- urine	
retrograde	RET-roh-grade	P/	retro- backward	Reversal of a normal flow; for example, back from the bladder into the ureters
		R/	-grade going	
urinalysis	you-rih-NAL-ih-sis	S/	-lysis to separate	Examination of urine to separate it into its elements and define their kind and/or quantity
		R/CF	urin/a- urine	

EXERCISES

A. Apply your knowledge *of medical language to this exercise. All the questions can be answered using terms from this spread. Circle the best answer.*

LO 13.1 and 13.6 *Apply*

1. An x-ray image taken during voiding: retrograde pyelogram   angiogram   cystourethrogram

2. Presence of glucose in urine: hematuria   polyuria   glycosuria

3. Urine collection method to test for proteinuria: catheterization   24 hour   clean catch

4. Reversal of normal flow: reflex   retrograde   regenerate

5. Excessive ketones in the blood, making it acid: ketosis   ketoacidosis   ketone

6. Separate urine into its elements: urinalysis   cystourethrogram   retrograde pyelogram

B. Demonstrate your knowledge *of abbreviations and the medical terms they represent. Write out in medical terms what each abbreviation represents.*

LO 13.3 and 13.6 *Remember*

1. KUB _____

2. UA _____

3. IVP _____

4. VCUG _____

C. Employ *the language of urology and match the correct diagnostic procedure in column 1 with the correct statement in column 2.*

LO 13.3, and 13.6 *Understand*

_____ 1. KUB   **A.** uses contrast material

_____ 2. cystoscopy   **B.** X-ray

_____ 3. renal angiogram   **C.** invasive procedure

_____ 4. CT scan   **D.** cross-sectional views

_____ 5. ultrasound imaging   **E.** noninvasive procedure

Lesson 13.2
(cont'd)
Urinary Tract Pharmacology
(LO 13.2 and 13.6)

The kidneys represent 0.5% of total body weight but receive approximately 25% of the total arterial blood pumped by the heart. When necessary, **diuretics** are prescribed to increase the output of urine in order to maintain homeostasis. There are several types of diuretics:

1. **Thiazides** are medium-potency diuretics used in mild heart failure and moderate hypertension. Examples are chlorothiazide (Diuril) and hydrochlorthiazide (HydroDiuril). A major side effect is loss of potassium.

2. **Loop diuretics** have a strong but brief diuresis and are the most potent diuretics available. The most commonly used is furosemide (Lasix), and it also has a major side effect of potassium loss.

3. **Potassium-sparing diuretics** such as spironolactone (Aldactone), which has been used since 1959 and is gradually being replaced by newer agents such as eplerenone (Inspra), are used for reducing cardiovascular risk following myocardial infarction. **Hyperkalemia** can be a side effect. All of these are not potent diuretics.

4. **Carbonic anhydrase inhibitors** such as acetazolamide (Diamox) are not in use as diuretics anymore, but they are used in open-angle glaucoma (*see Chapter 11*) and to prevent altitude sickness in mountain climbers.

5. An **osmotic diuretic,** such as mannitol (Osmitrol), is given intravenously and used occasionally to prevent renal failure or decrease intracranial pressure.

Alcohol also acts as a diuretic.

Uric acid, in the form of sodium urate crystals, contributes to the formation of kidney stones and produces the pain of gout when deposited in joints. **Uricosuric agents,** such as probenecid (Probalan), increase the excretion of uric acid by the kidneys and are used to prevent recurrences of kidney stones and to treat gout.

Medications used to treat incontinence include:

- **Anticholinergics,** which calm an overactive bladder and include oxybutynin (Ditropan), tolterodine (Detrol), and darifenacin (Enablex).

- **Antidepressants** imipramine (Tofranil) and duloxetine (Cymbalta) may be used to treat stress incontinence.

Word Analysis and Definition

WORD	PRONUNCIATION	ELEMENTS		DEFINITION
anticholinergic	AN-tee-koh-lih-NER-jik	S/ P/ R/ R/	-ic *pertaining to* anti- *against* -cholin- *choline* -erg- *work*	Antagonistic to parasympathetic nerve fibers
antidepressant	AN-tee-dee-PRESS-ant	S/ P/ R/	-ant *pertaining to* anti- *against* -depress- *press down*	An agent used to counteract depression
hyperkalemia	HIGH-per-kah-LEE-me-ah	S/ P/ R/	-emia *blood condition* hyper- *excess* -kal- *potassium*	An excessive amount of potassium in the blood
osmosis	os-MOH-sis	S/ R/	-sis *process* osmo- *push*	The passage of a solvent across a cell membrane
osmotic (adj)	os-MOT-ik	S/	-tic *pertaining to*	
potent	POH-tent		Latin *power*	Possessing strength, power
thiazide	THIGH-ah-zide	S/ R/	-ide *having a special quality* thiaz- *blue dye*	Abbreviated form of benzothiadiazide, a class of diuretic
uric acid uricosuric	YUR-ik ASS-id YUR-ih-koh-SU-rik	S/ R/CF	Latin *relating to urine* -suric *excess* uric/o *urine*	A chemical of white crystals poorly soluble in urine Pertaining to excessive amounts of uric acid in urine

EXERCISES

A. Deconstruct *the following medical terms into their elements and give the meaning of each term:*   **LO 13.1 and 13.6** *Analyze*

1. osmotic _____ / _____ / _____

                            P   R, R/CF   S

    Meaning: _____

    _____

2. vesicoureteral _____ / _____ / _____

                               P   R, R/CF   S

    Meaning: _____

    _____

3. antidepressant _____ / _____ / _____

                               P   R, R/CF   S

    Meaning: _____

    _____

4. hyperkalemia _____ / _____ / _____

                               P   R, R/CF   S

    Meaning: _____

    _____

5. reflux _____ / _____ / _____

                               P   R, R/CF   S

    Meaning: _____

    _____

Chapter Review exercises, along with additional practice items, are available in Connect!

The Male Reproductive System

The Essentials of the Language of the Male Reproductive System

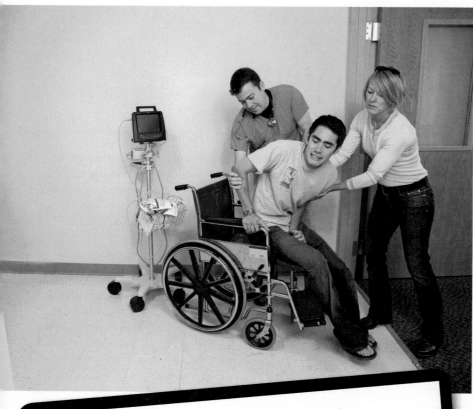

CHAPTER 14

Learning Outcomes

As you set up the next stage of Joseph's treatment, immediate clinical decisions will need to be made. You will have to communicate clearly with Dr. Helinski, other health professionals, the patient, and the patient's family. You will also need to document the patient's care. In order to participate effectively in this process, you must be able to:

LO 14.1 Use roots, combining forms, suffixes, and prefixes to construct and analyze (deconstruct) medical terms related to the male reproductive system.

LO 14.2 Spell and pronounce correctly medical terms related to the male reproductive system in order to communicate them with accuracy and precision in any health care setting.

LO 14.3 Define accepted abbreviations related to the male reproductive system.

LO 14.4 Describe the anatomy of the perineum, scrotum, testes, and spermatic cords and their functions, disorders, and treatments.

LO 14.5 Relate the anatomy and anatomical positions of the five accessory glands of the male reproductive system to their functions and disorders.

LO 14.6 Describe disorders of the prostate gland and their diagnosis and treatment.

LO 14.7 Relate the structure of the penis to its functions, disorders, and treatments.

LO 14.8 Explain the causes of male infertility and their treatments.

LO 14.9 Identify sexually transmitted diseases, their prevention, and treatments.

LO 14.10 Apply your knowledge of medical terms relating to the male reproductive system to documentation, medical records, and medical reports.

LO 14.11 Translate the medical terms relating to the male reproductive system into everyday language in order to communicate clearly with patients and their families.

Case Report 14.1

You are . . .

. . . an EMT-P working in the Emergency Department at Fulwood Medical Center.

You are communicating with . . .

. . . Joseph Davis, a 17-year-old high school senior, who has been brought in by his mother at 0400 hrs.

Joseph is complaining of **(c/o)** a sudden onset of pain in his left **testicle**, which began 3 hours earlier and woke him up. The pain is intense and has made him vomit. VS: T 99.2°F, P 88, R 15, BP 130/70. An examination reveals his left testicle to be enlarged, warm, and tender. His abdomen is normal to palpation.

At your request, Dr. Helinski, the emergency physician on duty, examines Joseph immediately. He diagnoses a **torsion** (twisting) of the patient's left testicle.

The health professionals involved in the diagnosis and treatment of problems with the male reproductive system include:

- Urologists, who are specialists in the diagnosis and treatment of diseases of the urinary system.
- Nurse practitioners, physicians' assistants, and technologists with special training and expertise also provide urologic patient care.

Lesson 14.1

The Male Reproductive System

Male Reproductive System
(LO 14.4, 14.5, and 14.7)

The **male reproductive organ system** *(Figure 14.1)* consists of the primary and secondary sex organs, and the accessory glands. These are categorized as follows:

1. The **primary sex organs,** or **gonads,** are the two **testes.**

2. The **secondary sex organs** include:

   a. The **penis;**

   b. The **scrotum;** and

   c. A system of ducts, including the **epididymis, ductus (vas) deferens,** and **urethra.**

3. The accessory glands include:

   a. The **prostate;**

   b. The **seminal vesicles;** and

   c. The **bulbourethral glands.**

Perineum (LO 14.4)

The external **genitalia** (the penis, scrotum, and testes) occupy the **perineum,** a diamond-shaped region between the thighs. The perineum borders the pubic symphysis anteriorly and the coccyx posteriorly *(Figure 14.2).* The anus is also in the perineum.

Scrotum (LO 14.4)

The scrotum is a skin-covered sac between the upper thighs. It is divided into two compartments. Each compartment contains a testis. The scrotum's function is to provide a cooler environment for the testes than that inside the body. **Sperm** are best produced and stored at a few degrees cooler than that of the male's internal body temperature.

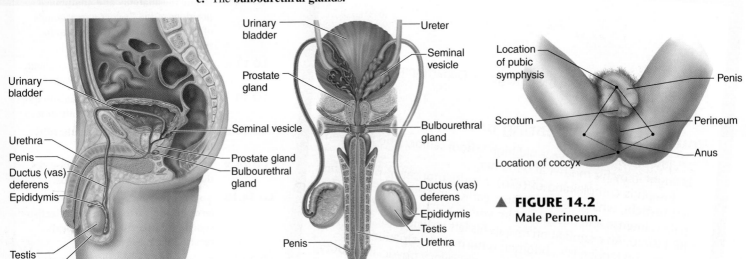

▲ **FIGURE 14.2**
Male Perineum.

▲ **FIGURE 14.1**
Male Reproductive System.
(a) Male pelvic cavity, midsagittal section.
(b) Male reproductive organs.

Word Analysis and Definition

S = Suffix   P = Prefix   R = Root   R/CF = Combining Form

WORD	PRONUNCIATION	ELEMENTS		DEFINITION
bulbourethral	BUL-boh-you-REE-thral	S/ R/CF R/	-al *pertaining to* bulb/o- *bulb* -urethr- *urethra*	Pertaining to the bulbous penis and urethra
ductus deferens *(same as* **vas deferens***)*	DUK-tus DEH-fuh-renz VAS		ductus, Latin *to lead* deferens, Latin *carry away* vas, Latin *vessel, canal*	Tube that receives sperm from the epididymis
epididymis	EP-ih-DID-ih-miss	P/ R/	epi- *above* -didymis *testis*	Coiled tube attached to testis
genitalia (Note: *Two suffixes*) genital (adj)	JEN-ih-TAY-lee-ah JEN-ih-tal	S/ S/ R/	-ia *condition* -al- *pertaining to* genit- *primary male or female sex organs*	External and internal organs of reproduction Pertaining to reproduction or to the male or female sex organs
gonad gonads (pl) gonadal	GO-nad GO-nadz	 S/	Greek *seed* -al *pertaining to*	Testis or ovary Pertaining to the testis or ovary
penis penile (adj)	PEE-nis PEE-nile	 S/ R/	Latin *tail* -ile *pertaining to* pen- *penis*	Conveys urine and semen to the outside Pertaining to the penis
perineum perineal (adj)	PER-ih-NEE-um PER-ih-NEE-al	 S/ R/	Greek *perineum* -al *pertaining to* perine- *perineum*	Area between the thighs, extending from the coccyx to the pubis Pertaining to the perineum
scrotum scrotal (adj)	SKRO-tum SKRO-tal	 S/ R/	Latin *scrotum* -al *pertaining to* scrot- *scrotum*	Sac containing the testes Pertaining to the scrotum
seminal vesicle	SEM-in-al VES-ih-kull	S/ R/ S/ R/	-al *pertaining to* semin- *semen* -le *small* vesic- *sac containing fluid*	Sac of the ductus deferens that produces seminal fluid
sperm spermatozoa (pl) spermatic (adj) spermatogenesis	SPERM SPER-mat-oh-ZOH-ah SPER-mat-ik SPER-mat-oh-JEN-eh-sis	 S/ R/CF S/ S/	Greek *seed* -zoa *animal* spermat/o- *sperm* -ic *pertaining to* -genesis *creation, formation*	Mature male sex cell Sperm (plural) Pertaining to sperm The process by which male germ cells differentiate into sperm
testicle testicular (adj) testis testes (pl)	TES-tih-kul tes-TICK-you-lar TES-tis TES-teez	 S/ R/	Latin *small testis* -ar *pertaining to* testicul- *testicle* Latin *testis*	One of the male reproductive glands Pertaining to the testicle Same as testicle
torsion	TOR-shun		Latin *to twist*	The act or result of twisting

EXERCISES

A. Review *the Case Report on the opening spread before answering the questions.*   **LO 14.4 and 14.10** *Understand*

1. What is the site of Joseph Davis's intense pain? _____

2. What is *palpation?* _____

3. What does *torsion* mean? _____

B. Documentation: *You could be working in the Emergency Department when this patient comes in. Take the information presented in Case Report 14.1 and document the case in the patient's record.*   **LO 14.4 and 14.10** *Apply*

1. This patient presented to the ED because of pain in his left _____.

2. Both _____ were examined, but the left _____ was enlarged, warm, and tender.

3. The emergency physician on duty diagnosed _____; patient will be scheduled for emergency surgery.

Testes and Spermatic Cord (LO 14.4)

Testes (LO 14.4)

Keynotes

- The sperm count of a 65-year-old man is approximately one-third of the count when he was 20.
- The spermatic cord can be palpated through the skin of the scrotum.

Abbreviation

BMR   basal metabolic rate

In the adult male, each testis is a small, oval organ that measures about 2 inches long and ¾ of an inch wide *(Figure 14.3)*. Each testis is covered by a serous membrane—the **tunica vaginalis**—which has outer and inner layers that are separated by serous fluid.

Inside the testis are some 250 lobules (small lobes); each contains three or four **seminiferous tubules,** which produce **semen.** Within these tubules are several layers of germ cells that are in the process of developing into sperm. Between the seminiferous tubules are the interstitial (occurring between tissues) cells. These cells produce hormones called **androgens.**

Testosterone is the major androgen produced by the interstitial cells of the testes. Its effects include the stimulation of the following activities:

1. **Spermatogenesis,** *(Figure 14.4)* which is responsible for testosterone levels peaking at age 20, then declining steadily to one-fifth of that level at age 80.

2. The development of the male secondary sex characteristics at puberty, which include:

    a. The enlargement of the testes, scrotum, and penis.

    b. The development of the pubic, axillary, body, and facial hair.

    c. The secretion of sebum in skin, which can result in acne *(Chapter 3)*.

3. A burst of growth at puberty, including an increased muscle mass, a higher basal metabolic rate **(BMR),** and a larger larynx (which deepens the voice).

4. Stimulating the brain to increase the male's **libido** (sex drive).

Spermatic Cord

(LO 14.4)

The blood vessels and nerves to the testes—which arise in the abdominal cavity—pass through the inguinal, or groin, canal, where they join with connective tissue. This forms the **spermatic cord** that suspends each testis in the scrotum *(Figure 14.3)*. The left testis is suspended lower than the right. Within the cord exist:

- an artery
- a **plexus** of veins
- nerves
- a thin muscle
- the ductus (vas) deferens into which sperm are deposited when they leave the testis

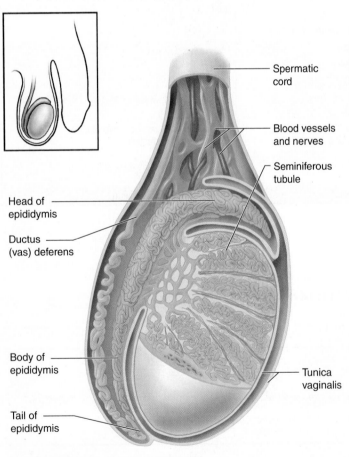

Spermatic cord

Blood vessels and nerves

Seminiferous tubule

Head of epididymis

Ductus (vas) deferens

Body of epididymis

Tail of epididymis

Tunica vaginalis

▲ **FIGURE 14.3**
The Testis and Associated Structures.

Germ cell (46 chromosomes)

First meiotic division

Homologous chromosomes pairing

Spermatids (23 chromosomes)

Sperm cells

▲ **FIGURE 14.4**
Spermatogenesis.

Word Analysis and Definition

S = Suffix   P = Prefix   R = Root   R/CF = Combining Form

WORD	PRONUNCIATION	ELEMENTS		DEFINITION
androgen	AN-droh-jen	S/ R/CF	-gen *create, produce* andr/o- *masculine*	Hormone that promotes masculine characteristics
libido	lih-BEE-doh		Latin *lust*	Sexual desire
plexus plexuses (pl)	PLEK-sus PLEK-sus-ez		Latin *braid*	A weblike network of joined nerves
semen seminiferous (adj)	SEE-men sem-ih-NIF-er-us	S/ R/ R/	Latin *seed* -ous *pertaining to* semin/i- *semen* -fer- *to bear, carry*	Penile ejaculate containing sperm and seminal fluid Pertaining to carrying semen
testosterone	tes-TOSS-ter-own	S/ R/CF	-sterone *steroid* test/o- *testis*	Powerful androgen produced by testes
tunica vaginalis	TYU-nih-kah vaj-ih-NAHL-iss	S/ R/	tunica, Latin *coat* -alis *pertaining to* vagin- *sheath, vagina*	Covering, particularly of a tubular structure The tunica vaginalis is the sheath of the testis and epididymis

EXERCISES

A. Write *the correct medical term to answer the question.*   **LO 14.2, 14.3, 14.4, and 14.10** *Understand*

1. What is the name of the serous membrane that covers the testis? _____

2. The term *seminiferous* pertains to: _____

3. What is another medical term for sex drive? _____

4. What does the abbreviation BMR mean? _____

5. What structure supports the testes? _____

B. Continue *using the language of the male reproductive system to complete the questions.*   **LO 14.2, 14.4, and 14.10** *Understand*

1. Which part of the male reproductive system produces semen? _____

2. What does *interstitial* mean? _____

3. What are the male hormones called? _____

4. What is the major male hormone, and where is it produced? _____ is produced in the _____.

5. What is another name for the "inguinal area"? _____

C. Meet lesson *and chapter objectives using the language of medicine to answer the following questions.*   **LO 14.2, 14.4, and 14.10** *Apply*

1. What does having a larger larynx do to the voice? _____

2. In the growing process, when does muscle mass begin to appear? _____

3. What separates the outer and inner layers of the tunica vaginalis? _____

4. Name the secondary sex characteristics in the male:

   a. _____

   b. _____

   c. _____

Sperm (LO 14.4)

A mature sperm has a pear-shaped head and a long tail. The sperm's head contains these three segments (*Figure 14.5*):

- The **nucleus,** which contains 23 chromosomes;
- The **cap,** which contains enzymes used to penetrate the egg; and
- The **basal body** of the tail.

The tail is further divided into three segments and is responsible for movement as the sperm swims up the female reproductive tract.

Case Report 14.1 (*continued*)

Joseph Davis presented with typical symptoms and signs of testicular torsion. The affected testis rapidly became painful, tender, swollen, and inflamed. Emergency surgery was performed, and the testis and cord were manually untwisted through an incision in the scrotum. The testis was stitched to surrounding tissues to prevent a recurrence of the torsion.

Disorders of the Testes (LO 14.4)

Testicular torsion is the twisting of a testis on its spermatic cord. The testicular artery in the twisted cord becomes blocked, and the blood supply to the testis is cut off. The condition occurs in men between puberty and age 25. In half the cases, it starts in bed at night, as it did for Joseph Davis in Case Report 14.1.

    Varicocele is a condition in which the veins in the spermatic cord become dilated and painful as varicose veins. If it is uncomfortable, it can be treated by surgically tying off the affected veins.

    Hydrocele is a collection of excess fluid in the space between the visceral and parietal layers of the tunica vaginalis of the testis (*Figure 14.6*). It is most common after age 40. The diagnosis can be confirmed by transillumination, (*Figure 14.6*), shining a bright light on the scrotal swelling to see the shape of the testis through the surrounding translucent excess fluid.

    Spermatocele is a collection of sperm in a sac formed in the epididymis, which is the sperm-containing tube attached to a testicle. It occurs in about 30% of men, is benign, and rarely causes symptoms. It does not require treatment unless it becomes uncomfortable.

    Cryptorchism occurs when a testis fails to descend from the abdomen into the scrotum before a boy is 12 months old. As undescended testicles have a higher risk of infertility and cancer, an **orchiopexy** is performed to bring the testis into the scrotum.

    Epididymitis is an inflammation of the epididymis; **epididymo-orchitis (orchitis)** is an inflammation of the epididymis and testis. Orchitis, an inflammation of the testis, is usually a consequence of epididymitis. In each of these cases, the inflammation is most commonly caused by a bacterial infection spreading from an infection in the urinary tract or prostate. These infections can also be caused by sexually transmitted diseases (**STDs**), like gonorrhea or chlamydia.

A viral cause of orchitis is **mumps.** In males past puberty who develop mumps, 30% will develop orchitis, and 30% of those will develop resulting testicular atrophy. A bilateral infection can result in **infertility.** Mumps is avoidable by immunization in childhood.

    Testicular cancer is the most common cancer in males aged 20-39 years. One of the first signs is often a lump in the testis, which may be found through self-examination of the testes. Metastasis is uncommon, but it can be seen in the lungs, in the abdominal and cervical lymph nodes, and occasionally in the brain. An **inguinal orchiectomy** is the usual treatment; if metastases are found, chemotherapy and radiotherapy can be used.

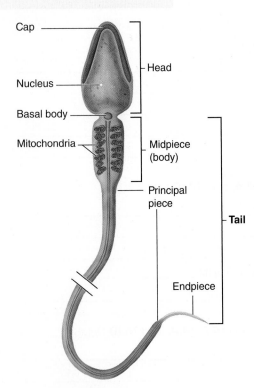

▲ **FIGURE 14.5**
Mature Sperm.

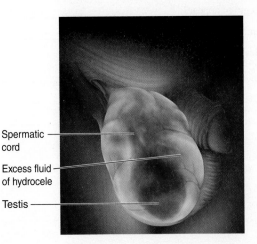

▶ **FIGURE 14.6**
Transillumination of Hydrocele Showing Testis and Spermatic Cord.

Word Analysis and Definition

S = Suffix P = Prefix R = Root R/CF = Combining Form

WORD	PRONUNCIATION	ELEMENTS		DEFINITION
cryptorchism	krip-**TOR**-kizm	S/ R/ R/	-ism *condition* crypt- *hidden* -orch- *testicle*	Failure of one or both testes to descend into the scrotum
epididymitis	EP-ih-did-ih-**MY**-tis	S/ R/	-itis *inflammation* epididym- *epididymis*	Inflammation of the epididymis
epididymo-orchitis *(same as* orchitis*)* (**Note:** *One of the two consecutive "i"s is not used.*)	ep-ih-**DID**-ih-moh-or-**KIE**-tis	S/ R/CF R/	-itis *inflammation* epididym/o- *epididymis* -orchi- *testicle*	Inflammation of the epididymis and testicle
hydrocele	**HIGH**-droh-seal	S/ R/CF	-cele *swelling* hydr/o- *water*	Collection of fluid in the space of the tunica vaginalis
inguinal	**IN**-gwin-al	S/ R/	-al *pertaining to* inguin- *groin*	Pertaining to the groin
orchiectomy	or-key-**ECK**-toe-me	S/ R/	-ectomy *surgical excision* orchi- *testicle*	Removal of one or both testes
orchiopexy	**OR**-key-oh-**PEK**-see	S/ R/CF	-pexy *surgical fixation* orchi/o- *testicle*	Surgical fixation of a testis in the scrotum
orchitis (**Note:** *One of the two consecutive "i"s is not used.*)	or-**KIE**-tis	S/	-itis *inflammation*	Inflammation of the testis
spermatocele	**SPER**-mat-oh-seal	S/ R/CF	-cele *swelling* spermat/o- *sperm*	Cyst of the epididymis that contains sperm
varicocele	**VAIR**-ih-koh-seal	S/ R/CF	-cele *swelling* varic/o- *varicosity*	Varicose veins of the spermatic cord

EXERCISES

A. Review *the Case Report 14.1 (continued) before answering the questions.* **LO 14.2, 14.4, and 14.10** *Understand*

1. What is the difference between a "symptom" and a "sign"?

   Symptom: _____

   Sign: _____

2. Name one symptom Joseph had when he presented to the Emergency Department. _____

3. Why was emergency surgery necessary for Joseph? _____

4. What is the medical term for the surgery that Joseph had? _____

5. Describe what the surgeon did to repair Joseph's condition. _____

B. Build your knowledge *of the language of the male reproductive system by correctly answering the questions regarding the elements in the following terms. Circle the best answer.* **LO 14.1 and 14.4** *Apply*

1. In the term *hydrocele,* the R/CF means:

   testis   water   sperm

2. In the term *cryptorchism,* the element *crypt* means:

   outside of   behind   hidden

3. In the term *orchiopexy,* the suffix means:

   removal   incision   fixation

4. In the term *epididymitis,* which element means inflammation?

   epi   epididym   itis

5. In the term *epididymo-orchitis,* the element *orch* means:

   threadlike   testicle   hidden

> **Study Hint**
>
> Before you attempt to answer the question, divide each term into its components with a slash. This will help you identify which element is referred to in the question.

Lesson 14.2

Spermatic Ducts, Accessory Glands, and Penis

Objectives

*The male prostate and urethra have both **urological** and **reproductive** functions, as the flow of urine and semen goes through both organs. Disorders of the prostate and urethra produce symptoms and signs that arise in both areas. The information provided in this lesson will enable you to use correct medical terminology to:*

14.2.1 Trace the pathway taken by a sperm cell from a testis to the sperm cell's ejaculation.

14.2.2 Identify the structure and functions of the prostate and other male accessory glands.

14.2.3 Describe the origins and functions of semen.

14.2.4 Discuss common disorders of the prostate gland.

14.2.5 Integrate the structures and functions of the penis and its disorders.

Keynotes

- Semen is derived from the secretions of several glands:
  - 5% comes from the testicles and epididymis (sperm).
  - 50% to 80%, from the seminal vesicles.
  - 15% to 33%, from the prostate gland.
  - 2% to 5%, from the bulbourethral glands.
- A normal sperm count is in the range of 75 to 150 million sperm per milliliter (mL) of semen. A normal ejaculation consists of 2 to 5 mL of semen.

Abbreviations

DRE	digital rectal examination
LCC-ST	Liaison Council on Certification for the Surgical Technologist
mL	milliliter

Case Report 14.2

You are . . .

. . . a surgical technologist (LCC-ST) working for urologist Phillip Johnson, MD, in the Urology Clinic at Fulwood Medical Center.

You are communicating with . . .

. . . Mr. Ronald Detrick, a 60-year-old man, who has been referred to the Urology Clinic.

Patient Interview

Mr. Detrick complains of having to get out of bed to urinate four or five times at night. He has difficulty starting urination, has a weak stream, and feels he is not emptying his bladder completely. He has lost interest in sex. His physical examination is unremarkable except that a digital rectal examination (DRE) reveals a diffusely enlarged **prostate** with no nodules.

Spermatic Ducts (LO 14.5)

As the sperm cells mature in the testes over a 60-day period, they move down the seminiferous tubules into the epididymis for storage. The epididymis adheres to the posterior side of the testis. It is a single-coiled duct or tube in which the sperm are stored for 12 to 20 days until they mature and become **motile** (capable of movement).

To be ejaculated, the sperm move into the ductus (vas) deferens, the **ejaculatory** duct, and finally the urethra to reach the outside of the body.

The ductus (vas) deferens is a muscular duct that travels up from the epididymis in the scrotum, passes behind the urinary bladder, and joins with the duct of the seminal vesicle to form the ejaculatory duct, which empties sperm and semen into the urethra.

Accessory Glands (LO 14.5)

The five accessory glands *(Figure 14.7)* are:

1. The two **seminal vesicles,** located on the posterior surface of the urinary bladder, hold fluid that mixes with the sperm in the vas deferens. The fluid is rich in sugar to provide nourishment for the sperm and has clotting properties that make the semen sticky.

2. The single **prostate gland** is close in size and shape to the average walnut. The prostate gland is located immediately below the bladder and anterior to the rectum. It surrounds the urethra and the ejaculatory duct. It is composed of 30 to 50 glands that open directly into the urethra; these glands secrete fluid that nourishes and protects sperm. During ejaculation, the prostate squeezes this fluid into the urethra to form part of semen.

3. The two **bulbourethral glands,** located one on either side of the membranous urethra. Each gland has a short duct leading into the spongy (penile) urethra. When sexually aroused, the glands produce a fluid that neutralizes any acidity in the urethra to make a more hospitable environment in which the sperm can travel.

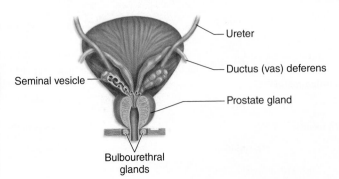

Ureter

Ductus (vas) deferens

Prostate gland

Seminal vesicle

Bulbourethral glands

◀ **FIGURE 14.7**
The five accessory glands of the male reproductive system.

WORD	PRONUNCIATION	ELEMENTS		DEFINITION
ejaculate (can be a verb or a noun)	ee-**JACK**-you-late	S/ R/	-ate *composed of, pertaining to* ejacul- *shoot out*	To expel suddenly; *or* the semen expelled in ejaculation
ejaculation (noun)	ee-**JACK**-you-**LAY**-shun	S/	-ation *process*	Process of expelling semen suddenly
ejaculatory (adj)	ee-**JACK**-you-lah-**TOR**-ee	S/	-atory *pertaining to*	Pertaining to ejaculation
motile	**MOH**-til	S/ R/	-ile *pertaining to* mot- *to move*	Capable of spontaneous movement
motility	moh-**TILL**-ih-tee	S/ R/	-ity *condition, state* motil- *to move*	The ability for spontaneous movement
prostate	**PROS**-tate (Note: *not* **PROS**-trate, *which means exhausted*)		Greek *one standing before*	Gland surrounding the beginning of the urethra
prostatic (adj)	pros-**TAT**-ik	S/ R/	-ic *pertaining to* prostat- *prostate*	Pertaining to the prostate

Study Hint

SEVEN UP is used to remember the pathway of sperm:

S = seminiferous tubules   N = nothing
E = epididymis   U = urethra
V = vas (ductus) deferens   P = penis
E = ejaculatory duct

EXERCISES

A. Review *the Case Report on this spread before answering the questions.*   **LO 14.2, 14.3, 14.5, and 14.10** *Understand*

1. What are Mr. Detrick's complaints? _____

2. What does the abbreviation *DRE* mean? _____

3. What did Mr. Detrick's DRE reveal? _____

4. What is a *nodule?* _____

5. What is responsible for Mr. Detrick's symptoms? _____

B. Writing practice: *Write a sentence that is not a definition for each of the following terms. Be sure to employ the correct form of the term in your sentence. Fill in the blanks.*   **LO 14.2, 14.5, and 14.10** *Apply*

1. *ejaculate*   (as a noun—thing):

_____

_____

2. *ejaculate*   (as a verb—action):

_____

_____

3. *ejaculatory*   (adjective):

_____

_____

Disorders of the Prostate Gland (LO 14.6)

Benign prostatic hyperplasia (BPH), also known as benign prostatic hypertrophy or **benign enlargement of the prostate (BEP)**—a noncancerous enlargement of the prostate—can cause symptoms starting around age 45; by age 80, some 90% of men have symptoms. This enlargement is one of **hyperplasia** (number of cells) rather than **hypertrophy** (size of cells), and it compresses the prostatic urethra to produce symptoms including:

- Difficulty starting and stopping the urine stream.
- **Nocturia** (excessive nighttime urination), **polyuria** (excessive urine production), and dysuria (difficulty or pain in urination).

Case Report 14.3 (continued)

Ronald Detrick was describing the symptoms listed above when he was referred to the Urology Clinic.

In some patients, surgical treatment by **transurethral** resection (**TURP**) relieves the symptoms. An endoscope called a **resectoscope** is inserted into the urethra and used to remove the tissue surrounding and compressing the urethra.

Prostatic cancer affects 10% of men over the age of 50, and its incidence is increasing. It forms hard nodules in the periphery of the gland and is often asymptomatic (produces no symptoms) in its early stages, as it does not compress the urethra.

Screening for prostatic cancer is performed using the following procedures:

- A **digital rectal exam (DRE),** which involves palpating the size and texture of the prostate by inserting a finger into the rectum.
  - A **prostate-specific antigen (PSA)** test, which measures the PSA level in the blood. Even though cancer can be present when the level is zero, the benefit of this test is that it can show whether levels rise rapidly over time. Some advisory groups now recommend against the use of PSA as a screen for prostate cancer because the benefits are limited and the harms in terms of unnecessary investigations and surgery for cancer are substantial.

▲ FIGURE 14.8
Vasectomy being performed showing a segment of the ductus deferens being removed.

- An **early prostate cancer antigen (EPCA-2)** test. This is more accurate than the PSA and is now in clinical trials.

Several treatment options involving radiotherapy are available for prostate cancer. **Brachytherapy** involves the insertion of small radioactive rods directly into the tumor. Sometimes, a **radical prostatectomy** is performed. This involves complete surgical removal of the prostate and surrounding tissues. A vaccine has been introduced that provides some extension of life in men with advanced prostate cancer.

Prostatitis is an inflammation of the prostate gland that causes groin pain and difficulty and discomfort when urinating.

Male Infertility (LO 14.8)

Infertility is the inability of a couple to conceive after one year of unprotected intercourse. **Male infertility is** the man's inability to produce or deliver fully functioning sperm. The main causes of male infertility are:

- Impaired sperm production, due to cryptorchidism, anorchism (absence of one or both testes), testicular trauma, testicular cancer, or orchitis after puberty.
- Impaired sperm delivery, due to infections and blockage of spermatic ducts.
- **Sperm disorders,** in which sperm are underdeveloped, abnormally shaped, unable to move properly, produced in abnormally low numbers (**oligospermia),** or not produced at all (**azoospermia).**
- **Varicoceles,** in which the dilated scrotal veins impair sperm production by preventing proper drainage of blood within the testes.
- Testosterone deficiency (**hypogonadism).** Phthalates in plastics and dioxins in paper are examples of environmental endocrine disrupters that can contribute to testosterone deficiency.

Each year, in the United States, half a million men choose to be made infertile (**sterile**) by having a **vasectomy** (*Figure 14.8*). Under local anesthesia, the ductus deferens is cut in two places, a 1-cm segment is removed, and the ends of the ductus deferens are cauterized and tied. The site of the surgery makes the man infertile but still able to produce and ejaculate seminal fluid.

Should a man choose to reverse his vasectomy, he can undergo a **vasovasostomy.** This is a microsurgical procedure that reverses a vasectomy by suturing back together the cut ends of the ductus deferens.

Word Analysis and Definition

S = Suffix   P = Prefix   R = Root   R/CF = Combining Form

WORD	PRONUNCIATION	ELEMENTS		DEFINITION
azoospermia	a-zoh-oh-**SPER**-me-ah	S/ P/ R/ R/	-ia *condition* a- *without* -zoo- *animal* -sperm- *seed*	Absence of living sperm in the semen
oligospermia	**OL**-ih-go-**SPER**-me-ah	P/	oligo- *too few*	Deficient numbers of sperm in the semen
brachytherapy	brah-kee-**THAIR**-ah-pee	P/ R/	brachy- *short* -therapy *treatment*	Radiation therapy in which the source of radiation is implanted in the tissue to be treated
hyperplasia	**HIGH**-per-**PLAY**-zee-ah	S/ P/ R/	-ia *condition* hyper- *excessive* -plas- *molding, formation*	Increase in the *number* of the cells in a tissue or organ
hypertrophy (Note: See Study Hint below.)	high-**PER**-troh-fee	S/	-trophy *development*	Increase in the *size* of the cells in a tissue or organ
hypogonadism	**HIGH**-poh-**GOH**-nad-izm	S/ P/ R/	-ism *condition* hypo- *deficient* -gonad- *testis or ovary*	Deficient gonad production of sperm, eggs, or hormones
infertility	in-fer-**TIL**-ih-tee	S/ P/ R/	-ity *condition* in- *not* -fertil- *able to conceive*	Failure to conceive
nocturia	nok-**TYU**-ree-ah	S/ P/ R/	-ia *condition* noct- *night* -ur- *urine*	Excessive urination at night
polyuria	pol-ee-**YOU**-ree-ah	S/ P/ R/	-ia *condition* poly- *excessive* -ur- *urine*	Excessive production of urine
prostatectomy	pros-tah-**TEK**-toe-me	S/ R/	-ectomy *surgical excision* prostat- *prostate*	Surgical removal of the prostate
prostatitis	pros-tah-**TIE**-tis	S/	-itis *inflammation*	Inflammation of the prostate
resectoscope	ree-**SEK**-toe-skope	S/ R/CF	-scope *instrument for viewing* resect/o- *cut off*	Endoscope for the transurethral removal of lesions
transurethral	**TRANS**-you-**REE**-thral	S/ P/ R/	-al *pertaining to* trans- *across, through* -urethr- *urethra*	Procedure performed through the urethra
vasectomy	vah-**SEK**-toe-me	S/ R/	-ectomy *surgical excision* vas- *duct*	Excision of a segment of the ductus deferens
vasovasostomy (vasectomy reversal)	**VAY**-soh-vay-**SOS**-toe-me	S/ R/CF	-stomy *new opening* vas/o- *duct*	Reanastomosis of the ductus deferens to restore the flow of sperm

EXERCISES

A. Review *the Case Report on this spread before answering the questions.* **LO 14.2, 14.6, and 14.10** *Apply*

1. Mr. Detrick presented to the Urology Clinic with nocturia, polyuria, and dysuria. Briefly define each term for your patient.

   nocturia: _____

   polyuria: _____

   dysuria: _____

2. Thinking of the meaning of the words *polyuria, nocturia,* and *oliguria,* what would the word *hematuria* mean? _____

Study Hint

Word association for **hypertrophy**:

Hypertrophy relates to an increase in **size**.

Remember that sports **trophies** come in all **sizes**.

B. Recognition: *As you become more familiar with elements (especially suffixes), you will be able to recognize medical terms that are procedures and diagnoses. Practice with the terms in the WAD box above. Fill in the blanks.* **LO 14.2, 14.8, and 14.10** *Remember*

1. List all the terms in the WAD that could be a possible diagnosis for a patient:

   _____

2. List all the terms in the WAD that are procedures:

   _____

3. What surgical procedure is the reversal of a vasectomy? _____

4. What is the medical term for testosterone deficiency? _____

5. What is another term for *infertile?* _____

Lesson 14.2
(cont'd)

- Erectile dysfunction occurs in some 20 million American men.
- Erectile dysfunction can be associated with diabetes, stroke, multiple sclerosis, hypertension, cigarette smoking, radiation therapy, drugs such as antidepressants and cholesterol-lowering medications, and loss of interest in one's sexual partner.

▲ FIGURE 14.9
Anatomy of the Penis.
(a) External anatomy.
(b) Cross-sectional view.

ED	erectile dysfunction
STD	sexually transmitted disease

Penis (LO 14.7)

The **penis** *(Figure 14.9(a))* is an important male external body structure, which is specifically designed to meet its two main functions:

- To enable urine to flow to the outside.
- To deposit semen in the female vagina around the cervix.

The external, visible part of the penis is composed of the **shaft** and the more sensitive **glans.** The external urethral meatus is located at the tip of the glans. The skin of the penis continues over the glans as the **prepuce,** otherwise known as the foreskin. A ventral fold of tissue called the **frenulum** attaches the foreskin to the glans.

The shaft of the penis contains these three **erectile vascular bodies** *(Figure 14.9(b)):*

- The paired **corpora cavernosa** (columns of erectile tissue found in the penis) are located dorsolaterally.
- The single **corpus spongiosum** is located inferiorly. It contains the urethra and goes on to form the glans.

Erection occurs when the corpora cavernosa fill with blood, causing the erectile bodies to distend and become rigid. It is a parasympathetic nervous system response to stimulation.

Ejaculation occurs when the sympathetic nervous system stimulates the smooth muscle of the ductus deferens, ejaculatory ducts, and the glands in the prostate to contract.

The Prepuce (Foreskin) and Urethra (LO 14.7)

The functions of the **prepuce** (foreskin) are to cover and protect the glans *(Figure 14.10(b)),* and to produce smegma. **Smegma** is a lubricant containing lipids, cell debris, and some natural antibiotics. Removal of the foreskin is called **circumcision** *(Figure 14.10(a)).*

Disorders of the Penis
(LO 14.7)

Disorders involving the penis range from minor injuries to STDs to cancer. These conditions are outlined below.

Trauma to the penis can vary from being caught in a pants' zipper to being fractured while erect during vigorous sexual intercourse.

Priapism is a persistent, painful erection that occurs when blood cannot escape from the erectile tissue. It can be caused by drugs like epinephrine, by blood clots, or by spinal cord injury.

Cancer of the penis occurs most commonly on the glans and is rare in circumcised men.

Sexually transmitted diseases (STDs) are discussed in detail in *Chapter 15.*

Erectile dysfunction (ED), or **impotence,** is the inability to have a satisfactory erection. Treatment is aimed at addressing any underlying disease.

Premature ejaculation is more common than erectile dysfunction. It occurs when a man ejaculates so quickly during intercourse that it causes distress or embarrassment to one or both partners.

Disorders of the Prepuce (LO 14.7)

- **Balanitis** is an infection of the glans and foreskin with bacteria or yeast.
- **Phimosis** is a condition in which the foreskin is tight because of a small opening and cannot be retracted over the glans for cleaning. It can lead to balanitis.
- **Paraphimosis** is a condition in which the retracted foreskin cannot be pulled forward to cover the glans.

Disorders of the Penile Urethra
(LO 14.7)

Urethritis is an inflammation of the urethra. It can be caused by bacteria, STDs, viruses, and chemical irritants from **spermicides** and contraceptive gels.

Urethral stricture is scarring that narrows the urethra. It results from infection or injury.

Hypospadias is a congenital defect in which the opening of the urethra is on the undersurface of the penis instead of at the head of the glans. It can be corrected surgically.

Epispadias is a congenital defect in which the opening of the urethra is on the dorsum of the penis.

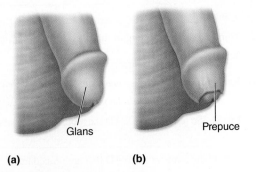

▲ FIGURE 14.10
Prepuce.
(a) Circumcised penis. (b) Uncircumcised penis.

Word Analysis and Definition

S = Suffix   P = Prefix   R = Root   R/CF = Combining Form

WORD	PRONUNCIATION	ELEMENTS		DEFINITION
balanitis	bal-ah-**NIE**-tis	S/ R/	-itis *inflammation* balan- *glans penis*	Inflammation of the glans and prepuce of the penis
cavernosa	kav-er-**NOH**-sah	S/ R/	-osa *like* cavern- *cave*	Resembling a cave
circumcision	ser-kum-**SIZH**-un	S/ P/ R/	-ion *action, condition* circum- *around* -cis- *to cut*	To remove part or all of the prepuce
corpus corpora (pl)	**KOR**-pus kor-**POR**-ah		Latin *body*	Major part of a structure
epispadias	ep-ih-**SPAY**-dee-as	S/ P/ R/	-ias *condition* epi- *above* -spad- *tear or cut*	Condition in which the urethral opening is on the dorsum of the penis
erectile	ee-**REK**-tile	S/ R/	-ile *pertaining to* erect- *to set up, straight*	Capable of erection or being distended with blood
erection	ee-**REK**-shun	S/	-ion *action, condition*	Distended and rigid state of an organ
frenulum	**FREN**-you-lum		Latin *small bridle*	Fold of mucous membrane between the glans and the prepuce
glans	GLANZ		Latin *acorn*	Head of the penis or clitoris
hypospadias	high-poh-**SPAY**-dee-as	S/ P/ R/	-ias *condition* hypo- *below* -spad- *tear or cut*	Urethral meatus on the underside of the penis
impotence	**IM**-poh-tence		Latin *inability*	Inability to achieve an erection
paraphimosis	**PAR**-ah-fih-**MOH**-sis	S/ P/ R/	-osis *condition* para- *abnormal* -phim- *muzzle*	Condition in which a retracted prepuce cannot be pulled forward to cover the glans
phimosis	fih-**MOH**-sis	S/ R/	-osis *condition* phim- *muzzle*	A condition where the prepuce cannot be retracted
prepuce (*same as* foreskin)	**PREE**-puce		Latin *foreskin*	Fold of skin that covers the glans penis
priapism	**PRY**-ah-pizm		Priapus, mythical Roman god of procreation	Persistent erection of the penis
smegma	**SMEG**-mah		Greek *ointment*	Oily material produced by the glans and prepuce
spermicide	**SPER**-mih-side	S/ R/CF	-cide *destroy* sperm/i- *sperm*	Agent that destroys sperm
spermicidal (adj)	sper-mih-**SIGH**-dal	S/	-al *pertaining to*	Pertaining to the killing of sperm; *or* destructive to sperm
spongiosum	spun-jee-**OH**-sum	S/ R/	-um *tissue* spongios- *sponge*	Spongelike tissue

EXERCISES

A. Language of urology: *Refine your knowledge of urological terminology by choosing the correct term to complete the statement. Circle the best choice. Be precise, and watch the spelling!* **LO 14.2 and 14.7** *Remember*

1. Condition in which a retracted prepuce cannot be pulled forward to cover the glans:

   hypospadias   phimosis   spongiosum   paraphimosis

2. To remove all or part of the prepuce:

   circumcision   circumscion   circummcision   circumsion

3. Skin that covers the glans penis:

   forskin   fourskin   forksin   foreskin

4. Fold of mucous membrane:

   frennulum   freeulum   freenulum   frenulum

Sexually Transmitted Diseases (STDs) (LO 14.3, and 14.9)

According to the Centers for Disease Control (CDC), 15 million new cases of sexually transmitted diseases (STDs) are reported annually in the United States. Adolescents and young adults have the greatest risk of contracting STDs.

Chlamydia is known as the "silent" disease because up to 75% of infected women and men have no symptoms. When there are signs, a vaginal or penile discharge and irritation with dysuria (difficult or painful urination) are common. Highly accurate urine tests and DNA probes are available for diagnosis. Treatment is with oral antibiotics. If left untreated, chlamydia can spread higher into the female reproductive tract and cause **pelvic inflammatory disease (PID)**. It can also be passed on to a newborn during childbirth and cause eye infections or pneumonia. For this reason, newborns receive antibiotic eyedrops.

Trichomoniasis ("trich") is caused by the parasite *Trichomonas vaginalis*. In women, it can produce a frothy yellow-green vaginal discharge with irritation and itching of the vulva. Because it is a "ping-pong" infection that goes back and forth between partners, both individuals should be treated.

Gonorrhea is spread by unprotected sex and can be passed on to a baby in childbirth, causing a serious eye infection. As with chlamydia, newborns receive antibiotic eyedrops to prevent eye infections from gonorrhea. Symptoms include a vaginal discharge, bleeding, and dysuria. Lab testing on a swab taken from the surface of the infected area can confirm the diagnosis. DNA probes are also available. Gonorrhea can be treated with a single dose of an antibiotic. However, it is developing resistance to antibiotics.

Syphilis is transmitted sexually and can spread through the bloodstream to every organ in the body. **Primary syphilis** begins 10 to 90 days after infection as an ulcer or **chancre** at the infection site. Four to ten weeks later, if the primary syphilis is not treated, **secondary syphilis** appears as a rash on the palms of the hands and the soles of the feet. Swollen glands and muscle and joint pain accompany the rash. **Tertiary syphilis** can occur years after the primary infection and cause permanent damage to the brain, with dementia.

Genital herpes simplex is a disease caused by the virus herpes simplex 2 **(HSV2)**. It manifests with painful genital sores *(Figure 14.11)*, which can recur throughout life *(Figures 14.11 and 14.12)*. There is no cure for genital herpes. Antiviral medications can provide a clinical benefit by limiting the **replication** of the virus. **Herpes of the newborn** *(Figure 14.12)* occurs when a pregnant woman with genital herpes sores delivers her baby vaginally and transmits the virus to the baby.

Human papilloma virus (HPV) causes genital warts in both men and women. HPV can also cause changes to the cells in the cervix. Some strains of the virus can increase a woman's risk for cervical cancer. More than 90% of abnormal **Pap** smears are caused by HPV infections. A vaccine is available that can prevent lasting infections with strains that cause cervical cancers and genital warts. The vaccine can be given to females aged 9 to 26, before they are sexually active. The vaccine can be given to males aged 9 to 26 years to reduce the likelihood of acquiring genital warts.

Molluscum contagiosum is a virus that can be sexually transmitted and produces small, shiny bumps that contain a milky-white fluid. They can disappear and reappear anywhere on the body.

Human immunodeficiency virus (HIV) is a virus that attacks the immune system and usually leads to **acquired immune deficiency syndrome (AIDS)**. HIV is carried in body fluids and transmitted during unprotected sex. Sharing needles can spread the virus. The virus can also pass from an infected pregnant woman to her unborn child, so she must take medications to protect the baby.

There is no cure for HIV or AIDS, but combinations of anti-HIV medications can be taken to stop the **replication** of the virus in the cells of the body, and to stop the progression of the disease. However, the development of resistance to the drugs is a problem.

HIV damages the immune system, allowing infections to develop that the body would normally cope with easily. These are **opportunistic infections** and include herpes simplex, candidiasis, syphilis, and tuberculosis **(TB)**.

Keynotes

- Three million cases of chlamydia are recognized annually in the United States and can be prevented by abstinence or by using a condom.
- Infection with gonorrhea can be prevented by abstinence or by using a condom.
- Three million cases of trichomoniasis occur annually in the United States and could be prevented by abstinence or by using a condom.

Abbreviations

AIDS	acquired immunodeficiency syndrome
CDC	Centers for Disease Control and Prevention
HIV	human immunodeficiency virus
HPV	human papilloma virus
HSV2	herpes simplex virus 2
Pap	Papanicolaou (test, stain)
PID	pelvic inflammatory disease
STD	sexually transmitted disease
TB	tuberculosis

Vesicles

▲ **FIGURE 14.11**
Genital Herpes Simplex in Male.

Herpes simplex vesicles

◀ **FIGURE 14.12**
Newborn Infant with Herpes Simplex.

Word Analysis and Definition

WORD	PRONUNCIATION		ELEMENTS	DEFINITION
acquired immuno-deficiency syndrome (AIDS)	ah-**KWIRED** **IM**-you-noh-dee-**FISH**-en-see **SIN**-drohm	S/ R/CF R/ P/ R/	acquired, Latin *obtain* -ency *condition* immun/o- *immune response* -defici- *lacking, inadequate* syn- *together* -drome *running*	Infection with the HIV virus Combination of signs and symptoms associated with a particular disease process
chancre	**SHAN**-ker		Latin *cancer*	Primary lesion of syphilis
chlamydia	klah-**MID**-ee-ah		Latin *cloak*	An STD caused by infection with *Chlamydia*, a species of bacteria
condom	**KON**-dom		Old English *sheath or cover*	A sheath or cover for the penis or vagina to prevent conception and infection
gonorrhea	gon-oh-**REE**-ah	S/ R/CF	-rrhea *flow, discharge* gon/o- *seed*	Specific contagious sexually transmitted infection
human immunodefi-ciency virus (HIV)	**HYU**-man **IM**-you-noh-dee-**FISH**-en-see **VIE**-rus	R/ S/ R/CF R/	human *human being* -ency *condition* immun/o- *immune response* -defici- *lacking, inadequate* virus, Latin *poison*	Etiologic agent of acquired immunodeficiency syndrome (AIDS)
human papilloma virus (HPV)	**HYU**-man pap-ih-**LOW**-mah **VIE**-rus	R/ S/ R/	human *human being* -oma *tumor* papill- *pimple* virus, Latin *poison*	Causes warts on the skin and genitalia and can increase the risk for cervical cancer
molluscum contagiosum (Note: "S" in "sum" added to enable word to flow.) (*modern word contagious*)	moh-**LUS**-kum kon-**TAY**-jee-oh-sum	S/ R/ R/CF	-um *structure* mollusc- *soft* contagi/o- *transmissible by contact*	STD caused by a virus
opportunistic infection (**Note:** *TWO suffixes*)	**OP**-or-tyu-**NIS**-tik in-**FEK**-shun	S/ S/ R/	-ic *pertaining to* -ist- *agent, specialist* opportun- *take advantage of*	An infection that causes disease when the immune system is compromised for other reasons
replication	rep-lih-**KAY**-shun	S/ R/	-ation *process of* replic- *reply*	Reproduction to produce an exact copy
syphilis	**SIF**-ih-lis		Principal character in a Latin poem	Sexually transmitted disease caused by a spirochete
Trichomonas trichomoniasis	trik-oh-**MOH**-nas **TRIK**-oh-moh-**NIE**-ah-sis	R/CF R/ S/ R/	trich/o- *hair* -monas *single unit* -iasis *condition* -mon- *single*	A parasite causing an STD Infection with *Trichomonas vaginalis*

EXERCISE

A. Construct *the correct medical term to match the definition that is given. Write the appropriate* **element on** *the line and the* **meaning** *of the element* **below** *the line.*   **LO 14.1, 14.2, and 14.9** *Apply*

1. Infection with *Trichomonas* _____ / _____ / _____

2. Reproduction of an exact copy _____ / _____ / _____

3. Infection that takes advantage of a compromised immune system

   _____ / _____ / _____

4. Contagious STD infection _____ / _____ / _____

5. Combination of signs and symptoms associated with a particular disease process

   _____ / _____ / _____

Chapter Review exercises, along with additional practice items, are available in Connect!

CHAPTER 15

The Female Reproductive System

The Essentials of the Languages of Gynecology and Obstetrics

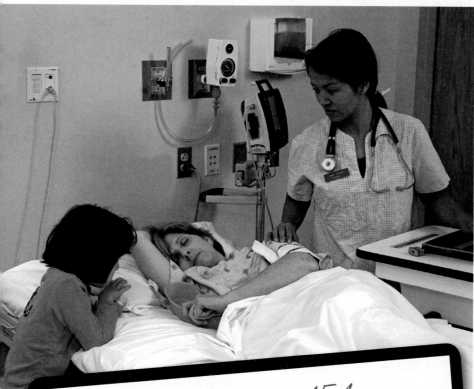

Case Report 15.1

You are . . .

. . . a licensed practical nurse (LPN) working in the Emergency Department at Fulwood Medical Center.

You are communicating with . . .

. . . Ms. Lara Baker, a 32-year-old single mother who works in the billing department of the medical center. You have been asked to take her vital signs. For the past couple of days, she has had muscle aches and a feeling of general uneasiness that she thought were due to her heavy menstrual period. In the past 3 hours, she has developed a severe headache with nausea and vomiting. A diffuse rash over her trunk that looks like sunburn is now spreading to her upper arms and thighs. VS: T 104.2°F, P 120 and irregular, R 20, BP 86/50. As you took her VS, you noted that she did not seem to understand where she was. She was unable to pass a urine specimen. For this patient, the treatment she receives in the next few minutes is vital for her survival. You have your supervising nurse and the emergency physician come to see her immediately. As you participate in this patient's care, clear communication among the team members is essential.

Learning Outcomes

As a health care professional in the area of gynecology and obstetrics, it's essential that you become familiar with not only the functions and structures of the female reproductive system, but also with its associated medical terminology. In order to provide patients with the best possible care, you will need to be able to:

LO 15.1 Use roots, combining forms, suffixes, and prefixes to construct and analyze (deconstruct) medical terms related to the female reproductive system.

LO 15.2 Spell and pronounce correctly medical terms related to the female reproductive system in order to communicate them with accuracy and precision in any health care setting.

LO 15.3 Define accepted abbreviations related to the female reproductive system.

LO 15.4 Relate the anatomy of the external genitalia and the female reproductive tract to their functions, disorders, and treatments.

LO 15.5 Identify the ovarian hormones and their relation to and use in menopause.

LO 15.6 Detail the causes of female infertility, their treatments, and the methods of contraception.

LO 15.7 Describe conception, implantation, and development of the embryo, fetus, and placenta during pregnancy, and their disorders.

LO 15.8 Explain the stages of delivery and the disorders of childbirth.

LO 15.9 Relate the structure of the breast to its disorders and to the development of lactation.

LO 15.10 Apply your knowledge of medical terms relating to the female reproductive system to documentation, medical records, and medical reports.

LO 15.11 Translate the medical terms relating to the female reproductive system into everyday language in order to communicate clearly with patients and their families.

The health professionals involved in the diagnosis and treatment of problems with the female reproductive system include:

- **Gynecologists** (GYN) are physicians who are specialists in diseases of the female reproductive tract.
- **Obstetricians** (OB) are physicians who are specialists in the care of women during pregnancy and childbirth.
- **Neonatologists** are physicians who are pediatric subspecialists in disorders of the newborn, particularly ill or premature infants.
- **Perinatologists** are physicians who are obstetric subspecialists in the care of the mother and fetus who are at higher-than-normal risk for complications.
- **Certified midwives/nurse-midwives** (CNM) are independent practitioners who provide care to mothers during pregnancy, delivery, and birth, and to mothers and newborn infants for 6 weeks after birth.
- **Obstetrical–gynecological nurse practitioners** (OB/GYN) are registered nurses who have acquired skills in the management of health and illness for women throughout their life cycle.

Objectives

*The female reproductive system is dormant or undeveloped until puberty, when the **ovaries** begin to secrete significant amounts of the sex hormones **estrogen** and **progesterone**. Then, the external genitalia become more prominent, pubic hair develops, the **vagina** becomes lubricated, and the breasts begin to enlarge. The information in this lesson will enable you to use correct medical terminology to:*

15.1.1 Describe the essential structures and functions of the external genitalia, vagina, and accessory glands.

15.1.2 Describe common disorders of the external genitalia and vagina.

Abbreviation

LPN	licensed practical nurse
(GYN)	Gynecologists
(OB)	Obstetricians
(OB/GYN)	Obstetrical–gynecological nurse practitioners
(CNM)	Certified midwives/nurse-midwives

Lesson 15.1

External Genitalia and Vagina

External Genitalia (LO 15.4)

The female external genitalia occupy most of the perineum and are collectively called the **vulva.** The structures of the vulva *(Figure 15.1a)* include the:

- **Mons pubis,** a mound of skin and adipose or fatty tissue overlying the symphysis pubis.
- **Labia majora,** a pair of thick folds of skin, connective tissue, and adipose tissue.
- **Labia minora,** a pair of thin folds of hairless skin immediately internal to the labia majora. Anteriorly, the labia minora join together to form the prepuce (hood) of the **clitoris.** The clitoris is a small erectile body capped with a glans. Posteriorly, these structures merge with the labia majora.
- **Vestibule,** the area enclosed by the labia minora. It contains the urinary and vaginal openings.

Deep into the labia majora on each side of the vaginal orifice (opening) is a pea-sized greater vestibular **(Bartholin)** gland *(Figure 15.1b)*. These glands secrete mucus to lubricate the vulva and vagina, and this secretion increases during sexual intercourse.

(a)   **(b)**

▲ **FIGURE 15.1**
Female Perineum and Vulva.
(a) Surface anatomy. (b) Subcutaneous structures.

Word Analysis and Definition

S = Suffix   P = Prefix   R = Root   R/CF = Combining Form

WORD	PRONUNCIATION		ELEMENTS	DEFINITION
cervix cervical (adj) (Note: *This term also means* pertaining to the neck region.)	**SER**-viks **SER**-vih-kal	S/ R/	Latin *neck* -al *pertaining to* cervic- *neck*	Lower part of the uterus Pertaining to the cervix
clitoris	**KLIT**-oh-ris		Greek *clitoris*	Erectile organ of the vulva
estrogen	**ES**-troh-jen	S/ R/CF	-gen *produce* estr/o *woman*	Generic term for hormones that stimulate female secondary sex characteristics
fornix fornices (pl)	**FOR**-niks **FOR**-nih-seez		Latin *a vault*	Arch-shaped, blind-ended part of the vagina behind and around the cervix
gynecology (GYN) gynecologist gynecologic (adj)	guy-nih-**KOL**-oh-jee guy-nih-**KOL**-oh-jist **GUY**-nih-koh-**LOJ**-ik	S/ R/CF S/ S/ R/CF R/	-logy *study of* gynec/o- *woman, female* -logist *one who studies, specialist* -ic *pertaining to* gynec/o- *woman, female* -log- *to study*	Medical specialty of diseases of the female reproductive tract Specialist in gynecology Pertaining to gynecology
hymen	**HIGH**-men		Greek *membrane*	Thin membrane partly occluding the vaginal orifice
labium labia (pl)	**LAY**-bee-um **LAY**-bee-ah		Greek *lip*	Fold of the vulva
majus majora (pl)	**MAY**-jus mah-**JOR**-ah		Latin *greater*	Bigger or greater; e.g., the labia majora
minus minora (pl)	**MY**-nus mih-**NOR**-ah		Latin *smaller*	Smaller or lesser; e.g., the labia minora
mons pubis	MONZ **PYU**-bis		mons, Latin *mountain* pubis, Latin *pubic bone*	Fleshy pad with pubic hair, overlying the pubic bone
ovary ovaries (pl) ovarian (adj)	**OH**-vah-ree **OH**-vah-reez oh-**VAIR**-ee-an	S/ R/	Latin *egg* -an *pertaining to* ovari- *ovary*	One of the paired female reproductive glands Pertaining to the ovary(ies)
progesterone (Note: *Two suffixes*)	pro-**JESS**-ter-own	S/ S/ P/ R/	-one *hormone, chemical substance* -er- *agent, one who does* pro- *before* -gest- *pregnancy*	Hormone that prepares the uterus for pregnancy
vagina vaginal (adj)	vah-**JIE**-nah **VAJ**-ih-nal	S/ R/	Latin *sheath* -al *pertaining to* vagin- *vagina*	The female genital canal extending from the uterus to the vulva Pertaining to the vagina
vulva vulvar (adj)	**VUL**-vah **VUL**-var	S/ R/	Latin *a wrapper or covering* -ar *pertaining to* vulv- *vulva*	Female external genitalia Pertaining to the vulva

EXERCISE

A. Review *the Case Report on the opening spread before answering the questions.*   **LO 15.2, 15.4, and 15.10** *Understand*

1. When Ms. Baker presented to the ED, what was her temperature? _____

2. What indicates that Ms. Baker was in a confused state of mind? _____

3. What is a "diffuse" rash? _____

4. What urinary symptom was Ms. Baker having? _____

5. List the rest of Ms. Baker's symptoms. _____

6. Is this a life-threatening emergency? _____

7. Which symptoms did Ms. Baker believe were caused by her heavy menstrual period? _____

Lesson 15.1 External Genitalia and Vagina   347

Lesson 15.1
(cont'd)

- Bacterial vaginosis is associated with increased risk of gonorrhea and HIV infection.
- Of all adult women, 75% have at least one genital yeast infection in their lifetimes.
- Ten million office visits annually are for vulvodynia.

Vagina (LO 15.4)

The **vagina,** or birth canal, is a fibromuscular tube that measures 4 to 5 inches long. It connects the vulva with the uterus *(Figure 15.2)* and has three main functions:

- To discharge menstrual fluid;
- To receive the penis and semen; and
- To deliver a baby.

The vagina is located between the rectum and the urethra. The urethra is embedded in the anterior wall of the vagina.

At its posterior end, the vagina extends beyond the **cervix** of the uterus and forms arch-shaped blind spaces called the anterior and posterior **fornices.** The lower end of the vagina contains numerous crosswise folds. These folds project into the vaginal opening to form the **hymen,** which stretches across the opening. The hymen contains one or two openings to allow menstrual fluid to escape.

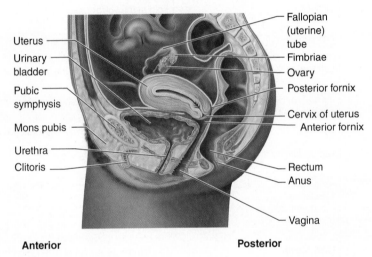

Anterior **Posterior**

▲ **FIGURE 15.2**
Female Reproductive Organs.

Disorders of the Vulva and Vagina (LO 15.4)

Bacterial vaginosis is the most common cause of **vaginitis** in women of childbearing age. The main symptom is an abnormal vaginal discharge with a fish-like odor. With bacterial vaginosis, different types of invading bacteria outnumber the vagina's normal bacteria. This disorder is diagnosed by a lab exam of a vaginal swab specimen, and it is treated with antibiotics.

Toxic shock syndrome is a life-threatening illness caused by toxins (poisons) circulating in the bloodstream. Bacteria in the vagina are encouraged to grow by the presence of a superabsorbent **tampon** that is not changed frequently *(see Case Report 15.1).* These bacteria produce toxins that are absorbed into the bloodstream. Other risk factors for toxic shock syndrome include skin wounds and surgery.

Vulvovaginal candidiasis is a common cause of genital itching or burning with a "cottage-cheese" vaginal discharge. It is caused by an overgrowth of the yeast fungus *Candida* and can occur after taking antibiotics. Treatment is with antifungal drugs.

Vulvovaginitis *(Figure 15.3)* can be caused by allergic and irritative agents found in vaginal hygiene products, spermicides, detergents, and synthetic underwear.

Vulvodynia is a chronic, severe pain around the vaginal orifice, which feels raw. Painful intercourse **(dyspareunia)** is common. The vulva may look normal or be slightly swollen. The etiology (cause) is unknown. Treatment varies from local anesthetics and creams to biofeedback therapy with exercises for the pelvic floor muscles. Surgical removal of the affected area **(vestibulectomy)** has been tried with variable results.

Vaginal cancers are uncommon, comprising only 1% to 2% of gynecologic malignancies. They can be effectively treated with surgery and radiation therapy.

Case Report 15.1 (continued)

Ms. Lara Baker presented to the Emergency Department with toxic shock syndrome. Because of her heavy period, she was using a superabsorbent tampon. She was admitted to intensive care. The tampon was removed and cultured. IV fluids and antibiotics were administered. Her kidney and liver functions were monitored. The causative organism was *Staphylococcus aureus.* She recovered well but had a second episode 6 months later.

Vulvovaginitis

◀ **FIGURE 15.3**
Patient with vulvovaginitis.

Word Analysis and Definition

WORD	PRONUNCIATION	ELEMENTS		DEFINITION
dyspareunia	dis-pah-**RUE**-nee-ah	S/ P/ R/	-ia *condition* dys- *painful* -pareun- *lying beside, sexual intercourse*	Pain during sexual intercourse
tampon	**TAM**-pon		French *plug*	Plug or pack in a cavity to absorb or stop bleeding
toxin	**TOK**-sin		Greek *poison*	Poisonous substance formed by a cell or organism
toxic	**TOK**-sick	S/ R/	-ic *pertaining to* tox- *poison*	Pertaining to a toxin
vaginosis	vah-jih-**NOH**-sis	S/ R/	-osis *condition* vagin- *vagina*	A disease of the vagina
vaginitis	vah-jih-**NIE**-tis	S/	-itis *inflammation*	Inflammation of the vagina
vestibulectomy	ves-tib-you-**LEK**-toe-me	S/ R/	-ectomy *surgical excision* vestibul- *entrance*	Surgical excision of the vulva
vulvodynia	vul-voh-**DIN**-ee-uh	S/ R/CF	-dynia *pain* vulv/o- *vulva*	Chronic vulvar pain
vulvovaginal	**VUL**-voh-**VAJ**-ih-nal	S/ R/CF R/	-al *pertaining to* vulv/o- *vulva* -vagin- *vagina*	Pertaining to the vulva and vagina
vulvovaginitis	**VUL**-voh-vaj-ih-**NIE**-tis	S/	-itis *inflammation*	Inflammation of the vulva and vagina

EXERCISES

A. Review *the Case Report on this spread before answering the questions.*   **LO 15.2, 15.4, and 15.10** *Understand*

1. What term in the diagnosis means *poison?* _____

2. Why was Ms. Baker admitted to the ICU? _____

3. Which other body systems could be affected by her toxic shock syndrome? _____

4. Is *Staphylococcus aureus* a viral or bacterial infection? _____

5. What term in the Case Report is your clue to the answer in #4? _____

6. What specific type of drug was administered by IV? _____

7. Did Ms. Baker have a transfusion or an infusion? _____

8. What harbored the staph infection? _____

9. How can toxic shock syndrome be prevented? _____

B. Suffixes in this WAD *box have appeared in many terms in previous chapters. Slash the medical term in the first column into elements to isolate the suffix. Define the meaning of the suffix, define the term in which it appears, write another term with a similar ending, and define that term. Fill in the chart.*   **LO 15.1, 15.2, and 15.4** *Remember*

Medical Term from WAD Above	Meaning of Suffix	Meaning of This Medical Term	Term from a Previous Chapter, with the Same Suffix	Meaning of That Medical Term
dyspareunia	1.	2.	3.	4.
vaginosis	5.	6.	7.	8.
vestibulectomy	9.	10.	11.	12.
vulvovaginal	13.	14.	15.	16.
vulvovaginitis	17.	18.	19.	20.

Lesson 15.2

Ovaries, Fallopian (Uterine) Tubes, and Uterus

*The primary female sex organs are the **ovaries**. The related internal accessory organs include a pair of **uterine tubes**, a **uterus**, and a vagina. Women are born with all the eggs **(ova)** that they will release in their lifetimes, but it is not until puberty that the eggs mature and start to leave the ovary. The ovarian hormones, estrogen and progesterone, are involved in puberty, **menstruation**, and **pregnancy**. These complex interactions are the core of the female human reproductive system and an essential part of understanding the human body. The information in this lesson will enable you to use correct medical terminology to:*

15.2.1 Describe the structure and functions of an ovary.

15.2.2 List the functions of estrogen and progesterone.

15.2.3 Explain the structures and functions of the ovaries, fallopian (uterine) tubes, and uterus.

15.2.4 Discuss common disorders of the ovaries, fallopian tubes, and uterus.

Abbreviations

CHES   certified health education specialist

GYN   gynecology

PCOS   polycystic ovarian syndrome

Case Report 15.2

You are ...

... a certified health education specialist **(CHES)** employed by Fulwood Medical Center.

You are communicating with ...

... Ms. Claire Marcos, a 21-year-old student referred to you by Anna Rusak, MD, a gynecologist. Ms. Marcos has been diagnosed with polycystic ovarian syndrome **(PCOS)**, and your task is to develop a program of self-care as part of her overall plan of therapy. From her medical record, you see that she presented with irregular, often-missed **menstrual** periods since the beginning of puberty; persistent acne; a loss of hair from the front of her scalp; and an inability to control her weight. She is 5 feet 4 inches tall and weighs 150 pounds. You are expected to counsel her about her self-care program involving exercise, diet, and the use of birth control medications.

Anatomy of the Female Reproductive Tract (LO 15.2 and 15.4)

Ovaries (LO 15.4)

Each **ovary** is an almond-shaped organ about 1 inch long and ½ inch in diameter. The ovaries are held in place by ligaments that attach them to the pelvic wall and uterus *(Figure 15.4)*. The ovaries' main functions are to:

- produce and release eggs and
- secrete hormones that affect puberty, menstruation, and pregnancy.

▶ **FIGURE 15.4**
Ovaries.
The ovaries are located on each side against the lateral walls of the pelvic cavity. The right fallopian (uterine) tube is retracted to reveal the ovarian ligament.

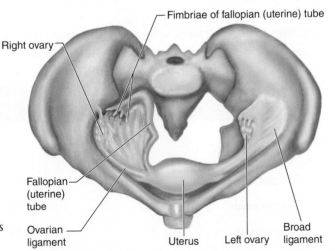

Word Analysis and Definition

S = Suffix   P = Prefix   R = Root   R/CF = Combining Form

WORD	PRONUNCIATION		ELEMENTS	DEFINITION
fallopian tubes (also called *uterine tubes*)	fah-**LOW**-pee-an		Gabrielle Fallopio, Italian anatomist, 1523–1562	Uterine tubes connected to the fundus of the uterus
menses (noun) menstruation (noun)	**MEN**-seez men-stru-**AY**-shun	S/ R/	Latin *month* -ation *process* menstru- *menses*	Monthly uterine bleeding Same as *menses*
menstruate (verb)	**MEN**-stru-ate	S/	-ate *composed of, pertaining to*	Act of menstruation
menstrual (adj)	**MEN**-stru-al	S/	-al *pertaining to*	Pertaining to menstruation
ovum ova (pl)	**OH**-vum **OH**-vah		Latin *egg*	Egg

EXERCISES

A. Review *the Case Report on this spread before answering the questions.*   **LO 15.2, 15.4, and 15.5** *Understand*

1. In her past medical history, what symptom did Ms. Marcos have relating to her menstrual period? _____

_____

2. What other symptoms does she have now? _____

3. What is Ms. Marcos being counseled about in relation to her condition? _____

4. What has been prescribed for Ms. Marcos? _____

5. What is the diagnosis for this patient? _____

B. Demonstrate *your knowledge of this chapter's medical vocabulary and circle the correct answer.*   **LO 15.2 and 15.4** *Apply*

1. Which term in the WAD has an element meaning *menses?*

   menstruate   fallopian   ova

2. Which term in the WAD refers to *egg?*

   menses   fallopian   ova

3. What other term means the same thing as *menses?*

   uterine   fallopian   menstruation

4. The plural of ovum is

   oval   oveas   ova

5. What is another name for the fallopian tubes?

   urinary tubes   uterine tubes   ureteral tubes

C. Meet lesson *and chapter objectives by describing the structure and functions of an ovary in the following questions.*   **LO 15.4 and 15.10** *Understand*

1. Structure:

_____

_____

2. Functions:

_____

_____

Lesson 15.2 Ovaries, Fallopian (Uterine) Tubes, and Uterus   351

Anatomy of the Female Reproductive Tract (continued)

Keynote

- Menarche cannot occur until a girl has at least 17% body fat.

Fallopian (Uterine) Tubes (LO 15.4)

Each **fallopian tube** is a canal about 4 inches long that extends from the uterus and opens to the abdominal cavity near an ovary. At the ovarian end, the outer third of the tube flares out into finger-like folds, each of which is called a **fimbria**. At ovulation, the **fimbriae** enclose the ovary *(Figure 15.5)*. The tubes' main functions are to enable sperm and eggs to meet and fertilize.

Uterus (LO 15.4)

The **uterus** is a thick-walled, muscular organ in the pelvic cavity. The main functions of the uterus are to cradle and nourish the fetus from conception to birth and to produce a woman's monthly menstrual flow (period). Anatomically, the uterus is divided into these three regions:

- The **fundus** is the broad, curved upper region between the lateral attachments of the fallopian (uterine) tubes;
- The **body** is the midportion; and
- The **cervix** is the cylindrical inferior portion that projects into the vagina.

The inner lining of the uterus is called the **endometrium;** the muscular layer is called the **myometrium.** The lower end of the uterine cavity communicates with the vagina through the cervical canal that has an external **os** (opening) into the vagina.

Ovarian Hormones (LO 15.5)

The ovaries of the sexually mature female secrete the hormones estrogen and progesterone.

Estrogens are produced in the ovarian follicles and their sexual functions are to:

1. Convert girls into sexually mature women through **thelarche, pubarche,** and **menarche;**
2. Regulate the menstrual cycle; and
3. Be involved in pregnancy when it occurs.

Progesterone is produced by the ovary's corpus luteum and also by the adrenal glands *(see Chapter 12)*. Its sexual functions are to:

1. Prepare the lining (endometrium) of the uterus for implantation of the egg *(Figure 15.5)*;
2. Inhibit lactation during pregnancy; and
3. Produce menstrual bleeding if pregnancy does not occur.

The ovaries also secrete small amounts of androgens, which are male hormones.

Sexual Cycle (LO 15.4 and 15.5)

The sexual cycle averages 28 days in length and includes the **menstrual** cycle. Physiologists recognize the beginning of the sexual cycle as **menstruation,** which occurs for the first 3 to 5 days. After menstruation, developing ovarian follicles mature, and one of them releases an oocyte around day 14. After this ovulation, the lining of the uterus hypertrophies, and the residual ovarian follicle becomes a secretory gland, which then **involutes** around day 26 to form an inactive scar called a **corpus luteum.** At this time, the arteries supplying the lining of the uterus contract. This leads to ischemia, tissue necrosis, and the start of menstruation.

▶ **FIGURE 15.5**
Female Reproductive Tract.

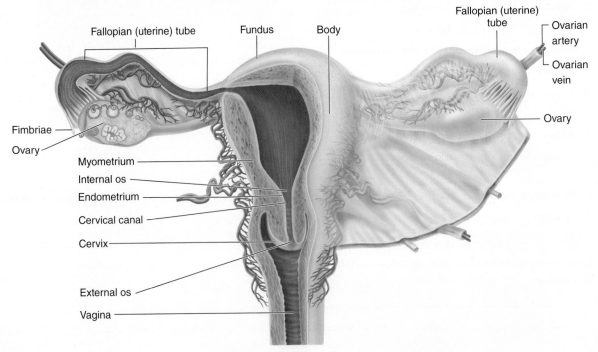

Fallopian (uterine) tube — Fundus — Body — Fallopian (uterine) tube — Ovarian artery — Ovarian vein — Ovary

Fimbriae — Ovary — Myometrium — Internal os — Endometrium — Cervical canal — Cervix — External os — Vagina

Word Analysis and Definition

S = Suffix   P = Prefix   R = Root   R/CF = Combining Form

WORD	PRONUNCIATION		ELEMENTS	DEFINITION
corpus luteum	KOR-puss LOO-tee-um		corpus Latin *body* luteum Latin *yellow*	Yellow structure formed at the site of a ruptured ovarian follicle
endometrium	en-doh-**ME**-tree-um	S/ P/ R/CF	-um *tissue* endo- *within, inside* -metr/i- *uterus*	Inner lining of the uterus
endometrial (adj)	en-doh-**ME**-tree-al	S/	-al *pertaining to*	Pertaining to the inner lining of the uterus
fallopian tubes (also called *uterine tubes*)	fah-**LOW**-pee-an		Gabrielle Fallopio, Italian anatomist, 1523–1562	Uterine tubes connected to the fundus of the uterus
fimbria fimbriae (pl)	**FIM**-bree-ah **FIM**-bree-ee		Latin *fringe*	Fringelike structure
fundus	**FUN**-dus		Latin *bottom*	The upper, rounded top of the uterus above the openings of the fallopian tubes
involution involute (verb)	in-voh-**LOO**-shun in-**VOH**-loot	S/ P/ R/	-ion *process* in- *in* -volut- *shrink*	A decrease in size.
menarche	meh-**NAR**-key	S/ R/	-arche *beginning* men- *month*	First menstrual period
myometrium	my-oh-**MEE**-tree-um	S/ R/CF R/CF	-um *tissue* my/o- *muscle* -metr/i- *uterus*	Muscle wall of the uterus
os	OS		Latin *mouth*	Opening into a canal; e.g., the cervix
pubarche	pyu-**BAR**-key	S/ R/	-arche *beginning* pub- *pubis*	Onset of development of pubic and axillary hair
thelarche	thee-**LAR**-key	S/ R/	-arche *beginning* thel- *breast, nipple*	Onset of breast development
uterus uterine (adj)	**YOU**-ter-us **YOU**-ter-in	S/ R/	Latin *womb* -ine *pertaining to* uter- *uterus*	Organ in which an egg develops into a fetus Pertaining to the uterus

EXERCISES

A. Meet lesson and chapter objectives *with the language of the female reproductive system. Fill in the blanks.*   **LO 15.2, 15.4, and 15.5** *Understand*

1. Which body cavity contains the uterus? _____

2. What is the main function of the fallopian tubes? _____

3. What two functions does the uterus have? _____

    _____

4. What does the os open into? _____

5. Where are estrogens produced? _____

6. Name one function of progesterone. _____

B. Choose *the correct pair of terms related to the question. Circle the correct answer.*   **LO 15.2, 15.4, and 15.5** *Remember*

1. Which two terms are structures inside the uterus?

   a. myocardium and pericardium

   b. perineum and periosteum

   c. endocardium and myocardium

   d. myometrium and endometrium

   e. sphincter and meatus

2. Name the regions of the uterus:

   a. fundus and os

   b. fundus, os, and body

   c. fundus, cervix, and body

   d. hypogastric, cervical, and fundus

   e. none of these is correct

3. Which pair of terms is associated with the production of progesterone?

   a. pubarche and menarche

   b. fundus and cervix

   c. adrenal glands and corpus luteum

   d. fornix and myometrium

   e. fimbriae and urethra

Lesson 15.3

Disorders of the Female Reproductive Tract

Case Report 15.2 (continued)

When Ms. Claire Marcos first presented in the gynecology clinic, Dr. Rusak examined her abdomen and pelvis. The doctor was able to palpate both enlarged ovaries on vaginal examination. A vaginal ultrasound scan showed multiple small cysts in each ovary. Dr. Rusack diagnosed Ms. Marcos with polycystic ovarian syndrome, and prescribed birth control pills because they contain estrogen and progesterone. The pills can correct the hormone imbalance, regulate Ms. Marcos' menses, and lower the level of testosterone to diminish her acne and hair loss problems.

Objectives

In order to care for a female patient who is experiencing reproductive tract disorders, you will need to effectively communicate with the patient, and with any of the other health care professionals involved in her case. The information provided in this lesson will enable you to use correct medical terminology to:

15.3.1 Describe common disorders of the ovaries, fallopian tubes, and uterus.

15.3.2 Identify the causes of and treatments for infertility.

15.3.3 Discuss different methods of contraception and their failure rates.

Keynotes

- The peak incidence of ovarian cancer is in the 50- and 60-year age groups.
- Oral contraceptives are 80% to 90% effective in relieving symptoms of PMS.

Abbreviations

GYN gynecology
PCOS polycystic ovarian syndrome
PMS premenstrual syndrome

Disorders of the Ovaries
(LO 15.4 and 15.5)

Ovarian Cysts (LO 15.4 and 15.5)

Ovarian cysts are fluid-filled sacs that can form, often during ovulation. They are usually benign and symptom-free unless they twist, bleed, or rupture.

Polycystic ovarian syndrome (PCOS), in which multiple follicular cysts form in both ovaries *(Figure 15.6)* is the disorder Ms. Marcos presented with. The repeated cyst formation prevents any eggs from maturing or being released, so ovulation does not occur and progesterone is not produced. Without progesterone, a female's menstrual cycle is irregular or absent.

Ovarian cysts produce androgens, which prevent ovulation and produce acne, the male-pattern hair loss

from the front of the scalp, and weight gain. Women with PCOS are also at increased risk for endometrial cancer, type 2 diabetes, high blood cholesterol, hypertension, and heart disease.

Ovarian cancer is the second most common gynecologic cancer after endometrial cancer. However, ovarian cancer accounts for more deaths than any other gynecologic cancer. Symptoms develop late in the disease process and are usually vague. Treatment is to surgically remove the tumor and administer chemotherapy. The 5-year survival rate is below 20%.

Primary amenorrhea occurs when a girl has not menstruated by age 16. This can occur with or without other signs of puberty.

Causes of primary amenorrhea include: drastic weight loss from malnutrition, dieting, bulimia, or anorexia nervosa; extreme exercise, as in some young gymnasts; extreme obesity; and chronic illness. Treatment is directed at the basic cause.

Secondary amenorrhea occurs when a woman who has menstruated normally misses three or more periods in a row and she is not pregnant or in her **menopause.**

The causes of secondary amenorrhea include: ovarian disorders, such as polycystic ovarian syndrome; excessive weight loss, low body fat percentage (e.g., as in gymnasts), or excessive exercise (e.g., as in marathon runners); and certain drugs, including antidepressants.

Primary dysmenorrhea, or **premenstrual syndrome (PMS)** refers to pain or discomfort associated with menstruation. The pain often begins 1 or 2 days before menses, peaks on the first day, and then slowly subsides.

▶ **FIGURE 15.6**
Polycystic Ovary.

Normal Ovary

Primary follicle
Secondary follicle
Mature follicle
Primordial follicle
Corpus albicans
Corpus luteum
Ovulation

Polycystic Ovary

Development stopped
Multiple immature follicles

Word Analysis and Definition

S = Suffix   P = Prefix   R = Root   R/CF = Combining Form

WORD	PRONUNCIATION	ELEMENTS		DEFINITION
amenorrhea	a-men-oh-**REE**-ah	S/ P/ R/CF	-rrhea *flow, discharge* a- *without* -men/o- *menses*	Absence or abnormal cessation of menstrual flow
dysmenorrhea	dis-men-oh-**REE**-ah	S/ P/ R/CF	-rrhea *flow, discharge* dys- *painful or difficult* men/o- *menses*	Painful and difficult menstruation
menopause (**Note:** *This term has no suffix, only a combining form and root.*)	**MEN**-oh-paws	R/ R/CF	-pause *cessation* men/o- *menses*	Permanent ending of menstrual periods
menopausal (adj)	**MEN**-oh-paws-al	S/	-al *pertaining to*	Pertaining to the menopause
polycystic	pol-ee-**SIS**-tik	S/ P/ R/	-ic *pertaining to* poly- *many* -cyst- *sac*	Composed of many cysts
premenstrual	pree-**MEN**-stru-al	S/ P/ R/	-al *pertaining to* pre- *before* -menstru- *menses*	Pertaining to the time immediately before the menses
primary	**PRY**-mair-ee		Latin *first*	The first disease or symptom, after which others may occur as complications
secondary	**SEK**-ond-air-ee		Latin *following or second*	Diseases or symptoms following a primary disease or symptom

EXERCISES

A. Review *the Case Report on this spread before answering the questions.*   **LO 15.2, 15.4, 15.5, and 15.10** *Understand*

1. What body cavity is formed by the abdomen and pelvis? _____

2. Explain the phrase *able to palpate.* _____

3. What was found on physical examination by the doctor? _____

4. What is the hormone content in Ms. Marcos's birth control pills? _____

5. What will her prescribed pills correct? _____
_____

6. What is the final diagnosis for Ms. Marcos? _____

B. Apply your knowledge *of the medical terminology for the female reproductive system by choosing the correct answer to each of the following questions. Circle the best choice.*   **LO 15.1, 15.4, and 15.5** *Apply*

1. The permanent ending of menstrual periods is:

menopause   dysmenorrhea   amenorrhea

2. *Premenstrual* happens:

before menses   after menses   in the middle of menses

3. The gynecologic malignancy that accounts for the most deaths is:

cervical cancer   breast cancer   ovarian cancer

4. Pick the term that contains a prefix, root, and suffix:

menopause   secondary   premenstrual

5. In the medical term *dysmenorrhea*, the prefix *dys* means:

without   first   painful

Keynote
- Residual scarring of the fallopian tube from salpingitis is a common cause of infertility.

Abbreviation

FUS	focused ultrasound surgery
PID	pelvic inflammatory disease
STD	sexually transmitted disease

Case Report 15.3

You are . . .

. . . a women's health nurse practitioner working with Anna Rusak, MD, a gynecologist at Fulwood Medical Center.

You are communicating with . . .

. . . Mrs. Carol Isbell, a 29-year-old woman c/o severe dysmenorrhea since the age of 15. Mrs. Isbell has been unable to conceive after 2 years of unprotected intercourse. She experiences severe, cramping lower abdominal pain for 2 days before, during, and 2 days after her periods, which are very heavy. She also has lower abdominal pain on intercourse. Her physical examination is unremarkable except that her pelvic examination shows several tender masses on each side of a normal-sized uterus. Dr. Rusak has also examined her and agreed with your diagnosis of endometriosis. Mrs. Isbell is to have an ultrasound examination.

▲ **FIGURE 15.7**
Prolapsed Uterus Protruding from the Vagina.

Fibroid
Wall of uterus
Cervix

◀ **FIGURE 15.8**
Large Single Fibroid in the Uterus.

Disorders of the Female Reproductive Tract (continued)

Disorders of the Uterus and Fallopian (Uterine) Tubes (LO 15.4)

Endometriosis is said to affect 1 in 10 American women of childbearing age. Here, the endometrium becomes implanted outside the uterus on the fallopian tubes, the ovaries, and the pelvic peritoneum. The displaced endometrium continues to go through its monthly cycle. It thickens and bleeds, leads to cysts and scar tissue, and produces pain. The cause of endometriosis is unknown. Treatment involves removing the abnormal tissue through laparoscopy.

Salpingitis is an inflammation of the fallopian (uterine) tubes and is part of pelvic inflammatory disease (**PID**). A bacterial infection, often from a sexually transmitted disease (**STD**), spreads from the vagina through the cervix and uterus. Symptoms are lower abdominal pain, fever, and a vaginal discharge. Treatment is with antibiotics.

Uterine Prolapse (LO 15.4)

The uterus is normally supported by the pelvic floor's muscles, ligaments, and connective tissue. However, a difficult childbirth, aging, obesity, lack of exercise, chronic coughing, and chronic constipation can weaken these tissues, causing the uterus to descend into the vaginal canal *(Figure 15.7)*. Uterine prolapse can be accompanied by prolapse of the bladder and anterior vaginal wall **(cystocele)**, or by prolapse of the rectum and posterior wall of the vagina **(rectocele).**

Treatment for uterine prolapse can be an individually fitted vaginal **pessary,** which is inserted into the vagina to support the uterus. Surgical procedures like sacral **colpopexy** (where a mesh patch is inserted into the pelvic floor), or vaginal **hysterectomy** (where the uterus is removed through the vagina) achieve good results.

Retroversion of the uterus is a normal variation, found in 20% of women. In retroversion, the body of the uterus is tipped backward instead of forward **(anteversion).** It can also be caused by lax pelvic muscles and ligaments, pelvic adhesions (scar tissue in the pelvis following salpingitis), or pelvic inflammatory disease. Retroversion by itself does not cause symptoms, and treatment is not usually necessary.

Uterine Fibroids (LO 15.4)

Uterine **fibroids** are noncancerous growths that appear during childbearing years. Three out of four women have them, but only one out of four women experiences their symptoms, which include **menorrhagia, metrorrhagia, polymenorrhea,** lower back pain, and pelvic pain.

Fibroids are also called **fibromyomas, leiomyomas,** or **myomas** *(Figure 15.8)*. They arise in the **myometrium** and produce a pale, firm, rubbery mass separate from the surrounding tissue. They vary in size from seedlings to large masses that distort the uterus. They can protrude into the uterine cavity, causing menorrhagia, or project outside the uterus and press on the bladder or rectum, thereby producing symptoms.

Treatment options are numerous and include watchful waiting, a **myomectomy,** and **focused ultrasound surgery (FUS). Hysterectomy** is a major surgery and is considered by many gynecologists as a last resort.

WORD	PRONUNCIATION	ELEMENTS		DEFINITION
anteversion	an-teh-**VER**-shun	S/ P/ R/	-ion *action, condition* ante- *forward* -vers- *turn*	Forward displacement or tilting of a structure (in this case, the uterus)
colpopexy	**KOL**-poh-peck-see	S/ R/CF	-pexy *surgical fixation* colp/o- *vagina*	Surgical fixation of the vaginal walls
cystocele	**SIS**-toh-seal	S/ R/CF	-cele *hernia* cyst/o- *bladder*	Hernia of the bladder into the anterior wall of the vagina
endometriosis	**EN**-doh-me-tree-**OH**-sis	S/ P/ R/CF	-osis *condition* endo- *within, inside* -metr/i- *uterus*	Endometrial tissue that functions outside the uterus
fibroid	**FIE**-broyd	S/ R/	-oid *resembling* fibr- *fiber*	Uterine tumor resembling fibrous tissue
fibromyoma	**FIE**-broh-my-**OH**-mah	S/ R/CF R/	-oma *tumor, mass* fibr/o- *fiber* -my- *muscle*	Benign neoplasm derived from smooth muscle and containing fibrous tissue
hysterectomy	his-ter-**EK**-toe-me	S/ R/	-ectomy *surgical excision* hyster- *uterus*	Surgical removal of the uterus
leiomyoma (also called *fibroid*)	**LIE**-oh-my-**OH**-mah	S/ R/CF R/	-oma *tumor, mass* lei/o- *smooth* -my- *muscle*	Benign neoplasm derived from smooth muscle
menorrhagia	men-oh-**RAY**-jee-ah	S/ R/CF	-rrhagia *flow, discharge* men/o- *menses*	Excessive menstrual bleeding
metrorrhagia	**MEH**-troh-**RAY**-jee-ah	S/ R/CF	-rrhagia *flow, discharge* metr/o- *uterus*	Irregular uterine bleeding between menses
myoma	my-**OH**-mah	S/ R/	-oma *tumor, mass* my- *muscle*	Benign tumor of muscle
myomectomy	my-oh-**MEK**-toe-me	S/ R/ R/	-ectomy *surgical excision* my- *muscle* -om- *tumor*	Surgical removal of a myoma
pessary	**PES**-ah-ree		Greek *an oval stone*	Appliance inserted into the vagina to support the uterus
polymenorrhea	**POL**-ee-men-oh-**REE**-ah	S/ P/ R/CF	-rrhea *flow* poly- *many, excessive* men/o- *menses*	More than normal frequency of menses
rectocele	**REK**-toe-seal	S/ R/CF	-cele *hernia* rect/o- *rectum*	Hernia of the rectum into the vagina
retroversion	reh-troh-**VER**-shun	S/ P/ R/	-ion *action, condition* retro- *backward* -vers- *turn*	Tipping backward of the uterus
salpingitis	sal-pin-**JIE**-tis	S/ R/	-itis *inflammation* salping- *tube*	Inflammation of the fallopian (uterine) tube
salpingectomy	sal-pin-**JEK**-toe-me	S/	-ectomy *surgical excision*	Surgical removal of a fallopian tube

EXERCISES

A. Review *the Case Report on this spread before answering the questions.* **LO 15.2, 15.4, and 15.10** *Understand*

1. What is *dysmenorrhea* in layperson's language? _____

2. Describe the symptoms Mrs. Isbell had with her monthly periods. _____

_____

3. What is shown on pelvic examination by Dr. Rusak? _____

4. What is the treatment for endometriosis? _____

5. What is *retroversion* in layperson's language? _____

6. What is *menorrhagia* in layperson's language? _____

Lesson 15.3 (cont'd) Disorders of the Female Reproductive Tract *(continued)*

Endometrial Cancer (LO 15.4)

Endometrial cancer is the fourth most common cancer in women, after lung, breast, and colon cancer. Each year, 40,000 new cases are diagnosed in the United States, mostly in women between ages 60 and 70. The most frequent symptom is vaginal bleeding after menopause. Surgery is the most prescribed treatment, which can involve a **total hysterectomy** (where the uterus and cervix are removed) or a **radical hysterectomy** (where the fallopian tubes and ovaries are removed along with the uterus). If the cancer has spread to other parts of the body, progesterone therapy, radiation therapy, and chemotherapy are used.

Cervical cancer is less common than endometrial cancer, but 50% of cervical cancer cases occur between ages 35 and 55. Some 10,000 new cases are diagnosed in the United States each year. Early cervical cancer produces no symptoms but may be found on a routine **Pap test.** In the **precancerous** stage, abnormal cells **(dysplasia)** are found only in the outer layer of the cervix. Thirteen types of human papilloma virus (HPV) can convert these **dysplastic** cells to cancer cells *(Figure 15.9).* A vaccine has been developed that appears to make people immune to two of the most common types of HPV. It has been licensed by the FDA for use in females aged 9 to 26.

Treatment depends on the stage of the cancer. In **preinvasive** cancer, when the cancer is only in the outer layer of the lining, the abnormal cells can be removed with a scalpel **(conization),** electrical current known as loop electrocautery excision procedure (LEEP), or laser beam. In an **invasive** stage, when the cancer has invaded the cervix and beyond, treatment can include a simple or radical hysterectomy, chemotherapy, and radiation therapy.

Normal cells   Dysplastic cells

LM 160×

▲ **FIGURE 15.9**
Abnormal Pap Smear with Dysplastic Cells.

Pap Test (LO 15.4)

In a Pap test, the doctor brushes cells from the cervix *(Figure 15.10).* These cells are smeared onto a slide or rinsed into a special liquid and sent to the laboratory for examination. The Pap test enables abnormal cells, precancerous or cancerous, to be detected. It is the most successful and accurate test for early detection of cervical cancer. A new FDA-approved test detects the DNA of the human papillomavirus in cells taken from the cervix. This can help identify women at high risk for developing cervical cancer, and it provides an additional tool to use in cervical cancer screening.

Other Causes of Abnormal Uterine Bleeding (LO 15.4)

Dysfunctional uterine bleeding is a term that's used when no cause can be found for a patient's menorrhagia. Treatment is with oral contraceptives. If that fails, **dilation and curettage (D & C)** may be effective. This procedure involves dilating the entrance to the uterus through the cervix so that a thin instrument can be inserted to scrape or suction away the lining of the uterus and take tissue samples. An alternative is endometrial **ablation,** in which a heat-generating tool or a laser removes or destroys the lining of the uterus and prevents or reduces menstruation. An endometrial ablation and hysterectomy can be used in women who have finished childbearing.

▲ **FIGURE 15.10**
Pap Smear Being Performed.

Menopause (LO 15.5)

Menopause is diagnosed when a woman has not menstruated for a year and is not pregnant. In this normal, natural, biological process of reproductive aging, levels of estrogen and progesterone start to decline around the age of 40, and most women stop menstruating between the ages of 45 and 55.

Without estrogen and progesterone, the uterus, vagina, and breasts atrophy, and more bone is lost than is replaced. Blood vessels constrict and dilate in response to changing hormone levels and can cause the characteristic menopausal "hot flashes."

Hormone replacement therapy (HRT), which involves taking medications containing the lacking female hormones, is no longer routinely recommended as a long-term replacement therapy for menopause. Studies have shown that its use increases the risk of heart disease, stroke, blood clots, and breast cancer.

Word Analysis and Definition

WORD	PRONUNCIATION	ELEMENTS		DEFINITION
ablation	ab-**LAY**-shun	S/ P/ R/	-ion *action, condition* ab- *away from* -lat- *to take*	Removal of tissue to destroy its function
conization	koh-ni-**ZAY**-shun	S/ R/	-ation *process* coniz- *cone*	Surgical excision of a cone-shaped piece of tissue
curettage	kyu-reh-**TAHJ**	S/ R/	-age *pertaining to* curett- *to cleanse*	Scraping the interior of a cavity
dysfunctional	dis-**FUNK**-shun-al	S/ P/ R/	-al *pertaining to* dys- *painful, difficult* -function- *perform*	Difficulty in performing
dysplasia	dis-**PLAY**-zee-ah	S/ P/ R/	-ia *condition* dys- *painful, difficult* -plas- *development, formation*	Abnormal tissue formation
dysplastic (adj)	dis-**PLAS**-tik	S/	-tic *pertaining to*	Pertaining to or showing abnormal tissue formation
menopause	**MEN**-oh-pawz	R/ R/CF	-pause *cessation* men/o- *menses*	Permanent ending of menstrual periods
menopausal (adj.)	**MEN**-oh-pawz-al	S/	-al *pertaining to*	Pertaining to the menopause
Pap test	PAP TEST		George Papanicolaou, Greek-U.S. physician, 1883–1962	Examination of cells taken from the cervix

EXERCISES

A. Deconstruct *the following medical terms into their elements with slashes. Be sure to write the identity of the element (P, R, CF, or S) under the line. Remember: Every element may not be present in every term. Space is provided for you to briefly define the term. Fill in the blanks.*
LO 15.1 and 15.4 *Analyze*

1. *ablation* _____ / _____ / _____

   Definition: _____

2. *dysfunctional* _____ / _____ / _____

   Definition: _____

3. *curettage* _____ / _____ / _____

   Definition: _____

4. *conization* _____ / _____ / _____

   Definition: _____

B. Patient education: *In language your patient can understand, explain to her the difference between:*   **LO 15.2, 15.4, 15.5, and 15.11** *Apply*

1. A total hysterectomy and a radical hysterectomy

   Total: _____

   Radical: _____

2. Explain to your patient the various treatment options available for endometrial cancer. _____
   _____
   _____

3. Your patient is asking you to explain what causes her "hot flashes." _____
   _____
   _____

Female Infertility and Contraception (LO 15.6)

Female Infertility (LO 15.6)

Infertility is the inability to become pregnant after 1 year of unprotected intercourse. It affects 10% to 15% of all couples. The causes of infertility include:

- The female factor alone in 35% of cases.
- The male factor alone in 30% of cases.
- Male and female factors in 20% of cases.
- Unknown factors in 15% of cases.

Causes of female infertility include scarring of the fallopian tubes, structural abnormalities of the uterus, and infrequent ovulation, all of which were addressed earlier in this chapter. Treatment is applied to any underlying cause arising from the results of the infertility evaluation.

Surgical procedures performed to initiate pregnancy include:

- **Intrauterine insemination,** in which sperm are inserted directly into the uterus via a special catheter.
- **In vitro fertilization (IVF),** in which eggs and sperm are combined in a laboratory dish and two to four resulting embryos are placed inside the uterus. This can result in twins or triplets.

Contraception (LO 15.5 and 15.6)

Contraception is the prevention of pregnancy. There are several common methods of contraception, including the approaches outlined below.

- **Behavioral methods:** These include **abstinence, coitus interruptus,** and the **rhythm method.** The latter two methods have a 20% failure rate.
- **Barrier methods:**
  - **Condoms** are available for males and females *(Figure 15.11)*. They have a 5% to 10% failure rate.
  - **Diaphragms** *(Figure 15.12)* and **cervical caps** consist of a latex or rubber dome that is inserted into the vagina and placed over the cervix. When used with a spermicide, they have a 5% to 10% failure rate.
  - **Spermicidal foams and gels** are inserted into the vagina. Used on their own, they have a 25% failure rate.
- **Intrauterine devices (IUDs):** These are T-shaped flexible plastic or copper devices inserted into the uterus and left in place for 1 to 4 years. The failure rate is less than 3%.
- **Hormonal methods:**
  - **Oral contraceptives** (birth control pills) utilize a mixture of estrogen and progesterone to prevent follicular development and ovulation. They have a 5% failure rate, usually due to inconsistent pill taking.
  - **Estrogen/progestin patches** deliver the hormones transdermally (through the skin). Their failure rate is below 1%.
  - **Injected progestins,** like Depo-Provera, are given by injection every 3 months. Their failure rate is below 1%.
  - **Implanted progestins,** like Norplant, are contained in porous silicone tubes that are inserted under the skin and slowly release the progestin for up to 5 years. Their failure rate is below 1%.
  - **Morning-after pills,** like Plan B, contain large doses of progestins to inhibit or delay ovulation. They are a backup when taken within 72 hours of unprotected intercourse. Their failure rate is around 10%.
  - **Mifepristone (RU486),** when taken with a prostaglandin, induces a miscarriage. It has an 8% failure rate.

Surgical Methods (LO 15.6)

- **Tubal ligation** ("getting your tubes tied") is performed with laparoscopy. Both fallopian tubes are cut, a segment is removed, and the ends are tied off and cauterized shut. The contraception failure rate is below 1%.

▲ **FIGURE 15.11**
Male and Female Condoms.

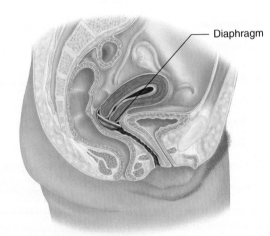

Diaphragm

▲ **FIGURE 15.12**
Diaphragm.

Word Analysis and Definition

S = Suffix   P = Prefix   R = Root   R/CF = Combining Form

WORD	PRONUNCIATION	ELEMENTS		DEFINITION
coitus postcoital (adj)	KOH-it-us post-KOH-ih-tal	S/ P/ R/	Latin come together -al pertaining to post- after -coit- sexual intercourse	Sexual intercourse After sexual intercourse
contraception	kon-trah-SEP-shun	S/ P/ R/	-ion action, condition contra- against -cept- receive	Prevention of pregnancy
contraceptive	kon-trah-SEP-tiv	S/	-ive quality of	An agent that prevents conception
diaphragm (Note: Also the term for the muscle that separates the thoracic and abdominal cavities.)	DIE-ah-fram		Greek partition or wall	A ring and dome-shaped material inserted into the vagina to prevent pregnancy
insemination	in-sem-ih-NAY-shun	S/ P/ R/	-ation process in- in -semin- semen	Introduction of semen into the vagina
inseminate (verb)	in-SEM-ih-nate	S/	-ate pertaining to	To introduce semen into the vagina
in vitro fertilization (IVF)	IN VEE-troh FER-til-ih-ZAY-shun	P/ S/ R/	in in vitro, Latin glass -ization process of creating fertil- able to conceive	Process of combining sperm and egg in a laboratory dish and placing resulting embryos inside the uterus
progestin	pro-JESS-tin	S/ P/ R/	-in substance pro- before -gest- produce, gestation	A synthetic form of progesterone

EXERCISES

A. Match the definitions in column 1 with the correct medical term in column 2. **Hint:** Be sure to use the correct form (noun, verb, adjective) of the term. Fill in the blanks.   **LO 15.6** Understand

_____ **1.** synthetic form of progesterone

_____ **2.** agent that prevents conception

_____ **3.** sexual intercourse

_____ **4.** introduction of semen into vagina

_____ **5.** having conceived

_____ **6.** egg and sperm in a lab dish

_____ **7.** ring and dome-shaped contraceptive device

A. diaphragm

B. pregnant

C. insemination

D. coitus

E. progestin

F. contraceptive

G. IVF

B. The following terms in the language of gynecology all appear in the text on contraception. Briefly define the following terms.
LO 15.2 and 15.6 Remember

1. injected _____

2. intrauterine _____

3. oral _____

4. implanted _____

5. spermicidal _____

6. transdermal _____

Lesson 15.4

Pregnancy

Objectives

For any health care professional involved in the care of a patient who is pregnant, it's necessary to be aware and informed of all aspects concerning pregnancy, childbirth, and their related conditions. The information in this lesson will enable you to use correct medical terminology to:

15.4.1 Describe conception and implantation.

15.4.2 Identify the characteristics of an embryo and **fetus.**

15.4.3 List the functions of the placenta.

15.4.4 Discuss the mechanisms of pregnancy (**PGY**) and childbirth and their common disorders.

Case Report 15.4

You are . . .

. . . an obstetric assistant (**OA**) employed by Garry Joiner, MD, an obstetrician at Fulwood Medical Center.

You are communicating with . . .

Mrs. Gloria Maggay, a 29-year-old housekeeper. Her last menstrual period was 8 weeks ago, and she has a positive home pregnancy test. This is her first pregnancy. She has breast tenderness and mild nausea. For the past 2 days, she has had some cramping, right-sided, lower abdominal pain and this morning had vaginal spotting. Her VS are T 99°F, P 80, R 14, BP 130/70. While you are waiting for Dr. Joiner to come and examine her, Mrs. Maggay complains of feeling faint and has a sharp, severe pain in the right side of her lower abdomen. Her pulse rate has increased to 92. You need to recognize what is happening and to use the correct medical terminology as you talk with Dr. Joiner.

Conception and Development (LO 15.7)

Conception (LO 15.7)

When released from the ovary, an egg takes 72 hours to travel to the uterus—but it must be **fertilized** within 12 to 24 hours to survive. Therefore, **fertilization** must take place in the distal third of the fallopian tube.

During unprotected intercourse, with male ejaculation, between 200 and 600 million sperm are deposited in the vagina near the cervix. The journey through the uterus into the fallopian tube takes about an hour. Some 2,000 to 3,000 sperm reach the egg. Several of these sperm penetrate the outer layers of the egg to clear the path for the one sperm that will penetrate all the way into the egg to **fertilize** it *(Figure 15.13)*. Once fertilized, the egg becomes a **zygote.**

Implantation (LO 15.7)

While still in the fallopian tube, the zygote divides; a fluid-filled cavity develops, and the zygote becomes a **blastocyst** (its first two weeks as a developing **embryo**). A week after fertilization, the blastocyst enters the uterine cavity and burrows into the endometrium, and **implantation** occurs. A group of cells in the blastocyst differentiate into the embryo. Other cells from the blastocyst, together with endometrial cells, form the **placenta.**

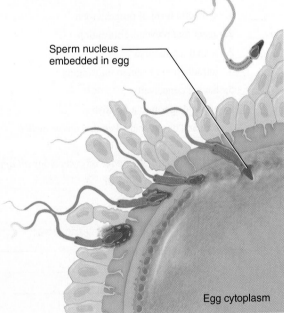

Sperm nucleus embedded in egg

Egg cytoplasm

▶ **FIGURE 15.13**
Fertilization.

Word Analysis and Definition

WORD	PRONUNCIATION	ELEMENTS		DEFINITION
blastocyst	**BLAS**-toe-sist	S/ R/CF	-cyst *cyst, bladder* blast/o- *germ or immaturecell*	First 2 weeks of the developing embryo
embryo	**EM**-bree-oh		Greek *a young one*	Developing organism from conception until the end of the second month
embryonic (adj)	em-bree-**ON**-ic	S/ R/	-ic *pertaining to* embryon- *embryo*	Pertaining to the embryo
fertilize (verb)	**FER**-til-ize		Latin *make fruitful*	Penetration of the oocyte by sperm
fertilization (noun)	**FER**-til-ih-**ZAY**-shun	S/ R/	-ation *process* fertiliz- *make fruitful*	Union of a male sperm and a female egg
fetus	**FEE**-tus		Latin *offspring*	Human organism from the end of the eighth week after conception to birth
fetal (adj)	**FEE**-tal	S/ R/	-al *pertaining to* fet- *fetus*	Pertaining to the fetus
implantation	im-plan-**TAY**-shun	S/ P/ R/	-ation *process* im- *in* -plant- *to plant, insert*	Attachment of a fertilized egg to the endometrium
placenta	plah-**SEN**-tah		Latin *a cake*	Organ that allows metabolic exchange between the mother and the fetus
zygote	**ZIGH**-goat		Greek *joined together*	Cell resulting from the union of the sperm and egg

EXERCISES

A. Review *the Case Report on this spread before answering the questions.*   **LO 15.2, 15.7, and 15.10** *Understand*

1. When was Mrs. Maggay's last menstrual period? _____

2. What are her presenting symptoms? _____

3. What has happened to her in the past two days? _____

4. What occurs while she is waiting for Dr. Joiner to examine her? _____

5. Which vital sign has increased? _____

6. Where is her sharp, severe pain now? _____

B. Meet lesson and chapter objectives *using the language of obstetrics.*   **LO 15.2, 15.7, and 15.10** *Understand*

1. Where does fertilization actually take place in the body? _____

2. Once fertilized, what is the new term for the egg and sperm? _____

3. During its first two weeks of development, the embryo is called the _____.

4. The entity in question #3 undergoes division into two separate entities called the _____ and the _____.

5. Attachment of the fertilized egg to the endometrium is called the _____.

C. Critical thinking: *What do you think could be happening to Mrs. Maggay based on her sudden, severe pain and the fact that she feels faint?*
   LO 15.2, 15.7, and 15.10 *Analyze*

1. _____

   _____

   _____

Lesson 15.4 Conception and Development *(continued)*

(cont'd) Placenta (LO 15.7)

Abbreviation

CVS   chorionic villus sampling

The placenta is a disc of tissue that increases in size as pregnancy proceeds *(Figure 15.14)*. The surface facing the fetus is smooth and gives rise to the **umbilical cord.** The surface attached to the uterine wall consists of treelike structures called **chorionic villi.** The cells of the villi keep the maternal and fetal circulations separate, but they are very thin and allow the exchange of gases, nutrients, and waste products.

The functions of the placenta are to:

- **Transport** nutrients and oxygen from the mother to the fetus;

- **Transport** nitrogenous wastes and carbon dioxide from the fetus to the mother, who can excrete them;

- **Transport** maternal antibodies and hormones to the fetus; and

- **Secrete** hormones like estrogen and progesterone.

Unfortunately, some undesirable matter and many medications can cross the placenta. These include: the HIV and rubella viruses; bacteria that cause syphilis; alcohol; nicotine and carbon monoxide from smoking; and drugs ranging from aspirin to heroin and cocaine. All of these can have detrimental effects on the fetus.

There are currently two common procedures that are performed during pregnancy to check the health of the fetus. Both **amniocentesis** (removal of amniotic fluid) and **chorionic villus sampling (CVS)** (where a sample of the chorionic villus cells is removed for a biopsy) test for chromosomal abnormalities and genetic birth defects.

▲ **FIGURE 15.14**
Embryo and Placenta at 13 Weeks.

Word Analysis and Definition

S = Suffix   P = Prefix   R = Root   R/CF = Combining Form

WORD	PRONUNCIATION	ELEMENTS		DEFINITION
amniocentesis	AM-nee-oh-sen-**TEE**-sis	S/ R/CF	-centesis *to puncture* amni/o- *amnion, fetal membrane*	Removal of amniotic fluid for diagnostic purposes
chorion chorionic (adj) chorionic villus	**KOH**-ree-on koh-ree-**ON**-ik **VILL**-us	S/ R/	Greek *membrane* -ic *pertaining to* chorion- *chorion* villus, Latin *shaggy hair*	The fetal membrane that forms the placenta Pertaining to the chorion Vascular process of the embryonic chorion to form the placenta
conception	kon-**SEP**-shun		Latin *something received*	Fertilization of the egg by sperm to form a zygote

EXERCISES

A. Precision in documentation *includes using the correct form (noun, verb, adjective) of the medical term. Practice precision in this written language of obstetrics. Fill in the blanks.*   **LO 15.2, 15.7, and 15.10** *Apply*

1. embryo   embryonic

In the _____ stage of gestation, the _____ forms in the first 8 weeks of human development.

2. chorionic   chorion

The _____ villi keep the maternal and fetal circulations separate. The _____ is the fetal membrane that forms the placenta.

Practice your precision in pronunciation, please!

B. Meet lesson objectives *and name the four functions of the placenta.*   **LO 15.2 and 15.7** *Remember*

1. _____

2. _____

3. _____

4. _____

C. Challenge your knowledge *of the language of obstetrics by answering the following questions.*   **LO 15.2 and 15.7** *Remember*

1. Where does the umbilical cord originate? _____

2. To what structure are the chorionic villi attached in the reproductive system? _____

3. What are the main functions of the villi? _____

_____

4. Name all the undesirable matter that can cross the placenta: _____

_____

5. Which two procedures can be performed during pregnancy to check the health of the fetus?

a. _____

b. _____

6. What two fetal problems are the procedures listed in question #5 looking for?

a. _____

b. _____

7. Why is the information gained in question #6 important to know early in pregnancy? _____

_____

Keynote

- Preeclampsia and eclampsia threaten the life of both mother and fetus.

Abbreviations

OR	operating room
POC	products of conception

Conception and Development (continued)

Embryo (LO 15.7)

The **embryonic period** occurs from week 2 until week 8. During this time, most of the embryo's external structures and internal organs are formed, together with the placenta, umbilical cord, **amnion** (the amniotic fluid-filled membrane around the fetus), and **chorion.** The amnion grows to envelop the embryo. At the eighth week, all the embryo's organ systems are present. The embryo is just over 1 inch long and is now officially a **fetus.**

Fetus (LO 15.7)

The fetal period lasts from the eighth week until birth. At the eighth week, the heart is beating. By the twelfth week, the bones have begun to calcify, and the external genitalia can be differentiated as male or female. In the fourth month, downy hair called **lanugo** appears on the body. In the fifth month, skeletal muscles become active, and the baby's movements are felt between 16 and 22 weeks of **gestation** *(Figure 15.15).* A protective substance called **vernix caseosa** covers the skin. In the sixth and seventh months, there is an increase in weight gain and body fat is deposited.

At 38 weeks, the baby is at full-term and ready for birth.

Gestation is divided into **trimesters:** The first trimester is up to week 12; the second from weeks 13 to 24; and the third from week 25 to birth.

▲ **FIGURE 15.15**
Developing Fetus at 20 Weeks.

Disorders of Pregnancy

(LO 15.7)

The paragraphs below explain the disorders in pregnancy that you will need to be familiar with when caring for a pregnant patient.

Ectopic Pregnancy

(LO 15.7)

In an **ectopic pregnancy,** there is an obstruction in the fallopian tube. As a result, the fertilized egg will be prevented from moving into the uterus. Instead, the egg will continue its development in the fallopian tube.

Case Report 15.4 *(continued)*

Mrs. Gloria Maggay's symptoms are indicative of an ectopic pregnancy. The sudden increase in pain and the rise in pulse rate can signal that the tube has ruptured and is hemorrhaging into the abdominal cavity. The gynecologist should see Mrs. Maggay immediately and take her to the operating room **(OR)** for laparoscopic surgery to stop the bleeding and evacuate the products of conception **(POC).**

Tubal disorders that cause ectopic pregnancy include previous salpingitis, pelvic inflammatory disease (PID), and endometriosis.

Preeclampsia and Eclampsia
(LO 15.7)

Preeclampsia is a sudden, abnormal increase in maternal blood pressure after the 20th week of pregnancy, with edema (swelling) of the face, hands, and feet. It is also accompanied by proteinuria (protein in the urine). Severe preeclampsia can lead to stroke, bleeding disorders, and death of the mother and fetus.

Eclampsia is a life-threatening condition, characterized by the signs and symptoms of preeclampsia, with the addition of convulsions. Management involves immediate admission to the hospital and control of the mother's blood pressure. The baby is delivered as soon as the mother is stabilized, regardless of its maturity.

Amniotic Fluid Abnormalities
(LO 15.7)

Amniotic fluid abnormalities occur in the second trimester, when the fetus breathes in and swallows amniotic fluid. This promotes development of the gastrointestinal tract and lungs. In the third trimester, the total amount of amniotic fluid is about 1 quart and is mostly fetal urine.

Oligohydramnios is a condition involving too little amniotic fluid. It is associated with an increase in the risk of birth defects and poor fetal growth. Its etiology is unknown.

Polyhydramnios is the opposite of oligohydramnios, and involves too much amniotic fluid. It causes abdominal discomfort and breathing difficulties for the mother. It is associated with **preterm delivery,** placental problems, and poor fetal growth.

Word Analysis and Definition

S = Suffix   P = Prefix   R = Root   R/CF = Combining Form

WORD	PRONUNCIATION		ELEMENTS	DEFINITION
amnion	AM-nee-on		Greek *membrane around fetus*	Membrane around the fetus that contains amniotic fluid
amniotic (adj)	am-nee-OT-ik	S/ R/CF	-tic *pertaining to* amni/o- *amnion, fetal membrane*	Pertaining to the amnion
ectopic	ek-TOP-ik	S/ R/	-ic *pertaining to* ectop- *on the outside, displaced*	Out of place, not in a normal position
gestation	jes-TAY-shun	S/ R/	-ion *action, condition* gestat- *pregnancy*	From conception to birth
gestational (adj)	jes-TAY-shun-al	S/	-al *pertaining to*	Pertaining to gestation
lanugo	la-NYU-go		Latin *wool*	Fine, soft hair on the fetal body
oligohydramnios	OL-ih-goh-high-DRAM-nee-os	R/CF R/ R/	oligo- *scanty, too little* -hydr- *water* -amnios *amnion*	Too little amniotic fluid
polyhydramnios	POL-ee-high-DRAM-nee-os	P/	poly- *many, excessive*	Too much amniotic fluid
preeclampsia	pree-eh-KLAMP-see-uh	S/ P/ R/	-ia *condition* pre- *before* -eclamps- *shining forth*	Hypertension, edema, and proteinuria during pregnancy
preterm (*same as* premature)	pree-TERM	P/ R/	pre- *before* -term *limit, end*	Baby delivered before 37 weeks of gestation
trimester	TRY-mes-ter		Latin *of 3 months' duration*	One-third of the length of a full-term pregnancy
vernix caseosa	VER-nicks kay-see-OH-sah		vernix, Latin *varnish* caseosa, Latin *cheese*	Cheesy substance covering the skin of the fetus

EXERCISES

A. Review *the Case Report on the opposite page before answering the questions.*   **LO 15.2, 15.7, and 15.10** *Understand*

1. "Mrs. Maggay has symptoms indicative of an ectopic pregnancy." What does that mean? _____
_____

2. Which two severe and sudden symptoms and signs may signal that her fallopian tube has ruptured? _____
_____

3. What is the treatment for Mrs. Maggay now? _____
_____

4. Name one tubal disorder that can cause an ectopic pregnancy._____
_____

B. Prefixes: *The WAD box contains prefixes that have appeared in previous chapters. In the chart below, the meaning of the prefix is given to you in the first column. List a term with that prefix from the WAD above, and give the meaning of the term. Then add another term with the same prefix from any previous chapter, and be sure to write its meaning as well. Fill in the chart.*   **LO 15.1** *Remember*

Meaning of Prefix	WAD Term with This Prefix	Meaning of This Term	Term from Previous Chapter	Meaning of Term from Previous Chapter
before	1.	2.	3.	4.
excessive	5.	6.	7.	8.
too little (scanty)	9.	10.	11.	12.

Lesson 15.4 (cont'd)

Disorders of Pregnancy (continued)

Abbreviation

GDM   gestational diabetes mellitus

Gestational Diabetes Mellitus (GDM) (LO 15.7)

In some pregnant women, the amount of insulin they can produce decreases and this leads to hyperglycemia. For the mother, gestational diabetes mellitus (**GDM**) increases the risk of preeclampsia and future type 2 diabetes. For the **neonate** (newborn child), it increases the risk of **perinatal** mortality, birth trauma, and **neonatal** hypoglycemia. Later in life, both mother and child are at increased risk for developing type 2 diabetes and obesity.

Hyperemesis Gravidarum (LO 15.7)

Eighty percent of pregnant women experience some degree of "morning sickness." It is at its worst between 2 and 12 weeks of pregnancy and resolves in the second trimester. For a few women, nausea is persistent, and vomiting is extreme and can lead to dehydration. This condition is called **hyperemesis gravidarum.** Severe cases may have to be admitted to the hospital for IV fluids.

Teratogenesis (LO 15.7)

Teratogenesis is the production of fetal abnormalities—**congenital malformations**—by a chemical agent affecting the mother during the early development of the fetus, while organs and structures are being formed. All medications readily cross the placenta. **Teratogens** include alcohol, isoretinoin (acne medication), valproic acid (an anticonvulsant), and the rubella virus.

Childbirth (LO 15.8)

Labor contractions begin about 30 minutes apart. They have to be intermittent because each contraction shuts down the maternal blood supply to the placenta and to the fetus. Labor pains are due to ischemia of the uterine muscle during contractions.

Labor is divided into three stages (*Figure 15.16*) each of which is usually longer in a **primipara** than in a **multipara**. Another term for pregnant is **gravid,** and a pregnant woman can be called **gravida.** A woman in her first pregnancy is called a **primigravida.**

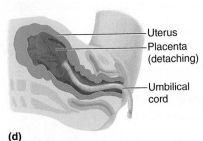

(a)
Placenta
Umbilical cord
Uterus
Cervix
Vagina

(b)
Pubic symphysis
Sacrum

(c)

(d)
Uterus
Placenta (detaching)
Umbilical cord

▲ **FIGURE 15.16**
The Stages of Childbirth.
(a) First stage: Early dilation.
(b) First stage: Late dilation.
(c) Second stage: Expulsion of the fetus.
(d) Third stage: Expulsion of the placenta.

First Stage—Dilation of the Cervix (LO 15.8)

This is the longest stage of labor. It can be a few minutes in a multipara to more than 1 day in a primipara. **Dilation** is the widening of the cervical canal to the same diameter as that of the baby's head (*Figure 15.16b*). At the same time that dilation occurs, the wall of the cervix becomes thinner—a process called **effacement.** During dilation, the fetal membranes rupture, and the "waters break" as amniotic fluid is released.

Second Stage—Expulsion of the Fetus (LO 15.8)

While the uterus continues to contract, the baby's head generates additional pain as it stretches the cervix and vagina. When the head reaches the vaginal opening and stretches the vulva, the head is said to be **crowning** and the baby can be delivered (*Figure 15.17*). Sometimes, this process can be helped by performing an **episiotomy** and making an incision in the perineum.

After the baby is delivered, blood in the placental vein is drained into the baby, and the umbilical cord is clamped in two places and cut between the two clamps.

Third Stage—Expulsion of the Placenta (LO 15.8)

After the baby is delivered, the uterus continues to contract. It pushes the placenta off the uterine wall and expels it from the vagina (*Figure 15.16d*).

Puerperium (LO 15.8)

The 6 weeks **postpartum** (after the birth) are called the **puerperium.** The uterus shrinks (**involution**) through self-digestion (**autolysis**) of uterine cells by their own enzymes. This generates a vaginal discharge called **lochia** that lasts about 10 days.

▲ **FIGURE 15.17**
Delivery of the Head.

Word Analysis and Definition

S = Suffix   P = Prefix   R = Root   R/CF = Combining Form

WORD	PRONUNCIATION	ELEMENTS		DEFINITION
autolysis	awe-**TOL**-ih-sis	P/ R/	auto- *self, same* -lysis *destruction*	Destruction of cells by enzymes within the cells
dilation	die-**LAY**-shun	S/ R/	-ion *process* dilat- *open out*	Stretching or enlarging an opening
effacement	ee-**FACE**-ment	S/ R/	-ment *resulting state* efface- *wipe out*	Thinning of the cervix in relation to labor
episiotomy	eh-piz-ee-**OT**-oh-me	S/ R/CF	-tomy *surgical incision* episi/o- *vulva*	Surgical incision of the vulva
gravid gravida	**GRAV**-id **GRAV**-ih-dah		Latin *pregnant* Latin *pregnant woman*	Pregnant A pregnant woman
hyperemesis	high-per-**EM**-eh-sis	P/ S/	hyper- *excessive* -emesis *vomiting*	Excessive vomiting
labor	**LAY**-bore		Latin *toil, suffering*	Process of expulsion of the fetus
lochia	**LOW**-kee-uh		Greek *relating to childbirth*	Vaginal discharge following childbirth
multipara	mul-**TIP**-ah-ruh	P/ R/	multi- *many* -para *to bring forth*	Woman who has given birth to two or more children
neonate neonatal (adj) (**Note:** *The "e" in the root is dropped because of the following vowel.*)	**NEE**-oh-nate **NEE**-oh-**NAY**-tal	R/CF R/ S/	neo- *new* -nate *born* -al *pertaining to*	A newborn infant Pertaining to the newborn infant or the newborn period
perinatal	per-ih-**NAY**-tal	S/ P/ R/	-al *pertaining to* peri- *around* -nat- *birth*	Around the time of birth
postpartum	post-**PAR**-tum	P/ R/	post- *after* -partum *childbirth, to bring forth*	After childbirth
primigravida	pree-mih-**GRAV**-ih-dah	P/ R/	primi- *first* -gravida *pregnancy*	A woman in her first pregnancy
primipara	pry-**MIP**-ah-ruh	P/ R/	primi- *first* -para *to bring forth*	Woman giving birth for the first time
puerperium (**Note:** *This term is composed of roots only.*)	pyu-er-**PER**-ee-um	R/ R/	puer- *child* -perium *a bringing forth*	Six-week period after birth in which the uterus involutes
teratogen teratogenic (adj) teratogenesis	**TER**-ah-toe-jen **TER**-ah-toe-**JEN**-ik **TER**-ah-toe-**JEN**-eh-sis	S/ R/CF S/ S/	-gen *create, produce* terat/o- *monster, malformed fetus* -ic *pertaining to* -esis *condition*	Agent that produces fetal deformities Capable of producing fetal deformities Process involved in producing fetal deformities

EXERCISES

A. Elements: *Several of these elements you have seen before, and you will certainly see them again in other terms. Learn an element once, and recognize it all the time. Circle the best answer to each question.* **LO 15.1, 15.7, and 15.8** *Understand*

1. The term that contains the prefix meaning *many* is:

   primipara   lochia   multipara

2. The term that contains the suffix meaning *incision* is:

   episiotomy   effacement   dilation

3. The term that contains the root meaning *destruction* is:

   autolysis   involution   effacement

4. The term that contains the root meaning *child* is:

   gravid   multipara   puerperium

Every newborn *(neonate)* is
either:

- Premature, less than 37
weeks' gestation;

- Full-term, between 37 and 42
weeks' gestation; or

- Post-term, longer than 42
weeks' gestation.

C-section	cesarean section
OB	obstetrics
PPH	postpartum hemorrhage
RDS	respiratory distress syndrome

Disorders of Childbirth
(LO 15.8)

Fetal distress, due to lack of oxygen, is an uncommon complication of labor, but it is detrimental if not recognized. During labor, there is electronic fetal heart monitoring. Treatment is to give the mother oxygen or increase IV fluids. If distress persists, the baby is delivered as quickly as possible by forceps extraction, vacuum extractor, or **cesarean section (C-section).**

An **abnormal position of the fetus** occurs at the beginning of labor if the baby is not a head-first **(vertex)** presentation facing rearward. Abnormal positions include:

- **Breech:** The buttocks present first *(Figure 15.18).*

- **Face:** The face, instead of the top of the head, presents first.

- **Shoulder:** The shoulder and upper back are trying to exit the uterus first.

If the baby cannot be turned into a vertex presentation, a C-section is usually performed.

In addition, other conditions can occur involving an abnormal placement of the baby's umbilical cord. In **prolapsed umbilical cord,** the cord precedes the baby down the birth canal. Pressure on the cord can cut off the baby's blood supply, which is still being provided through the umbilical arteries.

In **nuchal cord,** the cord is wrapped around the baby's neck during delivery. This occurs in 20% of deliveries.

Premature rupture of the membranes occurs in 10% of normal pregnancies and increases the risk of infection of the uterus and fetus.

Gestational Classification
(LO 15.8)

Prematurity occurs in about 8% of newborns. The earlier the baby is born, the more life-threatening problems occur.

Because their lungs are underdeveloped, premature babies can develop **respiratory distress syndrome**

(RDS), also called **hyaline membrane disease.** Their lungs are not mature enough to produce **surfactant,** a mixture of lipids and proteins that keeps the alveoli from collapsing. As a result, this prevents the respiratory exchange of oxygen and carbon dioxide.

An immature liver can impair the excretion of bilirubin (yellowish bile pigment) *(see Chapter 9),* and premature babies become jaundiced. High levels of bilirubin can produce **kernicterus,** in which deposits of bilirubin in the brain cause brain damage.

Postmaturity is much less common than prematurity. Its etiology is unknown, but the placenta begins to shrink, making it difficult to supply sufficient nutrients to the baby. For the baby, this leads to: hypoglycemia; loss of subcutaneous fat; dry, peeling skin; and, if oxygen is lacking, fetal distress. The baby can pass stools **(meconium)** into the amniotic fluid. In its distress, the baby can take deep gasping breaths and inhale the meconium fluid. This leads to **meconium aspiration syndrome** and respiratory difficulty at birth.

An **abortion** is the expulsion of an embryo or fetus from the uterus before the 20th week of gestation. It can be spontaneous (occurring from natural causes) or induced medically or surgically.

Placental Disorders (LO 15.8)

Placenta abruptio is the separation of the placenta from the uterine wall before delivery of the baby. The baby's oxygen supply is cut off, and fetal distress appears quickly. It is an **obstetric (OB)** emergency, and usually a **C-section** is performed.

Placenta previa is a low-lying placenta between the baby's head and the internal os of the cervix. It can cause severe bleeding during labor, and a C-section may be necessary.

In a **retained placenta,** all or part of the placenta and/or membranes remain behind in the uterus 30 minutes to an hour after the baby has been delivered. The result of a retained placenta is heavy uterine bleeding called **postpartum hemorrhage (PPH).** Manual removal of the retained placenta may be necessary under spinal, epidural, or general anesthesia *(Figure 15.19).*

▼ **FIGURE 15.18**
Breech Presentation.

◄ **FIGURE 15.19**
Placenta
(Afterbirth).

Umbilical cord

Placenta

Membranes

Placenta

Word Analysis and Definition

WORD	PRONUNCIATION	ELEMENTS		DEFINITION
abortion	ah-**BOR**-shun	S/ R/	-ion *action* abort- *fail at onset*	Spontaneous or induced expulsion of the embryo or fetus from the uterus at 20 weeks or less
breech	**BREECH**		Old English *trousers*	Buttocks-first presentation of the fetus at delivery
cesarean section (c-section)	seh-**ZAH**-ree-an **SEK**-shun		Roman law under the Caesars required that pregnant women who died be cut open and the fetus be extracted	Extraction of the fetus through an incision in the abdomen and uterine wall
kernicterus	ker-**NICK**-ter-us	R/ R/	kern- *nucleus* -icterus *jaundice*	Bilirubin staining of the basal nuclei of the brain
meconium	meh-**KOH**-nee-um		Greek *a little poppy*	The first bowel movement of the newborn
nuchal cord	**NYU**-kul **KORD**		nuchal, French *the back (nape) of the neck*	Loop(s) of umbilical cord around the fetal neck
placenta abruptio	plah-**SEN**-tah ab-**RUP**-she-oh		abruptio, Latin *to break off*	The premature detachment of the placenta
placenta previa	plah-**SEN**-tah **PREE**-vee-ah	P/ R/	pre- *before, in front of* -via *the way*	Condition in which the placenta is positioned between the fetus and the cervix
postmature	post-mah-**TYUR**	P/ R/	post- *after* -mature *ripe, ready*	Infant born after 42 weeks of gestation
postmaturity	post-mah-**TYUR**-ih-tee	S/	-ity *condition, state*	Condition of being postmature
premature (slang term "preemie")	pree-mah-**TYUR**	P/ R/	pre- *before* -mature *ripe, ready*	Occurring before the expected time
prematurity (same as *preterm*)	pree-mah-**TYUR**-ih-tee	S/	-ity *condition, state*	Condition of being premature
surfactant	sir-**FAK**-tant		*surface active agent*	A protein and fat compound that creates surface tension to hold the lung alveolar walls apart
vertex	**VER**-teks		Latin *whorl*	Topmost point of the vault of the skull

EXERCISES

A. Patient documentation: *Pick any two terms from the WAD, and use them to create your own patient documentation. You must be able to pronounce, spell, and define every term you use in your sentences as the instructor may ask you to read them aloud in class. Fill in the blanks.*
LO 15.2, 15.8, and 15.10 *Apply*

1. _____
   _____

2. _____
   _____

B. Meet lesson and chapter objectives *and apply the language of obstetrics to answer the following questions.*
LO 15.2, 15.3, 15.8, and 15.10 *Apply*

1. What is the result of a retained placenta? _____

2. What is a *spontaneous abortion?* _____

3. What are the other causes of abortion? _____

4. What is another medical term for RDS? _____

5. What is the function of a surfactant? _____

6. What is the medical term for normal presentation of the fetus? _____

Lesson 15.5

The Female Breast

You are ...

... a surgical technologist working with Charles Walsh, MD, a surgeon at Fulwood Medical Center.

You are communicating with ...

... Mrs. Victoria Post, a 62-year-old woman who has discovered a lump in her right breast. Mrs. Post found the lump in her right breast together with some lumps in her right armpit on self-examination. She had not examined her breasts for about 6 months. She began her menopause at age 52. Her mother and a sister died of breast cancer. Physical examination shows a 2-cm firm, painless lesion in the upper outer quadrant of her right breast, and several small, painless lymph nodes in her right axilla. Dr. Walsh has scheduled her for a biopsy of the breast lesion and for DNA testing.

Objectives

Until the relatively recent introduction of bottles filled with liquid supplied by cows or soybeans, the milk produced by the female breast was essential for the survival of the human species. Nourishment of the infant remains the breast's major function. It is important to complete your understanding of the female reproductive system by being able to use correct medical terminology to:

15.5.1 Describe the anatomy of the breast and the mammary gland.

15.5.2 Explain the physiology and mechanisms of lactation.

15.5.3 Discuss common disorders of the breast.

Keynote

- There is no relation between breast size and the ability to breastfeed.

Adipose tissue

Pectoralis major muscle

Lobe

Areola

Nipple

Lactiferous sinus

Lactiferous duct

▲ **FIGURE 15.20**
Anatomy of the Lactating Breast.

The Breast (LO 15.9)

Anatomy of the Breast (LO 15.9)

The female breasts can be both beautiful and functional. They help to give a woman her distinctive feminine shape, and, after childbirth, they provide natural nourishment for an infant. Each adult female breast has a **body** located over the pectoralis major muscle and an **axillary tail** extending toward the armpit. The **nipple** projects from the breast and contains multiple openings of the main milk ducts. The reddish-brown **areola** surrounds the nipple. The small bumps on its surface are called **areolar glands.** These are sebaceous glands whose secretions prevent chapping and cracking during breastfeeding.

The **nonlactating breast** consists mostly of adipose and connective tissues. It has a system of ducts that branch through the connective tissue and converge on the nipple.

Mammary Gland (LO 15.9)

When the **mammary** gland develops during pregnancy, it is divided into 15 to 20 lobes that contain the secretory **alveoli** that produce milk. The main milk ducts, called **lactiferous ducts** *(Figure 15.20)* drain each lobe immediately before opening onto the nipple.

Lactation (LO 15.9)

In late pregnancy, the secretory alveoli and lactiferous ducts contain **colostrum.** This is the first secretion from the breasts during pregnancy. Colostrum contains more protein but less fat than human milk. It also contains high levels of **immunoglobulins** *(see Chapter 7)* that give the infant protection from infections. Colostrum begins to be replaced by milk 2 or 3 days after the baby's birth, and this replacement is complete by day 5.

The essential stimulus to milk production is the baby's sucking. This stimulates the pituitary gland to produce **prolactin,** which in turn stimulates milk production, and **oxytocin** *(see Chapter 12)*, which causes milk to be ejected from the alveoli into the duct system.

After **lactation** completely stops, **involution** of the mammary gland occurs. The epithelial cells of the alveoli are lost through **apoptosis** (programmed cell death), the ducts shrink in size, and adipose and connective tissues return to be the major breast tissues.

Word Analysis and Definition

S = Suffix   P = Prefix   R = Root   R/CF = Combining Form

WORD	PRONUNCIATION	ELEMENTS		DEFINITION
apoptosis	AP-op-TOE-sis	P/ R/	apo- *separation from* -ptosis *drooping*	Programmed normal cell death
areola areolar (adj)	ah-REE-oh-lah ah-REE-oh-lar	 S/ R/	Latin *small area* -ar *pertaining to* areol- *areolar*	Circular reddish area surrounding the nipple Pertaining to the areola
colostrum	koh-LOSS-trum		Latin *foremilk*	The first breast secretion at the end of pregnancy
involution involute (verb)	in-voh-LOO-shun in-voh-LUTE	S/ P/ R/	-ion *action, condition* in- *in* -volut- *roll up, shrink*	Decrease in size
lactation (noun)	lak-TAY-shun	S/ R/	-ation *action, process of* lact- *milk*	Production of milk
lactate (verb) lactiferous (adj)	LAK-tate lak-TIF-er-us	S/ S/ R/	-ate *composed of, pertaining to* -ous *pertaining to* -ifer- *to bear, carry*	To produce milk Pertaining to or yielding milk
mammary	MAM-ah-ree	S/ R/	-ary *pertaining to* mamm- *breast*	Pertaining to the lactating breast
nipple	NIP-el		Old English *small nose*	Projection from the breast into which the lactiferous ducts open
oxytocin	OCK-see-TOE-sin	S/ R/ R/	-in *substance* oxy- *oxygen* -toc- *labor*	Pituitary hormone that stimulates the uterus to contract
prolactin	pro-LAK-tin	S/ P/ R/	-in *substance* pro- *before* -lact- *milk*	Pituitary hormone that stimulates the production of milk

EXERCISES

A. Review *the Case Report on this spread before answering the questions.*   **LO 15.2, 15.3, 15.9, and 15.10** *Understand*

1. Where did Mrs. Post find the lumps? _____

2. What important fact is in her history? _____

3. Why would Mrs. Post go to the doctor if the lumps in her breast and armpit were not causing her any pain? _____

4. Use an abbreviation to describe where the 2-cm lump was found. _____

5. Use the medical term to describe where the enlarged lymph nodes appeared. _____

B. Spelling *your documentation correctly is a mark of an educated professional. Read the following statements, and insert the correctly spelled term in the blanks.*   **LO 15.2, 15.9, and 15.10** *Apply*

1. The circular, reddish area surrounding the nipple is the *(aireola/areola)* _____.

2. After complete cessation of lactation, involution of the *(mamery/mammary)* _____ gland occurs.

3. Programmed cell death is known as *(apotosis/apoptosis)* _____.

4. The first breast secretion at the end of pregnancy is known as *(colestrium/colostrum)* _____.

C. Proofread *the following sentences for error in fact or spelling. Write the corrected sentences on the lines below.*   **LO 15.2, 15.9, and 15.10** *Apply*

1. The main milk ducts are called mammary ducts.

_____

2. The term *innvolution* means to decrease in size.

_____

3. The first secretion from the breasts during pregnancy is called meconium.

_____

- There is some disagreement whether routine mammograms should begin at age 40 or 50 and whether they should be performed annually or every 2 years.

BRCA1, BRCA2	breast cancer genes
BSE	breast self-examination
PMS	premenstrual syndrome

▲ **FIGURE 15.21**
Paget Disease of the Nipple Is Associated with Breast Cancer.

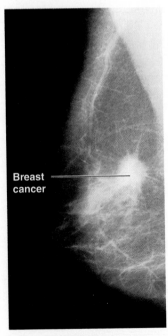

Breast cancer

▲ **FIGURE 15.22**
Mammogram Showing Breast Cancer.

Case Report 15.5 (continued)

Mrs. Victoria Post's biopsy confirmed that the lump was cancer. DNA testing showed the presence of the BRCA1 gene, which explained the occurrence of breast cancer in her mother and sister. Mrs. Post is to attend a consultation with her surgeon, Dr. Walsh, and her **geneticist**, Ingrid Hughes, MD, PhD, to determine what treatment should be undertaken. For example, because of her high risk of cancer, should she have her left breast, currently cancer-free, removed? With BRCA1, there is also a 20% to 40% risk of ovarian cancer. Therefore, should her ovaries also be removed?

Disorders of the Breast (LO 15.9)

Mastitis, an inflammation of the breast, can occur in association with breastfeeding if the nipple or areola is cracked or traumatized. **Mastalgia** (breast pain) is the most common benign breast disorder. This pain may be associated with breast tenderness or **PMS.**

Paget disease of the nipple presents as a scaling, crusting lesion of the nipple, sometimes with a discharge from the nipple *(Figure 15.21)*. It is indicative of an underlying cancer that must be the focus of diagnosis and treatment.

Nipple discharge, particularly if it is bloody and only from one breast, is an indication of an underlying disorder like breast cancer and should be investigated.

Fibroadenomas are confined, small, benign tumors that can be either cystic or solid, and can be multiple. These tumors can be surgically removed.

Fibrocystic breast disease presents as a dense, irregular, cobblestone consistency of the breast, often with intermittent breast discomfort. It occurs in over 60% of all women and is considered by many doctors as a normal condition.

Breast cancer affects one in eight women in their lifetimes. Risk factors include: a family history, particularly if a woman carries either the **BRCA1** or **BRCA2 gene;** the use of postmenopausal estrogen therapy; and an early menarche and late menopause.

Some breast cancers are discovered as a lump by the patient, which is why **monthly breast self-examinations (BSEs)** are important. Another 40% are discovered on routine **mammograms** *(Figure 15.22)*. Routine **mammography** reduces breast cancer mortality by 25% to 30%. Breast cancer rarely occurs in males.

Most breast cancers occur in the upper and outer quadrants of the breast. If cancer is suspected, a biopsy should be planned. Currently, it's common to perform a **stereotactic biopsy,** where a needle biopsy is done during mammography. Breast cancer can metastasize to the lymph nodes, lungs, liver, bones, brain, and skin. The surgical treatments available for breast cancer include:

- **Lumpectomy:** the tumor is removed and the surrounding breast tissue is preserved.
- Simple **mastectomy:** the breast with skin and the nipple is removed.
- Modified radical mastectomy: a simple mastectomy with lymph node dissection.
- Radical mastectomy: a modified mastectomy that includes the removal of lymph nodes and the pectoralis major muscle.

Additional radiotherapy and chemotherapy are also used.

Galactorrhea occurs when a woman produces milk when she's not breastfeeding. This can occur in association with hormone therapy, antidepressants, a pituitary gland tumor, and the use of street drugs like cocaine, heroin, and marijuana. In most cases, the milk production ceases with time.

Gynecomastia is an enlargement of the breast that can be unilateral or bilateral. It can occur in both sexes. It is usually associated with either liver disease, marijuana use, or drug therapy involving estrogens, calcium channel blockers, and **antineoplastic** drugs. Gynecomastia remits or disappears after the drug is withdrawn. Occasionally, cosmetic surgery is needed.

Word Analysis and Definition

S = Suffix   P = Prefix   R = Root   R/CF = Combining Form

WORD	PRONUNCIATION	ELEMENTS		DEFINITION
antineoplastic	AN-tee-nee-oh-PLAS-tik	S/ P/ R/CF R/	-tic *pertaining to* anti- *against* -ne/o- *new* -plas- *growth*	Pertaining to the prevention of the growth and spread of cancer cells
fibroadenoma	FIE-broh-ad-en-OH-muh	S/ R/CF R/	-oma *tumor* fibr/o- *fiber* -aden- *gland*	Benign tumor containing much fibrous tissue
fibrocystic disease	fie-broh-SIS-tik diz-EEZ	S/ R/CF R/	-ic *pertaining to* fibr/o- *fiber* -cyst- *cyst*	Benign breast disease with multiple tiny lumps and cysts
galactorrhea	gah-LAK-toe-REE-ah	S/ R/CF	-rrhea *flow* galact/o- *milk*	Abnormal flow of milk from the breasts
gene	JEEN		Greek *origin, birth*	Functional segment of DNA molecule
genetics	jeh-NET-iks	S/ R/	-ics *knowledge* genet- *origin*	Science of the inheritance of characteristics
geneticist (**Note:** *Two suffixes*)	jeh-NET-ih-sist	S/	-ist *specialist*	A specialist in genetics
gynecomastia	GUY-nih-koh-MAS-tee-ah	S/ R/CF R/	-ia *condition* gynec/o- *female* -mast- *breast*	Enlargement of the breast
lumpectomy	lump-ECK-toe-me	S/ R/	-ectomy *surgical excision* lump- *piece*	Removal of a lesion with preservation of surrounding tissue
mammogram	MAM-oh-gram	S/ R/CF	-gram *a record* mamm/o- *breast*	The record produced by x-ray imaging of the breast
mammography	mah-MOG-rah-fee	S/	-graphy *process of recording*	Process of x-ray examination of the breast
mastalgia	mass-TAL-jee-uh	S/ R/	-algia *pain* mast- *breast*	Pain in the breast
mastectomy	mass-TECK-toe-me	S/ R/	-ectomy *surgical excision* mast- *breast*	Surgical excision of the breast
mastitis	mass-TIE-tis	S/ R/	-itis *inflammation* mast- *breast*	Inflammation of the breast
Paget disease	PAJ-et diz-EEZ		Sir James Paget, 1814–1899, English surgeon	Scaling, crusting lesion of the nipple, often associated with an underlying cancer of the breast
stereotactic	STER-ee-oh-TAK-tic	S/ R/CF R/	-ic *pertaining to* stere/o- *three-dimensional* -tact- *orderly arrangement*	A precise three-dimensional method to locate a lesion

EXERCISES

A. Review *the Case Report on this spread before answering the questions.*   **LO 15.2, 15.9, and 15.10** *Understand*

1. Which diagnostic test confirmed the diagnosis of cancer for Mrs. Post? _____

2. What explains the occurrence of breast cancer in Mrs. Post's mother and sister? _____

3. What type of testing is used for genes? _____

4. What are some options for Mrs. Post's treatment plan? _____

B. Suffixes *always provide a big clue to the meaning of a medical term. Review all the terms in the WAD above, and then answer the following questions. All of these questions can be answered by analyzing the suffix in each term.*   **LO 15.1, 15.2, 15.9, and 15.10** *Analyze*

Which of the terms in this WAD means:

1. a condition of enlargement of the breast? _____

2. a glandular tumor? _____

3. process of an x-ray examination of the breast? _____

4. knowledge of the inheritance of characteristics? _____

5. an inflammation of the breast? _____

6. breast pain? _____

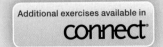

Additional exercises available in

Chapter Review exercises, along with additional practice items, are available in Connect!

Word Parts and Abbreviations

Note: For easy identification, the word parts in this appendix appear in the same colors as in the Word Analysis and Definition boxes: suffix, prefix, root, root/combining form. Any term that is used in the text in both root and combining form is shown only in this appendix as a combining form.

Word Part	Definition
a-	not, without
a-	variant of ad
ab-	away from
abdomin/o	abdomen
ability	competence
ablat	take away
-able	capable
abort	fail at onset, expel nonviable fetus
abras	scrape off
absorpt	to swallow, take in
ac-	toward
-ac	pertaining to
-acea	condition, remedy
acid/o	acid, low pH
acin	grape
acous	hearing
acr/o	peak, topmost, extremity, highest point
acromi/o	acromion
act	to do, perform, performance
activ	movement
acu	needle
acu-	sharp
acumin	to sharpen
ad-	to, toward, into
adapt	to adjust
-ade	process
aden/o	gland
adenoid	adenoid
adip	fat
adjust	alter
adjuv	give help
adolesc	beginning of adulthood
adren/o	adrenal gland

Word Part	Definition
aer/o	air, gas
affer	move toward the center
ag-	to
-age	pertaining to
agglutin	sticking together, clumping
-ago	disease
agon	to fight
-agon	to fight
agor/a	marketplace
-agra	severe pain
-al	pertaining to
alanine	an amino acid, protein synthesized in muscle
albicans	white
albin/o	white
albumin	albumin
ald/o	organic compound
-ale	pertaining to
alges	sensation of pain
-algia	pain, painful condition
aliment	nourishment
-alis	pertaining to
alkal	base
all/o	strange, other
allo-	strange, other
alopec-	baldness, mange
alpha-	first letter in the Greek alphabet
alveol	alveolus, air sac
-aly	condition
ambly-	dull
ambulat	to walk, walking
amin/o	nitrogen containing
-amine	nitrogen-containing substance

WORD PART	DEFINITION
ammon	ammonia
amni/o	amnion, fetal membrane
amnios	amnion
amph-	around
ampull	bottle-shaped
amput	to prune, cut off
amyl	starch
an-	not, lack of, without
-an	pertaining to
an/o	anus
ana-	away from, excessive
anabol	build up
analysis	process to study whole in terms of its parts
analyst	one who separates
anastom	provide a mouth
-ance	condition, state of
-ancy	state of
andr/o	male, masculine
aneurysm	dilation
angi/o	blood vessel, lymph vessel
angina	sore throat, chest pain radiating to throat
ankyl	stiff
-ant	forming, pertaining to
ant-	against
ante-	before, forward, in front of
anter	before, front part
anthrac	coal
anti-	against
aort	aorta
apo-	different from, separation from
appendic	appendix
apse	clasp
aqu-	water
-ar	pertaining to
arachn	cobweb, spider
-arche	beginning
areol	areola, small area
aria	air
-arian	one who is

WORD PART	DEFINITION
-aris	pertaining to
aroma	smell, sweet herb
array	place in order
arter	artery
arteri/o	artery
arteriosus	like an artery
arthr/o	joint
articul	joint
-ary	pertaining to
asbest	asbestos
ascit	fluid in the belly
-ase	enzyme
aspartate	an amino acid
aspergill	aspergillus
aspirat	to breathe on
assay	evaluate
assist	aid, help
asthm	asthma
astr/o	star
-ata	action, place, use
-ate	composed of, pertaining to
-ated	pertaining to a condition
atel	incomplete
ather/o	porridge, gruel, fatty substance
athet	without position, uncontrolled
-atic	pertaining to
-ation	a process
-ative	pertaining to, quality of
-ator	agent, instrument, person or thing that does something
-atory	pertaining to
atri/o	entrance, atrium
-atric	treatment
attent	awareness
attenu	to weaken
audi/o	hearing
audit	hearing
aur-	ear
auscult	listen to

S = Suffix   P = Prefix   R = Root   R/CF = Combining Form

Word Part	Definition
auto-	self, same
avail	useful
axill	armpit, axilla
ayur-	life
azot	nitrogen
-back	back, toward the starting point
bacteri/o	bacteria
balan	glans penis
bar	pressure
bari	weight
bas/o	base, opposite of acid
basal	deepest part
basil	base, support
be	life
behav	mental or motor activity
beta	second letter of Greek alphabet
bi-	two, twice, double
bi/o	life
-bil-	able
bil/i	bile
-blast	germ cell, immature cell
blast/o	germ cell, immature cell
blephar/o	eyelid
body	body, mass, substance
bov	cattle
brachi/o	arm
brachii	of the arm
brachy-	short
brady-	slow
bride	rubbish, rubble
bronch/i	bronchus
bronch/o	bronchus
brucell	pathologist David Bruce
buccinat	cheek
bulb/o	bulb
burs	bursa
calc/i	calcium
calcan	calcaneous
calcul	stone, little stone

Word Part	Definition
callos	thickening
calor	heat
canal	duct or channel
cancer	cancer
candid	*Candida*
capill	hairlike, capillary
capit	head
capn	carbon dioxide
caps	box, cover, shell
capsul	box
carb/o	carbon
carboxy	group of organic compounds
carcin/o	cancer
card	heart
cardi/o	heart
care	be responsible for
carotene	yellow-red pigment
carotid	large neck artery
carp/o	bones of the wrist
cartilag	cartilage
cata-	down
catabol	break down
catechol	tyrosine-containing
catheter	insert, catheter
caud	tail
cav	hollow space
cava	cave
cavern	cave
cec	cecum
-cele	cave, hernia, swelling
celi	abdomen
cellul	cell, small cell
cent-	hundred
-centesis	to puncture
centr/o	central
ceph	head
cephal/o	head
-cephalus	head
cephaly	condition of the head

WORD PART	DEFINITION
ceps	head
cept	to receive
cerebell	little brain, cerebellum
cerebr/o	brain
cerumin	cerumen
cervic	neck
cess	going forward
chancr	chancre
chem/o	chemical
chemic	chemical
-chete	hair
-chezia	pass a stool
chir/o	hand
chlor	green
chol/e	bile
cholangi	bile duct
cholecyst	gallbladder
choledoch/o	common bile duct
chondr/o	cartilage, rib, granule
chorion	chorion, membrane
chrom/o	color
chromat	color
chron/o	time
chym/o	chyme
-cidal	pertaining to killing
cide	to kill
cili	hairlike structure
circulat	circular route
circum-	around
cirrh	yellow
cis	to cut
cit/i	cell
-clast	break, break down
claudic	limp
claustr/o-	confined space
clav	clavicle
clave	lock
clavicul	clavicle
-cle	small

WORD PART	DEFINITION
clitor	clitoris
clon	cutting used for propagation, tumult
-clonus	violent action
co-	with, together
coagul/o	clot, clump
coarct	press together, narrow
cobal	cobalt
cocc	round bacterium
coccus	berry, spherical bacterium
cochle	cochlear
code	information system
cognit	thinking
coit	sexual intercourse
col-	with, together
col	colon
coll	collect, glue
coll/a	glue
colon/o	colon
coloniz	form a colony
colp/o	vagina
com	take care of
com-	with, together
comat	coma
combin	combine
comminut	break into pieces
commodat	adjust
compat	tolerate
compet	strive together
complex	woven together
compli	fulfill
compress	press together
compuls	drive, compel
con-	with, together
concav	arched, hollow
concept	become pregnant
concuss	shake or jar violently
condyl	knuckle
confus	bewildered
congest	accumulation of fluid

S = Suffix   P = Prefix   R = Root   R/CF = Combining Form

Word Part	Definition
coni	dust
coniz	cone
conjunctiv	conjunctiva
connect	join together
conscious	awareness
constip	press together
constrict	to narrow
contagi/o	transmissible by contact
contaminat/o	to corrupt, make unclean
contin	hold together
contra-	against
contract	draw together, pull together
contus	bruise
convalesc	recover
cor	heart
cori	skin
corne/o	cornea
coron	crown, coronary
corpor/e	body
corpus	body
cortic/o	cortex, cortisone
cortis	cortisone
cost	rib
crani/o	cranium, skull
crease	groove
creat	flesh
creatin	creatine
crete	to separate
cretin	cretin
crimin	distinguish
crine	secrete
crista	crest
-crit	to separate
cry/o	cold
crypt-	hidden
cub	cube
cubit	elbow
cubitus	elbow, ulna
cune/i	wedge

Word Part	Definition
cur	cleanse, cure
curat	to care for
curett	to cleanse
cursor	run
cusp	point
cutan/e	skin
cyan/o	dark blue
-cyst	cyst, bladder
cyst/o	bladder, sac, cyst
cysteine	an amino acid
cyt/o	cell
-cyte	cell
cyte	cell
dacry/o	tears, lacrimal duct
dai	day
de-	without, out of, removal, from
defec	clear out waste
defici	failure, lacking, inadequate
degenerat	deteriorate
deglutit	to swallow
del	visible
deliri	confusion, disorientation
delt	triangle
delus	deceive
dem	the people
demi-	half
dendr/o	treelike
dent	tooth
depend	rely on
depress	press down
derm/a	skin
-derma	skin
dermat/o	skin
dermis	skin
-desis	bind together, fixation of bone or joint
di-	two
dia-	complete
diabet	diabetes
diagnost	decision

Word Part	Definition
dialectic	argument
dialy	separate
diaphor	sweat
diaphragm/a	diaphragm
diastol	diastole, relaxation
dict	consent, surrender
didym/o	testis
didymis	testis
diet	a way of life
different	not identical
digest	to break down food
digit	finger or toe
dilat	open up, expand, widen
dips	thirst
dis-	apart, away from
discipl	understand
disciplin	disciple, instruction
dist	away from the center
-dium	appearance
diuret	increase urine output
diverticul	byroad
dorm	sleep
dors	back
dorsi	of the back
drome	running
drop	liquid globule
duce	to lead
ducer	to lead, leader
duct	to lead, lead
ductus	leading
duoden	twelve, duodenum
dur	dura
dura	hard
dwarf	miniature
dynam/o	power
-dynia	pain
dys-	bad, difficult, painful
e-	out of, from
-eal	pertaining to

Word Part	Definition
ease	normal function, freedom from pain
ec-	out, outside
ech/o	sound wave
echin	hedgehog
eclamps	shining forth
eco-	environment
-ectasis	dilation
-ectomy	excision, surgical excision
ectop	on the outside, displaced
eczem/a	eczema
-ed	pertaining to
edema	edema, swelling
-ee	person who is the object of an action
efface	wipe out
effer	move out from the center
effus	pour out
ejacul	shoot out
ejaculat	shoot out
elasma	plate
elect	choice
electr/o	electric, electricity
elimin	throw away, expel
-elle	small
-em	condition
em-	in, into
-ema	quality of, quantity of
emac/i	make thin
embol	plug
embryon	embryo, fertilized egg
emesis	vomiting
-emesis	to vomit, vomiting
emet	to vomit
emia	a blood condition
-emia	a blood condition
-emic	pertaining to a blood condition
emic	pertaining to a blood condition
emmetr-	measure
emuls	suspend in a liquid
en-	in

S = Suffix   P = Prefix   R = Root   R/CF = Combining Form

Word Part	Definition
-ence	forming, quality of, state of
enceph	brain
encephal/o	brain
encephaly	condition of the brain
-ency	condition, state of, quality of
end-	inside, within
endo-	inside, within
-ent	end result, pertaining to
enter/o	intestine
entery	condition of the intestine
enur	urinate
environ	surroundings
-eon	one who does
eosin/o	dawn
ependym	lining membrane
epi-	above, upon, over
epilept	seizure
epiphys/i	growth
episi/o	vulva
equi-	equal
equin	horse
equip	to fit out
-er	agent, one who does
erect	straight, to set up
erg/o	work
-ergy	process of working
-ery	process of
erysi-	red
erythemat	redness
erythr/o	red
-escent	process
-esis	condition
eso-	inward
esophag/e	esophagus
essent	existence
esthes	sensation, perception
esthet	sensation, perception
estr/o	woman
ethm	sieve

Word Part	Definition
eti/o	cause
-etic	pertaining to
-etics	pertaining to
-ette	little
eu-	good, normal
ex-	away from, out, out of
exacerbat	increase, aggravate
examin	test, examine
excis	cut out
excret	separate, discharge
exo-	outside, outward
expect	await
expir	breathe out
extra-	out of, outside
faci	face
factor	maker
farct	area of dead tissue
fasc/i	fascia
febr	fever
fec	feces
feed	to give food, nourish
femor	femur
fer	to bear, to carry
ferrit	iron
fertil	able to conceive
fertiliz	to make fruitful
fet/o	fetus
fibr/o	fiber, fibrous
fibrill	small fiber
fibrin/o	fibrin
fibul	fibula
-fication	remove
fida	split
field	definite area
filar	roundworm
filtr	strain through
fiss	split
fistul	tube, pipe
flammat	flame

S = Suffix   P = Prefix   R = Root   R/CF = Combining Form

Word Part	Definition
flat	flatus
flatul	excessive gas
flavin	yellow
flex	bend
fluid	flowing
fluo-	fluorine
fluor/o	flux, flow
flux	flow
foc	center, focus
follicul	follicle
foramin	opening, foramen
fore-	in front
-form	appearance of, resembling
format	to form
fract	break
fraction	small amount
free	free
frequ	repeated, often
front	front, forehead
fructos	fruit sugar
function	perform
fund/o	fundus
fung/i	fungus
fusion	to pour
galact/o	milk
gall	bile
gastr/o	stomach
gastrin	stomach hormone
gastrocnem	calf of leg
gemin	twin, double
gen/o	produce, create
-gen	create, produce, form
gen-	birth
-gene	production, give birth
gener	create, produce
genesis	origin, creation, production
-genesis	creation, origin, formation, source
genet	origin
-genic	creation, producing

Word Part	Definition
genit	bring forth, birth, primary male or female sex organ
genitor	offspring
ger	old age
geront/o	old age
gest	gestation, pregnancy, produce
gestat	gestation, pregnancy, to bear
gigant	giant
gingiv	gums
gland	gland
glauc	lens opacity, grey
gli/o	glue, supportive tissue of nervous system
-glia	glue, supportive tissue of nervous system
globin/o	protein
globul	globular, protein
glomerul/o	glomerulus
gloss/o	tongue
glott	mouth of windpipe
glottis	mouth of windpipe
gluc/o	glucose, sugar
glut	buttocks
glutin	glue, stick
glyc/o	glycogen, glucose, sugar
glycer	glycerol, sweet
gnath	jaw
gnose	use knowledge
gnosis	knowledge
gomph	bolt, nail
gon/o	seed
gonad/o	gonads, testes, or ovaries
gong	daily practice
-grade	going
graft	splice, transplant
-graft	tissue for transplant
graine	head pain
-gram	a record, recording
grand-	big
grand	big
granul/o	granule, small grain

S = Suffix   P = Prefix   R = Root   R/CF = Combining Form

Word Part	Definition
-graph	to record, write
-grapher	one who records
-graphy	process of recording
gravida	pregnant
gravis	serious
gru	to move
guan	dung
gurgit	flood
gynec/o	woman, female
habilitat	restore
hale	breathe
halit	breath
hallucin	imagination
hallux	big toe
hem/o	blood
hemangi/o	blood vessel
hemat/o	blood
heme	red iron-containing pigment
hemi-	half
hepar	liver
hepat/o	liver
herb/i	plant
herni/o	hernia, rupture
herp	blister
hetero-	different
hiat	opening
hist	derived from histidine
hist/o	tissue
holist	entire, whole
hom/i	man
home/o	the same
homo-	same, alike
hormon	chemical messenger, hormone
human	human being
humor	fluid
hyal	glass
hydr/o	water
hyp-	below
hyper-	above, beyond, excess, excessive

Word Part	Definition
hypn/o	sleep
hypo-	below, deficient, smaller, low, under
hyster/o	uterus
-ia	condition
-iac	pertaining to
-ial	pertaining to
-ian	one who does, specialist
-ias	condition
-iasis	abnormal condition
iatr	medical treatment, physician
-iatric	relating to medicine, medical knowledge
iatrics	medical knowledge
-iatrist	practitioner, one who treats
-iatry	treatment, field of medicine
-ibility	able to do
-ible	can do, able to
-ic	pertaining to
-ica	pertaining to
-ical	pertaining to
-ician	expert
-ics	knowledge
ict	seizure
icterus	jaundice
-id	having a particular quality, pertaining to
-ide	having a particular quality
idi/o	unknown, personal
ifer	to bear, carry
-ify	to become
-il	a thing
-ile	pertaining to
ile/o	ileum
ili/o	ilium (hip bone)
im-	in, not
imag	likeness
immun/o	immune, immune response, immunity
immune	protected from
immuniz	make immune
impair	worsen
impede	obstruct

Word Part	Definition
-imus	most
-in	substance, chemical compound
in-	not, into, in
incis	cut into
incub	sit on, lie on, hatch
index	to declare
-ine	pertaining to
infant	infant
infect	internal invasion, infection
infer	below, beneath
infest	invade, attack
inflammat	set on fire
inflat	blow up
infra-	below, beneath
-ing	quality of, doing
ingest	carry in
inguin	groin
inhal	breathe in
inhibit	repress
inject	force in
ino	sinew
insect/i	insect
insert	put together
inspir	breathe in
insul	island
integr	whole
integument	covering of the body
inter-	between
interstiti	space between tissues
intestin	gut, intestine
intra-	inside, within
intrins	on the inside
intus-	within
iod	violet, iodine
-ion	action, condition
-ior	pertaining to
-iosum	pertaining to
-ious	pertaining to
irrig	to water

Word Part	Definition
-is	belonging to, pertaining to
isch	to block
ischi	ischium
-ism	condition, process
-ismus	take action
iso-	equal
-ist	agent, specialist
-istic	pertaining to
-isy	inflammation
-ites	associated with
-ition	process
-itis	inflammation, infection
-ity	condition, state
-ium	structure
-ius	pertaining to
-ive	nature of, quality of, pertaining to
-iz	subject to
-ization	process of inserting or creating
-ize	action, affect in a specific way, policy
-ized	affected in a specific way
-izer	affects in a particular way, line of action
jejun	jejunum
jugul	throat
junct	joining together
juxta-	beside, near, close to
kal	potassium
kary/o	nucleus
kel/o	tumor
kerat	keratin, hard protein
kerat/o	cornea
kern	nucleus
ket/o	ketone
keton	ketone
ketone	organic compound
kin	motion
kinase	enzyme
kinesi/o	movement
kinet	motion
-kinin	move in

S = Suffix   P = Prefix   R = Root   R/CF = Combining Form

Word Part	Definition
klept/o	to steal
kyph/o	bent, humpback
labi	lip
labyrinth	inner ear
lacer	to tear
lacrim	tears, tear duct
lact	milk
lactat	secrete milk
lapar/o	abdomen in general
lapse	clasp, fall together
-lapse	fall together, slide
laryng/o	larynx
lash	end of whip
lat	to take
lateral	at the side
latiss	wide
-le	small
lei/o	smooth
-lemma	covering
-lepsy	seizure
lept	thin, small
-let	small
leuk/o	white
lex	word
librium	balance
ligament	ligament
ligat	tie up, tie off
lign	line
-ling	small
lingu	tongue
lip/o	fat
lipid	fat
lith/o	stone
liv	life, live
load	to carry
lob	lobe
locat	a place
log	to study
-logist	one who studies, specialist

Word Part	Definition
logous	relation
logy	study of
-logy	study of
longev	long life
lord/o	curve, swayback
lubric	make slippery
lucid	bright, clear
lumb	lower back, loin
lump	piece
lun	moon
lupus	wolf
-lus	small
lute	yellow
luxat	dislocate
ly	break down, separate
-ly	every
lymph/o	lymph, lymphatic system
lymphaden/o	lymph node
lymphangi/o	lymphatic vessels
lys/o	decompose, dissolve
lysis	destruction
-lysis	destruction, dissolve, separation
lyt	dissolve, destroy
-lyte	soluble
-lytic	relating to destruction
lyze	destruct, dissolve
macro-	large
macul	spot
magnet	magnet
mak	makes
-maker	one who makes
mal	bad, difficult, inadequate
mal-	bad, difficult
-malacia	abnormal softness
malign	harmful, bad
malleol	small hammer, malleolus
mamm/o	breast
man	frenzy, madness
man/o	pressure

387

Word Part	Definition
mandibul	mandible
-mania	frenzy, madness
manic	affected by frenzy
manipul	handful, use of hands
marker	sign
mast	breast
mastic	chew
mastoid	mastoid process
mater	mother
matern	mother
matur(e)	ripe, ready, fully developed
maxilla	maxilla
medi	middle
media	middle
mediastin/o	mediastinum
medic	medicine
medulla	middle
mega-	enormous
-megaly	enlargement
mei	lessening
mela	black
melan/o	melanin, black pigment
mellit	sweetened with honey
membran/o	cover, skin
men/o	menses, monthly, month
mening/o	meninges, membranes
menisc	crescent, meniscus
menstr/u	menses, occurring monthly
ment	mind, chin
-ment	action, state, resulting state
mere	part
mero-	partial
meso-	middle
meta-	after, beyond, subsequent to
metabol	change
-meter	measure, instrument to measure
metr/o	uterus
-metric	pertaining to measurement
-metrist	skilled in measurement

Word Part	Definition
-metry	process of measuring
mi-	derived from *hemi,* half
micr/o	small
micro-	small
mictur	pass urine
mid-	middle
mileusis	lathe
milli-	one-thousandth
miner	mines
mineral/o	inorganic material
miss	send
mit	thread
mito-	thread
mitr	having two points
mitt	send
mod	nature, form, method
molec	mass
mollusc	soft
mon	single
monas	single unit
monil	type of fungus
mono-	one, single
morbid	disease
morph/o	shape
mort	death
mot	move
motiv	move
muc/o	mucus, mucous membrane
mucosa	lining of a cavity
multi-	many
mune	in service
muscul/o	muscle
mut	silent
muta	genetic change
mutil	to maim
my/o	muscle
myc/o	fungus
myel/o	spinal cord, bone marrow
myelin	in the spinal cord, myelin

S = Suffix   P = Prefix   R = Root   R/CF = Combining Form

WORD PART	DEFINITION
myo-	to blink
myop	to blink
myos	muscle
myring/o	tympanic membrane, eardrum
myx-	mucus
narc/o	stupor
nas	nose
nat	born, birth
nate	born, birth
natr/i	sodium
natur/o	nature
ne/o	new
nebul	cloud
necr/o	death
neo-	new
nephr/o	kidney
nerv	nerve
-ness	quality, state
neur/o	nerve, nervous tissue
neutr/o	neutral
nici	lethal
nitr/o	nitrogen
noct-	night
noia	to think
nom	law
non-	no, not
nor-	normal
norm-	normal
nos/o	disease
nucle/o	nucleus
nucleol	small nucleus
nutri	nourish
nutrit	nourishment
o/o	egg
oblong	elongated
obsess	besieged by thoughts
obstetr	pregnancy and childbirth
occipit	back of head
occulta	hidden

WORD PART	DEFINITION
ocul/o	eye
-ode	way, road, path
odont	tooth
odyn/o	pain
-oid	resembling
-ol	alcohol, chemical, substance
-ola	small
-ole	small
olfact	smell
oligo-	scanty, too little
om/o	body, tumor
-oma	tumor, mass
onc/o	tumor
-one	chemical substance, hormone
onych/o	nail
ophthalm/o	eye
ophthalmos	eye
-opia	sight
opportun	take advantage of
-opsis	vision
-opsy	to view
opt/o	vision
optic	eye
-or	a doer, one who does, that which does something
or/o	mouth
orbit	orbit
orchi/o	testicle
ordin	arrange
orex	appetite
organ	organ, tool, instrument
orth/o	straight
orthot	correct
-orum	function of
-ory	having the function of
os	mouth
-osa	full of, like
-ose	full of
-osis	abnormal condition

Word Part	Definition
osmo	push
osmol	concentration
oss/e	bone
oste/o	bone
-osus	condition
ot/o	ear
-otomy	incision
-ous	pertaining to
ov/i	egg
ovari	ovary
ovul	ovum, egg
ox	oxygen
-oxia	oxygen condition
oxid	oxidize
oxy	oxygen
pace	step
palat	palate
palliat	reduce suffering
palm	palm
palpat	touch, stroke
palpit	throb
pan-	all
pancreat	pancreas
panto-	entire
papill/o	pimple
par-	abnormal, beside
para	to bring forth
para-	adjacent to, alongside, beside, abnormal
parasit	parasite
paresis	weakness
pareun	lying beside, sexual intercourse
pariet	wall
paroxysm	irritate; sudden, sharp attack
particul	little piece
partum	childbirth, to bring forth
pat	lie open
patell	patella
patent	lie open
-path	disease

Word Part	Definition
path/o	disease
pathet	suffering
-pathic	pertaining to a disease
pathy	disease, emotion
-pathy	disease
paus	cessation
pause	cessation
pector	chest
ped	child, foot
pedicul	louse
pelas	skin
pelv	pelvis
pen	penis
-penia	deficient, deficiency
peps	digestion
pepsin/o	pepsin
pept	digest
per-	through, intense
perforat	bore through
perfus	to pour
peri-	around
perine	perineum
peripher	external boundary, outer part, outer edge
periton/e	stretch over, peritoneum
perium	a bringing forth
perm/e	pass through
pes	foot
pesti	pest
petit	small
petit-	small
-pexy	fixation, surgical fixation
phaco-	lens
phag/o	to eat
phage	to eat
-phage	to eat
phagia	swallowing
-phagia	swallowing, eating
phalang/e	phalanx, finger, toe
pharmac/o	drug

S = Suffix   P = Prefix   R = Root   R/CF = Combining Form

WORD PART	DEFINITION
pharyng/o	pharynx
pharynx	pharynx, throat
phenol	benzene derivative
phenyl	chemical group
pheo-	gray
pher/o	to carry
-pheresis	removal
-phil	attraction
-phile	attraction
-philia	attraction
phim	muzzle
phleb/o	vein
phob	fear
-phobia	fear
phon/o	sound, voice
phor	bear, carry
phosphat	phosphorus
phot/o	light
phren	mind
phylac	protect
phylaxis	protection
-phyll	leaf
physema	blowing
physi/o	body
physis	growth
phyt/o	plant
pia	delicate
pituit	pituitary
pituitar	pituitary
plak	plate, plaque
plant	insert, plant
planus	flat surface
plas	molding, formation, growth
-plasia	formation
-plasm	something formed
plasm/o	to form
-plasty	formation, repair, surgical repair
plate	flat
pleg	paralysis

WORD PART	DEFINITION
plete	filled
pleur	pleura
plexy	stroke
-pnea	breathe
pneum/o	air, lung
pneumat	structure filled with air
pneumon	air, lung
pod	foot
-poiesis	to make
-poiet	the making
-poietin	the maker
poikilo-	irregular
point	to pierce
pol	pole
polio	gray matter
pollut	unclean
poly-	excessive, many, much
polyp	polyp
poplit/e	ham, back of knee
por/o	opening
post-	after
poster	back part
pract	efficient, practical
prand/i	breakfast
pre-	before, in front of
precis	accurate
pregn	with child, pregnant
presby	old man
press	press close, press down, squeeze
prevent	prevent
primi-	first
pro-	before, in front, projecting forward
proct/o	anus and rectum
product	lead forth
prolifer	bear offspring
pronat	bend down
prosta	prostate
prosthet	artificial part
prot/e	first

S = Suffix   P = Prefix   R = Root   R/CF = Combining Form

Word Part	Definition
protein	protein
proto-	first
provision	provide
proxim	nearest to the center
prurit	itch
pseudo-	false
psych/o	mind, soul
psyche	mind, soul
pteryg	wing
ptosis	drooping, falling
-ptosis	drooping
ptysis	spit
pub	pubis
puer	child
pulmon/o	lung
puls	to drive
pump	pump
punct	puncture
pupill-	pupil
pur	pus
purul	pus
py/o	pus
pyel/o	renal pelvis
pylor	gate, pylorus
pyr/o	fire, heat
pyrex	fever
pyrid	heat
quadrant	quadrant
quadri-	four
radi/o	radius, x-ray, radiation
radic	root
re-	again, back, backward
recept	receive
rect/o	rectum
reflex	bend back
refract	bend
regul	to rule, control
remiss	send back, give up
ren	kidney

Word Part	Definition
replic	reply
rescein	resin
resect/o	cut off
resid/u	left over, what is left over
resist	to withstand
respire/a	to breathe
restor	renew
resuscit	revive from apparent death
reticul	fine net, network
retin/o	retina
retinacul	hold back
retro-	backward
rhabd/o	rod shaped, striated
rheumat	a flow, rheumatism
rhin/o	nose
rhythm	rhythm
rib/o	like a rib
ribo	a sugar, pentose
ribo-	from ribose, a sugar
rigid	stiff
rose	rose
rotat	rotate
-rrhagia	excessive flow, discharge
-rrhaphy	suture
rrhea	flow, discharge
-rrhoid	flow
rrhyth	rhythm
rrhythm	rhythm
-rubin	rust colored
rumin	throat
sacchar	sugar
sacr/o	sacrum
sagitt	arrow
saliv	saliva
salping/o	fallopian tube, uterine tube
salpinx	trumpet
san	sound, healthy
sanit	health
sapon	soap

S = Suffix   P = Prefix   R = Root   R/CF = Combining Form

Word Part	Definition
sarc/o	flesh, muscle, sarcoma
satur	to fill
scapul	scapula
schiz/o	to split, cleave
scintill	spark
scler/o	hardness, white of eye
scoli/o	crooked
scope	instrument for viewing
-scope	instrument for viewing, instrument to examine
-scopy	to examine, to view
scorb	scurvy
scrot	scrotum
seb/o	sebum
sebac/e	wax
sebum	wax
secret	secrete, produce, separate
sect	cut off
sedat	to calm
sedent	sitting
segment	section
seiz	to grab
self	me, own individual
semi-	half
semin/i	semen
seminat	scatter seed
sen	old age
senesc	growing old
senil	senile
sens	feel
sensitiv	feeling
sensor/i	sensation, sensory
separat	move apart
seps	decay, infection
sept/o	septum, partition
ser/o	serum
serum	serum
sib	relative
-side	glycoside

Word Part	Definition
sigm	Greek letter "S"
silic	silicon, glass
simi	ape, monkey
simul	imitate
sin/o	sinus
sinus	sinus
sipid	flavor
-sis	abnormal condition, process
sit/u	place
skelet	skeleton
smear	spread
soc	partner
soci/o	society, social
soma	body
somat/o	body
-some	body
somn/o	sleep
son/o	sound
sorbit	fruit of a tree
sorpt	swallow
spad	tear or cut
spasm	spasm, sudden involuntary tightening
spast	tight
specif	species
sperm/i	sperm
spermat/o	sperm
sphen	wedge
spher/o	sphere
sphygm/o	pulse
spin/a	spine
spin/o	spine, spinal cord
spir/o	to breathe
spirat	breathe
spirit/u	spirit
spiro-	spiral, coil
splen/o	spleen
spongios	sponge
spor	spore
stable	steady

Word Part	Definition
stag	standing place
stalsis	constrict, constriction
staphyl/o	bunch of grapes
stasis	stagnate, to stand still
-stasis	stop, stand still, control
stat	stationary
-static	stopped, standing still
-statin	inhibit
stax	fall in drops
steat	fat
stein	stone
sten/o	narrow, contract
ster	solid, steroid
stere/o	three-dimensional
steril	sterile, make sterile
stern	chest, breastbone
-steroid	steroid
-sterol	steroid
-sterone	steroid
steth/o	chest
sthen	strength
stigmat	focus
stimul	excite, strengthen
stin	partition
stip	press
stiti	space
stoma	mouth
-stomy	new opening
stone	stone, pebble
storm	crisis
strab	squint
strat	layer
strept/o	twisted
strict	narrow
study	inquiry
su/i	self
sub-	below, under, underneath
suct	suck
suffic/i	enough

Word Part	Definition
sulf	sulfur
super	above, excessive
super-	above, excessive
supinat	bend backward
supplement	supply to remedy a deficiency
suppress	pressed under, push under
supra-	above
surfact	surface
surg	operate
suscept	to take up
-sylated	linked
sym-	together
symptomat	collection of symptoms
syn-	together
syndesm	bind together
synov	synovial membrane
syring/o	tube, pipe
system	the body as a whole
systol/e	contraction, systole
tachy-	rapid
tact	orderly arrangement
tag	touch
tain	hold
talip	ankle bone
tamin	touch
tampon	plug
tangent	touch
tars	ankle
tax	coordination
tempor/o	time, temple
ten/o	tendon
tendin	tendon
tens	pressure
-tensin	tense, taut
terat/o	monster, malformed fetus
term	limit, end
test/o	testis, testicle
testicul	testicle, testis
tetra-	four

S = Suffix   P = Prefix   R = Root   R/CF = Combining Form

Word Part	Definition
thalam	thalamus
thalamus	thalamus
thalass	sea
thel	breast, nipple
then	motion
thenar	palm
therap/o	healing, treatment
therapeut	healing, treatment
-therapist	one who treats
therapy	treatment
-therapy	treatment
therm/o	heat
thesis	arrange, place, organize
thet	arrange, place, organize
thi	sulfur
thora	chest
thorac/o	chest
thorax	chest
thromb/o	blood clot, clot
thym	thymus gland
thyr/o	thyroid
tibi	tibia
-tic	pertaining to
-tion	process, being
-tiz	pertaining to
toc	labor, birth
toler	endure
tom/o	cut, slice, layer
-tome	instrument to cut
-tomy	surgical incision
ton/o	pressure, tension
tonsil	tonsil
tonsill/o	tonsil
tope	part, location
topic	local
-tous	pertaining to
tox	poison
-toxic	able to kill
toxic/o	poison

Word Part	Definition
trache/o	trachea, windpipe
tract	draw, pull
tranquil	calm
trans-	across, through
traumat	wound, injury
tresia	a hole
tri-	three
trich/o	hair
-tripsy	crushing
-tripter	crusher
trochle	pulley
trop	turn, turning
troph	development, nourishment
trophy	development, nourishment
-tropic	a turning, change
-tropin	nourishing, stimulation
tryps	friction
tub	tube
tubercul	swelling, nodule, tuberculosis
tubul	small tube
tussis	cough
tympan/o	eardrum, tympanic membrane
-type	model, particular kind
typh	typhus
ulcer	a sore
-ule	little, small
-ulent	abounding in
uln	ulnar
ultra-	higher, beyond
-um	tissue, structure
umbilic	navel, umbilicus
un	one
un-	not
uni-	one
ur/o	urine, urinary system
-ure	process, result of
uresis	to urinate
uret	ureter, urine, urination
ureter/o	ureter

S = Suffix   P = Prefix   R = Root   R/CF = Combining Form

Word Part	Definition
urethr/o	urethra
-uria	urine
urin	urine
-us	pertaining to
uter/o	uterus
uve	uvea
uvul	uvula
vaccin	vaccine, giving a vaccine
vag	vagus nerve
vagin	sheath, vagina
valgus	turn out
valv	valve
varic/o	varicosity; dilated, tortuous vein
vas/o	blood vessel, duct
vascul	blood vessel
ved	knowledge
veget	plants
vegetat	growth
ven/a	vein
ven/o	vein
ventil	wind
ventr	belly
ventricul	ventricle
vers	turn
-version	change
vert	to turn
vertebr	vertebra
vesic	sac containing fluid
vestibul/o	vestibule, entrance
via	the way
violet	bluish purple
viril	masculine
virus	poison
viscer	internal organs
viscos	viscous, sticky
visu	sight
vita	life
voc	voice
vol	volume

Word Part	Definition
volunt	willing
volut	shrink, roll up
-volut	rolled up
vuls	tear, pull
vulv/o	vulva
whip	to swing
xanth	yellow
xeno-	foreign
-xis	condition
-yl	substance
zea-	to live
-zoa	animal
zyg	zygote
zygomat	cheekbone
zyme	fermenting, enzyme, transform

Abbreviations

ABBREVIATION	DEFINITION
µg	microgram; one-millionth of a gram
ʌ	increase/ above
v	decrease/ below
1°	primary
2°	secondary
Ab	antibody
ABGs	arterial blood gases
ABO	agents of biologic origin
ABO	a blood group system
AC	acromioclavicular
ACE	angiotensin-converting enzyme
ACL	anterior cruciate ligament
ACLS	advanced cardiac life support
ACTH	adrenocorticotropic hormone
AD	right ear
ADD	attention deficit disorder
ADH	antidiuretic hormone
ADHD	attention deficit hyperactivity disorder
ADL	activity of daily living
AED	automatic external defibrillator
Afib	atrial fibrillation
Ag	antigen
AIDS	acquired immunodeficiency syndrome
AKA	above-knee amputation
ALL	acute lymphocytic leukemia
ALS	amyotrophic lateral sclerosis
AMI	acute myocardial infarction
AMS	altered mental state
ANS	autonomic nervous system
AOM	acute otitis media
AP	anteroposterior
ARDS	adult respiratory distress syndrome
ARF	acute renal failure
ARF	acute respiratory failure
AROM	active range of motion

ABBREVIATION	DEFINITION
AS	left ear
ASD	atrial septal defect
ASD	autism spectrum disorder
ASHD	arteriosclerotic heart disease
AU	both ears
AV	atrioventricular
AVM	arteriovenous malformation
BBB	blood brain barrier
BD	brain death
BEP	benign enlargement of the prostate
BKA	below-knee amputation
BM	bowel movement
BMD	bone mineral density
BMR	basal metabolic rate
BOM	bilateral otitis media
BP	blood pressure
BPD	borderline personality disorder
BPH	benign prostatic hyperplasia
BPPV	benign paroxysmal positional vertigo
BRCA1	genetic mutation responsible for breast and ovarian cancer (**br**east **ca**ncer 1)
BRCA2	genetic mutation responsible for breast cancer (**br**east **ca**ncer 2)
BSE	bovine spongiform encephalopathy
BSE	breast self-examination
C1	first cervical vertebra
C5	fifth cervical vertebra or nerve
C7	seventh cervical vertebra
CA	cancer
CABG	coronary artery bypass graft
CAD	coronary artery disease
CAO	chronic airway obstruction
CAPD	continuous ambulatory peritoneal dialysis
CBC	complete blood count
CBT	cognitive-behavioral therapy

ABBREVIATION	DEFINITION
CD	conduct disorder
CDC	Centers for Disease Control and Prevention
CF	cystic fibrosis
CHD	congenital heart disease
CHES	certified health education specialist
CHF	congestive heart failure
CJD	Creutzfeldt–Jakob disease
CK	creatine kinase
CKD	chronic kidney disease
CMA	certified medical assistant
CMV	cytomegalovirus
CNA	certified nurse assistant
CNS	central nervous system
c/o	complains of
CO_2	carbon dioxide
COPD	chronic obstructive pulmonary disease
COT	certified occupational therapist
COTA	certified occupational therapist assistant
CP	cerebral palsy
CPAP	continuous positive airway pressure
CPR	cardiopulmonary resuscitation
CPT	cognitive processing therapy
CRF	chronic renal failure
CRH	corticoreleasing hormone
CRP	C-reactive protein
C-section	cesarean section
CSF	cerebrospinal fluid
CT	computed tomography
CVA	cerebrovascular accident
CVP	central venous pressure
CVS	cardiovascular system
CVT	cardiovascular technologist
CXR	chest x-ray
D & C	dilation and curettage
DASH	dietary approaches to stop hypertension
DEXA	dual-energy x-ray absorptiometry
DI	diabetes insipidus
DIC	disseminated intravascular coagulation
DID	dissociative identity disorder

ABBREVIATION	DEFINITION
DIFF	differential white blood cell count
DJD	degenerative joint disease
DKA	diabetic ketoacidosis
dL	deciliter; one-tenth of a liter
DM	diabetes mellitus
DMD	Duchenne muscular dystrophy
DNA	deoxyribonucleic acid
DNR	do not resuscitate
DO	Doctor of Osteopathy
DRE	digital rectal examination
DSM-IV	*Diagnostic and Statistical Manual of Mental Disorders,* Fourth Edition
DVT	deep vein thrombosis
EBV	Epstein–Barr virus
ECG	electrocardiogram
ECT	electroconvulsive therapy
ED	emergency department
ED	erectile dysfunction
EEG	electroencephalogram
EKG	electrocardiogram
EMG	electromyography
EMT	emergency medical technician
EMT-P	emergency medical technician-paramedic
EPCA-2	early prostate cancer antigen-2
ER	emergency room
ERT	estrogen replacement therapy
ESR	erythrocyte sedimentation rate
ESRD	end-stage renal disease
ESWL	extracorporeal shock wave lithotripsy
FAS	fetal alcohol syndrome
FDA	U.S. Food and Drug Administration
FEV1	forced expiratory volume in 1 second
FSH	follicle-stimulating hormone
FTD	fronto-temporal dementia
FTT	failure to thrive
FUS	focused ultrasound surgery
FVC	forced vital capacity
Fx	fracture
g	gram

ABBREVIATION	DEFINITION
GAD	generalized anxiety disorder
GDM	gestational diabetes mellitus
GERD	gastroesophageal reflux disease
GFR	glomerular filtration rate
GH	growth hormone, somatotrophin
GHRH	growth hormone-releasing hormone
GI	gastrointestinal
GI	glycemic index
GL	glycemic load
GnRH	gonadotrophin-releasing hormone
GTT	glucose tolerance test
GYN	gynecology
HAV	hepatitis A virus
Hb	hemoglobin
Hb A1c	glycosylated hemoglobin A-one-C
HBOT	hyperbaric oxygen therapy
HBV	hepatitis B virus
HCG	human chorionic gonadotropin
HCl	hydrochloric acid
Hct	hematocrit
HCV	hepatitis C virus
HDL	high-density lipoprotein
HDN	hemolytic disease of the newborn
Hgb	hemoglobin
HIPAA	Health Insurance Portability and Accountability Act
HIV	human immunodeficiency virus
HMD	hyaline membrane disease
HPI	history of present illness
HPV	human papilloma virus
HRT	hormone replacement therapy
HSV	herpes simplex virus
HSV-1	herpes simplex virus, type 1
HTN	hypertension
HUS	hemolytic uremic syndrome
IBS	irritable bowel syndrome
ICD	implantable cardioverter/defibrillator
IDDM	insulin-dependent diabetes mellitus
Ig	immunoglobulin
IgA	immunoglobulin A

ABBREVIATION	DEFINITION
IgD	immunoglobulin D
IgE	immunoglobulin E
IgG	immunoglobulin G
IgM	immunoglobulin M
IM	intramuscular
INR	international normalized ratio
ITP	idiopathic (immunologic) thrombocytopenic purpura
IU	international unit(s)
IUD	intrauterine device
IV	intravenous
IVC	inferior vena cava
IVF	in vitro fertilization
IVP	intravenous pyelogram
JRA	juvenile rheumatoid arthritis
KUB	x-ray of abdomen to show kidneys, ureters, and bladder
LADA	latent autoimmune diabetes in adults
LASER	light amplification by stimulated emission of radiation
LCC-ST	certified surgical technologist
LD	learning disability
LDL	low-density lipoprotein
LFT	liver function test
LH	luteinizing hormone
LLQ	left lower quadrant
LOC	loss of consciousness
LPN	licensed practical nurse
LUQ	left upper quadrant
LVN	licensed vocational nurse
mcg	microgram; one-millionth of a gram
MCP	metacarpophalangeal
MCS	minimally conscious state
MCV	mean corpuscular volume
MD	Doctor of Medicine
mg	milligram
MI	myocardial infarction
mL	milliliter
mm^3	cubic millimeter
MOAB	monoclonal antibody
MODY	mature onset diabetes of the young

ABBREVIATION	DEFINITION
MONA	morphine, oxygen, nitroglycerine, and aspirin
MPD	multiple personality disorder
MRA	magnetic resonance angiography
MRI	magnetic resonance imaging
mRNA	messenger RNA
MRSA	methicillin-resistant *Staphylococcus aureus*
MS	multiple sclerosis
MSA	myositis specific antibody
NCI	National Cancer Institute
NIDDM	non-insulin-dependent diabetes mellitus
NIH	National Institutes of Health
NKA	no known allergies
NO	nitric oxide
NRDS	neonatal respiratory distress syndrome
NSAID	nonsteroidal anti-inflammatory drug
O_2	oxygen
OA	obstetric assistant
OA	osteoarthritis
OB	obstetrics
OCD	obsessive compulsive disorder
OD	Doctor of Osteopathy
OD	right eye
ODD	oppositional defiant disorder
OGTT	oral glucose tolerance test
OME	otitis media with effusion
OR	operating room
OS	left eye
OSHA	Occupational Safety and Health Administration
OT	occupational therapy
OT	ophthalmic technician
OT	oxytocin
OTC	over the counter
OU	both eyes
P	pulse rate
PA	pernicious anemia
PA	posteroanterior
PaO_2	partial pressure of arterial oxygen
Pap	Papanicolaou (Pap test, Pap smear)

ABBREVIATION	DEFINITION
PAT	paroxysmal atrial tachycardia
PCL	posterior cruciate ligament
PCOS	polycystic ovarian syndrome
PDA	patent ductus arteriosus
PDD-NOS	pervasive developmental disorder, not otherwise specified
PDT	postural drainage therapy
PE tube	pressure equalization tube
PEEP	positive end-expiratory pressure
PEFR	peak expiratory flow rate
PERRLA	pupils equal, round, reactive to light, and accommodation
PET	positron emission tomography
PFTs	pulmonary function tests
PGY	pregnancy
pH	hydrogen ion concentration
PhD	Doctor of Philosophy
PID	pelvic inflammatory disease
PIP	proximal interphalangeal
PKD	polycystic kidney disease
PMDD	premenstrual dysphoric disorder
PMNL	polymorphonuclear leukocyte
PM&R	physical medicine and rehabilitation
PMS	premenstrual syndrome
PNB	pulseless, nonbreather
PNS	peripheral nervous system
PO	by mouth
POC	products of conception
polio	poliomyelitis
PPH	postpartum hemorrhage
PPS	postpolio syndrome
p.r.n, PRN	when necessary
PSA	prostate-specific antigen
PT	physical therapy, physical therapist
PT	physiotherapy
PT	prothrombin time
PTA	physical therapy assistant
PTCA	percutaneous transluminal coronary angioplasty
PTH	parathyroid hormone
PTSD	posttraumatic stress disorder

ABBREVIATION	DEFINITION
PTT	partial thromboplastin time
PVC	premature ventricular contractions
PVD	peripheral vascular disease
PVS	persistent vegetative state
q.4.h.	every 4 hours
q.i.d.	four times each day
R	respiration rate
RA	rheumatoid arthritis
RBC	red blood cell
RDA	recommended dietary allowance
RDS	respiratory distress syndrome
Rh	Rhesus
Rho-GAM	Rhesus immune globulin
RICE	rest, ice, compression, and elevation
RLQ	right lower quadrant
RN	registered nurse
RNA	ribonucleic acid
ROM	range of motion
RU-486	mifepristone
RUQ	right upper quadrant
SA	sinoatrial
SAD	seasonal affective disorder
SARS	severe acute respiratory syndrome
SBS	shaken baby syndrome
SC	subcutaneous
SCI	spinal cord injury
SET	self-examination of the testes
SFD	small for date
SG	specific gravity
SGA	small for gestational age
SI	sacroiliac
SIDS	sudden infant death syndrome
SLE	systemic lupus erythematosus
SOB	short(ness) of breath
SP	standard precautions
SSRI	selective serotonin reuptake inhibitor
STAT	immediately
STD	sexually transmitted disease
SVC	superior vena cava

ABBREVIATION	DEFINITION
T	temperature
T1	first thoracic vertebra or nerve
T3	triiodothyronine
T4	tetraiodothyronine (thyroxine)
TB	tuberculosis
TBI	traumatic brain injury
TENS	transcutaneous electrical nerve stimulation
THR	total hip replacement
TIA	transient ischemic attack
t.i.d.	(Latin *ter in die*) three times a day
TMJ	temporomandibular joint
TN	trigeminal neuralgia
TNM	**t**umor-**n**ode-**m**etastasis staging system for cancer
TOF	tetralogy of Fallot
tPA	tissue plasminogen activator
TRH	thyrotrophin-releasing hormone
TSH	thyroid-stimulating hormone
TTM	trichotillomania
TTN	transient tachypnea of the newborn
TTP	thrombotic thrombocytopenic purpura
TURP	transurethral resection of the prostate
UA	urinalysis
UP	universal precautions
URI	upper respiratory infection
USDA	U.S. Department of Agriculture
UTI	urinary tract infection
UV	ultraviolet
VEP	visual evoked potential
Vfib	ventricular fibrillation
VS	vital signs
VSD	ventricular septal defect
V-tach	ventricular tachycardia
vWD	von Willebrand disease
vWF	von Willebrand factor
WAD	Word Analysis and Definition (box)
WBC	white blood cell; white blood (cell) count
WNL	within normal limits
WNV	West Nile virus

Diagnostic and Therapeutic Procedures

A compilation of the diagnostic and therapeutic procedural terms used in this book.

A

abdominoplasty Esthetic operation on the abdominal wall (tummy tuck).

ablation Removal of tissue to destroy its function.

activated partial thromboplastin time (APTT) Blood test used to monitor the dose of heparin, an anticoagulant.

adenoidectomy Surgical removal of the adenoid tissue.

alignment Process of bringing the ends of a fractured bone at the break back opposite each other so that they fit together as they did in the original bone.

ambulatory Surgery or any other care provided without an overnight stay in a medical facility.

ambulatory blood pressure monitor Device that provides a record of blood pressure readings over a 24-hour period as patients go about their daily activities.

amniocentesis Removal of amniotic fluid for diagnostic purposes.

amputation Process of removing a limb, part of a limb, a breast, or other projecting part.

anastomosis Surgically made union between two tubular structures.

angiogram Radiographic image of arteries or veins after injection of contrast material.

angiography The process of obtaining an angiogram.

angioplasty Reopening of a blood vessel by surgery.

anoscopy Examination of the anus and lower rectum with a rigid instrument.

Apgar score Evaluation of a newborn's status.

appendectomy Surgical removal of the appendix.

arterial blood gases The measurement of the levels of oxygen and carbon dioxide in the blood—a good indicator of respiratory function.

arteriography X-ray visualization of an artery after injection of contrast material.

arthrocentesis Aspiration of fluid from a joint; used to establish a diagnosis by laboratory examination of the fluid, drain off infected fluid, or insert medication such as local corticosteroids.

arthrodesis Fixation or stiffening of a joint by surgery.

arthrography X-ray of a joint after injection of a contrast medium into the joint to make the inside details of the joint visible.

arthroplasty Replacement of a joint with a prosthesis.

arthroscopy Procedure performed using an arthroscope to examine the internal compartments of a joint or perform a surgical procedure such as debridement, removal of damaged tissue, or repair of torn ligaments.

aspiration Removal by suction of fluid or gas from a body cavity.

atherectomy Surgical removal of atheroma from a blood vessel.

audiometer Electronic device that generates sounds in different frequencies and intensities to test for hearing loss.

auscultation Diagnostic method of listening to body sounds with a stethoscope.

autograft Graft removed from the patient's own skin.

automatic external defibrillator (AED) Device that sends an electric shock to the heart to stop the heart and allow a normal contraction rhythm to resume.

B

bariatric surgery Surgical treatment of obesity.

barium meal Ingestion of barium sulfate to study the distal esophagus, stomach, and duodenum on x-ray.

barium swallow Ingestion of barium sulfate, a contrast material, to show details of the pharynx and esophagus on x-ray.

biopsy Removal of tissue from a living person for laboratory examination.

blepharoplasty Correction of defects in the eyelids.

bone marrow aspiration or biopsy Use of a needle to remove bone marrow cells.

bone mineral density (BMD) Screening test for osteoporosis using a dual-energy x-ray absorptiometry (DEXA) scan.

brace Appliance to support a part of the body in its correct position.

brachytherapy Radiation therapy in which the source of irradiation is implanted in the tissue to be treated.

bronchoscopy Examination of the interior of the tracheobronchial tree with an endoscope.

C

cannula Tube inserted into a blood vessel or cavity as a channel for fluid or gas.

cardiac catheterization Procedure that detects patterns of pressures and blood flows in the heart. A thin tube is guided into the heart under x-ray guidance after being inserted into a vein or artery.

cardiac stress testing Exercise tolerance test that raises the heart rate and monitors the effect on cardiac function.

cardiopulmonary resuscitation Attempt to restore cardiac and pulmonary function.

cardioversion Restoration of a normal heart rhythm by electrical shock. Also called *defibrillation*.

catheterization Introduction of a catheter.

cerebral angiography Injection of a radiopaque dye into the blood vessels of the neck and brain to detect blood vessels that are partially or completely blocked, aneurysms, or arteriovenous malformations.

cerebral arteriography Procedure used to determine the site of bleeding in hemorrhagic strokes, enabling surgery to be performed to stop the bleed or to clip off the aneurysm.

chest x-ray Radiograph image of the chest that can be taken in anteroposterior (AP), posteroanterior (PA), lateral, and sometimes oblique and lateral decubitus positions.

cholangiography Use of a contrast medium to radiographically visualize the bile ducts.

cholecystectomy Surgical removal of the gallbladder.

cholelithotomy Surgical removal of a gallstone(s).

circumcision Removal of part or all of the prepuce of the penis.

clean-catch, midstream urine specimen Sample collected after the external urethral meatus is cleaned. The first part of the urine stream is not collected, and the sterile collecting vessel is introduced into the urinary stream to collect the last part.

clot-busting drugs Drugs injected within a few hours of an MI or thrombotic stroke to dissolve the thrombus. Also called *thrombolytic drugs.*

cognitive behavioral therapy (CBT) A form of psychotherapy that emphasizes the role of thoughts and attitudes in one's feelings and behaviors.

cognitive processing therapy (CPT) Uses a variety of techniques in psychotherapy such as self-discovery and self-instruction.

colonoscopy Examination of the inside of the colon by endoscopy.

colostomy Artificial opening from the colon to the outside of the body.

colpopexy Surgical fixation of a relaxed and prolapsed vagina to the anterior abdominal wall.

computed tomography (CT) Scan in which images of sections of the body are generated by a computer synthesis of x-rays obtained in many different directions in a given plane.

conization Surgical excision of a cone-shaped piece of tissue, e.g., from the outer lining of the cervix.

constant positive airway pressure (CPAP) Attempt to keep alveoli open by maintaining a positive pressure in the airways. A mask is fitted over the nose and mouth and attached to a ventilator.

continuous ambulatory peritoneal dialysis (CAPD) Dialysis performed by the patient at home through an implanted peritoneal catheter, usually 4 times a day, 7 days a week.

continuous cycling peritoneal dialysis Use of a machine to automatically infuse dialysis solution into and out of the abdominal cavity through a peritoneal catheter during sleep.

coronary angiogram Injection of a contrast dye during cardiac catheterization to identify coronary artery blockages.

coronary artery bypass surgery (CABG) Procedure in which healthy blood vessels harvested as a graft from the leg, chest, or arm are used to bypass (detour) the blood around blocked coronary arteries.

cryosurgery Use of liquid nitrogen or argon gas in a probe to freeze and kill abnormal tissue.

curette Scoop-shaped instrument for scraping or removing new growths (or earwax).

cystoscopy Insertion of a pencil-thin, flexible, tubelike telescope through the urethra into the bladder to examine directly the lining of the bladder and to take a biopsy if needed.

cystourethrogram X-ray image during voiding to show the structure and function of the bladder and urethra.

D

debridement Removal of injured or necrotic tissue.

defibrillation Restoration of uncontrolled twitching of cardiac muscle fibers to a normal rhythm.

dermabrasion Removal of upper layers of the skin using a high-powered rotating brush.

dermascope An instrument that shines a light on the skin and magnifies a lesion for better diagnostic viewing.

dialysis Artificial method of removing waste materials and excess fluid from blood.

digital rectal examination (DRE) Palpation of the rectum and prostate gland with an index finger.

dilation and curettage (D & C) Dilation of the cervix so that a thin instrument can be inserted to scrape away the lining of the uterus and take tissue samples.

dipstick Plastic strip bearing paper squares of reagent—the most cost-effective method of screening urine. After the stick is dipped in the urine specimen, the color change in each segment of the dipstick is compared to a color chart on the container. Dipsticks can screen for pH, specific gravity, protein, blood, glucose, ketones, bilirubin, nitrite, and leukocyte esterase.

Doppler ultrasound Diagnostic instrument that sends an ultrasonic beam into the body.

E

early morning urine collection Process used to determine the ability of the kidneys to concentrate urine following overnight dehydration.

echocardiography Ultrasound recording of heart function.

echoencephalography Use of ultrasound in the diagnosis of intracranial lesions.

electrocardiogram Record of the electrical signals of the heart.

electrocardiography Interpretation of electrocardiograms.

electroconvulsive therapy (ECT) Passage of electric current through the brain to produce convulsions and treat persistent depression.

electroencephalography Recording of the electrical activity of the brain.

electromyography Recording of electrical activity in muscle.

endarterectomy Surgical removal of plaque from an artery.

endometrial ablation Use of a heat-generating tool or a laser to remove or destroy the lining of the uterus and prevent or reduce menstruation.

endoscope An instrument for the examination of the interior of a hollow or tubular organ.

endoscopy Use of an endoscope to examine the interior of a tubular or hollow organ and perform a biopsy, remove polyps (polypectomy), and coagulate bleeding lesions.

enema Injection of fluid into the rectum and lower bowel.

enteroscopy Examination of the lining of the digestive tract.

episiotomy Surgical incision in the perineum to dilate the opening of the vagina.

evoked responses Use of stimuli for vision, sound, and touch to activate specific areas of the brain and measure their responses with EEG. This provides information about how that specific area of the brain is functioning.

excision Surgical removal of part or all of a structure or organ.

excisional biopsy Removal of a tumor with a surrounding margin of normal tissue.

external fixation Method of maintaining the alignment of a fractured bone by immobilizing the bone through the use of plaster casts, splints, traction, and external fixators such as steel rods and pins.

extracorporeal shock wave lithotripsy (ESWL) Process in which a machine called a *lithotripter* produces shock waves that crumble renal or ureteral stones into small pieces that can pass down the ureter.

F

fasciectomy Surgical removal of fascia.

fecal occult blood test Diagnostic procedure that detects the presence of blood not visible to the naked eye. Trade name: *Hemoccult* test.

fistulectomy Surgical excision of a fistula.

fistulotomy Surgical enlargement or opening up of a fistula.

flexible endoscopy Use of a flexible, slim fiber-optic instrument that transmits light and sends back images to the observer.

forceps extraction Assisted delivery of a baby by an instrument that grasps the head of the baby.

fundoscopy Examination of the retina with an ophthalmoscope.

G

gastroscopy Endoscopic examination of the inside of the stomach.

gavage To feed by a stomach tube.

gingivectomy Surgical removal of diseased gum tissue.

H

heart transplant Surgery in which the heart of a recently deceased person (donor) is transplanted to the recipient after the recipient's diseased heart has been removed.

Hemoccult test Trade name for *fecal occult blood test*.

hemodialysis Process that filters blood through an artificial kidney machine (dialyzer).

hemorrhoidectomy Surgical removal of hemorrhoids.

herniorrhaphy Surgical repair of a hernia.

heterograft Graft from a nonhuman species. Also called *xenograft*.

Holter monitor Continuous ECG recorded on a tape cassette for at least 24 hours as a person works, plays, and rests.

homocysteine Amino acid in the blood. Elevated levels are related to a higher risk of CAD, stroke, and peripheral vascular disease.

homograft Skin graft from another person or a cadaver. Also called *allograft*.

hysterectomy Surgical removal of the uterus.

I

ileostomy Artificial opening from the ileum to the outside of the body.

implantable cardioverter/defibrillator (ICD) Implanted device that senses abnormal rhythms and gives the heart a small electrical shock to return the rhythm to normal.

incision Cut or surgical wound.

internal fixation Use of tissue-compatible materials such as stainless steel and titanium to stabilize fractured bony parts, enabling the patient to return to function more quickly and reducing the incidence of nonunion and malunion (improper healing). The types of internal fixation are wires used as sutures to "sew" the bone fragments together; plates that extend along both or all fragments of bone and are held in place by screws; rods inserted through the medullary cavity of both fragments to align the bones; and screws that can be used on their own as well as with plates.

intradermal injection Introduction of a short, thin needle into the epidermis, thus raising a small wheal. This site is used for allergy and tuberculosis (TB) testing.

intramuscular (IM) injection Use of a long needle that penetrates the epidermis, dermis, and hypodermis to reach into the muscles underneath. Some antibiotics and immunizations are given by this route.

intrauterine insemination Insertion of sperm directly into the uterus via a special catheter to initiate pregnancy.

intravenous pyelogram (IVP) Procedure in which a contrast material containing iodine is injected intravenously and its progress through the urinary tract is then recorded on a series of rapid radiological images.

intubation Insertion of a tube into a canal, hollow organ, or cavity, e.g., into the trachea for anesthesia or control of ventilation.

in vitro fertilization (IVF) Process of combining sperm and egg in a laboratory dish and placing the resulting embryos inside the uterus.

Ishihara color system Test for color vision defects.

J

Jaeger reading card Chart containing type in different sizes of print for testing near vision.

K

keratomileusis Procedure that cuts and shapes the cornea.

keratoplasty Corneal graft or transplant.

keratotomy Incision through the cornea.

kidney transplant Surgery in which the kidney of a donor is transplanted to a recipient; provides a better quality of life than kidney dialysis, if a suitable donor can be found.

KUB X-ray of the abdomen to show **k**idneys, **u**reters, and **b**ladder.

L

laparoscopy Examination of the contents of the abdomen using an endoscope, which can also be used to perform surgery and take samples for biopsy.

laryngoscopy Use of a hollow tube with a light and camera to visualize or operate on the larynx.

laser surgery Use of a concentrated, intense narrow beam of electromagnetic radiation for surgery. (*laser:* **l**ight **a**mplification by **s**imulated **e**mission of **r**adiation.)

LASIK Acronym for laser-assisted in situ keratomileusis.

lipectomy Surgical removal of fatty tissue.

lipid profile Group of blood tests that help determine the risk of CAD and comprise total cholesterol; high-density lipoprotein (HDL), or "good cholesterol"; low-density lipoprotein (LDL), or "bad cholesterol"; and triglycerides.

liposuction Surgical removal of fatty tissue using suction.

lobectomy Surgical removal of a lobe of a structure, for example, a lobe of a lung.

lumbar puncture Use of a hollow needle to remove CSF so that it can be examined in the laboratory. Also called *spinal tap.*

lumpectomy Removal of a lesion with preservation of surrounding tissue.

lymphadenectomy Surgical removal of a lymph gland(s).

lymphangiogram Radiographic images of lymph vessels and nodes following injection of contrast material.

M

magnetic resonance angiography (MRA) Method of visualizing vessels that contain flowing structures by producing a contrast between them and stationary structures.

magnetic resonance imaging (MRI) Diagnostic technique that creates detailed images of structures and tissues in various planes without exposing patients to radiation as in conventional radiography or computed tomography.

mammogram Record produced by x-ray imaging of the breast.

mammoplasty Surgical reshaping of the breasts.

mastectomy Surgical excision of the breast.

mechanical ventilation Process by which gases are moved into and out of the lungs via a ventilator that is set to meet the respiratory requirements of the patient.

mediastinoscopy Examination of the mediastinum using an endoscope inserted through an incision in the suprasternal notch.

myomectomy Surgical removal of a uterine myoma (fibroid).

myringotomy Incision through the tympanic membrane; e.g., for the placement of pressure equalization (PE) tubes to allow an effusion to drain.

N

nebulizer Device used to deliver liquid medicine in a fine mist.

nephrectomy Surgical removal of a kidney.

nephrolithotomy Incision into the kidney for removal of a stone.

nephroscopy Examination of the pelvis of the kidney.

nerve conduction studies Studies that measure the speed at which motor or sensory nerves conduct impulses.

nuclear imaging of the heart Use of an injection of a radioactive substance in association with a cardiac stress test to assess cardiac function.

O

ophthalmoscopy Examination of the retina using an ophthalmoscope.

orchiopexy Surgical fixation of a testis in the scrotum.

ostomy Artificial opening into a tubular structure, for example, ileostomy and colostomy.

otoscopy Examination of the ear using an otoscope.

P

pacemaker Device that regulates cardiac electrical activity. The device generates electronic signals carried along thin, insulated wires to the heart muscle.

palpation Examination with the fingers and hands.

panendoscopy Visual examination of the inside of the esophagus, stomach, and upper duodenum using a flexible fiber-optic endoscope.

Pap test Examination of cells taken from the cervix.

parathyroidectomy Surgical removal of the parathyroid glands.

peak flow meter Instrument used to record the greatest flow of air that can be sustained for 10 milliseconds on forced expiration, the peak expiratory flow rate (PEFR). It is of value in following the course of asthma and in postoperative care to monitor the return of lung function after anesthesia.

percutaneous nephrolithotomy Insertion of a nephroscope through the skin to locate and remove a renal pelvic or ureteral stone.

percutaneous transluminal coronary angioplasty (PTCA) Procedure in which a balloon-tipped catheter is guided to the site of the blockage and inflated to expand the artery from the inside by compressing the plaque against the walls of the artery.

percutaneous transthoracic needle aspiration Insertion of a needle with a cutting chamber through an intercostal space to hook a specimen of parietal pleura for laboratory examination.

peritoneal dialysis Procedure in which a dialysis solution is infused into and drained out of the abdominal cavity through a small, flexible, implanted catheter.

phacoemulsification To break down and remove the lens of the eye using an ultrasound needle.

phlebotomy Process of taking blood from a vein.

photocoagulation Use of a laser beam to form a clot or destroy abnormal capillaries. In the eye, this slows the pace of the visual loss in macular degeneration.

phototherapy Treatment using light rays.

pneumonectomy Surgical removal of a lung.

polypectomy Excision or removal of a polyp.

polysomnography Test to monitor brain waves, muscle tension, eye movement, and oxygen levels in the blood as the patient sleeps.

positive end expiratory pressure (PEEP) Technique in ventilation to keep the alveoli from collapsing in adult and neonatal respiratory distress syndromes.

positron emission tomography (PET) Scan that shows the uptake and distribution of substances such as sugar in tissues to locate abnormal, often malignant, structures.

postural drainage therapy (PDT) Treatment that involves positioning and tilting the patient so that gravity promotes drainage of secretions from lung segments. Chest percussion (tapping) on the chest wall can help loosen, mobilize, and drain the retained secretions.

proctoscopy Examination of the inside of the anus and rectum by endoscopy.

prostatectomy Surgical removal of part or all of the prostate.

prosthesis Manufactured substitute for a missing part of the body.

prothrombin time (PT) Test used to monitor the dose of Coumadin, an anticoagulant. It is reported as an *international normalized ratio (INR)* instead of in seconds.

psychotherapy Treatment of psychiatric disorders based on verbal and nonverbal interventions with the patient.

pulmonary rehabilitation Therapeutic restoration of lung function that includes education, breathing exercises and retraining, exercises for the upper and lower extremities, and psychosocial support.

pulse oximeter Sensor placed on the finger to measure the oxygen saturation of the blood.

pyelogram X-ray image of the renal pelvis and ureters.

Q

quadrantectomy Surgical excision of a quadrant of the breast.

R

radical hysterectomy Surgical removal of the fallopian tubes and ovaries as well as the uterus.

radical mastectomy Complete surgical removal of all breast tissue, the pectoralis major muscle, and associated lymph nodes.

radical prostatectomy Complete surgical removal of the prostate and surrounding tissues.

random urine collection Process in which a sample is taken with no precautions regarding contamination. It is often used for collecting samples for drug testing. "Pee into a cup."

reduction Procedure in which the distal segment of a fractured bone is pulled back into alignment with the proximal segment. Anesthesia may be used.

rehabilitation Therapeutic restoration of an ability to function as before after disease, illness, or injury.

renal angiogram X-ray with contrast material used to assess blood flow to the kidneys.

resection Removal of a specific part of an organ or structure.

retrograde pyelogram Injection of contrast material through a urinary catheter into the ureters to locate stones and other obstructions.

rhinoplasty Surgical procedure to alter the size or shape of the nose.

Rinne test Test for a conductive hearing loss.

S

salpingectomy Surgical removal of a fallopian tube.

sclerotherapy Injection of a solution into a vein to thrombose it.

segmentectomy Surgical excision of a segment of a tissue or organ.

sigmoidoscopy Endoscopic examination of the sigmoid colon.

Snellen letter chart Test for acuity of distant vision.

sphygmomanometer Instrument for measuring arterial blood pressure.

spinal tap Placement of a needle through an intervertebral space into the subarachnoid space to withdraw CSF.

spirometer Device used to measure the volume of air that a patient moves in and out of the respiratory system.

splenectomy Surgical removal of the spleen.

staging Process of determining the extent of the distribution of a neoplasm. The TNM (tumor-node-metastasis) staging system can be used.

stent placement Procedure in which a wire mesh tube, or stent, is placed inside the vessel to reduce the likelihood that an occluded artery will close up again. Some stents (drug-eluting stents) are covered with a special medication to help keep the artery open.

sterilization Process of making sterile.

stethoscope Instrument for listening to cardiac, respiratory, and other sounds.

stoma Artificial opening.

subcutaneous (SC) injection Injection in which a needle pierces the epidermis and dermis to reach the hypodermis (subcutaneous) layer. This site is used for insulin injections and for some immunizations.

suprapubic transabdominal needle aspiration of the bladder Procedure used with newborns and small infants to obtain a pure sample of urine.

suture Process or material that brings together the edges of a wound to enhance tissue healing. Also, a form of fibrous joint to unite two bones.

T

thoracentesis Insertion of a needle through an intercostal space to remove fluid from a pleural effusion for laboratory study or to relieve pressure. Also called *pleural tap.*

thoracoscopy Examination of the pleural cavity with an endoscope.

thoracotomy Incision through the chest wall.

thymectomy Surgical removal of the thymus gland.

thyroidectomy Surgical removal of the thyroid gland.

tomography Radiographic image of a selected slice of tissue.

tonometry Measurement of intraocular pressure.

tonsillectomy Surgical removal of the tonsils.

tracheal aspiration Procedure in which a soft catheter is passed into the trachea to allow brushings and washings to remove cells and secretions from the trachea and main bronchi for diagnostic study.

tracheostomy Insertion of a tube into the windpipe to assist breathing.

tracheotomy The process of making an incision into the trachea.

traction Gentle but continuous application of a pulling force that can align a fracture, reduce muscle spasm, and relieve pain.

transdermal application Administration of some medications through the skin by an adhesive transdermal patch that is applied to the skin. The medication diffuses across the epidermis and enters the blood vessels in the dermis. Contraceptive hormones, analgesics, and antinausea/seasickness medications are examples.

transplant The tissue or organ used or the transfer of tissue from one person to another.

transthoracic Going through the chest wall.

tubal ligation Surgery, using laparoscopy, in which both fallopian tubes are cut, a segment is removed, and the ends are tied off and cauterized shut.

24-hour urine collection Process that determines the amount of protein being excreted daily and estimates the kidneys' filtration ability.

tympanostomy Surgically created new opening in the tympanic membrane to allow fluid to drain from the middle ear.

U

ultrasonography Delineation of deep structures using sound waves.

ureteroscopy Examination of the ureter. A small flexible ureteroscope is passed through the urethra and bladder into the ureter. Devices can be passed through the endoscope to remove or fragment stones.

urinalysis (microscopic) Analysis of the solids deposited by centrifuging a specimen of urine. It can reveal RBCs, WBCs, and renal tubular epithelial cells stuck together to form casts (cylindrical molds of cells) in nephrotic syndrome.

urinalysis (U/A) Examination of urine to separate it into its elements and define their kind and/or quantity. A routine urinalysis in the laboratory can include tests for color, clarity, pH, specific gravity, protein, glucose, ketones, and leukocyte esterase (indicator of infection).

urine culture Culture taken from a clean-catch urine specimen. It is the definitive test for a urinary tract infection.

vasectomy Excision of a segment of the ductus deferens to interrupt the flow of sperm.

vasovasostomy Microsurgical procedure to suture back together the cut ends of the ductus deferens to restore the flow of sperm. Also called *vasectomy reversal*.

venogram Radiograph of veins after injection of radiopaque contrast material.

vestibulectomy Surgical excision of the vulva.

voiding cystourethrogram (VCUG) Imaging in which a contrast material is inserted into the bladder through a catheter and x-rays are taken during voiding.

Weber test Test for sensorineural hearing loss.

xenograft Graft from a nonhuman species. Also called *heterograft*.

Pharmacology

A compilation of pharmacologic terms used in this book.

A

acetaminophen Analgesic (reduces response to pain) and antipyretic (reduces fever).

adrenaline (1) Hormone produced by the adrenal medulla that boosts the supply of oxygen and glucose to the brain and increases heart rate and output. (2) Drug used to treat cardiac arrest and dysrhythmias and relieve bronchospasm in asthma. Also called *epinephrine*.

allergen Substance producing a hypersensitivity (allergic) reaction. Examples are animal fur and dander, penicillins, and foods such as eggs, milk, and wheat.

alpha-glucosidase inhibitors Block the breakdown of starches in the intestine.

analgesic Substance that reduces or relieves the response to pain without producing loss of consciousness. Examples are aspirin and other NSAIDs, acetaminophen, and codeine.

androgen Hormone that promotes masculine characteristics. An example is testosterone.

anesthetic Agent that causes absence of feeling or sensation. Examples of local anesthetics are lidocaine and novocaine; examples of general anesthetics are nitrous oxide, thiopental, and ketamine.

antacid Agent that neutralizes the acidity of stomach contents. Examples are aluminum hydroxide, magnesium hydroxide, and calcium carbonate.

antiarrhythmic Agents that restore normal heart rate and rhythm.

antibiotic Substance that has the capacity to inhibit the growth of or destroy bacteria and other microorganisms. Examples are penicillin, erythromycin, cefotaxime, and flucloxacillin.

anticholinergics Agents antagonistic to parasympathetic nerve fibers.

anticoagulant Substance that prevents clotting. Examples are heparin and Coumadin (warfarin).

antidepressants A class of drugs that alleviate the symptoms of depression.

antidiabetic drugs Medications used to treat diabetes. Those given orally include metformin, acarbose, and thiazolidinediones, such as troglitazone. Insulin is given by injection or inhaled.

antidiuretic Agent that decreases urine production. Examples are vasopressin, amiloride, and chlorpropamide.

antiepileptic Agent capable of preventing or arresting epilepsy. Examples are phenobarbitol, phenytoin, and valproate.

antifungal agents can be purchased over the counter and include 1% clotrimazole (Lomotrin, Mycelex) and 1% terbinafine (Lamisil).

antihistamine Agent used to treat allergic symptoms because of its action antagonistic to histamine. Examples are benadryl, diphenhydramine, and cimetidine.

anti-inflammatory Agent that reduces inflammation by acting on the body's responses, without affecting the causative agent. Examples are corticosteroids and aspirin.

antimicrobial Agent used to destroy or prevent multiplication of organisms. (See *antibiotic*.)

antineoplastic Agent that prevents the growth and spread of cancer cells. Examples are methotrexate, fluorouracil, and cyclophosphamide.

antipruritic Medication against itching. Examples are calamine lotion, hydrocortisone cream applied topically, and diphenhydramine (Benadryl) taken orally.

antipyretic Agent that reduces fever. Examples are aspirin and acetaminophen.

antiseptic Agent that reduces the number of microorganisms in different situations. Examples are alcohol, chlorhexidine, and providone-iodine.

anxiolytics Class of drugs that relieve the symptoms of anxiety.

atropine Agent used to dilate the pupils.

B

benzothiazide Diuretic that increases the excretion of sodium and potassium with an accompanying volume of water.

beta blocker Agent used in the treatment of a variety of cardiovascular diseases. Examples are propanalol and acebutolol.

biguanides Agents that decrease glucose production in the liver.

bronchodilator Agent that relaxes the smooth muscles of the bronchioles. Examples are theophylline; beta-2 agonists, such as salbutamol and terbutaline; and anticholinergics, such as ipratropium bromide.

C

calcium channel blocker Agent that decreases the force of contraction of the myocardium, dilates coronary arteries, and reduces blood pressure. Examples are amlodipine and verapamil.

chemotherapy Treatment using chemical agents, usually in relation to neoplastic disease. Examples are platinum compounds such as cisplatin or paraplatin.

chronotropic Agents that alter the heart rate.

cleansing agents Soaps, shampoos, and detergents that are used to clean wounds and abrasions or to remove crusts and scales.

coagulant Substance that causes clotting. Thrombin and fibrin glue are used surgically to treat bleeding.

contraceptive Agent that prevents conception. Examples are condoms, diaphragms, and birth control pills using a mixture of estrogen and progesterone.

corticosteroids Hormones produced by the adrenal cortex. Examples are cortisol and aldosterone.

cortisol One of the glucocorticoids produced by the adrenal cortex; has anti-inflammatory effects. Also called *hydrocortisone*.

creams Water-based emulsions with a cooling and soothing effect that are cosmetically well tolerated.

D

decongestant An agent that reduces the swelling and fluid in the nose and sinuses. Examples are pseudoephedrine and phenylephrine.

depressant Substance that diminishes activity, sensation, or tone, particularly in relation to the nervous system. Examples are alcohol, barbiturates, and benzodiazepines.

disease-modifying drug Agent that has partial success in slowing down the accumulation of disabilities in a specific disease process. Examples in multiple sclerosis (MS) include interferons and mitoxantrone.

disinfectant Agent used to destroy pathogenic and other microorganisms on nonliving surfaces. Examples are alcohol, hydrogen peroxide, and hypochlorites.

diuretic Agent that increases urine output. Examples are furosemide, hydrochlorthiazide, spironolactone, and mannitol.

dopamine Chemical neurotransmitter in some specific areas of the brain.

E

epinephrine (1) Hormone produced by the adrenal medulla that boosts the supply of oxygen and glucose to the brain and increases heart rate and output. (2) Drug used to treat cardiac arrest and dysrhythmias and relieve bronchospasm in asthma. Also called *adrenaline.*

estrogen Generic term for hormones that stimulate female secondary sex characteristics.

F

fluorescein Dye that produces a vivid green color under a blue light; used to diagnose corneal abrasions and foreign bodies in the eye.

G

gels Jelly-like watery suspension using a chemical gelling agent for insoluble drugs such as corticosteroids and retinoids.

H

histamine Compound liberated in tissues as a result of injury or an immune response.

hydrocortisone Potent glucocorticoid with anti-inflammatory properties. Also called *cortisol.*

I

immunization Treatment with an agent designed to protect susceptible people from a communicable disease, such as agents that protect against the childhood diseases of measles, rubella, and pertussis.

inotropic Agents that change the force of ventricular contraction.

insulin Hormone produced by the islet cells of the pancreas that promotes glucose use. Injectable insulin preparations are classified by their speed of action.

L

lidocaine Ocular local anesthetic.

loop diuretic Promotes evacuation of urine in the kidney.

M

melatonin Hormone formed and secreted by the pineal gland during darkness. Serotonin is a precursor. It assists in the control of daily body rhythms, stimulates the immune system, and is an antioxidant.

morphine Derivative of opium used as an analgesic or sedative.

mucolytic Agent that attempts to break up mucus to allow it to be cleared more effectively from the airways. Examples are guaifenesin (common in over-the-counter cough medications), potassium iodide, and *N*-acetylcysteine (taken through a nebulizer).

mydriatic Agent that dilates the pupils of the eye.

N

narcotic Drug derived from opium. Examples are heroin, morphine, codeine, and demerol.

neurotransmitter Chemical that crosses a synapse to stimulate or inhibit another neuron or the cell of a muscle or gland. Examples are norepinephrine, serotonin, and dopamine.

O

ointments Agents that contain no water and are oil-based to provide an occlusive layer to retain water in the skin; they are used to treat chronic, dry, and scaly conditions.

opiate Drug derived from opium. Examples are morphine, codeine, heroin, and demerol.

osmotic diuretic Promotes evacuation of water and electrolytes in the kidney.

oxygen Gas given by nasal cannula or by mask and intubation to relieve hypoxia. Patients with severe, chronic COPD can be attached to a portable cylinder of oxygen.

P

pharmacist Person licensed by the state to prepare and dispense drugs.

pharmacology Science of the preparation, uses, and effects of drugs.

pharmacy Facility licensed to prepare and dispense drugs.

placebo Inert, medicinally inactive compound with no intrinsic therapeutic value.

progesterone Hormone used to correct abnormalities of menstruation, and as a contraceptive.

prostaglandin Hormone present in many tissues; first isolated from the prostate gland.

psychedlic A class of drugs that enhance sensory experiences and consciousness.

psychoactive Agent able to alter mood, behavior, and/or cognition. Examples include narcotics, stimulants, antidepressants, and hallucinogens.

R

retinoids Keratolytic agents applied for psoriasis, acne, and photo damage.

S

saline Salt solution, usually sodium chloride.

selective serotonin reuptake inhibitors Class of drugs that prevent the reuptake of serotonin and are used in the treatment of depression.

somatotropin Hormone of the anterior pituitary gland that stimulates the growth of body tissues. Also called *growth hormone (GH).*

spermicide Agent that destroys sperm. Examples are nonoxynol-9 and benzalkonium chloride.

sterilization Elimination of all microorganisms by high-pressure steam (autoclave), dry heat (oven), or radiation.

steroid Large family of chemical substances found in many drugs, hormones, and body components.

stimulant Agent that excites or strengthens. Examples include caffeine, nicotine, and cocaine.

sulfonylureas Agents that stimulate the beta cells of the pancreas to produce more insulin.

surfactant Protein and fat compound that creates surface tension to hold the lung alveolar walls apart.

T

teratogen Agent that produces fetal abnormalities—congenital malformations—while organs and structures are being formed. (All medications readily cross the placenta.) Examples include alcohol, isoretinoin (acne medication), valproic acid (anticonvulsant), and the rubella virus.

testosterone The major androgen that promotes development of male sex characteristics.

thrombolytic Agent injected within a few hours of a myocardial infarction (MI) or stroke to dissolve the thrombus causing the arterial blockage. Examples are streptokinase and tissue plasminogen activator (tPA). Also called *clot-busting drug.*

thyroxine Thyroid hormone T4, tetraiodothyronine.

topical Medication applied to the skin to obtain a local effect. Examples are ointments, creams, gels, lotions, patches, and sprays.

toxin Poisonous substance formed by a living cell or organism. Examples are venom from bee stings, snake bites, and jellyfish stings.

triamcinalone Synthetic corticosteroid.

V

vaccine Agent used to generate immunity and composed of the antigenic components of a killed or attenuated microorganism or its inactivated toxins. See *immunization.*

vasopressin Synthetic hormone causing contraction of smooth muscle.

vitamin Essential organic substance necessary in small amounts for normal cell function.

W

warfarin Anticoagulant; also used as rat poison. Trade name: *Coumadin.*

A

abdomen (**AB**-doh-men) Part of the trunk between the thorax and the pelvis.

abdominal (ab-**DOM**-in-al) Pertaining to the abdomen.

abdominopelvic (ab-**DOM**-ih-no-**PEL**-vik) Pertaining to the abdomen and pelvis.

abdominoplasty (ab-**DOM**-ih-noh-plas-tee) Surgical removal of excess subcutaneous fat from the abdominal wall (tummy tuck).

abduction (ab-**DUCK**-shun) Action of moving away from the midline.

abductor (ab-**DUCK**-tor) Muscle that moves the thigh away from the midline.

ablation (ab-**LAY**-shun) Removal of tissue to destroy its function.

abortion (ah-**BOR**-shun) Spontaneous or induced expulsion of the fetus from the uterus at 20 weeks or less.

abrasion (ah-**BRAY**-zhun) Area of skin or mucous membrane that has been scraped off.

abruptio (ab-**RUP**-she-oh) Placenta abruptio is the premature detachment of the placenta.

absorb (ab-**SORB**). To take in.

absorption (ab-**SORP**-shun) Uptake of nutrients and water by cells in the GI tract.

accessory (ak-**SESS**-oh-ree) A muscle or nerve that is auxiliary to a more major structure.

accommodate (ah-**KOM**-oh-date) To adapt to meet a need.

accommodation (ah-kom-oh-**DAY**-shun) The act of adjusting something to make it fit the needs; for example, the lens of the eye adjusts itself.

accommodative (ah-kom-oh-**DAY**-tiv) Pertaining to accommodation.

acetabulum (ass-eh-**TAB**-you-lum) The cup-shaped cavity of the hip bone that receives the head of the femur to form the hip joint.

acetaminophen (ah-seat-ah-**MIN**-oh-fen) Medication that is an analgesic and an antipyretic.

acetone (**ASS**-eh-tone) Ketone that is found in blood, urine, and breath when diabetes mellitus is out of control.

Achilles tendon (ah-**KILL**-eeze) A tendon formed from gastrocnemius and soleus muscles and inserted into the calcaneus bone. Also called *calcaneal tendon.*

achondroplasia (a-kon-droh-**PLAY**-zee-ah) Condition with abnormal conversion of cartilage into bone, leading to dwarfism.

acne (**AK**-nee) Inflammatory disease of sebaceous glands and hair follicles.

acoustic (ah-**KYU**-stik) Pertaining to hearing.

acquired immunodeficiency syndrome (AIDS) (ah-**KWIRED IM**-you-noh-dee-**FISH**-en-see **SIN**-drohm) Infection with the HIV.

acromegaly (ak-roe-**MEG**-ah-lee) Enlargement of the head, face, hands, and feet due to excess growth hormone in an adult.

acromioclavicular (AC) (ah-**CROW**-mee-oh-klah-**VICK**-you-lar) The joint between the acromion and the clavicle.

acromion (ah-**CROW**-mee-on) Lateral end of the scapula, extending over the shoulder joint.

active (**AK**-tiv) Causing action or change.

activities of daily living (ADLs) (ak-**TIV**-ih-teez of **DAY**-lee **LIV**-ing) Daily routines for mobility, personal care, bathing, dressing, eating, and moving.

activity (ak-**TIV**-ih-tee) A goal-directed human action.

acute (ah-**KYUT**) Disease of sudden onset.

adapt (a-**DAPT**) To adjust to different conditions.

adaptation (ad-ap-**TAY**-shun) Change in the function or structure of an organ to meet new conditions.

addict (**ADD**-ikt) One who cannot live without a substance or practice.

addiction (ah-**DIK**-shun) Habitual psychologic and physiologic dependence on a substance or practice.

Addison disease (**ADD**-ih-son diz-**EEZ**) An autoimmune disease leading to decreased production of adrenocortical steroids.

adduction (ah-**DUCK**-shun) Action of moving toward the midline.

adductor (ah-**DUCK**-tor) Muscle that moves the thigh toward the midline.

adenocarcinoma (**ADD**-eh-noh-kar-sih-**NOH**-mah) A cancer arising from glandular epithelial cells.

adenoid (**ADD**-eh-noyd) Single mass of lymphoid tissue in the midline at the back of the throat.

adenoidectomy (**ADD**-eh-noy-**DEK**-toh-me) Surgical removal of the adenoid tissue.

adipose (**ADD**-ih-pose) Containing fat.

adolescence (ad-oh-**LESS**-ence) Stage that begins with puberty and ends with physical maturity.

adolescent (ad-oh-**LESS**-ent) Pertaining to adolescence or a person in that stage.

adrenal gland (ah-**DREE**-nal GLAND) The suprarenal gland on the upper pole of each kidney.

adrenaline (ah-**DREN**-ah-lin) One of the catecholamines. Also called *epinephrine.*

adrenocortical (ah-**DREE**-noh-**KOR**-tih-kal) Pertaining to the cortex of the adrenal gland.

adrenocorticotropic (ah-**DREE**-noh-**KOR**-tih-koh-**TROH**-pik) Hormone of the anterior pituitary that stimulates the cortex of the adrenal gland to produce its own hormones.

afferent (**AFF**-eh-rent) Moving toward a center; for example, nerve fibers conducting impulses to the spinal cord and brain.

aged (**A**-jid) Having lived to an advanced age.

agenesis (a-**JEN**-eh-sis) Failure to develop any organ or any part.

agglutinate (ah-**GLUE**-tin-ate) Stick together to form clumps.

agglutination (ah-glue-tih-**NAY**-shun) Process by which cells or other particles adhere to each other to form clumps.

aging (**A**-jing) The process of human maturation and decline.

agranulocyte (a-**GRAN**-you-loh-site) A white blood cell without any granules in its cytoplasm.

aldosterone (al-**DOS**-ter-own) Mineralocorticoid hormone of the adrenal cortex.

alignment (a-**LINE**-ment) Having a structure in its correct position relative to other structures.

alimentary (al-ih-**MEN**-tar-ee) Pertaining to the digestive tract.

alimentary canal (al-ih-**MEN**-tar-ee kah-**NAL**) Digestive tract.

allergen (**AL**-er-jen) Substance producing a hypersensitivity (allergic) reaction.

allergenic (al-er-**JEN**-ik) Pertaining to the capacity to produce an allergic reaction.

allergic (ah-**LER**-jik) Pertaining to or suffering from an allergy.

allergy (**AL**-er-jee) Hypersensitivity to an allergen.

alloimmune (**AL**-oh-im-**YUNE**) Immune reaction directed against foreign tissue.

alopecia (al-oh-**PEE**-shah) Partial or complete loss of hair, naturally or from medication.

alveolus (al-**VEE**-oh-lus) Terminal element of the respiratory tract where gas exchange occurs. Plural *alveoli*.

Alzheimer disease (**AWLZ**-high-mer diz-**EEZ**) Common form of dementia.

amblyopia (am-blee-**OH**-pee-ah) Failure or incomplete development of the pathways of vision to the brain.

ambulatory (**AM**-byu-**LAY**-tor-ee) Surgery or any other care provided without an overnight stay in a medical facility.

amenorrhea (a-men-oh-**REE**-ah) Absence or abnormal cessation of menstrual flow.

amino acid (ah-**ME**-no **ASS**-id) The basic building block for protein.

ammonia (ah-**MOAN**-ih-ah) Toxic breakdown product of amino acids (proteins).

amniocentesis (**AM**-nee-oh-sen-**TEE**-sis) Removal of amniotic fluid for diagnostic purposes.

amnion (**AM**-nee-on) Membrane around the fetus that contains amniotic fluid.

amniotic (am-nee-**OT**-ik) Pertaining to the amnion.

ampulla (am-**PULL**-ah) Dilated portion of a canal or duct.

amputation (am-pyu-**TAY**-shun) Process of removing a limb, a part of a limb, a breast, or some other projecting part. Verb *amputate*.

amputee (**AM**-pyu-tee) A person with an amputation.

amylase (**AM**-il-ase) One of a group of enzymes that breaks down starch.

amyotrophic (a-my-oh-**TROH**-fik) Pertaining to muscular atrophy.

anabolism (an-**AB**-oh-lizm) The buildup of complex substances in the cell from simpler ones as a part of metabolism.

anal (**A**-nal) Pertaining to the anus.

analgesia (an-al-**JEE**-zee-ah) State in which pain is reduced.

analgesic (an-al-**JEE**-zic) Substance that produces analgesia.

anaphylactic (**AN**-ah-fih-**LAK**-tik) Pertaining to anaphylaxis.

anaphylaxis (**AN**-ah-fih-**LAK**-sis) Immediate severe allergic response.

anastomosis (ah-**NAS**-toh-**MOH**-sis) A surgically made union between two tubular structures. Plural *anastomoses*.

androgen (**AN**-droh-jen) Hormone that promotes masculine characteristics.

anemia (ah-**NEE**-me-ah) Decreased number of red blood cells.

anemic (ah-**NEE**-mik) Pertaining to or suffering from anemia.

anencephaly (**AN**-en-**SEF**-ah-lee) Born without cerebral hemispheres.

anesthesia (an-es-**THEE**-zee-ah) Complete loss of sensation.

anesthesiologist (**AN**-es-thee-zee-**OL**-oh-jist) Medical specialist in anesthesia.

anesthesiology (**AN**-es-thee-zee-**OL**-oh-jee) Medical specialty related to anesthesia.

anesthetic (an-es-**THET**-ik) Agent that causes absence of feeling or sensation.

aneurysm (**AN**-yur-izm) Circumscribed dilation of an artery or cardiac chamber.

angiogram (**AN**-jee-oh-gram) Radiograph obtained after injection of radiopaque contrast material into blood vessels.

angiography (an-jee-**OG**-rah-fee) Radiography of vessels after injection of contrast material.

angioplasty (**AN**-jee-oh-**PLAS**-tee) Recanalization of a blood vessel by surgery.

anomaly (ah-**NOM**-ah-lee) Structural abnormality present at birth.

anorectal junction (A-no-**RECK**-tal **JUNK**-shun) Junction between the anus and the rectum.

anorexia (an-oh-**RECK**-see-ah) Without an appetite; *or* having an aversion to food.

anoxia (an-**OCK**-see-ah) Without oxygen.

anoxic (an-**OCK**-sik) Pertaining to or suffering from a lack of oxygen.

antacid (ant-**ASS**-id) Agent that neutralizes the acidity of stomach contents.

antagonist (an-**TAG**-oh-nist) An opposing structure, agent, disease, or process.

antagonistic (an-**TAG**-oh-nist-ik) Having an opposite function.

antecubital (an-teh-**KYU**-bit-al) In front of the elbow.

anterior (an-**TEER**-ee-or) Front surface of body; situated in front.

anteversion (an-teh-**VER**-zhun) Forward displacement or tilting of a structure.

anthracosis (an-thra-**KOH**-sis) Lung disease caused by the inhalation of coal dust.

anthrax (**AN**-thraks) A severe, malignant infectious disease.

antibiotic (**AN**-tih-bye-**OT**-ik) A substance that has the capacity to inhibit growth of and destroy bacteria and other microorganisms.

antibody (**AN**-tee-body) Protein produced in response to an antigen. Plural *antibodies*.

anticoagulant (**AN**-tee-koh-**AG**-you-lant) Substance that prevents clotting.

antidiuretic (**AN**-tih-die-you-**RET**-ik) An agent that decreases urine production.

antidiuretic hormone (ADH) (**AN**-tih-die-you-**RET**-ik **HOR**-mohn) Posterior pituitary hormone that decreases urine output by acting on the kidney. Also called *vasopressin*.

antiepileptic (**AN**-tih-epi-**LEP**-tik) A pharmacologic agent capable of preventing or arresting epilepsy.

antigen (**AN**-tee-jen) Substance capable of triggering an immune response.

antihistamine (**AN**-tih-**HISS**-tah-mean) Drug used to treat allergic symptoms because of its action antagonistic to histamine.

antimicrobial (**AN**-tee-my-**KROH**-bee-al) Agent to destroy or prevent multiplication of organisms.

antineoplastic (**AN**-tee-nee-oh-**PLAS**-tik) Pertaining to the prevention of the growth and spread of cancer cells.

antipruritic (**AN**-tee-pru-**RIT**-ik) Medication against itching.

antipyretic (**AN**-tee-pie-**RET**-ik) Agent that reduces fever.

antisepsis (an-tee-**SEP**-sis) Inhibiting the growth of infectious agents.

antiseptic (an-tee-**SEP**-tik) An agent or substance capable of affecting antisepsis.

antiserum (an-tee-**SEER**-um) Serum taken from another human or animal that has antibodies to a disease. Also called *immune serum.*

antisocial personality disorder (**AN**-tee-**SOH**-shall per-son-**AL**-ih-tee dis-**OR**-der) Chronic violation of the rights of others.

antrum (**AN**-trum) A closed cavity.

anuria (an-**YOU**-ree-ah) Absence of urine production.

anus (**A**-nus) Terminal opening of the digestive tract through which feces are discharged.

anxiety (ang-**ZI**-eh-tee) Distress and dread caused by fear.

aorta (a-**OR**-tuh) Main trunk of the systemic arterial system.

aortic (a-**OR**-tik) Pertaining to the aorta.

apex (**A**-peks) Tip or end; for example, of the cone-shaped heart.

Apgar score (**AP**-gar SKOR) Evaluation of a newborn's status.

aphthous (**AF**-thus) Painful small oral ulcers (canker sores).

apnea (**AP**-nee-ah) Absence of spontaneous respiration.

apoptosis (**AP**-op-**TOE**-sis) Programmed normal cell death.

appendicitis (ah-pen-dih-**SIGH**-tis) Inflammation of the appendix.

appendicular (**AP**-en-**DICK**-you-lar) Relating to the limbs, e.g., the appendicular skeleton.

appendix (ah-**PEN**-dicks) Small blind projection from the pouch of the cecum.

aqueous humor (**AK**-we-us **HEW**-mor) Watery liquid in the anterior and posterior chambers of the eye.

arachnoid mater (ah-**RACK**-noyd **MAY**-ter) Weblike middle layer of the three meninges.

areola (ah-**REE**-oh-luh) Circular reddish area surrounding the nipple.

areolar (ah-**REE**-oh-lar) Pertaining to the areola.

arrhythmia (a-**RITH**-me-ah) Condition when the heart rhythm is abnormal.

arteriography (ar-teer-ee-**OG**-rah-fee) X-ray visualization of an artery after injection of contrast material.

arteriole (ar-**TIER**-ee-ole) Small terminal artery leading into the capillary network.

arteriosclerosis (ar-**TIER**-ee-oh-skler-**OH**-sis) Hardening of the arteries.

arteriosclerotic (ar-**TIER**-ee-oh-skler-**OT**-ik) Pertaining to or suffering from arteriosclerosis.

artery (**AR**-ter-ee) Thick-walled blood vessel carrying blood away from the heart.

arthritis (ar-**THRI**-tis) Inflammation of a joint or joints.

arthrocentesis (**AR**-throw-sen-**TEE**-sis) Withdrawal of fluid from a joint through a needle.

arthrodesis (ar-throw-**DEE**-sis) Fixation or stiffening of a joint by surgery.

arthrography (ar-**THROG**-rah-fee) X-ray of a joint taken after the injection of a contrast medium into the joint.

arthroplasty (**AR**-throw-plas-tee) Surgery to restore, as far as possible, the function of a joint.

arthroscope (**AR**-thro-skope) Endoscope used to examine the interior of a joint.

arthroscopy (ar-**THROS**-koh-pee) Visual examination of the interior of a joint.

articulate (ar-**TIK**-you-late) Two separate bones have formed a joint.

articulation (ar-tik-you-**LAY**-shun) A joint.

asbestosis (as-bes-**TOE**-sis) Lung disease caused by the inhalation of asbestos particles.

ascites (ah-**SIGH**-teez) Accumulation of fluid in the abdominal cavity.

asepsis (a-**SEP**-sis) Absence of living pathogenic organisms.

Asperger syndrome (**AHS**-per-ger **SIN**-drohm) Developmental disorder of children.

aspiration (**AS**-pih-**RAY**-shun) Removal by suction of fluid or gas from a body cavity. Verb *aspirate.*

asthma (**AZ**-mah) Episodes of breathing difficulty due to narrowed or obstructed airways.

asthmatic (az-**MAT**-ik) Suffering from or pertaining to asthma.

astigmatism (ah-**STIG**-maht-izm) Inability to focus light rays that enter the eye in different planes.

asymptomatic (**A**-simp-toe-**MAT**-ik) Without any symptoms experienced by the patient.

asystole (a-**SIS**-toe-lee) Absence of contractions of the heart.

ataxia (a-**TAK**-see-ah) Inability to coordinate muscle activity, leading to jerky movements.

ataxic (a-**TAK**-sik) Pertaining to or suffering from ataxia.

atelectasis (at-el-**ECK**-tah-sis) Collapse of part of a lung.

atherectomy (ath-er-**EK**-toe-me) Surgical removal of atheroma.

atheroma (ath-er-**ROE**-mah) Lipid deposit in the lining of an artery.

atherosclerosis (**ATH**-er-oh-skler-**OH**-sis) Atheroma in arteries.

athetoid (**ATH**-eh-toyd) Resembling or suffering from athetosis.

athetosis (ath-eh-**TOE**-sis) Slow, writhing involuntary movements.

atonic (a-**TOHN**-ik) Without normal muscular tone.

atopic (a-**TOP**-ik) Pertaining to an allergy.

atopy (**AT**-oh-pee) State of hypersensitivity to an allergen—allergic.

atresia (a-**TREE**-zee-ah) Congenital absence of a normal opening or lumen.

atrial (**A**-tree-al) Pertaining to the atrium.

atrioventricular (AV) (**A**-tree-oh-ven-**TRICK**-you-lar) Pertaining to both the atrium and the ventricle.

atrium (**A**-tree-um) Chamber where blood enters the heart on both right and left sides. Plural *atria.*

atrophy (**A**-troh-fee) Wasting or diminished volume of a tissue or organ.

atropine (**AT**-ro-peen) Pharmacologic agent used to dilate pupils.

attenuate (ah-**TEN**-you-ate) Weaken the ability of an organism to produce disease.

audiologist (aw-dee-**OL**-oh-jist) Specialist in evaluation of hearing function.

audiology (aw-dee-**OL**-oh-jee) Study of hearing disorders.

audiometer (aw-dee-**OM**-eh-ter) Instrument to measure hearing.

audiometric (**AW**-dee-oh-**MET**-rik) Pertaining to the measurement of hearing.

auditory (**AW**-dih-tor-ee) Pertaining to the sense or the organs of hearing.

aura (**AWE**-rah) Sensory experience preceding an epileptic seizure or a migraine headache.

auricle (**AW**-ri-kul) The shell-like external ear.

auscultation (aws-kul-**TAY**-shun) Diagnostic method of listening to body sounds with a stethoscope.

autism (**AWE**-tizm) Developmental disorder of children.

autistic (awe-**TIS**-tik) Pertaining to autism.

autoantibody (awe-toe-**AN**-tee-bod-ee) Antibody produced in response to an antigen from the host's own tissue.

autograft (**AWE**-toe-graft) A graft using tissue taken from the same individual who is receiving the graft.

autoimmune (awe-toe-im-**YUNE**) Immune reaction directed against a person's own tissue.

autologous (awe-**TOL**-oh-gus) Blood transfusion with the same person as donor and recipient.

autolysis (awe-**TOL**-ih-sis) Destruction of cells by enzymes within the cells.

autonomic (awe-toh-**NOM**-ik) Self-governing visceral motor division of the peripheral nervous system.

autopsy (**AWE**-top-see) Examination of the body and organs of a dead person to determine the cause of death.

avascular (a-**VAS**-cue-lar) Without a blood supply.

avulsion (a-**VUL**-shun) Forcible separation or tearing away, often of a tendon from bone.

axial (**AK**-see-al) Relating to the head and trunk, e.g., the axial skeleton.

axilla (**AK**-sill-ah) Medical name for the armpit. Plural *axillae*.

axillary (**AK**-sill-air-ee) Pertaining to the armpit.

axon (**ACK**-son) Single process of a nerve cell carrying nervous impulses away from the cell body.

azoospermia (a-zoh-oh-**SPER**-me-ah) Absence of living sperm in the semen.

azotemia (a-zo-**TEE**-me-ah) Excess nitrogenous waste products in the blood.

B

bacterial (bak-**TEER**-ee-al) Pertaining to bacteria.

bacterium (bak-**TEER**-ee-um) A unicellular (single-cell), simple, microscopic organism. Plural *bacteria*.

balanitis (bal-ah-**NIE**-tis) Inflammation of the glans and prepuce of the penis.

bariatric (bar-ee-**AT**-rik) Treatment of obesity.

basilar (**BAS**-ih-lar) Pertaining to the base of a structure.

basophil (**BAY**-so-fill) A basophil's granules attract basic blue stain in the laboratory.

Bell palsy (BELL **PAWL**-zee) Paresis, or paralysis, of one side of the face.

biceps brachii (BYE-sepz **BRAY**-key-eye) A muscle of the arm that has two heads or points of origin on the scapula.

bicuspid (by-**KUSS**-pid) Having two points. A bicuspid heart valve has two flaps; a bicuspid (premolar) tooth has two points.

bifid (**BI**-fid) Separated into two parts.

bilateral (by-**LAT**-er-al) On two sides; for example, in both ears.

bile (BILE) Fluid secreted by the liver into the duodenum.

bile acids (BILE **AH**-sids) Steroids synthesized from cholesterol.

biliary (**BILL**-ee-air-ree) Pertaining to bile or the biliary tract.

bilirubin (bill-ee-**RU**-bin) Bile pigment formed in the liver from hemoglobin.

binge eating (BINJ **EE**-ting) Eating with periods of excessive intake.

biopsy (**BI**-op-see) Removing tissue from a living person for laboratory examination.

bipolar disorder (bi-**POH**-lar dis-**OR**-der) A mood disorder with alternating episodes of depression and mania.

bladder (**BLAD**-er) Hollow sac that holds fluid, for example, urine or bile.

blastocyst (**BLAS**-toe-sist) First 2 weeks of the developing embryo.

blepharitis (blef-ah-**RYE**-tis) Inflammation of the eyelid.

blepharoplasty (**BLEF**-ah-roh-**PLAS**-tee) Surgical repair of the eyelid.

blepharoptosis (**BLEF**-ah-**ROP**-toe-sis) Drooping of the upper eyelid.

blood-brain barrier (BBB) (BLUD BRAYN **BAIR**-ee-er) A selective mechanism that protects the brain from toxins and infections.

bolus (**BOH**-lus) Single mass of a substance.

botulism (**BOT**-you-lizm) Food poisoning caused by the neurotoxin produced by *Clostridium botulinum*.

bovine spongiform encephalopathy (**BO**-vine **SPON**-jee-form en-sef-ah-**LOP**-ah-thee) Disease of cattle that can be transmitted to humans, causing Creutzfeldt-Jakob disease. Also called *mad cow disease*.

bowel (**BOUGH**-el) Another name for *intestine*.

brace (BRACE) Appliance to support a part of the body in its correct position.

brachial (**BRAY**-kee-al) Pertaining to the arm.

brachialis (**BRAY**-kee-al-is) Muscle that lies underneath the biceps and is the strongest flexor of the forearm.

brachioradialis (**BRAY**-kee-oh-**RAY**-dee-al-is) Muscle that helps flex the forearm.

brachytherapy (brah-kee-**THAIR**-ah pee) Radiation therapy in which the source of radiation is implanted in the tissue to be treated.

bradycardia (brad-ee-**KAR**-dee-ah) Slow heart rate (below 60 beats per minute).

bradypnea (brad-ip-**NEE**-ah) Slow breathing.

brainstem (**BRAYN**-stem) Comprises the thalamus, pineal gland, pons, fourth ventricle, and medulla oblongata.

breech (BREECH) Buttocks-first presentation of the fetus at delivery.

broad-spectrum (broad-**SPECK**-trum) An antibiotic with a wide range of activity against a variety of organisms.

bronchiectasis (brong-key-**ECK**-tah-sis) Chronic dilation of the bronchi following inflammatory disease and obstruction.

bronchiole (**BRONG**-key-ole) Increasingly smaller subdivisions of bronchi.

bronchiolitis (brong-key-oh-**LYE**-tis) Inflammation of the small bronchioles.

bronchitis (bron-**KI**-tis) Inflammation of the bronchi.

bronchoconstriction (**BRONG**-koh-kon-**STRIK**-shun) Reduction in the diameter of a bronchus.

bronchodilator (**BRONG**-koh-die-**LAY**-tor) Agent that increases the diameter of a bronchus.

bronchogenic (**BRONG**-koh-**JEN**-ik) Arising from a bronchus.

bronchopneumonia (**BRONG**-koh-new-**MOH**-nee-ah) Acute inflammation of the walls of smaller bronchioles with spread to lung parenchyma.

bronchoscope (**BRONG**-koh-skope) Endoscope used for bronchoscopy.

bronchoscopy (brong-**KOS**-koh-pee) Examination of the interior of the tracheobronchial tree with an endoscope.

bronchus (**BRONG**-kuss) One of two subdivisions of the trachea. Plural *bronchi*.

bulbourethral (**BUL**-boh-you-**REE**-thral) Pertaining to the bulbous penis and urethra.

bulimia (buh-**LEEM**-ee-ah) Episodic bouts of excessive eating with compensatory throwing up.

bulla (**BULL**-ah) Bubble-like dilated structure. Plural *bullae*.

bundle of His (**BUN**-del of HISS) Pathway for electrical signals to be transmitted to the ventricles.

bunion (**BUN**-yun) A swelling at the base of the big toe.

bursa (**BURR**-sah) A closed sac containing synovial fluid. Plural *bursae*.

bursitis (burr-**SIGH**-tis) Inflammation of a bursa.

C

cadaver (kah-**DAV**-er) A dead body or corpse.

calcaneal (kal-**KAY**-knee-al) Pertaining to the calcaneus.

calcaneus (kal-**KAY**-knee-us) Bone of the tarsus that forms the heel.

calcitonin (kal-sih-**TONE**-in) Thyroid hormone that moves calcium from blood to bones.

calculus (**KAL**-kyu-lus) Small stone. Plural *calculi*.

callus (**KAL**-us) Bony tissue that forms at a fracture site early in healing.

calyx (**KAY**-licks) Funnel-shaped structure. Plural *calyces*.

cancellous (**KAN**-seh-lus) Bone that has a spongy or lattice-like structure.

cancer (**KAN**-ser) General term for a malignant neoplasm.

Candida (**KAN**-did-ah) A yeastlike fungus.

Candida albicans (**KAN**-did-ah **AL**-bih-kanz) The most common form of *Candida*.

candidiasis (can-dih-**DIE**-ah-sis) Infection with the yeastlike fungus *Candida*. Also called *thrush*.

canker (**KANG**-ker) Nonmedical term for an aphthous ulcer. Also called *mouth ulcer*.

cannula (**KAN**-you-lah) Tube inserted into a blood vessel or cavity as a channel for fluid.

capillary (**KAP**-ih-lair-ee) Minute blood vessel between the arterial and venous systems.

capsular (**KAP**-syu-lar) Pertaining to a capsule.

capsule (**KAP**-syul) Fibrous tissue layer surrounding a joint or other structure.

carbohydrate (kar-boh-**HIGH**-drate) Group of organic food compounds that includes sugars, starch, glycogen, and cellulose.

carbuncle (**KAR**-bunk-ul) Infection of many furuncles in a small area, often on the back of the neck.

carcinogen (kar-**SIN**-oh-jen) Cancer-producing agent.

carcinogenesis (kar-**SIN**-oh-**JEN**-eh-sis) Origin and development of cancer.

carcinoma (kar-sih-**NOH**-mah) A malignant and invasive epithelial tumor.

carcinoma in situ (kar-sih-**NOH**-mah in **SIGH**-too) Carcinoma that has not invaded surrounding tissues.

cardiac (**KAR**-dee-ak) Pertaining to the heart.

cardiogenic (**KAR**-dee-oh-**JEN**-ik) Of cardiac origin.

cardiologist (**KAR**-dee-**OL**-oh-jist) A medical specialist in the diagnosis and treatment of disorders of the heart (cardiology).

cardiology (**KAR**-dee-**OL**-oh-jee) Medical specialty of diseases of the heart.

cardiomegaly (**KAR**-dee-oh-**MEG**-ah-lee) Enlargement of the heart.

cardiomyopathy (**KAR**-dee-oh-my-**OP**-ah-thee) Disease of the heart muscle, the myocardium.

cardiopulmonary resuscitation (**KAR**-dee-oh-**PUL**-moh-nary ree-sus-ih-**TAY**-shun) The attempt to restore cardiac and pulmonary function.

cardiovascular (**KAR**-dee-oh-**VAS**-kyu-lar) Pertaining to the heart and blood vessels.

cardioversion (**KAR**-dee-oh-**VER**-zhun) Restoration of a normal heart rhythm by electric shock. Also called *defibrillation*.

caries (**KARE**-eez) Bacterial destruction of teeth.

carotid (kah-**ROT**-id) Main artery of the neck.

carotid endarterectomy (kah-**ROT**-id **END**-ar-ter-**EK**-toe-me) Surgical removal of diseased lining from the carotid artery to leave a smooth lining and restore blood flow.

carpal (**KAR**-pal) Pertaining to the wrist.

carpus (**KAR**-pus) Collective term for the eight carpal bones of the wrist.

cartilage (**KAR**-tih-lage) Nonvascular, firm connective tissue found mostly in joints.

catabolism (kah-**TAB**-oh-lizm) Breakdown of complex substances into simpler ones as a part of metabolism.

cataplexy (**KAT**-ah-plek-see) Sudden loss of muscle tone with brief paralysis.

cataract (**KAT**-ah-ract) Complete or partial opacity of the lens.

catecholamine (kat-eh-**COAL**-ah-meen) Major element in the stress response; includes epinephrine and norepinephrine.

catheter (**KATH**-eh-ter) Hollow tube to allow passage of fluid into or out of a body cavity, organ, or vessel.

catheterization (**KATH**-eh-ter-ih-**ZAY**-shun) Introduction of a catheter.

catheterize (**KATH**-eh-teh-**RIZE**) To introduce a catheter.

caudal (**KAW**-dal) Pertaining to or nearer to the tailbone.

cautery (**KAW**-ter-ee) Agent or device used to burn or scar a tissue.

cavernosa (kav-er-**NOH**-sah) Resembling a cave.

cavity (**KAV**-ih-tee) Hollow space or body compartment. Plural *cavities*.

cecal (**SEE**-kal) Pertaining to the cecum.

cecum (**SEE**-kum) Blind pouch that is the first part of the large intestine.

celiac (**SEE**-lee-ack) Relating to the abdominal cavity.

celiac disease (**SEE**-lee-ak diz-**EEZ**) Disease caused by sensitivity to gluten.

cell (SELL) The smallest unit of the body capable of independent existence.

cellular (SELL-you-lar) Pertaining to a cell.

cellulitis (SELL-you-LIE-tis) Infection of subcutaneous connective tissue.

cephalic (seh-FAL-ik) Pertaining to or nearer to the head.

cerebellum (ser-eh-BELL-um) The most posterior area of the brain, located between the midbrain and the cerebral hemispheres.

cerebral (SER-ee-bral) Pertaining to the cerebral hemispheres or the brain.

cerebrospinal (SER-ee-broh-SPY-nal) Pertaining to the brain and spinal cord.

cerebrospinal fluid (CSF) (SER-ee-broh-SPY-nal FLU-id) Fluid formed in the ventricles of the brain that surrounds the brain and spinal cord.

cerebrum (SER-ee-brum) Cerebral hemispheres.

cerumen (seh-ROO-men) Waxy secretion of the ceruminous glands of the external ear.

ceruminous (seh-ROO-mih-nus) Pertaining to cerumen.

cervical (SER-vih-kal) Pertaining to the cervix or to the neck region.

cervix (SER-viks) The lower part of the uterus.

cesarean section (seh-ZAH-ree-an SEK-shun) Extraction of the fetus through an incision in the abdomen and uterine wall. Also called *C-section*.

chancre (SHAN-ker) Primary lesion of syphilis.

chemotherapy (KEY-moh-THAIR-ah-pee) Treatment using chemical agents.

chiasm (KYE-asm) X-shaped crossing of the two optic nerves at the base of the brain. Alternative term *chiasma*.

chickenpox (CHICK-en-pocks) Acute, contagious viral disease. Also called *varicella*.

chiropractic (kye-roh-PRAK-tik) Diagnosis, treatment, and prevention of mechanical disorders of the musculoskeletal system.

chiropractor (kye-roh-PRAK-tor) Practitioner of chiropractic.

chlamydia (klah-MID-ee-ah) An STD caused by an infection with *Chlamydia*, a species of bacteria.

cholangiography (KOH-lan-jee-OG-rah-fee) Use of a contrast medium to radiographically visualize the bile ducts.

cholecystectomy (KOH-leh-sis-TECK-toe-me) Surgical removal of the gallbladder.

cholecystitis (KOH-leh-sis-TIE-tis) Inflammation of the gallbladder.

choledocholithiasis (KOH-leh-DOH-koh-li-THIGH-ah-sis) Presence of a gallstone in the common bile duct.

cholelithiasis (KOH-leh-lih-THIGH-ah-sis) Condition of having bile stones (gallstones).

cholelithotomy (KOH-leh-lih-THOT-oh-me) Surgical removal of a gallstone(s).

cholesteatoma (KOH-less-tee-ah-TOE-mah) Yellow, waxy tumor arising in the middle ear.

cholesterol (koh-LESS-ter-ol) Formed in liver cells; is the most abundant steroid in tissues and circulates in the plasma attached to proteins of different densities.

chorea (kor-EE-ah) Involuntary, irregular spasms of limb and facial muscles.

choreic (kor-EE-ik) Pertaining to or suffering from chorea.

chorion (KOH-ree-on) The fetal membrane that forms the placenta.

chorionic (koh-ree-ON-ik) Pertaining to the chorion.

chorionic villus (koh-ree-ON-ik VILL-us) Vascular process of the embryonic chorion to form the placenta.

choroid (KOR-oid) Region of the retina and uvea.

chromosome (KROH-moh-sohm) Body in the nucleus that contains DNA and genes.

chronic (KRON-ik) A persistent, long-term disease.

chyle (KYLE) A milky fluid that results from the digestion and absorption of fats in the small intestine.

chyme (KYME) Semifluid, partially digested food passed from the stomach into the duodenum.

cilium (SILL-ee-um) Hairlike motile projection from the surface of a cell. Plural *cilia*.

circulation (SER-kyu-LAY-shun) Continuous movement of blood through the heart and blood vessels.

circumcision (ser-kum-SIZH-un) To remove part or all of the prepuce.

circumduct (ser-kum-DUCKT) To move an extremity in a circular motion.

circumduction (ser-kum-DUCK-shun) Movement of an extremity in a circular motion.

cirrhosis (sir-ROE-sis) Extensive fibrotic liver disease.

claudication (klaw-dih-KAY-shun) Intermittent leg pain and limping.

clavicle (KLAV-ih-kul) Curved bone that forms the anterior part of the pectoral girdle.

clavicular (klah-VICK-you-lar) Pertaining to the clavicle.

cleft lip (KLEFT LIP) Congenital defect of the upper lip.

cleft palate (KLEFT PAL-ate) Congenital defect of the palate.

clitoris (KLIT-oh-ris) Erectile organ of the vulva.

clonic (KLON-ik) State of rapid successions of muscular contractions and relaxations.

closed fracture (KLOSD FRAK-chur) A bone is broken but the skin over it is intact.

Clostridium botulinum (klos-TRID-ee-um bot-you-LIE-num) Bacterium that causes food poisoning.

clot (KLOT) The mass of fibrin and cells that is produced in a wound.

coagulant (koh-AG-you-lant) Substance that causes clotting.

coagulate (koh-AG-you-late) Form a clot.

coagulation (koh-ag-you-LAY-shun) The process of blood clotting.

coagulopathy (koh-ag-you-LOP-ah-thee) Disorder of blood clotting. Plural *coagulopathies*.

coarctation (koh-ark-TAY-shun) Constriction, stenosis, particularly of the aorta.

coccyx (KOK-sicks) Small tailbone at the lower end of the vertebral column.

cochlea (KOK-lee-ah) An intricate combination of passages; used to describe the inner ear.

cochlear (KOK-lee-ar) Pertaining to the cochlea.

cognition (kog-NIH-shun) Process of acquiring knowledge through thinking, learning, and memory.

cognitive-behavioral therapy (CBT) (KOG-nih-tiv be-HAYV-yur-al THAIR-ah-pee) Psychotherapy that emphasizes thoughts and attitudes in one's behavior.

coitus (**KOH**-it-us) Sexual intercourse.

colic (**KOL**-ik) Spasmodic, crampy pains in the abdomen.

colitis (koh-**LIE**-tis) Inflammation of the colon.

collagen (**KOLL**-ah-jen) Major protein of connective tissue, cartilage, and bone.

collateral (koh-**LAT**-er-al) Situated at the side, often to bypass an obstruction.

Colles fracture (**KOL**-ez **FRAK**-chur) Fracture of the distal radius at the wrist.

colloid (**COLL**-oyd) Liquid containing suspended particles.

colon (**KOH**-lon) The large intestine, extending from the cecum to the rectum.

colostomy (koh-**LOSS**-toe-me) Artificial opening from the colon to the outside of the body.

colostrum (koh-**LOSS**-trum) The first breast secretion at the end of pregnancy.

colpopexy (**KOL**-poh-peck-see) Surgical fixation of the vagina.

coma (**KOH**-mah) State of deep unconsciousness.

comatose (**KOH**-mah-toes) In a state of coma.

comedo (**KOM**-ee-doh) A whitehead or blackhead caused by too much sebum and too many keratin cells blocking the hair follicle. Plural *comedones*.

comminuted fracture (**KOM**-ih-nyu-ted **FRAK**-chur) A fracture in which the bone is broken into small pieces.

competent (**KOM**-peh-tent) Capable of performing a task or function.

complement (**KOM**-pleh-ment) Group of proteins in the serum that finish off the work of antibodies to destroy bacteria and other cells.

complete fracture (kom-**PLEET FRAK**-chur) A bone is fractured into two separate pieces.

compliance (kom-**PLY**-ance) Measure of the capacity of a chamber or hollow viscus (e.g., the lungs) to expand; *or* consistency and accuracy with which a patient follows a treatment regimen.

compression (kom-**PRESH**-un) Squeeze together to increase density and/or decrease a dimension of a structure.

compression fracture (kom-**PRESH**-un **FRAK**-chur) Fracture of a vertebra causing loss of height of the vertebra.

compulsion (kom-**PUL**-shun) Uncontrollable impulses to perform an act repetitively.

compulsive (kom-**PUL**-siv) Possessing uncontrollable impulses to perform an act repetitively.

conception (kon-**SEP**-shun) Fertilization of the egg by sperm to form a zygote.

concha (**KON**-kah) Shell-shaped bone on the medial wall of the nasal cavity. Plural *conchae*.

concussion (kon-**KUSH**-un) Mild brain injury.

condom (**KON**-dom) A sheath or cover for the penis or vagina to prevent conception and infection.

conductive hearing loss (kon-**DUK**-tiv) Hearing loss caused by lesions in the outer ear or middle ear.

condyle (**KON**-dile) Large, smooth, rounded expansion of the end of a bone where it forms a joint with another bone.

confusion (kon-**FEW**-zhun) Mental state in which environmental stimuli are not processed appropriately.

congenital (kon-**JEN**-ih-tal) Present at birth, either inherited or due to an event during gestation up to the moment of birth.

conization (koh-ni-**ZAY**-shun) Surgical excision of a cone-shaped piece of tissue.

conjunctiva (kon-junk-**TIE**-vah) Inner lining of the eyelids.

conjunctival (kon-junk-**TIE**-val) Pertaining to the conjunctiva.

conjunctivitis (kon-junk-tih-**VI**-tis) Inflammation of the conjunctiva.

connective tissue (koh-**NECK**-tiv **TISH**-you) The supporting tissue of the body.

consciousness (**KON**-shus-ness) The state of being aware of and responsive to the environment.

constipation (kon-stih-**PAY**-shun) Hard, infrequent bowel movements.

constrict (kon-**STRIKT**) To become or make narrow.

constriction (kon-**STRIK**-shun) A narrowed portion of a structure.

contagious (kon-**TAY**-jus) Infection can be transmitted from person to person or from a person to a surface to a person.

contaminate (kon-**TAM**-in-ate) To cause the presence of an infectious agent to be on any surface or in any substance.

contamination (**KON**-tam-ih-**NAY**-shun) Presence of an infectious agent on a surface or in substances.

contraception (kon-trah-**SEP**-shun) Prevention of pregnancy.

contraceptive (kon-trah-**SEP**-tiv) An agent that prevents conception.

contract (kon-**TRAKT**) Draw together or shorten.

contracture (kon-**TRAK**-chur) Muscle shortening due to spasm or fibrosis.

contrecoup (**KON**-treh-koo) Injury to the brain at a point directly opposite the point of original contact.

contusion (kon-**TOO**-zhun) Hemorrhage into a tissue (bruising), including the brain.

convulsion (kon-**VUL**-shun) Alternative name for seizure.

cor pulmonale (**KOR** pul-moh-**NAH**-lee) Right-sided heart failure arising from chronic lung disease.

cornea (**KOR**-nee-ah) The central, transparent part of the outer coat of the eye covering the iris and pupil.

corneal (**KOR**-nee-al) Pertaining to the cornea.

coronal (**KOR**-oh-nal) Pertaining to the vertical plane dividing the body into anterior and posterior portions.

coronal plane (**KOR**-oh-nal **PLAIN**) Vertical plane dividing the body into anterior and posterior portions.

coronary circulation (**KOR**-oh-nair-ee **SER**-kyu-**LAY**-shun) Blood vessels supplying the heart.

corpus (**KOR**-pus) Major part of a structure. Plural *corpora*.

corpus albicans (**KOR**-pus **AL**-bih-kanz) An atrophied corpus luteum.

corpus callosum (**KOR**-pus kah-**LOW**-sum) Bridge of nerve fibers connecting the two cerebral hemispheres.

corpus luteum (**KOR**-pus **LOO**-teh-um) Yellow structure formed at the site of a ruptured ovarian follicle.

corpuscle (**KOR**-pus-ul) A blood cell.

cortex (**KOR**-teks) Outer portion of an organ, such as bone; gray covering of cerebral hemispheres. Plural *cortices*.

cortical (**KOR**-tih-cal) Pertaining to a cortex.

corticosteroid (**KOR**-tih-koh-**STAIR**-oyd) A hormone produced by the adrenal cortex.

corticotropin (**KOR**-tih-koh-TROH-pin) Pituitary hormone that stimulates the cortex of the adrenal gland to secrete corticosteroids.

cortisol (**KOR**-tih-sol) One of the glucocorticoids produced by the adrenal cortex; has anti-inflammatory effects. Also called *hydrocortisone*.

coryza (koh-**RYE**-zah) Viral inflammation of the mucous membrane of the nose. Also called *acute rhinitis*.

coup (KOO) Injury to the brain occurring directly under the skull at the point of contact.

coxa (**COCK**-sah) Hipbone. Plural *coxae*.

cranial (**KRAY**-nee-al) Pertaining to the cranium.

craniofacial (**KRAY**-nee-oh-**FAY**-shal) Pertaining to both the face and the cranium.

cranium (**KRAY**-nee-um) The skull.

cretin (**KREH**-tin) A person with severe congenital hypothyroidism.

cretinism (**KREH**-tin-izm) Condition of severe congenital hypothyroidism.

Creutzfeldt-Jakob disease (**KROITS**-felt **YAK**-op diz-**EEZ**) Progressive incurable neurologic disease caused by infectious prions.

cricoid (**CRY**-koyd) Ring-shaped cartilage in the larynx.

crista ampullaris (**KRIS**-tah am-**PULL**-air-is) Mound of hair cells and gelatinous material in the ampulla of a semicircular canal.

Crohn disease (**KRONE** diz-**EEZ**) Narrowing and thickening of terminal small bowel. Also called *regional enteritis*.

croup (KROOP) Infection of the upper airways in children, characterized by a barking cough. Also called *laryngotracheobronchitis*.

cruciate (**KRU**-she-ate) Shaped like a cross.

cryosurgery (cry-oh-**SUR**-jer-ee) Use of liquid nitrogen or argon gas in a probe to freeze and kill abnormal tissue.

cryptorchism (krip-**TOR**-kizm) Failure of one or both testes to descend into the scrotum.

curettage (kyu-reh-**TAHJ**) Scraping the interior of a cavity.

curette (kyu-**RET**) Scoop-shaped instrument for scraping the interior of a cavity or removing new growths.

Cushing syndrome (**KUSH**-ing **SIN**-drohm) Hypersecretion of cortisol (hydrocortisone) by the adrenal cortex.

cutaneous (kyu-**TAY**-nee-us) Pertaining to the skin.

cuticle (**KEW**-tih-cul) Nonliving epidermis at the base of the fingernails and toenails.

cyanosis (sigh-ah-**NO**-sis) Blue discoloration of the skin, lips, and nail beds due to low levels of oxygen in the blood.

cyanotic (sigh-ah-**NOT**-ik) Pertaining to or marked by cyanosis.

cyst (SIST) An abnormal, fluid-containing sac.

cystic (**SIS**-tik) Relating to a cyst.

cystic fibrosis (CF) (**SIS**-tik fie-**BROH**-sis) Genetic disease in which excessive viscid mucus obstructs passages, including bronchi.

cystitis (sis-**TIE**-tis) Inflammation of the urinary bladder.

cystocele (**SIS**-toh-seal) Hernia of the bladder into the vagina.

cystoscope (**SIS**-toh-skope) An endoscope inserted to view the inside of the bladder.

cystoscopy (sis-**TOS**-koh-pee) Using a cystoscope to examine the inside of the urinary bladder.

cystourethrogram (sis-toh-you-**REETH**-roe-gram) X-ray image during voiding to show the structure and function of the bladder and urethra.

cytologist (**SIGH**-tol-oh-jist) Specialist in the structure, chemistry, and pathology of the cell.

cytology (**SIGH**-tol-oh-jee) Study of the cell.

cytoplasm (**SIGH**-toh-plazm) Clear, gelatinous substance that forms the substance of a cell except for the nucleus.

cytotoxic (sigh-toh-**TOX**-ik) Destructive to cells.

D

dandruff (**DAN**-druff) Scales in hair from shedding of the epidermis.

death (DETH) Total and permanent cessation of all vital functions.

debridement (day-**BREED**-mon) The removal of injured or necrotic tissue.

decongestant (dee-con-**JESS**-tant) Agent that reduces the swelling and fluid in the nose and sinuses.

decubitus ulcer (de-**KYU**-bit-us **UL**-ser) Sore caused by lying down for long periods of time.

defecation (def-eh-**KAY**-shun) Evacuation of feces from the rectum and anus.

defect (**DEE**-fect) An absence, malformation, or imperfection.

defective (dee-**FEK**-tiv) Imperfect.

defibrillation (de-fib-rih-**LAY**-shun) Restoration of uncontrolled twitching of cardiac muscle fibers to normal rhythm.

defibrillator (de-fib-rih-**LAY**-tor) Instrument for defibrillation.

deformity (de-**FOR**-mih-tee) A permanent structural deviation from the normal.

degenerative (dee-**JEN**-er-a-tiv) Relating to the deterioration of a structure.

deglutition (dee-glue-**TISH**-un) The act of swallowing.

dehydration (dee-high-**DRAY**-shun) Process of losing body water.

delirium (de-**LIR**-ee-um) Acute altered state of consciousness with agitation and disorientation; condition is reversible.

deltoid (**DEL**-toyd) Large, fan-shaped muscle connecting the scapula and clavicle to the humerus.

delusion (dee-**LOO**-zhun) Fixed, unyielding false belief held despite strong evidence to the contrary.

dementia (da-**MEN**-sha) Chronic, progressive, irreversible loss of intellectual and mental functions.

demyelination (dee-**MY**-eh-lin-**A**-shun) Process of losing the myelin sheath of a nerve fiber.

dendrite (**DEN**-dright) Branched extension of the nerve cell body that receives nervous stimuli.

dental (**DEN**-tal) Pertaining to the teeth.

dentine (**DEN**-tin) Dense, ivory-like substance located under the enamel in a tooth. (Also spelled *dentin*.)

dentist (**DEN**-tist) Legally qualified specialist in dentistry.

dentistry (**DEN**-tis-tree) Evaluation, diagnosis, prevention, and treatment of conditions of the oral cavity and associated structures.

deoxyribonucleic acid (DNA) (dee-**OCK**-see-rye-boh-nyu-**KLEE**-ik **ASS**-id) Source of hereditary characteristics found in chromosomes.

dependence (dee-**PEN**-dense) The state of needing or relying on someone or something else.

dependent (dee-**PEN**-dent) Having to rely on someone else.

depressant (de-**PRESS**-ant) Substance that diminishes activity, sensation, or tone.

depression (de-**PRESS**-shun) Mental disorder with feelings of deep sadness and despair.

dermabrasion (der-mah-**BRAY**-zhun) Removal of upper layers of skin by rotary brush.

dermal (**DER**-mal) Pertaining to the skin.

dermascope (**DER**-mah-skope) Instrument that shines a light on the skin and magnifies a lesion.

dermatitis (der-mah-**TYE**-tis) Inflammation of the skin.

dermatologic (der-mah-toh-**LOJ**-ik) Pertaining to the skin and dermatology.

dermatologist (der-mah-**TOL**-oh-jist) Medical specialist in diseases of the skin.

dermatology (der-mah-**TOL**-oh-jee) Medical specialty concerned with disorders of the skin.

dermatomyositis (**DER**-mah-toe-my-oh-**SIGH**-tis) Inflammation of the skin and muscles.

dermis (**DER**-miss) Connective tissue layer of the skin beneath the epidermis.

detoxification (dee-**TOKS**-ih-fih-**KAY**-shun) Remove poison from a tissue or substance.

diabetes insipidus (dye-ah-**BEE**-teez in-**SIP**-ih-dus) Excretion of large amounts of dilute urine as a result of inadequate ADH production.

diabetes mellitus (dye-ah-**BEE**-teez **MEL**-ih-tus) Metabolic syndrome caused by absolute or relative insulin deficiency and/or insulin ineffectiveness.

diabetic (dye-ah-**BET**-ik) Pertaining to or suffering from diabetes.

diagnose (die-ag-**NOSE**) To make a diagnosis.

diagnosis (die-ag-**NO**-sis) The determination of the cause of a disease. Plural *diagnoses.*

diagnostic (die-ag-**NOS**-tik) Pertaining to or establishing a diagnosis.

dialysis (die-**AL**-ih-sis) An artificial method of filtration to remove excess waste materials and water from the body.

diaphoresis (**DIE**-ah-foh-**REE**-sis) Sweat or perspiration.

diaphoretic (**DIE**-ah-foh-**RET**-ic) Pertaining to sweat or perspiration.

diaphragm (**DIE**-ah-fram) A ring and dome-shaped material inserted into the vagina to prevent pregnancy; *or* the muscular sheet separating the abdominal and thoracic cavities.

diaphragmatic (**DIE**-ah-frag-**MAT**-ik) Pertaining to the diaphragm.

diaphysis (die-**AF**-ih-sis) The shaft of a long bone.

diarrhea (die-ah-**REE**-ah) Abnormally frequent and loose stools.

diastasis (die-**ASS**-tah-sis) Separation of normally joined parts.

diastole (die-**AS**-toe-lee) Dilation of heart cavities, during which they fill with blood.

diastolic (die-as-**TOL**-ik) Pertaining to diastole.

differential (dif-er-**EN**-shal) A differential white blood cell count lists percentages of the different leukocytes in a blood sample.

diffuse (di-**FUSE**) To disseminate or spread out.

diffusion (di-**FYU**-zhun) The means by which small particles move between tissues.

digestion (die-**JESS**-shun) Breakdown of food into elements suitable for cell metabolism.

digestive (die-**JEST**-iv) Pertaining to digestion.

digital (**DIJ**-ih-tal) Pertaining to a finger or toe.

dilate (**DIE**-late) To perform or undergo dilation.

dilation (die-**LAY**-shun) Stretching or enlarging an opening or a structure.

diphtheria (dif-**THEER**-ee-ah) Disease with a thick, membranous (leathery) coating of the pharynx.

diplegia (die-**PLEE**-jee-ah) Paralysis of all four limbs, with the two legs affected most severely.

dipstick (**DIP**-stick) Strip of plastic or paper bearing squares of reagents that change color in the presence of abnormal chemicals in the urine.

disability (dis-ah-**BILL**-ih-tee) Diminished capacity to perform certain activities or functions.

discipline (**DIS**-ih-plin) Training for proper conduct or action.

disease (diz-**EEZ**) A disorder of body functions, systems, or organs.

disinfectant (dis-in-**FEK**-tant) Agent that disinfects.

disinfection (dis-in-**FEK**-shun) Process of destruction of microorganisms by chemical agents.

dislocation (dis-low-**KAY**-shun) Completely out of joint.

displaced fracture (dis-**PLAYSD FRAK**-chur) A fracture in which the fragments are separated and are not in alignment.

disseminate (dih-**SEM**-in-ate) Widely scattered throughout the body or an organ.

dissociative identity disorder (di-**SO**-see-ah-tiv eye-**DEN**-tih-tee dis-**OR**-der) Part of an individual's personality is separated from the rest, leading to multiple personalities.

distal (**DISS**-tal) Situated away from the center of the body.

diuresis (die-you-**REE**-sis) Excretion of large volumes of urine.

diuretic (die-you-**RET**-ik) Agent that increases urine output.

diverticulitis (**DIE**-ver-tick-you-**LIE**-tis) Inflammation of the diverticula.

diverticulosis (**DIE**-ver-tick-you-**LOW**-sis) Presence of a number of small pouches in the wall of the large intestine.

diverticulum (die-ver-**TICK**-you-lum) A pouchlike opening or sac from a tubular structure (e.g., gut). Plural *diverticula.*

dopamine (**DOH**-pah-meen) Neurotransmitter in specific small areas of the brain.

Doppler (**DOP**-ler) Diagnostic instrument that sends an ultrasonic beam into the body.

Doppler ultrasonography (**DOP**-ler **UL**-trah-soh-**NOG**-rah-fee) Detects direction, velocity, and turbulence of blood flow; used in workup of stroke patients.

dormant (**DOOR**-mant) Inactive.

dorsal (**DOOR**-sal) Pertaining to the back or situated behind.

dorsum (**DOOR**-sum) Upper, posterior, or back surface.

Down syndrome (**DOWN SIN**-drome) A syndrome with variable abnormalities associated with three copies of chromosome 21.

Duchenne muscular dystrophy (**DOO**-shen **MUSS**-kyu-lar **DISS**-troh-fee) Symmetrical weakness and wasting of pelvic, shoulder, and proximal limb muscles.

ductus arteriosus (DUK-tus ar-TEER-ih-OH-sus) Fetal vessel that connects the descending aorta with the left pulmonary artery.

ductus deferens (DUK-tus DEH-fuh-renz) Tube that receives sperm from the epididymis. Also known as *vas deferens*.

duodenal (du-oh-DEE-nal) Pertaining to the duodenum.

duodenum (du-oh-DEE-num) The first part of the small intestine; approximately 12 finger-breadths (9 to 10 inches) in length.

dura mater (DYU-rah MAY-ter) Hard, fibrous outer layer of the meninges.

dysentery (DIS-en-tare-ee) Disease with diarrhea, bowel spasms, fever, and dehydration.

dysfunctional (dis-FUNK-shun-al) Difficulty in functioning.

dyslexia (dis-LEK-see-ah) Impaired reading and writing ability below the person's level of intelligence.

dyslexic (dis-LEK-sik) Pertaining to or suffering from dyslexia.

dysmenorrhea (dis-men-oh-REE-ah) Painful and difficult menstruation.

dyspareunia (dis-pah-RUE-nee-ah) Pain during sexual intercourse.

dyspepsia (dis-PEP-see-ah) "Upset stomach," epigastric pain, nausea, and gas.

dysphagia (dis-FAY-jee-ah) Difficulty in swallowing.

dysphoria (dis-FOR-ee-ah) Psychiatric mood disorder.

dysplasia (dis-PLAY-zee-ah) Abnormal tissue formation.

dysplastic (dis-PLAS-tik) Pertaining to or showing abnormal tissue formation.

dyspnea (disp-NEE-ah) Difficulty breathing.

dyspneic (disp-NEE-ik) Pertaining to or suffering from difficulty in breathing.

dysrhythmia (dis-RITH-me-ah) An abnormal heart rhythm.

dysuria (dis-YOU-ree-ah) Difficulty or pain with urination.

E

echocardiography (EK-oh-kar-dee-OG-rah-fee) Ultrasound recording of heart function.

echoencephalography (EK-oh-en-sef-ah-LOG-rah-fee) Use of ultrasound in the diagnosis of intracranial lesions.

eclampsia (ek-LAMP-see-uh) Convulsions in a patient with preeclampsia.

ectopic (ek-TOP-ik) Out of place, not in a normal position.

eczema (EK-zeh-mah) Inflammatory skin disease, often with a serous discharge.

eczematous (ek-ZEM-ah-tus) Pertaining to or marked by eczema.

edema (ee-DEE-mah) Excessive accumulation of fluid in cells and tissues.

edematous (ee-DEM-ah-tus) Pertaining to or marked by edema.

effacement (ee-FACE-ment) Thinning of the cervix in relation to labor.

efferent (EFF-eh-rent) Moving away from a center; for example, conducting nerve impulses away from the brain or spinal cord.

effusion (eh-FYU-zhun) Collection of fluid that has escaped from blood vessels into a cavity or tissues.

ejaculate (ee-JACK-you-late) To expel suddenly; *or* the semen expelled in ejaculation.

ejaculation (ee-JACK-you-LAY-shun) Process of expelling semen suddenly.

ejaculatory (ee-JACK-you-LAY-tor-ee) Pertaining to ejaculation.

elective (e-LEK-tiv) Surgery or a procedure that is not urgent or vital.

electrocardiogram (ECG or EKG) (ee-LEK-troh-KAR-dee-oh-gram) Record of the electrical signals of the heart.

electrocardiograph (ee-LEK-troh-KAR-dee-oh-graf) Machine that makes the electrocardiogram.

electrocardiography (ee-LEK-troh-kar-dee-OG-rah-fee) Interpretation of electrocardiograms.

electroconvulsive therapy (ECT) (ee-LEK-troh-kon-VUL-siv THAIR-ah-pee) Passage of electric current through the brain to produce convulsions and treat persistent depression.

electrode (ee-LEK-trode) A device for conducting electricity.

electroencephalogram (EEG) (ee-LEK-troh-en-SEF-ah-low-gram) Record of the electrical activity of the brain.

electroencephalograph (ee-LEK-troh-en-SEF-ah-low-graf) Device used to record the electrical activity of the brain.

electroencephalography (ee-LEK-troh-en-SEF-ah-LOG-rah-fee) The process of recording the electrical activity of the brain.

electrolyte (ee-LEK-troh-lite) Substance that, when dissolved in a suitable medium, forms electrically charged particles.

electromyogram (ee-LEK-troh-MY-oh-gram) Recording of electric currents associated with muscle action.

electromyography (ee-LEK-troh-my-OG-rah-fee) Recording of electrical activity in muscle.

electroneurodiagnostic (ee-LEK-troh-NYUR-oh-die-ag-NOS-tik) Pertaining to the use of electricity in the diagnosis of a neurologic disorder.

elimination (e-lim-ih-NAY-shun) Removal of waste material from the digestive tract.

emaciated (ee-MAY-see-AY-ted) Pertaining to or suffering from emaciation.

emaciation (ee-may-see-AY-shun) Abnormal thinness.

embolus (EM-boh-lus) Detached piece of thrombus, a mass of bacteria, quantity of air, or foreign body that blocks a blood vessel.

embryo (EM-bree-oh) Developing organism from conception until the end of the second month.

embryology (em-bree-OL-oh-jee) Science of the origin and early development of an organism.

embryonic (em-bree-ON-ic) Pertaining to the embryo.

emesis (EM-eh-sis) Vomit.

emmetropia (emm-eh-TROH-pee-ah) Normal refractive condition of the eye.

empathy (EM-pah-thee) Ability to place yourself into the feelings, emotions, and reactions of another person.

emphysema (em-fih-SEE-mah) Dilation of respiratory bronchioles and alveoli.

empyema (EM-pie-EE-mah) Pus in a body cavity, particularly in the pleural cavity.

emulsify (ee-MUL-sih-fye) Break up into very small droplets to suspend in a solution (emulsion).

emulsion (ee-MUL-shun) The system that contains small droplets suspended in a liquid.

enamel (ee-**NAM**-el) Hard substance covering a tooth.

encephalitis (en-**SEF**-ah-**LIE**-tis) Inflammation of brain cells and tissues.

encephalocele (en-**SEF**-ah-loh-seal) Congenital defect of the cranium with herniation of brain tissue.

encephalomyelitis (en-**SEF**-ah-loh-**MY**-eh-**LIE**-tis) Inflammation of the brain and spinal cord.

encephalopathy (en-sef-ah-**LOP**-ah-thee) Any disorder of the brain.

encopresis (en-koh-**PREE**-sis) Repeated soiling with feces.

endarterectomy (**END**-ar-ter-**EK**-toe-me) Surgical removal of plaque from an artery.

endemic (en-**DEM**-ik) Pertaining to a disease always present in a community.

endocardial (en-doh-**KAR**-dee-al) Pertaining to the endocardium.

endocarditis (**EN**-doh-kar-**DIE**-tis) Inflammation of the lining of the heart.

endocardium (en-doh-**KAR**-dee-um) The inside lining of the heart.

endocrine (**EN**-doh-krin) A gland that produces an internal or hormonal substance.

endocrinologist (**EN**-doh-krih-**NOL**-oh-jist) A medical specialist in endocrinology.

endocrinology (**EN**-doh-krih-**NOL**-oh-jee) Medical specialty concerned with the production and effects of hormones.

endometrial (en-doh-**ME**-tree-al) Pertaining to the inner lining of the uterus.

endometriosis (**EN**-doh-me-tree-**OH**-sis) Endometrial tissue outside the uterus.

endometrium (en-doh-**ME**-tree-um) Inner lining of the uterus.

endorphin (en-**DOR**-fin) A natural substance in the brain that simulates opium.

endoscope (**EN**-doh-skope) Instrument to examine the inside of a tubular or hollow organ.

endoscopy (en-**DOS**-koh-pee) The use of an endoscope.

endotracheal (en-doh-**TRAY**-kee-al) Pertaining to being inside the trachea.

enema (**EN**-eh-mah) An injection of fluid into the rectum.

enteric (en-**TEHR**-ik) Pertaining to the intestine.

enteroscope (**EN**-ter-oh-**SKOPE**) Slender, tubular instrument with light source and camera to visualize the digestive tract.

enteroscopy (en-ter-**OSS**-koh-pee) The examination of the lining of the digestive tract.

enuresis (en-you-**REE**-sis) Bedwetting; urinary incontinence.

enzyme (**EN**-zime) Protein that induces changes in other substances.

eosinophil (ee-oh-**SIN**-oh-fill) An eosinophil's granules attract a rosy-red color on staining.

epicardial (ep-ih-**KAR**-dee-al) Pertaining to the epicardium.

epicardium (ep-ih-**KAR**-dee-um) The outer layer of the heart wall.

epicondyle (ep-ih-**KON**-dile) Projection above the condyle for attachment of a ligament or tendon.

epidemic (ep-ih-**DEM**-ik) Pertaining to an outbreak in a community of a disease or a health-related behavior.

epidermal (ep-ih-**DER**-mal) Pertaining to the epidermis.

epidermis (ep-ih-**DER**-miss) Top layer of the skin.

epididymis (ep-ih-**DID**-ih-miss) Coiled tube attached to the testis.

epididymitis (ep-ih-did-ih-**MY**-tis) Inflammation of the epididymis.

epididymoorchitis (ep-ih-**DID**-ih-moh-or-**KIE**-tis) Inflammation of the epididymis and testicle. Also called *orchitis*.

epidural (ep-ih-**DYU**-ral) Above the dura.

epidural space (ep-ih-**DYU**-ral SPASE) Space between the dura mater and the wall of the vertebral canal.

epigastric (ep-ih-**GAS**-trik) Pertaining to the abdominal region above the stomach.

epigastrium (ep-ih-**GAS**-tri-um) The abdominal region above the stomach.

epiglottis (ep-ih-**GLOT**-is) Leaf-shaped plate of cartilage that shuts off the larynx during swallowing.

epiglottitis (ep-ih-glot-**EYE**-tis) Inflammation of the epiglottis.

epilepsy (**EP**-ih-**LEP**-see) Chronic brain disorder due to paroxysmal excessive neuronal discharges.

epileptic (**EP**-ih-**LEP**-tik) Pertaining to or suffering from epilepsy.

epinephrine (ep-ih-**NEF**-rin) Main catecholamine produced by the adrenal medulla. Also called *adrenaline*.

epiphysial (ep-ih-**FIZ**-ee-al) Pertaining to an epiphysis.

epiphysial plate (eh-ih-**FIZ**-ee-al PLATE) Layer of cartilage between the epiphysis and the metaphysis where bone growth occurs.

epiphysis (ep-ih-**FI**-sis) Expanded area at the proximal and distal ends of a long bone to provide increased surface area for attachment of ligaments and tendons.

episiotomy (eh-piz-ee-**OT**-oh-me) Surgical incision of the vulva.

epispadias (ep-ih-**SPAY**-dee-as) Condition in which the urethral opening is on the dorsum of the penis.

epistaxis (ep-ih-**STAK**-sis) Nosebleed.

epithelium (ep-ih-**THEE**-lee-um) Tissue that covers surfaces or lines cavities.

equilibrium (ee-kwi-**LIB**-ree-um) Being evenly balanced.

erectile (ee-**REK**-tile) Capable of erection or being distended with blood.

erection (ee-**REK**-shun) Distended and rigid state of an organ.

erosion (ee-**ROE**-zhun) Form a shallow ulcer in the lining of a structure.

erythroblast (eh-**RITH**-ro-blast) Precursor to a red blood cell.

erythroblastosis (eh-**RITH**-roh-blas-**TOH**-sis) Condition of many immature red cells in blood.

erythrocyte (eh-**RITH**-roh-site) A red blood cell.

erythropoiesis (eh-**RITH**-roh-poy-**EE**-sis) The formation of red blood cells.

erythropoietin (eh-**RITH**-roh-**POY**-ee-tin) Protein secreted by the kidney that stimulates red blood cell production.

eschar (**ESS**-kar) The burnt, dead tissue lying on top of third-degree burns.

Escherichia coli (esh-eh-**RIK**-ee-ah **KOH**-lie) Organism in the intestine; releases an exotoxin that can cause diarrhea.

esophageal (ee-**SOF**-ah-**JEE**-al) Pertaining to the esophagus.

esophagitis (ee-**SOF**-ah-**JI**-tis) Inflammation of the lining of the esophagus.

esophagus (ee-**SOF**-ah-gus) Tube linking the pharynx to the stomach.

esotropia (es-oh-**TROH**-pee-ah) Turning the eye inward toward the nose.

estrogen (**ES**-troh-jen) Generic term for hormones that stimulate female secondary sex characteristics.

ethmoid (**ETH**-moyd) Bone that forms the back of the nose and encloses numerous air cells.

etiology (ee-tee-**OL**-oh-jee) The study of the causes of a disease.

eupnea (yoop-**NEE**-ah) Normal breathing.

eustachian tube (you-**STAY**-shun TYUB) Tube that connects the middle ear to the nasopharynx. Also called *auditory tube.*

euthyroid (you-**THIGH**-royd) Normal thyroid function.

eversion (ee-**VER**-zhun) Turning outward.

evert (ee-**VERT**) To turn outward.

evolve (ee-**VOLV**) To develop gradually.

Ewing sarcoma (**YOU**-ing sar-**KOH**-mah) A malignant neoplasm of bone.

exacerbation (ek-zas-er-**BAY**-shun) Period when there is an increase in the severity of a disease.

exanthem (ek-**ZAN**-them) Skin eruption or rash occurring as the outward sign of a viral or bacterial disease.

excision (ek-**SIZH**-un) Surgical removal of part or all of a structure.

excoriate (eks-**KOR**-ee-ate) To scratch.

excoriation (eks-**KOR**-ee-**AY**-shun) Scratch mark.

excrete (eks-**KREET**) To pass waste products of metabolism out of the body.

excretion (eks-**KREE**-shun) Removal of waste products of metabolism out of the body.

exhale (**EKS**-hail) Breathe out.

exocrine (**EK**-soh-krin) A gland that secretes substances outwardly through excretory ducts.

exophthalmos (ek-sof-**THAL**-mos) Protrusion of the eyeball.

exotropia (ek-soh-**TROH**-pee-ah) Turning the eye outward away from the nose.

expectorate (ek-**SPEK**-toh-rate) Cough up and spit out mucus from the respiratory tract.

expiration (**EKS**-pih-**RAY**-shun) Breathe out.

extension (eks-**TEN**-shun) Straighten a joint to increase its angle.

extracorporeal (**EKS**-tra-kor-**POH**-ree-al) Outside the body.

extravasate (eks-**TRAV**-ah-sate) To ooze out from a vessel into the tissues.

extrinsic (eks-**TRIN**-sik) Any muscle located entirely on the outside of the structure under consideration; for example, the eye.

F

facies (**FASH**-eez) Facial features and expressions.

fallopian tubes (fah-**LOW**-pee-an) Uterine tubes connected to the fundus of the uterus.

Fallot (fah-**LOW**) First described the tetralogy of congenital heart defects.

fascia (**FASH**-ee-ah) Sheet of fibrous connective tissue.

fasciectomy (fash-ee-**EK**-toe-me) Surgical removal of fascia.

fasciitis (fash-ee-**EYE**-tis) Inflammation of fascia.

fasciotomy (fash-ee-**OT**-oh-me) An incision through a band of fascia, usually to relieve pressure on underlying structures.

febrile (**FEB**-ril or **FEB**-rile) Pertaining to or suffering from fever.

fecal (**FEE**-kal) Pertaining to feces.

feces (**FEE**-seez) Undigested, waste material discharged from the bowel.

femoral (**FEM**-oh-ral) Pertaining to the femur.

femur (**FEE**-mur) The thigh bone.

fertilization (**FER**-til-eye-**ZAY**-shun) Union of a male sperm and a female egg.

fertilize (**FER**-til-ize) Penetration of the egg by sperm.

fetal (**FEE**-tal) Pertaining to the fetus.

fetalis (fee-**TAH**-lis) Erythroblastosis fetalis is a hemolytic disease of the newborn.

fetus (**FEE**-tus) Human organism from the end of the eighth week after conception to birth.

fever (**FEE**-ver) Increased body temperature that is a physiologic response to disease.

fibrillation (fi-brih-**LAY**-shun) Uncontrolled quivering or twitching of the heart muscle.

fibrin (**FIE**-brin) Stringy protein fiber that is a component of a blood clot.

fibrinogen (fie-**BRIN**-oh-jen) Precursor of fibrin in blood-clotting process.

fibroadenoma (**FIE**-broh-ad-en-**OH**-muh) Benign tumor containing much fibrous tissue.

fibroblast (**FIE**-broh-blast) Cell that forms collagen fibers.

fibrocystic disease (fie-broh-**SIS**-tik diz-**EEZ**) Benign breast disease with multiple tiny lumps and cysts.

fibroid (**FIE**-broyd) Uterine tumor resembling fibrous tissue.

fibromyalgia (fie-broh-my-**AL**-jee-ah) Pain in the muscle fibers.

fibromyoma (**FIE**-broh-my-**OH**-mah) Benign neoplasm derived from smooth muscle and containing fibrous tissue.

fibrosis (fie-**BROH**-sis) Repair of dead tissue cells by formation of fibrous tissue.

fibrotic (fie-**BROT**-ik) Pertaining to or affected by fibrosis.

fibula (**FIB**-you-lah) The smaller of the two bones of the lower leg.

fibular (**FIB**-you-lar) Pertaining to the fibula.

filter (**FIL**-ter) Porous substance used to separate liquids or gases from particulate matter; *or* to subject a substance to the action of a filter.

filtrate (**FIL**-trate) That which has passed through a filter.

filtration (fil-**TRAY**-shun) Process of passing liquid through a filter.

fimbria (**FIM**-bree-ah) A fringelike structure on the surface of a cell or microorganism. Plural *fimbriae.*

fissure (**FISH**-ur) Deep furrow or cleft. Plural *fissures.*

fistula (**FIS**-tyu-lah) Abnormal passage. Plural *fistulae* or *fistulas.*

flank (FLANK) Side of the body between pelvis and ribs.

flatulence (**FLAT**-you-lence) Excessive amount of gas in the stomach and intestines.

flatus (**FLAY**-tus) Gas or air expelled through the anus.

flex (FLEKS) To bend a joint so that the two parts come together.

flexion (**FLEK**-shun) Bend a joint to decrease its angle.

flexor (**FLEK**-sor) Muscle or tendon that flexes a joint.

flexure (**FLEK**-shur) A bend in a structure.

flora (**FLO**-rah) Microrganisms covering the exterior and interior surfaces of a healthy animal.

fluorescein (flor-**ESS**-ee-in) Dye that produces a vivid green color under a blue light to diagnose corneal abrasions and foreign bodies.

follicle (**FOLL**-ih-kull) Spherical mass of cells containing a cavity; *or* a small cul-de-sac, such as a hair follicle.

follicular (fo-**LIK**-you-lar) Pertaining to a follicle.

foramen (fo-**RAY**-men) An opening through a structure. Plural *foramina.*

forceps extraction (**FOR**-seps ek-**STRAK**-shun) Assisted delivery of the baby by an instrument that grasps the head of the baby.

foreskin (**FOR**-skin) Skin that covers the glans penis.

fornix (**FOR**-niks) Arch-shaped, blind-ended part of the vagina behind and around the cervix. Plural *fornices.*

fovea centralis (**FOH**-vee-ah sen-**TRAH**-lis) Small pit in the center of the macula that has the highest visual acuity.

frenulum (**FREN**-you-lum) Fold of mucous membrane between the glans and the prepuce.

frontal (**FRON**-tal) Vertical plane dividing the body into anterior and posterior portions.

function (**FUNK**-shun) The ability of an organ or tissue to perform its special work.

fundoscopic (fun-doh-**SKOP**-ik) Pertaining to fundoscopy.

fundoscopy (fun-**DOS**-koh-pee) Examination of the fundus (retina) of the eye.

fundus (**FUN**-dus) Part farthest from the opening of a hollow organ.

fungicide (**FUN**-ji-side) Agent to destroy fungi.

fungus (**FUN**-gus) General term used to describe yeasts and molds. Plural *fungi.*

G

galactorrhea (gah-**LAK**-toe-**REE**-ah) Abnormal flow of milk from the breasts.

gallbladder (**GAWL**-blad-er) Receptacle on the inferior surface of the liver for storing bile.

gallstone (**GAWL**-stone) Hard mass of cholesterol, calcium, and bilirubin that can be formed in the gallbladder and bile duct.

ganglion (**GANG**-lee-on) Collection of nerve cells outside the brain and spinal cord; *or* a fluid-filled cyst. Plural *ganglia.*

gastric (**GAS**-trik) Pertaining to the stomach.

gastrin (**GAS**-trin) Hormone secreted in the stomach that stimulates secretion of HCl and increases gastric motility.

gastritis (gas-**TRY**-tis) Inflammation of the lining of the stomach.

gastrocnemius (gas-trok-**NEE**-me-us) Major muscle in back of the lower leg (the calf).

gastroenteritis (**GAS**-troh-en-ter-**I**-tis) Inflammation of the stomach and intestines.

gastroenterologist (**GAS**-troh-en-ter-**OL**-oh-jist) Medical specialist in gastroenterology.

gastroenterology (**GAS**-troh-en-ter-**OL**-oh-gee) Medical specialty of the stomach and intestines.

gastroesophageal (**GAS**-troh-ee-sof-ah-**JEE**-al) Pertaining to the stomach and esophagus.

gastrointestinal (GI) (**GAS**-troh-in-**TESS**-tin-al) Pertaining to the stomach and intestines.

gastroscope (**GAS**-troh-skope) Endoscope for examining the inside of the stomach.

gastroscopy (gas-**TROS**-koh-pee) Endoscopic examination of the stomach.

gavage (guh-**VAHZH**) To feed by a stomach tube.

gene (JEEN) Functional segment of DNA molecule.

geneticist (jeh-**NET**-ih-sist) A specialist in genetics.

genetics (jeh-**NET**-iks) Science of the inheritance of characteristics.

genital (**JEN**-ih-tal) Relating to reproduction or to the male or female sex organs.

genitalia (**JEN**-ih-**TAY**-lee-ah) External and internal organs of reproduction.

geriatrician (jer-ee-ah-**TRISH**-an) Medical specialist in the process and problems of aging.

geriatrics (jer-ee-**AT**-riks) Medical specialty that deals with the problems of aging.

gerontologist (jer-on-**TOL**-oh-jist) Medical specialist in the process and general problems of aging.

gerontology (jer-on-**TOL**-oh-jee) Study of the process and problems of aging.

gestation (jes-**TAY**-shun) From conception to birth.

gestational (jes-**TAY**-shun-al) Pertaining to gestation.

gigantism (**JI**-gan-tizm) Abnormal height and size of the entire body.

gingiva (**JIN**-jih-vah) Tissue surrounding the teeth and covering the jaw.

gingival (**JIN**-jih-val) Pertaining to the gingiva.

gingivectomy (jin-jih-**VEC**-toe-me) Surgical removal of diseased gum tissue.

gingivitis (jin-jih-**VI**-tis) Inflammation of the gums.

glans (GLANZ) Head of the penis or clitoris.

glaucoma (glau-**KOH**-mah) Increased intraocular pressure.

glia (**GLEE**-ah) Connective tissue that holds a structure together.

glial (**GLEE**-al) Pertaining to glia or neuroglia.

glioma (gli-**OH**-mah) Tumor of a glial cell.

glomerulonephritis (glo-**MER**-you-low-nef-**RYE**-tis) Infection of the glomeruli of the kidney.

glomerulus (glo-**MER**-you-lus) Plexus of capillaries; part of a nephron. Plural *glomeruli.*

glossodynia (gloss-oh-**DIN**-ee-ah) Painful, burning tongue.

glossopharyngeal (**GLOSS**-oh-fah-**RIN**-jee-al) Ninth (IX) cranial nerve, supplying the tongue and pharynx.

glottis (**GLOT**-is) Vocal apparatus of the larynx.

glucagon (**GLU**-kah-gon) Pancreatic hormone that supports blood glucose levels.

glucocorticoid (glu-co-**KOR**-tih-koyd) Hormone of the adrenal cortex that helps regulate glucose metabolism.

gluconeogenesis (**GLU**-koh-nee-oh-**JEN**-eh-sis) Formation of glucose from noncarbohydrate sources.

glucose (**GLU**-kose) The final product of carbohydrate digestion and the main sugar in the blood.

gluteal (**GLU**-tee-al) Pertaining to the buttocks.

gluten (**GLU**-ten) Insoluble protein found in wheat, barley, and oats.

gluteus (**GLU**-tee-us) Refers to one of three muscles in the buttocks.

glycogen (**GLYE**-koh-gen) The body's principal carbohydrate reserve, stored in the liver and skeletal muscle.

glycogenolysis (**GLYE**-koh-jen-oh-**LYE**-sis) Conversion of glycogen to glucose.

glycosuria (**GLYE**-koh-**SYU**-ree-ah) Presence of glucose in urine.

glycosylated hemoglobin (Hb A1c) (**GLYE**-koh-sih-lay-ted **HE**-moh-**GLOW**-bin) Hemoglobin A fraction linked to glucose; used as an index of glucose control.

goiter (**GOY**-ter) Enlargement of the thyroid gland.

gomphosis (gom-**FOE**-sis) Joint formed by a peg and socket. Plural *gomphoses.*

gonad (**GO**-nad) Testis or ovary. Plural *gonads.*

gonadotropin (**GO**-nad-oh-**TROH**-pin) Any hormone that stimulates gonad function.

gonorrhea (gon-oh-**REE**-ah) Specific contagious sexually transmitted infection.

grade (**GRAYD**) In cancer pathology, a classification of the rate of growth of cancer cells.

graft (**GRAFT**) Transplantation of living tissue.

grand mal (**GRAHN MAL**) Old name for generalized tonic-clonic seizure.

granulation (gran-you-**LAY**-shun) New fibrous tissue formed during wound healing.

granulocyte (**GRAN**-you-loh-site) A white blood cell that contains multiple small granules in its cytoplasm.

granulosa cell (gran-you-**LOW**-sah SELL) Cell lining the ovarian follicle.

Graves disease (**GRAVZ** diz-**EEZ**) Hyperthyroidism with toxic goiter.

gravid (**GRAV**-id) Pregnant.

gravida (**GRAV**-ih-dah) A pregnant woman.

gray matter (**GRAY MATT**-er) Regions of the brain and spinal cord occupied by cell bodies and dendrites.

greenstick fracture (**GREEN**-stik **FRAK**-chur) A fracture in which one side of the bone is partially broken and the other side is bent. Occurs mostly in children.

groin (**GROYN**) Crease where the thigh joins the abdomen.

Guillain-Barré syndrome (**GEE**-yan bah-**RAY SIN**-drom) Disorder in which the body makes antibodies against myelin, disrupting nerve conduction.

gurney (**GURR**-knee) A stretcher on wheels used to transport hospital patients.

gynecologic (**GUY**-nih-koh-**LOJ**-ik) Pertaining to gynecology.

gynecologist (guy-nih-**KOL**-oh-jist) Specialist in gynecology.

gynecology (guy-nih-**KOL**-oh-jee) Medical specialty of diseases of the female.

gynecomastia (**GUY**-nih-koh-**MAS**-tee-ah) Enlargement of the breast.

gyrus (**JI**-rus) Rounded elevation on the surface of the cerebral hemispheres. Plural *gyri.*

H

hairline fracture (**HAIR**-line **FRAK**-chur) A fracture without separation of the fragments.

halitosis (hal-ih-**TOE**-sis) Bad odor of the breath.

hallucination (hah-loo-sih-**NAY**-shun) Perception of an object or event when there is no such thing present.

hallux valgus (**HAL**-uks **VAL**-gus) Deviation of the big toe toward the lateral side of the foot.

Hashimoto disease (hah-shee-**MOH**-toe diz-**EEZ**) Autoimmune disease of the thyroid gland. Also called *Hashimoto thyroiditis.*

Haversian canals (hah-**VER**-shan ka-**NALS**) Vascular canals in bone. Also called *central canals.*

Heberden node (**HEH**-ber-den NOHD) Bony lump on the terminal phalanx of the fingers in osteoarthritis.

hemangioma (he-**MAN**-jee-oh-mah) Abnormal mass of proliferating blood vessels.

hematemesis (he-mah-**TEM**-eh-sis) Vomiting of red blood.

hematocrit (Hct) (**HE**-mat-oh-krit) Percentage of red blood cells in the blood.

hematologist (he-mah-**TOL**-oh-jist) Specialist in hematology.

hematology (he-mah-**TOL**-oh-jee) Medical specialty of disorders of the blood.

hematoma (he-mah-**TOE**-mah) Collection of blood that has escaped from the blood vessels into surrounding tissues. Also called *bruise.*

hematuria (he-mah-**TYU**-ree-ah) Blood in the urine.

heme (**HEEM**) The iron-based component of hemoglobin that carries oxygen.

hemiparesis (**HEM**-ee-pah-**REE**-sis) Weakness of one side of the body.

hemiplegia (hem-ee-**PLEE**-jee-ah) Paralysis of one side of the body.

hemiplegic (hem-ee-**PLEE**-jik) Pertaining to or suffering from hemiplegia.

Hemoccult test (**HEEM**-o-kult TEST) Trade name for a fecal occult blood test.

hemodialysis (**HE**-moh-die-**AL**-ih-sis) An artificial method of filtration to remove excess waste materials and water directly from the blood.

hemodynamics (**HE**-moh-die-**NAM**-iks) The science of the flow of blood through the circulation.

hemoglobin (**HE**-moh-**GLOW**-bin) Red-pigmented protein that is the main component of red blood cells.

hemoglobinopathy (**HE**-moh-**GLOW**-bin-**OP**-ah-thee) Disease caused by the presence of an abnormal hemoglobin in the red blood cells.

hemolysis (he-**MOL**-ih-sis) Destruction of red blood cells so that hemoglobin is liberated.

hemolytic (he-moh-**LIT**-ik) Pertaining to the process of destruction of red blood cells.

hemophilia (he-moh-**FILL**-ee-ah) An inherited disease from a deficiency of clotting factor VIII.

hemoptysis (he-**MOP**-tih-sis) Bloody sputum.

hemorrhage (**HEM**-oh-raj) To bleed profusely.

hemorrhoid (**HEM**-oh-royd) Dilated rectal vein producing painful anal swelling. Plural *hemorrhoids.*

hemorrhoidectomy (**HEM**-oh-royd-**EK**-toh-me) Surgical removal of hemorrhoids.

hemostasis (he-moh-**STAY**-sis) Control of or stopping bleeding.

hemothorax (he-moh-**THOR**-ax) Blood in the pleural cavity.

heparin (**HEP**-ah-rin) An anticoagulant secreted particularly by liver cells.

hepatic (hep-**AT**-ik) Pertaining to the liver.

hepatitis (hep-ah-**TIE**-tis) Inflammation of the liver.

hernia (**HER**-nee-ah) Protrusion of a structure through the tissue that normally contains it.

herniate (**HER**-nee-ate) To protrude.

herniation (her-nee-**AY**-shun) Protrusion of an anatomical structure from its normal location.

herniorrhaphy (**HER**-nee-**OR**-ah-fee) Repair of a hernia.

herpes simplex virus (HSV) (**HER**-peez **SIM**-pleks **VIE**-rus) Manifests with painful, watery blisters on the skin and mucous membranes.

herpes zoster (**HER**-peez **ZOS**-ter) Painful eruption of vesicles that follows a nerve root on one side of the body. Also called *shingles*.

heterograft (**HET**-er-oh-graft) A graft using tissue taken from another species. Also called *xenograft*.

hiatal (high-**AY**-tal) Pertaining to a hernia.

hiatus (high-**AY**-tus) An opening through a structure.

hilum (**HIGH**-lum) The site where the nerves and blood vessels enter and leave an organ. Plural *hila*.

histamine (**HISS**-tah-mean) Compound liberated in tissues as a result of injury or an allergic response.

histologist (his-**TOL**-oh-jist) Specialist in histology.

histology (his-**TOL**-oh-jee) Study of the structure and function of cells, tissues, and organs.

Hodgkin lymphoma (**HOJ**-kin lim-**FOH**-mah) Marked by chronic enlargement of lymph nodes spreading to other nodes in an orderly way.

holistic (ho-**LIS**-tik) Pertaining to the care of the whole person in physical, mental, emotional, and spiritual dimensions.

homeostasis (hoh-mee-oh-**STAY**-sis) Maintaining the stability of a system or the body's internal environment.

homograft (**HOH**-moh-graft) Skin graft from another person or a cadaver.

hordeolum (hor-**DEE**-oh-lum) Abscess in an eyelash follicle. Also called *stye*.

hormonal (hor-**MOHN**-al) Pertaining to a hormone.

hormone (**HOR**-mohn) Chemical formed in one tissue or organ and carried by the blood to stimulate or inhibit a function of another tissue or organ.

Horner syndrome (**HOR**-ner **SIN**-drome) Disorder of the sympathetic nerves to the face and eye.

hospice (**HOS**-pis) Provides care to the dying and their families.

human immunodeficiency virus (HIV) (**HYU**-man **IM**-you-noh-dee-**FISH**-en-see **VIE**-rus) Etiologic agent of acquired immunodeficiency syndrome (AIDS).

human papilloma virus (HPV) (**HYU**-man pap-ih-**LOW**-mah **VIE**-rus) Causes warts on the skin and genitalia and can increase the risk for cervical cancer.

humerus (**HYU**-mer-us) Single bone of the upper arm.

humoral immunity (**HYU**-mor-al ihm-**YUNE**-ih-tee) Defense mechanism arising from antibodies in the blood.

Huntington disease (**HUN**-ting-ton diz-**EEZ**) Progressive inherited, degenerative, incurable neurologic disease. Also called *Huntington chorea*.

hyaline (**HIGH**-ah-line) Cartilage that looks like frosted glass and contains fine collagen fibers.

hyaline membrane disease (**HIGH**-ah-line **MEM**-brain diz-**EEZ**) Respiratory distress syndrome of the newborn.

hydrocele (**HIGH**-droh-seal) Collection of fluid in the space of the tunica vaginalis.

hydrocephalus (high-droh-**SEF**-ah-lus) Excess CSF in the cerebral ventricles; may cause enlarged head.

hydrochloric acid (HCl) (high-droh-**KLOR**-ik **ASS**-id) The acid of gastric juice.

hydrocortisone (high-droh-**KOR**-tih-sohn) Potent glucocorticoid with anti-inflammatory properties. Also called *cortisol*.

hydronephrosis (**HIGH**-droh-neh-**FROH**-sis) Dilation of the pelvis and calyces of a kidney.

hydronephrotic (**HIGH**-droh-neh-**FROT**-ik) Pertaining to or suffering from hydronephrosis.

hymen (**HIGH**-men) Thin membrane partly occluding the vaginal orifice.

hyperactivity (**HIGH**-per-ac-**TIV**-ih-tee) Excessive restlessness and movement.

hypercalcemia (**HIGH**-per-cal-**SEE**-me-ah) Excessive level of calcium in the blood.

hypercapnia (**HIGH**-per-**KAP**-nee-ah) Abnormal increase of carbon dioxide in the arterial bloodstream.

hyperemesis (high-per-**EM**-eh-sis) Excessive vomiting.

hyperflexion (high-per-**FLEK**-shun) Flexion of a limb or part beyond the normal limits.

hyperglycemia (**HIGH**-per-gly-**SEE**-me-ah) High level of glucose (sugar) in blood.

hyperglycemic (**HIGH**-per-gly-**SEE**-mik) Pertaining to or having hyperglycemia.

hyperimmune globulin (**HIGH**-per-im-**YUNE GLOB**-youlin) Immunoglobulin prepared from serum of people with a high antibody titer to a specific antigen.

hyperkalemia (**HIGH**-per-kah-**LEE**-me-ah) High level of potassium in the blood.

hypernatremia (**HIGH**-per-nah-**TREE**-me-ah) High level of sodium in the blood.

hyperopia (high-per-**OH**-pee-ah) Able to see distant objects but unable to see close objects.

hyperosmolar (**HIGH**-per-os-**MOH**-lar) Marked hyperglycemia without ketoacidosis.

hyperparathyroidism (**HIGH**-per-para-**THIGH**-royd-izm) Excessive production of parathyroid hormone.

hyperplasia (**HIGH**-per-**PLAY**-zee-ah) Increase in the number of cells in a tissue or organ.

hyperpnea (high-perp-**NEE**-ah) Deeper and more rapid breathing than normal.

hyperpyrexia (**HIGH**-per-pie-**REK**-see-ah) Extremely high body temperature or fever.

hypersecretion (**HIGH**-per-seh-**KREE**-shun) Excessive secretion (of mucus or enzymes or waste products).

hypersensitivity (**HIGH**-per-sen-sih-**TIV**-ih-tee) Exaggerated abnormal reaction to an allergen.

hypersplenism (high-per-**SPLEN**-izm) Condition in which the spleen removes blood components at an excessive rate.

hypertension (**HIGH**-per-**TEN**-shun) Persistent high arterial blood pressure.

hypertensive (**HIGH**-per-**TEN**-siv) Pertaining to or suffering from high blood pressure.

hyperthyroidism (high-per-**THIGH**-royd-izm) Excessive production of thyroid hormones.

hypertrophy (high-**PER**-troh-fee) Increase in size, but not in number, of an individual tissue element.

hypochondriac (high-poh-**KON**-dree-ack) A person who exaggerates the significance of symptoms.

hypochromic (high-poh-**CROW**-mik) Pale in color, as in RBCs when hemoglobin is deficient.

hypodermic (high-poh-**DER**-mik) Pertaining to the hypodermis.

hypodermis (high-poh-**DER**-miss) Tissue layer of skin below the dermis.

hypogastric (high-poh-**GAS**-trik) Abdominal region below the stomach.

hypoglossal (high-poh-**GLOSS**-al) Twelfth (XII) cranial nerve, supplying muscles of the tongue.

hypoglycemia (**HIGH**-poh-gly-**SEE**-me-ah) Low level of glucose (sugar) in the blood.

hypoglycemic (**HIGH**-poh-gly-**SEE**-mik) Pertaining to or suffering from low blood sugar.

hypogonadism (**HIGH**-poh-**GOH**-nad-izm) Deficient gonad production of sperm or eggs or hormones.

hypokalemia (**HIGH**-poh-kah-**LEE**-me-ah) Low level of potassium in the blood.

hyponatremia (**HIGH**-poh-nah-**TREE**-me-ah) Low level of sodium in the blood.

hypoparathyroidism (**HIGH**-poh-par-ah-**THIGH**-royd-izm) Deficient production of parathyroid hormone.

hypophysis (high-**POF**-ih-sis) Another name for *pituitary gland.*

hypopituitarism (**HIGH**-poh-pih-**TYU**-ih-tah-rizm) Condition of one or more deficient pituitary hormones.

hypospadias (high-poh-**SPAY**-dee-as) Urethral opening more proximal than normal on the ventral surface of the penis.

hypotension (**HIGH**-poh-**TEN**-shun) Persistent low arterial blood pressure.

hypotensive (**HIGH**-poh-**TEN**-siv) Pertaining to or suffering from low blood pressure.

hypothalamic (high-poh-thal-**AM**-ik) Pertaining to the hypothalamus.

hypothalamus (high-poh-**THAL**-ah-muss) An area of gray matter lying below the thalamus.

hypothenar eminence (high-poh-**THAY**-nar **EM**-in-nens) The fleshy mass at the base of the little finger.

hypothermia (high-poh-**THER**-me-ah) Very low core body temperature.

hypothyroidism (high-poh-**THIGH**-royd-izm) Deficient production of thyroid hormones.

hypovolemic (**HIGH**-poh-vo-**LEE**-mik) Decreased blood volume in the body.

hypoxia (high-**POCK**-see-ah) Below-normal levels of oxygen in tissues, gases, or blood.

hypoxic (high-**POCK**-sik) Deficient in oxygen.

hysterectomy (his-ter-**EK**-toe-me) Surgical removal of the uterus.

I

ictal (**IK**-tal) Pertaining to, or a condition caused by, a stroke or epilepsy.

idiopathic (**ID**-ih-oh-**PATH**-ik) Pertaining to a disease of unknown etiology.

ileocecal (**ILL**-ee-oh-**SEE**-cal) Pertaining to the junction of the ileum and cecum.

ileocecal sphincter (**ILL**-ee-oh-**SEE**-cal **SFINK**-ter) A band of muscle that encircles the junction of the ileum and cecum.

ileoscopy (ill-ee-**OS**-koh-pee) Endoscopic examination of the ileum.

ileostomy (ill-ee-**OS**-toe-me) Artificial opening from the ileum to the outside of the body.

ileum (**ILL**-ee-um) Third portion of the small intestine.

iliac (**ILL**-ee-ack) A structure related to the ilium (pelvic bone).

ilium (**ILL**-ee-um) Large wing-shaped bone at the upper and posterior part of the pelvis. Plural *ilia.*

immune (im-**YUNE**) Protected from an infectious disease.

immune serum (im-**YUNE SEER**-um) Serum taken from another human or animal that has antibodies to a disease. Also called *antiserum.*

immunity (im-**YUNE**-ih-tee) State of being protected.

immunization (**IM**-you-nih-**ZAY**-shun) Administration of an agent to provide immunity.

immunize (**IM**-you-nize) To make resistant to an infectious disease.

immunodeficiency (**IM**-you-noh-dee-**FISH**-en-see) Failure of the immune system.

immunoglobulin (**IM**-you-noh-**GLOB**-you-lin) Specific protein evoked by an antigen. All antibodies are immunoglobulins.

immunologist (im-you-**NOL**-oh-jist) Medical specialist in immunology.

immunology (im-you-**NOL**-oh-jee) The science and practice of immunity and allergy.

immunosuppression (**IM**-you-noh-suh-**PRESH**-un) Failure of the immune system caused by an outside agent.

impacted (im-**PAK**-ted) Immovably wedged, as with earwax blocking the external canal.

impacted fracture (im-**PAK**-ted **FRAK**-chur) A fracture in which one bone fragment is driven into the other.

impairment (im-**PAIR**-ment) The state of being worse, weaker, or damaged.

impetigo (im-peh-**TIE**-go) Infection of the skin producing thick, yellow crusts.

implant (im-**PLANT**) To insert material into tissues; *or* the material inserted into tissues.

implantable (im-**PLAN**-tah-bul) A device that can be inserted into tissues.

implantation (im-plan-**TAY**-shun) Attachment of a fertilized egg to the endometrium.

impotence (**IM**-poh-tence) Inability to achieve an erection.

impulsive (im-**PUL**-siv) Inability to resist performing inappropriate actions.

in situ (IN **SIGH**-tyu) In the correct place.

in utero (IN **YOU**-ter-oh) Within the womb; not yet born.

in vitro fertilization (IVF) (en **VEE**-troh **FER**-til-eye-**ZAY**-shun) Process of combining sperm and egg in a laboratory dish and placing the resulting embryos inside the uterus.

inattention (**IN**-ah-**TEN**-shun) Lack of concentration and direction.

incision (in-**SIZH**-un) A cut or surgical wound.

incompetence (in-**KOM**-peh-tense) Failure of valves to close completely.

incomplete fracture (in-kom-**PLEET FRAK**-chur) A fracture that does not extend across the bone, as in a hairline fracture.

incontinence (in-**KON**-tin-ence) Inability to prevent discharge of urine or feces.

incontinent (in-**KON**-tin-ent) Denoting incontinence.

incubation (in-kyu-**BAY**-shun) Process to develp an infection.

incus (**IN**-cuss) Middle one of the three ossicles in the middle ear; shaped like an anvil.

independence (in-dee-**PEN**-dense) The state of being able to think and act for oneself.

independent (in-dee-**PEN**-dent) Pertaining to the ability to think and act for oneself.

indigestion (in-dee-**JESS**-chun) Symptoms resulting from difficulty in digesting food.

infancy (**IN**-fan-see) The first year of life.

infant (**IN**-fant) Child in the first year of life.

infarct (in-**FARKT**) Area of cell death resulting from blockage of its blood supply.

infarction (in-**FARKT**-shun) Sudden blockage of an artery.

infect (in-**FEKT**) To invade an organism by a microorganism.

infection (in-**FEK**-shun) Invasion of the body by disease-producing microorganisms.

infectious (in-**FEK**-shus) Capable of being transmitted to a person; *or* a disease caused by the action of a microorganism.

inferior (in-**FEER**-ee-or) Situated below.

infertility (in-fer-**TIL**-ih-tee) Failure to conceive.

infestation (in-fes-**TAY**-shun) Act of being invaded on the skin by a troublesome other species, such as a parasite.

inflammation (in-flah-**MAY**-shun) A complex of cell and chemical reactions in response to an injury or a chemical or biologic agent.

inflammatory (in-**FLAM**-ah-tor-ee) Causing or affected by inflammation.

influenza (in-flew-**EN**-zah) An acute, viral infection of upper and lower respiratory tracts.

infusion (in-**FYU**-zhun) Introduction intravenously of a substance other than blood.

ingestion (in-**JES**-chun) Intake of food, either by mouth or through a nasogastric tube.

inguinal (**ING**-gwin-ahl) Pertaining to the groin.

inhale (**IN**-hail) Breathe in.

insanity (in-**SAN**-ih-tee) Nonmedical term for a person unable to be responsible for his or her actions.

insecticide (in-**SEK**-tih-side) Agent to destroy insects.

inseminate (in-**SEM**-ih-nate) To introduce semen into the vagina.

insemination (in-sem-ih-**NAY**-shun) The introduction of semen into the vagina.

insertion (in-**SIR**-shun) The insertion of a muscle is the attachment of a muscle to a more movable part of the skeleton, as distinct from the origin.

inspiration (in-spih-**RAY**-shun) Breathe in.

instability (in-stah-**BIL**-ih-tee) Abnormal tendency of a joint to partially or fully dislocate.

insufficiency (in-suh-**FISH**-en-see) Lack of completeness of function; for example, for a heart valve to fail to close properly.

insulin (**IN**-syu-lin) A hormone produced by the islet cells of the pancreas.

integument (in-**TEG**-you-ment) Organ system that covers the body, the skin being the main organ within the system.

integumentary (in-**TEG**-you-**MENT**-ah-ree) Pertaining to the covering of the body.

interatrial (**IN**-ter-**AY**-tree-al) Between the atria of the heart.

intercostal (**IN**-ter-**KOS**-tal) The space between two ribs.

intermittent (**IN**-ter-**MIT**-ent) Alternately ceasing and beginning again.

internist (in-**TER**-nist) A physician trained in internal medicine.

interosseous (in-ter-**OSS**-ee-us) A structure between bones; for example, muscles.

interphalangeal (**IN**-ter-fay-**LAN**-jee-al) Finger or toe joint between two phalanges.

interstitial (in-ter-**STISH**-al) Pertaining to spaces between cells in a tissue or organ.

interventricular (**IN**-ter-ven-**TRIK**-you-lar) Between the ventricles of the heart.

intervertebral (**IN**-ter-**VER**-teh-bral) The space between two vertebrae.

intestinal (in-**TESS**-tin-al) Pertaining to the intestine.

intestine (in-**TESS**-tin) The digestive tube from stomach to anus.

intolerance (in-**TOL**-er-ance) Inability of the small intestine to digest and dispose of a particular dietary substance.

intracameral (in-trah-**CAM**-er-al) Introduction of an agent into the anterior chamber of the eye.

intracellular (in-trah-**SELL**-you-lar) Within the cell.

intracranial (in-trah-**KRAY**-nee-al) Within the cranium (skull).

intradermal (in-trah-**DER**-mal) Within the epidermis.

intramuscular (in-trah-**MUSS**-kew-lar) Within the muscle.

intraocular (in-trah-**OCK**-you-lar) Pertaining to the inside of the eye.

intrathecal (**IN**-trah-**THEE**-kal) Within the subarachnoid or subdural space.

intrauterine (**IN**-trah-**YOU**-ter-ine) Inside the uterine cavity.

intravenous (**IN**-trah-**VEE**-nus) Through a vein.

intravitreal (in-trah-**VIT**-ree-al) Introduction of an agent into the vitreous body of the eye.

intrinsic (in-**TRIN**-sik) Any muscle located entirely within (inside) the structure under consideration; for example, muscles inside the vocal cords or the eye.

intrinsic factor (in-**TRIN**-sik **FAK**-tor) Makes the absorption of vitamin B_{12} happen.

intubation (IN-tyu-**BAY**-shun) Insertion of a tube into the trachea.

intussusception (IN-tuss-sus-**SEP**-shun) The slipping of one part of the bowel inside another to cause obstruction.

inversion (in-**VER**-zhun) Turning inward.

invert (in-**VERT**) Turn inward.

involuntary (in-**VOL**-un-tay-ree) Not under control of the will.

involute (in-**VOH**-loot) Regressive changes in a tissue.

involution (in-voh-**LOO**-shun) Decrease in size.

iodine (**EYE**-oh-dine or **EYE**-oh-deen) Chemical element, the lack of which causes thyroid disease.

iris (**EYE**-ris) Colored portion of the eye with the pupil in its center.

irrigation (ih-rih-**GAY**-shun) Use of water to remove wax out of the external ear canal.

ischemia (is-**KEY**-me-ah) Lack of blood supply to tissue.

ischemic (is-**KEY**-mik) Pertaining to or affected by the lack of blood supply to tissue.

ischial (**IS**-key-al) Pertaining to the ischium.

ischium (**IS**-key-um) Lower and posterior part of the hip bone. Plural *ischia.*

Ishihara color system (ish-ee-**HAR**-ah) Test for color vision defects.

islet cells (**EYE**-let SELLZ) Hormone-secreting cells of the pancreas.

islets of Langerhans (**EYE**-lets of **LAHNG**-er-hahnz) Areas of pancreatic cells that produce insulin and glucagon.

isotope (**I**-so-tope) Radioactive element used in diagnostic procedures.

J

Jaeger reading cards (**YA**-ger) Type of different sizes for testing near vision.

jaundice (**JAWN**-dis) Yellow staining of tissues with bile pigments, including bilirubin.

jejunal (je-**JEW**-nal) Pertaining to the jejeunum.

jejunum (je-**JEW**-num) Segment of small intestine between the duodenum and the ileum.

K

Kaposi sarcoma (kah-**POH**-see sar-**KOH**-mah) A skin cancer seen in AIDS patients.

keloid (**KEY**-loyd) Raised, irregular, lumpy scar due to excess collagen fiber production during healing of a wound.

keratin (**KER**-ah-tin) Protein found in the skin, nails, and hair.

keratoconjunctivitis (**KER**-ah-toe-con-**JUNGK**-tih-**VI**-tis) Inflammation of the cornea and conjunctiva.

keratomileusis (**KER**-ah-toe-my-**LOO**-sis) Cuts and shapes the cornea.

keratotomy (**KER**-ah-**TOT**-oh-mee) Incision in the cornea.

kernicterus (ker-**NICK**-ter-us) Bilirubin staining of the basal nuclei of the brain.

ketoacidosis (**KEY**-toe-ass-ih-**DOE**-sis) Excessive production of ketones, making the blood acid.

ketone (**KEY**-tone) Chemical formed in uncontrolled diabetes or in starvation.

ketosis (key-**TOE**-sis) Excess production of ketones.

kidney (**KID**-nee) Organ of excretion.

kyphosis (ki-**FOH**-sis) A normal posterior curve of the thoracic spine that can be exaggerated in disease.

kyphotic (ki-**FOT**-ik) Pertaining to or suffering from kyphosis.

L

labium (**LAY**-bee-um) Fold of the vulva. Plural *labia.*

labor (**LAY**-bore) Process of expulsion of the fetus.

labyrinth (**LAB**-ih-rinth) The inner ear.

labyrinthitis (**LAB**-ih-rin-**THI**-tis) Inflammation of the inner ear.

laceration (lass-eh-**RAY**-shun) A tear of the skin.

lacrimal (**LAK**-rim-al) Pertaining to tears; *or* bone that forms the medial wall of the orbit.

lactase (**LAK**-tase) Enzyme that breaks down lactose (milk sugar) to glucose and galactose.

lactate (**LAK**-tate) To produce milk.

lactation (lak-**TAY**-shun) Production of milk.

lacteal (**LAK**-tee-al) A lymphatic vessel carrying chyle away from the intestine.

lactiferous (lak-**TIF**-er-us) Pertaining to or yielding milk.

lactose (**LAK**-toes) The disaccharide found in cow's milk.

lanugo (la-**NYU**-go) Fine, soft hair on the fetal body.

laparoscope (**LAP**-ah-roh-skope) Instrument (endoscope) used for viewing the abdominal contents.

laparoscopic (**LAP**-ah-roh-**SKOP**-ik) Pertaining to laparoscopy.

laparoscopy (lap-ah-**ROS**-koh-pee) Examination of the contents of the abdomen using an endoscope.

laryngeal (lah-**RIN**-jee-al) Pertaining to the larynx.

laryngitis (lah-rin-**JEYE**-tis) Inflammation of the larynx.

laryngopharynx (lah-**RIN**-go-**FAH**-rinks) Region of the pharynx below the epiglottis that includes the larynx.

laryngoscope (lah-**RING**-oh-skope) Hollow tube with a light and camera used to visualize or operate on the larynx.

laryngotracheobronchitis (lah-**RING**-oh-**TRAY**-kee-oh-brong-**KIE**-tis) Inflammation of the larynx, trachea, and bronchi. Also called *croup.*

larynx (**LAH**-rinks) Organ of voice production.

laser surgery (**LAY**-zer **SUR**-jer-ee) Use of a concentrated, intense narrow beam of electromagnetic radiation for surgery.

lateral (**LAT**-er-al) Situated at the side of a structure.

latissimus dorsi (lah-**TISS**-ih-muss **DOOR**-sigh) The widest (broadest) muscle in the back.

leiomyoma (**LIE**-oh-my-**OH**-mah) Benign tumor derived from smooth muscle.

lens (LENZ) Transparent refractive structure behind the iris.

lentigo (len-**TIH**-go) Age spot; small, flat, brown-black spot in the skin of older people. Plural *lentigines.*

leptin (**LEP**-tin) Hormone secreted by adipose tissue.

lesion (**LEE**-zhun) Pathologic change or injury in a tissue.

lethargy (**LETH**-ar-jee) Abnormal drowsiness in depth, length, or time. Adj *lethargic*.

leukemia (loo-**KEE**-mee-ah) Disease when the blood is taken over by white blood cells and their precursors.

leukemic (loo-**KEE**-mik) Pertaining to or affected by leukemia.

leukocyte (**LOO**-koh-site) Another term for a white blood cell. Alternative spelling *leucocyte*.

leukocytosis (**LOO**-koh-sigh-**TOE**-sis) An excessive number of white blood cells.

leukopenia (loo-koh-**PEE**-nee-ah) A deficient number of white blood cells.

libido (lih-**BEE**-doh) Sexual desire.

life expectancy (LIFE eck-**SPEK**-tan-see) Statistical determination of the number of years an individual is expected to live.

life span (LIFE SPAN) The age that a person reaches.

ligament (**LIG**-ah-ment) Band of fibrous tissue connecting two structures.

limbic (**LIM**-bic) Array of nerve fibers surrounding the thalamus.

linear fracture (**LIN**-ee-ar **FRAK**-chur) A fracture running parallel to the length of the bone.

lipase (**LIE**-paze) Enzyme that breaks down fat.

lipectomy (lip-**ECK**-toe-me) Surgical removal of adipose tissue.

lipid (**LIP**-id) General term for all types of fatty compounds; for example, cholesterol, triglycerides, and fatty acids.

lipoprotein (**LIP**-oh-pro-teen) Bonding of molecules of fat and protein.

liposuction (**LIP**-oh-suck-shun) Surgical removal of adipose tissue using suction.

lithotripsy (**LITH**-oh-trip-see) Crushing stones by sound waves.

lithotripter (**LITH**-oh-trip-ter) Machine that generates sound waves.

liver (**LIV**-er) Body's largest organ, located in the right upper quadrant of the abdomen.

lobar (**LOW**-bar) Pertaining to a lobe.

lobe (LOBE) Subdivision of an organ or other part.

lobectomy (low-**BECK**-toe-me) Surgical removal of a lobe.

lochia (**LOW**-kee-uh) Vaginal discharge following childbirth.

longevity (lon-**JEV**-ih-tee) Duration of life beyond the normal expectation.

Loop of Henle (LOOP of **HEN**-lee) Part of the renal tubule where reabsorption occurs.

lordosis (lore-**DOH**-sis) A normal forward curvature of the lumbar spine that can be exaggerated in disease.

lordotic (lore-**DOT**-ik) Pertaining to or suffering from lordosis.

louse (LOWSE) Parasitic insect. Plural *lice*.

lumbar (**LUM**-bar) Region in the back and sides between the ribs and pelvis.

lumen (**LOO**-men) The interior space of a tubelike structure.

lumpectomy (lump-**ECK**-toe-me) Removal of a lesion with preservation of surrounding tissue.

luteal (**LOO**-tee-al) Pertaining to a corpus luteum.

lutein (**LOO**-tee-in) Yellow pigment.

luteum (**LOO**-tee-um) Corpus luteum is the yellow (lutein) body formed after an ovarian follicle ruptures.

lymph (**LIMF**) A clear fluid collected from body tissues and transported by lymph vessels to the venous circulation.

lymphadenectomy (lim-**FAD**-eh-**NECK**-toe-me) Surgical excision of a lymph node(s).

lymphadenitis (lim-**FAD**-eh-neye-tis) Inflammation of a lymph node(s).

lymphadenopathy (lim-**FAD**-eh-**NOP**-ah-thee) Any disease process affecting a lymph node.

lymphangiogram (lim-**FAN**-jee-oh-gram) Radiographic images of lymph vessels and nodes following injection of contrast material.

lymphatic (lim-**FAT**-ic) Pertaining to lymph or the lymphatic system.

lymphedema (**LIMF**-eh-**DEE**-mah) Tissue swelling due to lymphatic obstruction.

lymphocyte (**LIM**-foh-site) Small white blood cell with a large nucleus.

lymphoid (**LIM**-foyd) Resembling lymphatic tissue.

lymphoma (lim-**FOH**-mah) Any neoplasm of lymphatic tissue.

M

macrocyte (**MACK**-roh-site) Large red blood cell.

macrocytic (mack-roh-**SIT**-ik) Pertaining to a macrocyte.

macrophage (**MACK**-roh-fayj) Large white blood cell that removes bacteria, foreign particles, and dead cells.

macula lutea (**MACK**-you-lah **LOO**-tee-ah) Yellowish spot on the back of the retina; contains the fovea centralis.

macule (**MACK**-yul) Small, flat spot or patch on the skin.

majus (**MAY**-jus) Bigger or greater; for example, labium majus. Plural *majora*.

malabsorption (mal-ab-**SORP**-shun) Inadequate gastrointestinal absorption of nutrients.

malformation (**MAL**-for-**MAY**-shun) Failure of proper or normal development.

malfunction (mal-**FUNK**-shun) Inadequate or abnormal function.

malignancy (mah-**LIG**-nan-see) State of being malignant.

malignant (mah-**LIG**-nant) Tumor that invades surrounding tissues and metastasizes to distant organs.

malleus (**MAL**-ee-us) Outer (lateral) one of the three ossicles in the middle ear; shaped like a hammer.

malnutrition (mal-nyu-**TRISH**-un) Inadequate nutrition from poor diet or inadequate absorption of nutrients.

malunion (mal-**YOU**-nee-un) The two bony ends of a fracture fail to heal together in the correct position.

mammary (**MAM**-ah-ree) Relating to the lactating breast.

mammogram (**MAM**-oh-gram) The record produced by x-ray imaging of the breast.

mammography (mah-**MOG**-rah-fee) The process of x-ray examination of the breast.

mammoplasty (**MAM**-oh-plas-tee) Surgical reshaping of the breast.

mandible (**MAN**-di-bel) Lower jawbone.

mandibular (man-**DIB**-you-lar) Pertaining to the mandible.

mania (**MAY**-nee-ah) Mood disorder with hyperactivity, irritability, and rapid speech.

manic (**MAN**-ik) Pertaining to or suffering from mania.

marrow (**MAH**-roe) Fatty, blood-forming tissue in the cavities of long bones.

mastalgia (mass-**TAL**-jee-uh) Pain in the breast.

mastectomy (mass-**TECK**-toe-me) Surgical excision of the breast.

masticate (**MASS**-tih-kate) To chew.

mastication (mass-tih-**KAY**-shun) The process of chewing.

mastitis (mass-**TIE**-tis) Inflammation of the breast.

mastoid (**MASS**-toyd) Small bony protrusion immediately behind the ear.

maternal (mah-**TER**-nal) Pertaining to or derived from the mother.

matrix (**MAY**-triks) Substance that surrounds and protects cells, is manufactured by the cells, and holds them together.

maturation (mat-you-**RAY**-shun) Process to achieve full development.

mature (mah-**TYUR**) Fully developed.

maxilla (mak-**SILL**-ah) Upper jawbone, containing right and left maxillary sinuses.

maxillary (**MAK**-sih-lair-ee) Pertaining to the maxilla.

maximus (**MAKS**-ih-mus) The gluteus maximus muscle is the largest muscle in the body, covering a large part of each buttock.

meatal (me-**AY**-tal) Pertaining to a meatus.

meatus (me-**AY**-tus) The external opening of a passage.

meconium (meh-**KOH**-nee-um) The first bowel movement of the newborn.

medial (**ME**-dee-al) Nearer to the middle of the body.

mediastinal (**ME**-dee-ass-**TIE**-nal) Pertaining to the mediastinum.

mediastinoscopy (**ME**-dee-ass-tih-**NOS**-koh-pee) Examination of the mediastinum using an endoscope.

mediastinum (**ME**-dee-ass-**TIE**-num) Area between the lungs containing the heart, aorta, venae cavae, esophagus, and trachea.

medius (**ME**-dee-us) The gluteus medius muscle is partly covered by the gluteus maximus.

medulla (meh-**DULL**-ah) Central portion of a structure surrounded by cortex.

medulla oblongata (meh-**DULL**-ah ob-lon-**GAH**-tah) Most posterior subdivision of the brainstem; continuation of the spinal cord.

medullary (**MED**-ul-ah-ree) Pertaining to a medulla.

meiosis (my-**OH**-sis) Two rapid cell divisions, resulting in half the number of chromosomes.

melanin (**MEL**-ah-nin) Black pigment found in the skin, hair, and retina.

melanoma (mel-ah-**NO**-mah) Malignant neoplasm formed from cells that produce melanin.

melatonin (mel-ah-**TONE**-in) Hormone formed by the pineal gland.

melena (mel-**EN**-ah) The passage of black, tarry stools.

membrane (**MEM**-brain) Thin layer of tissue covering a structure or cavity.

membranous (**MEM**-brah-nus) Pertaining to a membrane.

menarche (meh-**NAR**-key) First menstrual period.

Ménière disease (men-**YEAR** diz-**EEZ**) Disorder of the inner ear with acute attacks of tinnitus, vertigo, and hearing loss.

meninges (meh-**NIN**-jeez) Three-layered covering of the brain and spinal cord.

meningitis (men-in-**JIE**-tis) Inflammation of the meninges.

meningocele (meh-**NIN**-goh-seal) Protrusion of the meninges from the spinal cord or brain through a defect in the vertebral column or cranium.

meningococcal (meh-**NING**-goh-**KOK**-al) Pertaining to the *meningococcus* bacterium.

meningomyelocele (meh-nin-goh-**MY**-el-oh-seal) Protrusion of the spinal cord and meninges through a defect in the vertebral arch of one or more vertebrae.

meniscectomy (**MEN**-ih-**SEK**-toh-me) Excision (cutting out) of all or part of a meniscus.

meniscus (meh-**NISS**-kuss) Disc of cartilage between the bones of a joint; for example, in the knee joint. Plural *menisci*.

menopausal (**MEN**-oh-pawz-al) Pertaining to the menopause.

menopause (**MEN**-oh-pawz) Permanent ending of menstrual periods.

menorrhagia (men-oh-**RAY**-jee-ah) Excessive menstrual bleeding.

menses (**MEN**-seez) Monthly uterine bleeding.

menstrual (**MEN**-stru-al) Pertaining to menstruation.

menstruate (**MEN**-stru-ate) The act of menstruation.

menstruation (men-stru-**AY**-shun) Synonym of *menses*.

mesentery (**MESS**-en-ter-ree) A double layer of peritoneum enclosing the abdominal viscera.

metabolic (met-ah-**BOL**-ik) Pertaining to metabolism.

metabolic acidosis (met-ah-**BOL**-ik ass-ih-**DOE**-sis) Decreased pH in the blood and body tissues as a result of an upset in metabolism.

metabolism (meh-**TAB**-oh-lizm) The constantly changing physical and chemical processes occurring in the cell that are the sum of anabolism and catabolism.

metacarpal (**MET**-ah-**KAR**-pal) The five bones between the carpus and the fingers.

metacarpophalangeal (**MET**-ah-**KAR**-poh-fay-**LAN**-jee-al) The articulations (joints) between the metacarpal bones and the phalanges.

metastasis (meh-**TAS**-tah-sis) Spread of a disease from one part of the body to another. Plural *metastases*.

metastasize (meh-**TAS**-tah-size) To spread to distant parts.

metastatic (meh-tah-**STAT**-ik) Pertaining to the character of cells that can metastasize.

metatarsal (**MET**-ah-**TAR**-sal) Pertaining to the metatarsus.

metatarsus (**MET**-ah-**TAR**-sus) The five parallel bones of the foot between the tarsus and the phalanges.

metrorrhagia (**MEH**-troh-**RAY**-jee-ah) Irregular uterine bleeding between menses.

microbe (**MY**-krohb) Short for *microorganism*.

microcephalic (**MY**-kroh-seh-**FAL**-ik) Pertaining to or suffering from a small head.

microcephaly (**MY**-kroh-**SEF**-ah-lee) An abnormally small head.

microcyte (**MY**-kroh-site) Small red blood cell.

microcytic (my-kroh-**SIT**-ik) Pertaining to a small cell.

microorganism (**MY**-kroh-**OR**-gan-izm) Any organism too small to be seen by the naked eye.

microscope (**MY**-kroh-skope) Instrument for viewing something small that cannot be seen in detail by the naked eye.

microscopic (**MY**-kroh-**SKOP**-ik) Visible only with the aid of a microscope.

micturate (**MIK**-choo-rate) Pass urine.

micturition (mik-choo-**RISH**-un) Act of passing urine.

migraine (**MY**-grain) Paroxysmal severe headache confined to one side of the head.

mineral (**MIN**-er-al) Inorganic compound usually found in the earth's crust.

mineralocorticoid (**MIN**-er-al-oh-**KOR**-tih-koyd) Hormone of the adrenal cortex that influences sodium and potassium metabolism.

minimus (**MIN**-ih-mus) The gluteus minimus is the smallest of the gluteal muscles and lies under the gluteus medius.

minus (**MY**-nus) Smaller or lesser; for example, labium minus. Plural *minora.*

miosis (my-**OH**-sis) Constriction of the pupil.

mitochondrion (my-toe-**KON**-dree-on) Organelle that generates, stores, and releases energy for cell activities. Plural *mitochondria.*

mitosis (my-**TOE**-sis) Cell division that creates two identical cells, each with 46 chromosomes.

mitral (**MY**-tral) Shaped like the headdress of a Catholic bishop.

modify (**MOD**-ih-fie) Change the form or qualities of something.

molar (**MO**-lar) One of six teeth in each jaw that grind food.

mole (MOLE) Benign localized area of melanin-producing cells.

molecule (**MOLL**-eh-kyul) Very small particle.

molluscum contagiosum (moh-**LUS**-kum kon-**TAY**-jee-**OH**-sum) STD caused by a virus.

monocyte (**MON**-oh-site) Large white blood cell with a single nucleus.

mononeuropathy (**MON**-oh-nyu-**ROP**-ah-thee) Disorder affecting a single nerve.

mononucleosis (**MON**-oh-nyu-klee-**OH**-sis) Presence of large numbers of specific, diagnostic mononuclear leukocytes.

monoplegia (**MON**-oh-**PLEE**-jee-ah) Paralysis of one limb.

monoplegic (**MON**-oh-**PLEE**-jik) Pertaining to or suffering from monoplegia.

mons pubis (MONZ **PYU**-bis) Fleshy pad with pubic hair, overlying the pubic bone.

morbidity (mor-**BID**-ih-tee) The frequency of the appearance of a disease.

morphine (**MOR**-feen) Derivative of opium used as an analgesic or sedative.

mortality (mor-**TAL**-ih-tee) Death rate.

motile (**MOH**-til) Capable of spontaneous movement.

motility (moh-**TILL**-ih-tee) The ability for spontaneous movement.

motor (**MOH**-tor) Structures of the nervous system that send impulses out to cause muscles to contract or glands to secrete.

mouth (MOWTH) External opening of a cavity or canal.

mucin (**MYU**-sin) Protein element of mucus.

mucocutaneous (**MYU**-koh-kyu-**TAY**-nee-us) Junction of skin and mucous membrane; for example, the lips.

mucolytic (**MYU**-koh-**LIT**-ik) Agent capable of dissolving or liquefying mucus.

mucosa (myu-**KOH**-sah) Lining of a tubular structure that secretes mucus. Another name for *mucous membrane.*

mucous (**MYU**-kus) Pertaining to mucus or the mucosa.

mucus (**MYU**-kus) Sticky secretion of cells in mucous membranes.

multipara (mul-**TIP**-ah-ruh) Woman who has given birth to two or more children.

murmur (**MUR**-mur) Abnormal heart sound heard with a stethoscope when a valve closes or opens abnormally.

muscle (**MUSS**-el) A tissue consisting of contractile cells.

musculoskeletal (**MUSS**-kyu-loh-**SKEL**-eh-tal) Pertaining to the muscles and the bony skeleton.

mutation (myu-**TAY**-shun) Change in the chemistry of a gene.

mute (MYUT) Unable or unwilling to speak.

mutism (**MYU**-tizm) Absence of speech.

myasthenia gravis (my-as-**THEE**-nee-ah **GRA**-vis) Disorder of fluctuating muscle weakness.

mydriasis (mih-**DRY**-ah-sis) Dilation of the pupil.

myelin (**MY**-eh-lin) Material of the sheath around the axon of a nerve.

myelitis (**MY**-eh-**LIE**-tis) Inflammation of the spinal cord.

myelocele (**MY**-eh-low-seal) Protrusion of the spinal cord through a defect in the vertebral arch.

myelomeningocele (**MY**-eh-low-meh-**NING**-oh-seal) Protrusion of the spinal cord and meninges through a defect in the vertebral arch of one or more vertebrae.

myocardial (my-oh-**KAR**-dee-al) Pertaining to heart muscle.

myocarditis (**MY**-oh-kar-**DIE**-tis) Inflammation of the heart muscle.

myocardium (my-oh-**KAR**-dee-um) All the heart muscle.

myoma (my-**OH**-mah) Benign tumor of muscle.

myomectomy (my-oh-**MEK**-toe-me) Surgical removal of a myoma (fibroid).

myometrium (my-oh-**MEE**-tree-um) Muscle wall of the uterus.

myopathy (my-**OP**-ah-thee) Any disease of muscle.

myopia (my-**OH**-pee-ah) Able to see close objects but unable to see distant objects.

myositis (my-oh-**SIGH**-tis) Inflammation of muscle tissue.

myringotomy (mir-in-**GOT**-oh-me) Incision in the tympanic membrane.

myxedema (miks-eh-**DEE**-muh) Nonpitting, waxy edema of the skin in hypothyroidism.

N

narcissism (**NAR**-sih-sizm) A state of relating everything to oneself.

narcissistic (**NAR**-sih-**SIS**-tik) Relating everything to oneself.

narcolepsy (**NAR**-koh-lep-see) Involuntary falling asleep.

narcotic (nar-**KOT**-ik) Drug derived from opium or any drug with effects similar to those of opium derivatives.

nares (**NAH**-rees) Nostril. Plural *nares.*

nasal (**NAY**-zal) Pertaining to the nose.

nasogastric (**NAY**-zoh-**GAS**-trik) Pertaining to the nose and stomach.

nasolacrimal duct (**NAY**-zoh-**LAK**-rim-al DUKT) Passage from the lacrimal sac to the nose.

nasopharyngeal (**NAY**-zoh-fah-**RIN**-jee-al) Pertaining to the nasopharynx.

nasopharynx (**NAY**-zoh-**FAH**-rinks) Region of the pharynx at the back of the nose and above the soft palate.

natal (**NAY**-tal) Pertaining to birth.

nebulizer (**NEB**-you-liz-er) Device used to deliver liquid medicine in a fine mist.

necrosis (neh-**KROH**-sis) Pathologic death of cells or tissue.

necrotic (neh-**KROT**-ik) Pertaining to or affected by necrosis.

necrotizing fasciitis (neh-kroh-**TIZE**-ing fash-ee-**EYE**-tis) Inflammation of fascia producing death of the tissue.

neonatal (**NEE**-oh-**NAY**-tal) Pertaining to the newborn infant or the newborn period.

neonate (**NEE**-oh-nate) A newborn infant.

neonatologist (**NEE**-oh-nay-**TOL**-oh-jist) Medical specialist in disorders of the newborn.

nephrectomy (nef-**REK**-toe-me) Surgical removal of a kidney.

nephritis (nef-**RY**-tis) Inflammation of the kidney.

nephroblastoma (**NEF**-roh-blas-**TOE**-mah) Cancerous kidney tumor of childhood. Also known as *Wilms tumor.*

nephrolithiasis (**NEF**-roe-lih-**THIGH**-ah-sis) Presence of a kidney stone.

nephrolithotomy (**NEF**-roe-lih-**THOT**-oh-me) Incision for removal of a kidney stone.

nephrologist (nef-**ROL**-oh-jist) Medical specialist in disorders of the kidney.

nephrology (nef-**ROL**-oh-jee) Medical specialty of diseases of the kidney.

nephron (**NEF**-ron) Filtration unit of the kidney; glomerulus + renal tubule.

nephropathy (nef-**ROP**-ah-thee) Any disease of the kidney.

nephroscope (**NEF**-roe-skope) Endoscope to view the inside of the kidney.

nephroscopy (nef-**ROS**-koh-pee) To examine the kidney.

nephrosis (nef-**ROH**-sis) Same as *nephrotic syndrome.*

nephrotic syndrome (nef-**ROT**-ik **SIN**-drome) Glomerular disease with marked loss of protein. Also called *nephrosis.*

nerve (NERV) A cord of nerve fibers bound together by connective tissue.

nervous (**NER**-vus) Pertaining to a nerve or the nervous system; *or* easily excited or agitated.

nervous system (**NER**-vus **SIS**-tem) The whole, integrated nerve apparatus.

neural (**NYU**-ral) Pertaining to nervous tissue.

neuralgia (nyu-**RAL**-jee-ah) Pain in the distribution of a nerve.

neuroglia (nyu-**ROG**-lee-ah) Connective tissue holding nervous tissue together.

neurohypophysis (**NYU**-roh-high-**POF**-ih-sis) Posterior lobe of the pituitary gland.

neurologic (**NYU**-roh-**LOJ**-ik) Pertaining to the nervous sytem.

neurologist (nyu-**ROL**-oh-jist) Medical specialist in disorders of the nervous system.

neurology (nyu-**ROL**-oh-jee) Medical specialty of disorders of the nervous system.

neuroma (nyu-**ROH**-mah) Any tumor arising from cells in the nervous system.

neuromuscular (**NYU**-roh-**MUSS**-kyu-lar) A junction where a nerve supplies muscle tissue.

neuron (**NYU**-ron) Technical term for a nerve cell; consists of the cell body with its dendrites and axons.

neuropathy (nyu-**ROP**-ah-thee) Any disorder affecting the nervous system.

neurosurgeon (**NYU**-roh-**SUR**-jun) One who operates on the nervous system.

neurosurgery (**NYU**-roh-**SUR**-jer-ee) Operating on the nervous system.

neurotoxin (**NYU**-roh-tock-sin) Agent that poisons the nervous system.

neurotransmitter (**NYU**-roh-trans-**MIT**-er) Chemical agent that relays messages from one nerve cell to the next.

neutropenia (**NEW**-troh-**PEE**-nee-ah) A deficiency of neutrophils.

neutrophil (**NEW**-troh-fill) A neutrophil's granules take up (purple) stain equally, whether the stain is acid or alkaline.

neutrophilia (**NEW**-troh-**FILL**-ee-ah) An increase in neutrophils.

nevus (**NEE**-vus) Congenital lesion of the skin. Plural *nevi.*

nipple (**NIP**-el) Projection from the breast into which the lactiferous ducts open.

nitrite (**NI**-trite) Chemical formed in urine by *E. coli* and other microorganisms.

nitrogenous (ni-**TRO**-jen-us) Containing or generating nitrogen.

nocturia (nok-**TYU**-ree-ah) Excessive urination at night.

node (NOHD) A circumscribed mass of tissue.

nonunion (non-**YOU**-nee-un) Total failure of healing of a fracture.

norepinephrine (**NOR**-ep-ih-**NEFF**-rin) Catecholamine hormone of the adrenal gland that is a parasympathetic neurotransmitter. Also called *noradrenaline.*

nosocomial (noh-soh-**KOH**-mee-al) Acquired while in the hospital.

nuchal cord (**NYU**-kul KORD) Loop(s) of umbilical cord around the fetal neck.

nuclear (**NYU**-klee-ar) Pertaining to a nucleus.

nucleolus (nyu-**KLEE**-oh-lus) Small mass within the nucleus.

nucleus (**NYU**-klee-us) Functional center of a cell or structure.

nutrient (**NYU**-tree-ent) A substance in food required for normal physiologic function.

nutrition (nyu-**TRISH**-un) The study of food and liquid requirements for normal function of the human body.

nystagmus (nis-**TAG**-mus) Fast uncontrollable movements of the eye in any direction.

O

obesity (oh-**BEE**-sih-tee) Excessive amount of fat in the body.

oblique fracture (ob-**LEEK FRAK**-chur) A diagonal fracture across the long axis of the bone.

obsession (ob-**SESH**-un) Persistent, recurrent, uncontrollable thoughts or impulses.

obsessive (ob-**SES**-iv) Possessing persistent, recurrent, uncontrollable thoughts or impulses.

obstetrician (ob-steh-**TRISH**-un) Medical specialist in obstetrics.

obstetrics (OB) (ob-**STET**-ricks) Medical specialty for the care of women during pregnancy and the postpartum period.

occipital (ock-**SIP**-it-al) The back of the skull.

occipital lobe (ock-**SIP**-it-al LOBE) Posterior area of the cerebral hemispheres.

occlude (oh-**KLUDE**) To close, plug, or completely obstruct.

occlusion (oh-**KLU**-zhun) A complete obstruction.

occult (oh-**KULT**) Not visible on the surface, hidden.

occult blood (oh-**KULT** BLUD) Blood that cannot be seen in the stool but is positive on a fecal occult blood test.

occupational (**OCK**-you-**PAY**-shun-al) A disorder resulting from exposure to an agent during performance of one's work.

ocular (**OCK**-you-lar) Pertaining to the eye.

olfaction (ol-**FAK**-shun) Sense of smell.

olfactory (ol-**FAK**-toh-ree) Related to the sense of smell.

oligohydramnios (**OL**-ih-goh-high-**DRAM**-nee-os) Too little amniotic fluid.

oligospermia (**OL**-ih-go-**SPER**-me-ah) Too few sperm in the semen.

oliguria (ol-ih-**GYUR**-ee-ah) Scanty production of urine.

omentum (oh-**MEN**-tum) Membrane that encloses the bowels.

onychomycosis (oh-nih-koh-my-**KOH**-sis) Condition of a fungus infection in a nail.

oocyte (**OH**-oh-site) Female egg cell.

oogenesis (oh-oh-**JEN**-eh-sis) Development of a female egg cell.

open fracture (**OH**-pen **FRAK**-chur) The skin over the fracture is broken.

ophthalmia neonatorum (off-**THAL**-me-ah ne-oh-nay-**TOR**-um) Conjunctivitis of the newborn.

ophthalmic (off-**THAL**-mik) Pertaining to the eye.

ophthalmologist (off-thal-**MALL**-oh-jist) Medical specialist in ophthalmology.

ophthalmology (off-thal-**MALL**-oh-jee) Diagnosis and treatment of diseases of the eye.

ophthalmoscope (off-**THAL**-moh-skope) Instrument for viewing the retina.

ophthalmoscopic (**OFF**-thal-moh-**SKOP**-ik) Pertaining to the use of an ophthalmoscope.

ophthalmoscopy (**OFF**-thal-**MOS**-koh-pee) The process of viewing the retina.

opiate (**OH**-pee-ate) A drug derived from opium.

opportunistic (**OP**-or-tyu-**NIS**-tik) An organism or a disease in a host with lowered resistance.

opportunistic infection (**OP**-or-tyu-**NIS**-tik in-**FEK**-shun) An infection that causes disease when the immune system is compromised for other reasons.

optic (**OP**-tik) The eye or vision; *or* second (II) cranial nerve, which carries visual information.

optical (**OP**-tih-kal) Pertaining to the eye or vision.

optometrist (op-**TOM**-eh-trist) Someone skilled in the measurement of vision but who cannot treat eye diseases or prescribe medication.

optometry (op-**TOM**-eh-tree) The profession of the measurement of vision.

oral (**OR**-al) Pertaining to the mouth.

orbit (**OR**-bit) The bony socket that holds the eyeball.

orbital (**OR**-bit-al) Pertaining to the orbit.

orchiectomy (or-key-**ECK**-toe-me) Removal of one or both testes.

orchiopexy (**OR**-key-oh-**PEK**-see) Surgical fixation of a testis in the scrotum.

orchitis (or-**KIE**-tis) Inflammation of the testis. Also called *epididymoorchitis.*

organ (**OR**-gan) Structure with specific functions in a body system.

organelle (**OR**-gah-nell) Part of a cell having specialized function(s).

organism (**OR**-gan-izm) Any whole, living individual animal or plant.

orifice (**OR**-ih-fis) Any opening or aperture.

origin (**OR**-ih-gin) Fixed source of a muscle at its attachment to bone.

oropharyngeal (**OR**-oh-fah-**RIN**-jee-al) Pertaining to the oropharynx.

oropharynx (**OR**-oh-**FAH**-rinks) Region at the back of the mouth between the soft palate and the tip of the epiglottis.

orthopedic (or-tho-**PEE**-dik) Pertaining to the correction and cure of deformities and diseases of the musculoskeletal system; originally, most of the deformities treated were in children. Also spelled *orthopaedic.*

orthopedist (or-tho-**PEE**-dist) Specialist in orthopedics.

orthopnea (or-**THOP**-nee-ah) Difficulty in breathing when lying flat.

orthopneic (or-**THOP**-nee-ik) Pertaining to or affected by orthopnea.

orthotic (or-**THOT**-ik) Orthopedic appliance to correct an abnormality.

orthotist (or-**THOT**-ist) Maker and fitter of orthopedic appliances.

os (OSS) Opening into a canal; for example, the cervix.

ossicle (**OSS**-ih-kel) A small bone, particularly relating to the three bones in the middle ear.

osteoarthritis (**OSS**-tee-oh-ar-**THRI**-tis) Chronic inflammatory disease of the joints, with pain and loss of function.

osteoblast (**OSS**-tee-oh-blast) Bone-forming cell.

osteocalcin (**OSS**-tee-oh-**KAL**-sin) A hormone produced by bone cells.

osteocyte (**OSS**-tee-oh-site) A bone-maintaining cell.

osteogenesis imperfecta (**OSS**-tee-oh-**JEN**-eh-sis im-per-**FEK**-tah) Inherited condition when bone formation is incomplete, leading to fragile, easily broken bones.

osteogenic sarcoma (**OSS**-tee-oh-**JEN**-ik sar-**KOH**-mah) Malignant tumor originating in bone-producing cells.

osteomalacia (**OSS**-tee-oh-mah-**LAY**-she-ah) Soft, flexible bones lacking in calcium (rickets).

osteomyelitis (**OSS**-tee-oh-my-eh-**LIE**-tis) Inflammation of bone tissue.

osteopath (**OSS**-tee-oh-path) Practitioner of osteopathy.

osteopathy (**OSS**-tee-**OP**-ah-thee) Medical practice based on maintaining the balance of the body.

osteopenia (**OSS**-tee-oh-**PEE**-nee-ah) Decreased calcification of bone.

osteoporosis (**OSS**-tee-oh-poh-**ROE**-sis) Condition in which the bones become more porous, brittle, and fragile and more likely to fracture.

ostomy (**OSS**-toe-me) Artificial opening into a tubular structure.

otitis media (oh-**TIE**-tis **ME**-dee-ah) Inflammation of the middle ear.

otolith (**OH**-toe-lith) A calcium particle in the vestibule of the inner ear.

otologist (oh-**TOL**-oh-jist) Medical specialist in diseases of the ear.

otology (oh-**TOL**-oh-jee) Study of the function and diseases of the ear.

otorhinolaryngologist (oh-toe-rye-no-lah-rin-**GOL**-oh-jist) Ear, nose, and throat medical specialist.

otosclerosis (**OH**-toe-sklair-**OH**-sis) Hardening at the junction of the stapes and oval window that causes loss of hearing.

otoscope (**OH**-toe-skope) Instrument for examining the ear.

otoscopic (**OH**-toe-**SKOP**-ik) Pertaining to examination with an otoscope.

otoscopy (oh-**TOS**-koh-pee) Examination of the ear.

ovarian (oh-**VAIR**-ee-an) Pertaining to the ovary(ies).

ovary (**OH**-vah-ree) One of the paired female egg-producing glands. Plural *ovaries.*

ovulate (**OV**-you-late) Release the oocyte from a follicle.

ovulation (**OV**-you-**LAY**-shun) Release of an oocyte from a follicle.

ovum (**OH**-vum) Egg. Also called *oocyte.* Plural *ova.*

oxygen (**OCK**-see-jen) The gas essential for life.

oxyhemoglobin (**OCK**-see-he-moh-**GLOW**-bin) Hemoglobin in combination with oxygen.

oxytocin (**OCK**-see-**TOE**-sin) Pituitary hormone that stimulates the uterus to contract.

P

pacemaker (**PACE**-may-ker) Device that regulates cardiac electrical activity.

palate (**PAL**-ate) Roof of the mouth.

palatine (**PAL**-ah-tine) Bone that forms the hard palate and parts of the nose and orbits.

palliative care (**PAL**-ee-ah-tiv **KAIR**) To relieve symptoms and pain without curing.

pallor (**PAL**-or) Paleness of the skin.

palm (PAHLM) Flat or anterior surface of the hand.

palmar (**PAHL**-mar) Pertaining to the palm.

palpate (**PAL**-pate) To examine with the fingers and hands.

palpation (pal-**PAY**-shun) Examination with the fingers and hands.

palpitation (pal-pih-**TAY**-shun) Forcible, rapid beat of the heart felt by the patient.

palsy (**PAWL**-zee) Paralysis or paresis from brain damage.

pancreas (**PAN**-kree-as) Lobulated gland, the head of which is tucked into the curve of the duodenum.

pancreatic (**PAN**-kree-**AT**-ik) Pertaining to the pancreas.

pancreatitis (**PAN**-kree-ah-**TIE**-tis) Inflammation of the pancreas.

pancytopenia (**PAN**-site-oh-**PEE**-nee-ah) Deficiency of all types of blood cells.

pandemic (pan-**DEM**-ik) Pertaining to a disease attacking the population of a very large area.

panendoscopy (pan-en-**DOS**-koh-pee) A visual examination of the inside of the esophagus, stomach, and upper duodenum using a flexible fiber-optic endoscope.

panhypopituitarism (pan-**HIGH**-poh-pih-**TYU**-ih-tah-rizm) Deficiency of all the pituitary hormones.

Pap test (PAP) Examination of cells taken from the cervix.

papilla (pah-**PILL**-ah) Any small projection. Plural *papillae.*

papilledema (pah-pill-eh-**DEE**-mah) Swelling of the optic disc in the retina.

papillomavirus (pap-ih-**LOH**-mah-vi-rus) Virus that causes warts and is associated with cancer.

papule (**PAP**-yul) Small, circumscribed elevation on the skin.

para (**PAH**-rah) Abbreviation for number of deliveries.

paralysis (pah-**RAL**-ih-sis) Loss of voluntary movement.

paralytic (par-ah-**LYT**-ik) Suffering from paralysis.

paralyze (**PAR**-ah-lyze) To make incapable of movement.

paranasal (**PAR**-ah-**NAY**-zal) Adjacent to the nose.

paranoia (par-ah-**NOY**-ah) Presence of persecutory delusions.

paranoid (**PAR**-ah-noyd) Having delusions of persecution.

paraphimosis (**PAR**-ah-fih-**MOH**-sis) Condition in which a retracted prepuce cannot be pulled forward to cover the glans.

paraplegia (par-ah-**PLEE**-jee-ah) Paralysis of both lower extremities.

paraplegic (par-ah-**PLEE**-jik) Pertaining to or suffering from paraplegia.

parasite (**PAR**-ah-site) An organism that attaches itself to, lives on or in, and derives its nutrition from another species.

parasitic (par-ah-**SIT**-ik) Pertaining to a parasite.

parasympathetic (par-ah-sim-pah-**THET**-ik) Division of the autonomic nervous system; has opposite effects of the sympathetic division.

parathyroid (par-ah-**THIGH**-royd) Endocrine glands embedded in the back of the thyroid gland.

paraurethral (**PAR**-ah-you-**REE**-thral) Situated around the urethra.

parenchyma (pah-**RENG**-kih-mah) Characteristic functional cells of a gland or organ that are supported by the connective tissue framework.

parenteral (pah-**REN**-ter-al) Giving medication by any means other than the gastrointestinal tract.

paresis (par-**EE**-sis) Partial paralysis (weakness).

paresthesia (par-es-**THEE**-ze-ah) An abnormal sensation; for example, tingling, burning, prickling. Plural *parasthesias.*

parietal (pah-**RYE**-eh-tal) Pertaining to the outer layer of the pericardium and the wall of any body cavity; *or* the two bones forming the sidewalls and roof of the cranium.

parietal lobe (pah-**RYE**-eh-tal LOBE) Area of the brain under the parietal bone.

Parkinson disease (**PAR**-kin-son diz-**EEZ**) Disease of muscular rigidity, tremors, and a masklike facial expression.

paronychia (par-oh-**NICK**-ee-ah) Infection alongside the nail.

parotid (pah-**ROT**-id) Parotid gland is the salivary gland beside the ear.

paroxysmal (par-ock-**SIZ**-mal) Occurring in sharp, spasmodic episodes.

particle (**PAR**-tih-kul) A small piece of matter.

particulate (par-**TIK**-you-late) Relating to a fine particle.

passive (**PASS**-iv) Not active.

patella (pah-**TELL**-ah) Thin, circular bone in front of the knee joint and embedded in the patellar tendon. Also called *kneecap.* Plural *patellae.*

patellar (pah-**TELL**-ar) Pertaining to the patella.

patent (**PAY**-tent) Open.

patent ductus arteriosus (**PAY**-tent **DUK**-tus ar-ter-ee-**OH**-sus) An open, direct channel between the aorta and the pulmonary artery.

pathogen (**PATH**-oh-jen) A disease-causing microorganism.

pathogenic (path-oh-**JEN**-ik) Causing disease.

pathologic fracture (path-oh-**LOJ**-ik **FRAK**-chur) Fracture occurring at a site already weakened by a disease process, such as cancer.

pathologist (pa-**THOL**-oh-jist) A specialist in pathology.

pathology (pa-**THOL**-oh-jee) Medical specialty dealing with the structural and functional changes of a disease process or the cause, development, and structural changes in disease.

pectoral (**PEK**-tor-al) Pertaining to the chest.

pectoral girdle (**PEK**-tor-al **GIR**-del) Incomplete bony ring that attaches the upper limb to the axial skeleton.

pectoralis (**PEK**-tor-ah-lis) Pertaining to the chest.

pedal (**PEED**-al) Pertaining to the foot.

pediatrician (**PEE**-dee-ah-**TRISH**-an) Medical specialist in pediatrics.

pediatrics (pee-dee-**AT**-riks) Medical specialty of treating children during development from birth through adolescence.

pediculosis (peh-dick-you-**LOH**-sis) An infestation with lice.

peer (PEER) A person at the same level or standing.

pelvic (**PEL**-vik) Pertaining to the pelvis.

pelvis (**PEL**-viss) A basin-shaped ring of bones, ligaments, and muscles at the base of the spine; *or* a basin-shaped cavity, as in the pelvis of the kidney.

penile (**PEE**-nile) Pertaining to the penis.

penis (**PEE**-nis) Conveys urine and semen to the outside.

pepsin (**PEP**-sin) Enzyme produced by the stomach that breaks down protein.

pepsinogen (pep-**SIN**-oh-jen) Converted by HCl in stomach to pepsin.

peptic (**PEP**-tik) Relating to the stomach and duodenum.

percutaneous (**PER**-kyu-**TAY**-nee-us) Passage through the skin.

perforated (**PER**-foh-ray-ted) Punctured with one or more holes.

perforation (per-foh-**RAY**-shun) A hole through the wall of a structure.

perfuse (per-**FYUSE**) To force blood to flow through a lumen or a vascular bed.

perfusion (per-**FYU**-zhun) The act of perfusing.

pericardial (per-ih-**KAR**-dee-al) Pertaining to the pericardium.

pericarditis (**PER**-ih-kar-**DIE**-tis) Inflammation of the pericardium, the covering of the heart.

pericardium (per-ih-**KAR**-dee-um) A double layer of membranes surrounding the heart.

perimetrium (per-ih-**ME**-tree-um) The covering of the uterus; part of the peritoneum.

perinatal (per-ih-**NAY**-tal) Around the time of birth.

perineal (**PER**-ih-**NEE**-al) Pertaining to the perineum.

perineum (**PER**-ih-**NEE**-um) Area between the thighs, extending from the coccyx to the pubis.

periodontal (**PER**-ee-oh-**DON**-tal) Around a tooth.

periodontics (**PER**-ee-oh-**DON**-tiks) Branch of dentistry specializing in disorders of tissues around the teeth.

periodontist (**PER**-ee-oh-**DON**-tist) Specialist in periodontics.

periodontitis (**PER**-ee-oh-don-**TIE**-tis) Inflammation of tissues around a tooth.

periorbital (per-ee-**OR**-bit-al) Pertaining to tissues around the orbit.

periosteal (**PER**-ee-**OSS**-tee-al) Pertaining to the periosteum.

periosteum (**PER**-ee-**OSS**-tee-um) Fibrous membrane covering a bone.

peripheral (peh-**RIF**-er-al) Pertaining to the periphery or external boundary.

peripheral vision (peh-**RIF**-er-al **VIZH**-un) Ability to see objects as they come into the outer edges of the visual field.

peristalsis (per-ih-**STAL**-sis) Waves of alternate contraction and relaxation of the muscle wall of a tube; for example, of the intestinal wall to move food along the digestive tract.

peritoneal (**PER**-ih-toe-**NEE**-al) Pertaining to the peritoneum.

peritoneum (**PER**-ih-toe-**NEE**-um) Membrane that lines the abdominal cavity.

peritonitis (**PER**-ih-toe-**NIE**-tis) Inflammation of the peritoneum.

pernicious anemia (per-**NISH**-us ah-**NEE**-me-ah) Chronic anemia due to lack of vitamin B_{12}.

pertussis (per-**TUSS**-is) Infectious disease with a spasmodic, intense cough ending on a whoop (stridor). Also called *whooping cough.*

pes planus (PES **PLAY**-nuss) A flat foot with no plantar arch.

pessary (**PES**-ah-ree) Appliance inserted into the vagina to support the uterus.

petechia (peh-**TEE**-kee-ah) Pinpoint capillary hemorrhagic spot in the skin. Plural *petechiae.*

petit mal (peh-**TEE** MAL) Old name for absence seizures.

phacoemulsification (**FAKE**-oh-ee-**MUL**-sih-fih-**KAY**-shun) Breaking down and sucking out a cataract with an ultrasonic needle.

phagocyte (**FAG**-oh-site) Blood cell that ingests and destroys foreign particles and cells.

phagocytic (fag-oh-**SIT**-ik) Pertaining to a phagocyte.

phagocytosis (**FAG**-oh-sigh-**TOE**-sis) Process of ingestion and destruction.

phalanx (**FAY**-lanks) A bone of a finger or toe. Plural *phalanges.*

pharmacist (**FAR**-mah-sist) Person licensed by the state to prepare and dispense drugs.

pharmacology (far-mah-**KOLL**-oh-jee) Science of the preparation, uses, and effects of drugs.

pharmacy (**FAR**-mah-see) Facility licensed to prepare and dispense drugs.

pharyngeal (fah-**RIN**-jee-al) Pertaining to the pharynx.

pharyngitis (fah-rin-**JIE**-tis) Inflammation of the pharynx.

pharynx (**FAH**-rinks) Tube from the back of the nose to the larynx.

phimosis (fih-**MOH**-sis) Prepuce cannot be retracted.

phlebitis (fleh-**BIE**-tis) Inflammation of a vein.

phlebotomist (fleh-**BOT**-oh-mist) Person skilled in taking blood from veins.

phlebotomy (fleh-**BOT**-oh-me) Taking blood from a vein.

phlegm (FLEM) Abnormal amounts of mucus expectorated from the respiratory tract.

phobia (**FOH**-bee-ah) Pathologic fear or dread.

photocoagulation (**FOH**-toe-koh-**AG**-you-**LAY**-shun) Using light (laser beam) to form a clot.

photophobia (foh-toe-**FOH**-bee-ah) Fear of the light because it hurts the eyes.

photophobic (foh-toe-**FOH**-bik) Pertaining to or suffering from photophobia.

photoreceptor (**FOH**-toe-ree-**SEP**-tor) A photoreceptor cell receives light and converts it into electrical impulses.

photosensitive (**FOH**-toe-**SEN**-sih-tiv) Abnormally sensitive to light.

photosensitivity (**FOH**-toe-sen-sih-**TIV**-ih-tee) Light produces pain in the eye.

phototherapy (foh-toe-**THAIR**-ah-pee) Treatment using light rays.

physiatrist (fizz-**I**-ah-trist) A physician who specilizes in physical medicine and rehabilitation.

physiatry (fizz-**I**-ah-tree) Physical medicine.

physical (**FIZZ**-ih-kal) Relating to the body.

pia mater (**PEE**-ah **MAY**-ter) Delicate inner layer of the meninges.

pica (**PIE**-kah) Eating substances not considered to be food.

pineal (**PIN**-ee-al) Pertaining to the pineal gland.

pink eye Conjunctivitis.

pinna (**PIN**-ah) Another name for *auricle*. Plural *pinnae*.

pitting edema (ee-**DEE**-mah) An indentation made by a finger in an edematous area persists for a long time.

pituitary (pih-**TYU**-ih-tar-ee) Pertaining to the pituitary gland.

placebo (plah-**SEE**-boh) An inert compound with no innate therapeutic value.

placenta (plah-**SEN**-tah) Organ that allows metabolic interchange between the mother and the fetus.

placenta abruptio (plah-**SEN**-tah ab-**RUP**-she-oh) Premature detachment of the placenta.

placenta previa (plah-**SEN**-tah **PREE**-vee-ah) Placenta obstructing the fetus during delivery.

plaque (PLAK) Patch of abnormal tissue.

plasma (**PLAZ**-mah) Fluid, noncellular component of blood.

platelet (**PLAYT**-let) Cell fragment involved in the clotting process. Also called *thrombocyte*.

pleura (**PLUR**-ah) Membrane covering the lungs and lining the ribs in the thoracic cavity. Plural *pleurae*.

pleural (**PLUR**-al) Pertaining to the pleura.

pleurisy (**PLUR**-ih-see) Inflammation of the pleura.

plexus (**PLEK**-sus) A weblike network of joined nerves. Plural *plexuses*.

pneumoconiosis (**NEW**-moh-koh-nee-**OH**-sis) Fibrotic lung disease caused by the inhalation of different dusts.

pneumonectomy (**NEW**-moh-**NECK**-toe-me) Surgical removal of a lung.

pneumonia (new-**MOH**-nee-ah) Inflammation of the lung parenchyma (tissue).

pneumonitis (new-moh-**NI**-tis) Synonym for *pneumonia*.

pneumothorax (new-moh-**THOR**-ax) Air in the pleural cavity of the chest.

podiatrist (poh-**DIE**-ah-trist) Practitioner of podiatry.

podiatry (poh-**DIE**-ah-tree) The diagnosis and treatment of disorders and injuries of the foot.

poliomyelitis (**POE**-lee-oh-**MY**-eh-lie-tis) Inflammation of the gray matter of the spinal cord, leading to paralysis of the limbs and muscles of respiration. Abbreviation *polio*.

pollutant (poh-**LOO**-tant) Substance that makes an environment unclean or impure.

pollution (poh-**LOO**-shun) Condition that is unclean, impure, and a danger to health.

polycystic (pol-ee-**SIS**-tik) Composed of many cysts.

polycythemia vera (**POL**-ee-sigh-**THEE**-me-ah **VEH**-rah) Chronic disease with bone marrow hyperplasia, increase in number of RBCs, and increase in blood volume.

polydipsia (pol-ee-**DIP**-see-ah) Excessive thirst.

polyhydramnios (**POL**-ee-high-**DRAM**-nee-os) Too much amniotic fluid.

polymenorrhea (**POL**-ee-men-oh-**REE**-ah) More than normal frequency of menses.

polymorphonuclear (**POL**-ee-more-foh-**NEW**-klee-ahr) White blood cell with a multilobed nucleus.

polymyositis (**POL**-ee-my-oh-**SIGH**-tis) Inflammation of a number of voluntary muscles simultaneously.

polyneuropathy (**POL**-ee-nyu-**ROP**-ah-thee) Disorder affecting many nerves.

polyp (**POL**-ip) Any mass of tissue that projects outward.

polypectomy (pol-ip-**ECK**-toh-mee) Excision or removal of a polyp.

polyphagia (pol-ee-**FAY**-jee-ah) Excessive eating.

polyposis (pol-ee-**POH**-sis) Presence of several polyps.

polysomnography (**POL**-ee-som-**NOG**-rah-fee) Test to monitor brain waves, muscle tension, eye movement, and oxygen levels in the blood as the patient sleeps.

polyuria (pol-ee-**YOU**-ree-ah) Excessive production of urine.

pons (PONZ) Part of the brainstem.

popliteal (pop-**LIT**-ee-al) Pertaining to the back of the knee.

popliteal fossa (pop-**LIT**-ee-al **FOSS**-ah) The hollow at the back of the knee.

portal vein (**POR**-tal) The vein that carries blood from the intestines to the liver.

postcoital (post-**KOH**-ih-tal) After sexual intercourse.

posterior (pos-**TEER**-ee-or) Pertaining to the back surface of the body; situated behind.

postictal (post-**IK**-tal) Transient neurologic deficit after a seizure.

postmature (post-mah-**TYUR**) Infant born after 42 weeks of gestation.

postmaturity (post-mah-**TYUR**-ih-tee) Condition of being postmature.

postmortem (post-**MOR**-tem) Examination of the body and organs of a dead person to determine the cause of death.

postnatal (post-**NAY**-tal) After the birth.

postpartum (post-**PAR**-tum) After childbirth.

postpolio syndrome (PPS) (post-**POE**-lee-oh **SIN**-drome) Progressive muscle weakness in a person previously affected by polio.

postprandial (post-**PRAN**-dee-al) Following a meal.

posttraumatic (post-traw-**MAT**-ik) Occurring after and caused by trauma.

Pott fracture (POT **FRAK**-shur) Fracture of the lower end of the fibula, often with fracture of the tibial malleolus.

precancerous (pree-**KAN**-ser-us) Lesion from which cancer can develop.

precipitate labor (pree-**SIP**-ih-tate **LAY**-bore) A very rapid labor and delivery.

precursor (pree-**KUR**-sir) Cell or substance formed earlier in the development of the cell or substance.

preeclampsia (pree-eh-**KLAMP**-see-uh) Hypertension, edema, and proteinuria during pregnancy.

preemie (**PREE**-me) Slang for *premature baby.*

pregnancy (**PREG**-nan-see) State of being pregnant.

pregnant (**PREG**-nant) Having conceived.

prehypertension (pree-**HIGH**-per-**TEN**-shun) Precursor to hypertension.

premature (pree-mah-**TYUR**) Occurring before the expected time; for example, an infant born before 37 weeks of gestation.

prematurity (pree-mah-**TYUR**-ih-tee) Condition of being premature.

premenstrual (pree-**MEN**-stru-al) Pertaining to the time immediately before the menses.

prenatal (pree-**NAY**-tal) Before birth.

prepatellar (pree-pah-**TELL**-ar) In front of the patella.

prepuce (**PREE**-puce) Fold of skin that covers the glans penis. Same as *foreskin.*

presbyopia (prez-bee-**OH**-pee-ah) Difficulty in nearsighted vision occurring in middle and old age.

preterm (**PREE**-term) Baby delivered before 37 weeks of gestation. Also called *premature.*

previa (**PREE**-vee-ah) Anything blocking the fetus during its birth; for example, an abnormally situated placenta, *placenta previa.*

priapism (**PRY**-ah-pizm) Persistent erection of the penis.

primary (**PRY**-mah-ree) The first of a disease or symptom, after which others may occur as complications arise.

primigravida (pry-mih-**GRAV**-ih-dah) First pregnancy.

primipara (pry-**MIP**-ah-ruh) Woman giving birth for the first time.

prion (**PREE**-on) Small infectious protein particle.

proctitis (prok-**TIE**-tis) Inflammation of the lining of the rectum.

proctoscopy (prok-**TOSS**-koh-pee) Examination of the inside of the anus by endoscopy.

progesterone (pro-**JESS**-ter-own) Hormone that prepares the uterus for pregnancy.

progestin (pro-**JESS**-tin) A synthetic form of progesterone.

prognathism (**PROG**-nah-thizm) Condition of a forward-projecting jaw.

prognosis (prog-**NO**-sis) Forecast of the probable future course and outcome of a disease.

prolactin (pro-**LAK**-tin) Pituitary hormone that stimulates the production of milk.

prolapse (pro-**LAPS**) A sinking down of an organ or tissue.

proliferate (pro-**LIF**-eh-rate) To increase in number through reproduction.

pronate (**PRO**-nate) Rotate the forearm so that the surface of the palm faces posteriorly in the anatomical position.

pronation (pro-**NAY**-shun) Process of lying face down or of turning a hand or foot with the volar (palm or sole) surface down.

prone (PRONE) Lying face down, flat on your belly.

prophylactic (pro-fih-**LAK**-tik) The act or the agent that prevents a disease.

prophylaxis (pro-fih-**LAK**-sis) Prevention of disease.

prostaglandin (**PROS**-tah-**GLAN**-din) Hormone present in many tissues but first isolated from the prostate gland.

prostate (**PROS**-tate) Organ surrounding the urethra at the base of the male urinary bladder.

prostatectomy (pros-tah-**TEK**-toe-me) Surgical removal of the prostate.

prostatic (pros-**TAT**-ik) Pertaining to the prostate.

prostatitis (pros-tah-**TIE**-tis) Inflammation of the prostate.

prosthesis (**PROS**-thee-sis) Manufactured substitute for a missing part of the body.

prosthetic (pros-**THET**-ik) Pertaining to a prosthesis.

prostrate (pros-**TRAYT**) To lay flat or to be overcome by physical weakness and exhaustion.

prostration (pros-**TRAY**-shun) To be lying flat or to be overcome by physical weakness and exhaustion.

protease (**PRO**-tee-ase) Group of enzymes that break down protein.

protein (**PRO**-teen) Class of food substances based on amino acids.

proteinuria (pro-tee-**NYU**-ree-ah) Presence of protein in urine.

prothrombin (pro-**THROM**-bin) Protein formed by the liver and converted to thrombin in the blood-clotting mechanism.

proton pump inhibitor (**PRO**-ton PUMP in-**HIB**-ih-tor) Agent that blocks the enzyme system in the lining of the stomach that produces gastric acid.

provisional diagnosis (pro-**VIZH**-un-al die-ag-**NO**-sis) A temporary diagnosis pending further examination or testing.

proximal (**PROK**-sih-mal) Situated nearest the center of the body.

pruritic (proo-**RIT**-ik) Itchy.

pruritus (proo-**RYE**-tus) Itching.

psoriasis (so-**RYE**-ah-sis) Rash characterized by reddish, silver-scaled patches.

psychedelic (sigh-keh-**DEL**-ik) An agent that intensifies sensory perception.

psychiatric (sigh-kee-**AH**-trik) Pertaining to psychiatry.

psychiatrist (sigh-**KIGH**-ah-trist) Licensed medical specialist in psychiatry.

psychiatry (sigh-**KIGH**-ah-tree) Diagnosis and treatment of mental disorders.

psychologic (sigh-koh-**LOJ**-ik) Pertaining to psychology.

psychological (sigh-koh-**LOJ**-ik-al) Pertaining to psychology.

psychologist (sigh-**KOL**-oh-jist) One who studies and becomes a specialist in psychology.

psychology (sigh-**KOL**-oh-jee) Study of the behavior of the human mind.

psychopath (**SIGH**-koh-path) Person with antisocial personality disorder.

psychosis (sigh-**KOH**-sis) Disorder causing mental disruption and loss of contact with reality.

psychosocial (**SIGH**-koh-**SOH**-shal) Involving both the mind and various social and community aspects of life.

psychosomatic (**SIGH**-koh-soh-**MAT**-ik) Disorders of the body influenced by the mind.

psychotic (sigh-**KOT**-ik) Pertaining to or affected by psychosis.

ptosis (**TOE**-sis) Sinking down of the upper eyelid or an organ.

pubarche (pyu-**BAR**-key) Development of pubic and axillary hair.

puberty (**PYU**-ber-tee) Process of maturing from child to young adult.

pubic (**PYU**-bik) Pertaining to the pubis.

pubis (**PYU**-bis) Alternative name for *pubic bone.*

puerperium (pyu-er-**PER**-ee-um) Six-week period after birth in which the uterus involutes.

pulmonary (**PULL**-moh-**NAR**-ee) Pertaining to the lungs.

pulmonologist (**PULL**-moh-**NOL**-oh-jist) Specialist in treating disorders of the lungs.

pulmonology (**PULL**-moh-**NOL**-oh-jee) Study of the lungs, or the medical specialty of disorders of the lungs.

pulp (PULP) Dental pulp is the connective tissue in the cavity in the center of the tooth.

pupil (**PYU**-pill) The opening in the center of the iris that allows light to reach the lens. Plural *pupillae.*

pupillary (**PYU**-pill-ah-ree) Pertaining to the pupil.

purge (PURJ) Consciously throw up or cause bowel evacuation.

Purkinje fibers (per-**KIN**-jee **FI**-berz) Network of nerve fibers in the myocardium.

purpura (**PUR**-pyu-rah) Skin hemorrhages that are red initially and then turn purple.

purulent (**PURE**-you-lent) Showing or containing a lot of pus.

pustule (**PUS**-tyul) Small protuberance on the skin that contains pus.

pyelitis (pie-eh-**LYE**-tis) Inflammation of the renal pelvis.

pyelogram (**PIE**-el-oh-gram) X-ray image of renal pelvis and ureters.

pyelonephritis (**PIE**-eh-loh-neh-**FRY**-tis) Inflammation of the kidney and renal pelvis.

pyloric (pie-**LOR**-ik) Pertaining to the pylorus.

pylorus (pie-**LOR**-us) Exit area of the stomach.

pyorrhea (pie-oh-**REE**-ah) Purulent discharge.

pyrexia (pie-**REK**-see-ah) An abnormally high body temperature or fever.

pyromania (pie-roh-**MAY**-nee-ah) Morbid impulse to set fires.

Q

quadrant (**KWAD**-rant) One-quarter of a circle; *or* one of four regions of the surface of the abdomen.

quadrantectomy (kwad-ran-**TEK**-toe-me) Surgical excision of a quadrant of the breast.

quadriceps femoris (**KWAD**-rih-seps **FEM**-or-is) An anterior thigh muscle with four heads.

quadriplegia (kwad-rih-**PLEE**-jee-ah) Paralysis of all four limbs.

quadriplegic (kwad-rih-**PLEE**-jik) Pertaining to or suffering from quadriplegia.

R

radial (**RAY**-dee-al) Pertaining to the forearm or to any of the structures (artery, vein, nerve) named after it; *or* diverging in all directions from any given center.

radiation (ray-dee-**AY**-shun) To spread out.

radiologic (**RAY**-dee-oh-**LOJ**-ik) Pertaining to radiology.

radiologist (ray-dee-**OL**-oh-jist) Medical specialist in the use of x-rays and other imaging techniques.

radiology (ray-dee-**OL**-oh-jee) Study of medical imaging.

radius (**RAY**-dee-us) The forearm bone on the thumb side.

rale (RAHL) Crackle heard through a stethoscope when air bubbles through liquid in the lungs. Plural *rales.*

rash (RASH) Skin eruption.

rectocele (**RECK**-toe-seal) Hernia of the rectum into the vagina.

rectum (**RECK**-tum) Terminal part of the colon from the sigmoid to the anal canal.

reduction (ree-**DUCK**-shun) Restore a structure to its normal position.

reflex (**REE**-fleks) An involuntary response to a stimulus.

reflux (**REE**-fluks) Backward flow.

refract (ree-**FRAKT**) Make a change in the direction of, or bend, a ray of light.

refraction (ree-**FRAKT**-shun) The bending of light.

regenerate (ree-**JEN**-eh-rate) Reconstitution of a lost part.

regeneration (ree-**JEN**-eh-**RAY**-shun) The process of reconstitution.

regulate (**REG**-you-late) To control the way in which a process progresses.

regulation (**REG**-you-**LAY**-shun) Control of the way in which a process progresses.

regurgitate (ree-**GUR**-jih-tate) To flow backward; for example, blood through a heart valve.

regurgitation (ree-gur-jih-**TAY**-shun) Expel contents of the stomach into the mouth, short of vomiting.

rehabilitation (**REE**-hah-bill-ih-**TAY**-shun) Therapeutic restoration of an ability to function as before.

remission (ree-**MISH**-un) Period when there is a lessening or absence of the symptoms of a disease.

renal (**REE**-nal) Pertaining to the kidney.

replication (rep-lih-**KAY**-shun) Reproduction to produce an exact copy.

reproduction (ree-pro-**DUK**-shun) The process by which organisms produce offspring.

reproductive (ree-pro-**DUK**-tiv) Pertaining to reproduction.

resection (ree-**SEK**-shun) Removal of a specific part of an organ or structure.

resectoscope (ree-**SEK**-toe-skope) Endoscope for transurethral removal of lesions of the prostate.

residual (reh-**ZID**-you-al) Pertaining to anything left over.

resistance (reh-**ZIS**-tants) Ability of an organism to withstand the effects of an antagonistic agent.

resistant (reh-**ZIS**-tant) Able to resist.

respiration (**RES**-pih-**RAY**-shun) Process of breathing; fundamental process of life used to exchange oxygen and carbon dioxide.

respirator (**RES**-pih-**RAY**-tor) Another name for *ventilator.*

respiratory (**RES**-pih-rah-tor-ee) Pertaining to respiration.

retention (ree-**TEN**-shun) Holding back in the body what should normally be discharged (e.g., urine).

retina (**RET**-ih-nah) Light-sensitive innermost layer of the eyeball.

retinal (**RET**-ih-nal) Pertaining to the retina.

retinoblastoma (**RET**-in-oh-blas-**TOE**-mah) Malignant neoplasm of primitive retinal cells.

retinoids (**RET**-ih-noydz) Keratolytic agents applied for psoriasis, acne, and photodamage.

retinopathy (ret-ih-**NOP**-ah-thee) Any disease of the retina.

retrograde (**RET**-roh-grade) Reversal of a normal flow; for example, back from the bladder into the ureters.

retroversion (reh-troh-**VER**-zhun) Tipping backward of the uterus.

retroverted (**REH**-troh-vert-ed) Tilted backward.

retrovirus (**REH**-troh-vie-rus) Virus with an RNA core.

rhesus factor (**REE**-sus **FAK**-tor) An antigen on the surface of red blood cells of Rh +ve individuals. First discovered in Rhesus monkeys.

rheumatic (ru-**MA**-tik) Pertaining to or affected by rheumatism.

rheumatism (**RU**-ma-tizm) Pain in various parts of the musculoskeletal system.

rheumatoid arthritis (RA) (**RU**-mah-toyd ar-**THRI**-tis) Disease of connective tissue, with arthritis as a major manifestation.

rhinitis (rye-**NIE**-tis) Inflammation of the nasal mucosa. Also called *coryza*.

rhinoplasty (**RYE**-no-plas-tee) Surgical procedure to change size or shape of the nose.

rhonchus (**RONG**-kuss) Wheezing sound heard on auscultation of the lungs; made by air passing through a constricted lumen. Plural *rhonchi*.

ribonucleic acid (RNA) (**RYE**-boh-nyu-**KLEE**-ik **ASS**-id) Information carrier from DNA in the nucleus to an organelle to produce protein molecules.

ribosome (**RYE**-boh-sohm) Structure in the cell that assembles amino acids into protein.

rickets (**RICK**-ets) Disease due to vitamin D deficiency, producing soft, flexible bones.

rigidity (ri-**JID**-ih-tee) Increased muscle tone at rest.

Rinne test (**RIN**-eh) Test for conductive hearing loss.

root (ROOT) Fundamental or beginning part of a structure.

rooting (**RUE**-ting) A neonatal reflex to turn toward the nipple and open the mouth when a nipple is placed on the cheek.

rosacea (roh-**ZAY**-she-ah) Persistent erythematous rash of the central face.

rotator cuff (roh-**TAY**-tor CUFF) Part of the capsule of the shoulder joint.

rumination (roo-min-**NAY**-shun) To bring back food into the mouth to chew over and over.

rupture (**RUP**-tyur) Break or tear of any organ or body part.

S

sacral (**SAY**-kral) Pertaining to or in the neighborhood of the sacrum.

sacroiliac joint (say-kroh-**ILL**-ih-ak JOINT) The joint between the sacrum and the ilium.

sacrum (**SAY**-crum) Segment of the vertebral column that forms part of the pelvis.

sagittal (**SAJ**-ih-tal) Vertical plane through the body dividing it into right and left portions.

saline (**SAY**-leen) Salt solution, usually sodium chloride.

saliva (sa-**LIE**-vah) Secretion in the mouth from salivary glands.

salivary (**SAL**-ih-var-ee) Pertaining to saliva.

salpingectomy (sal-pin-**JEK**-toe-me) Surgical excision of a fallopian tube.

salpingitis (sal-pin-**JIE**-tis) Inflammation of the uterine tube.

saphenous (**SAPH**-ih-nus) Relating to the saphenous vein in the thigh.

sarcoidosis (sar-koy-**DOH**-sis) Granulomatous lesions of the lungs and other organs; cause is unknown.

sarcoma (sar-**KOH**-mah) A malignant tumor originating in connective tissue.

sarcopenia (sar-koh-**PEE**-nee-ah) Progressive loss of muscle mass and strength with aging.

saturated fatty acid (**SATCH**-you-ray-ted **FAT**-ee **ASS**-id) Lipid that is incapable of absorbing any more hydrogen.

scab (SKAB) Crust that forms over a wound or sore during healing.

scabies (**SKAY**-beez) Skin disease produced by mites.

scald (SKAWLD) Burn from contact with hot liquid or steam.

scapula (**SKAP**-you-lah) Shoulder blade. Plural *scapulae*.

scapular (**SKAP**-you-lar) Pertaining to the scapula.

scar (SKAR) Fibrotic seam that forms when a wound heals.

schizophrenia (skitz-oh-**FREE**-nee-ah) Disorder of perception, thought, emotion, and behavior.

Schwann cell (SHWANN SELL) Connective tissue cell of the peripheral nervous system that forms a myelin sheath.

sclera (**SKLAIR**-ah) Fibrous outer covering of the eyeball and the white of the eye.

scleral (**SKLAIR**-al) Pertaining to the sclera.

scleritis (sklair-**RI**-tis) Inflammation of the sclera.

scleroderma (sklair-oh-**DERM**-ah) Thickening and hardening of the skin due to new collagen formation.

sclerose (skleh-**ROSE**) To harden or thicken.

sclerosis (skleh-**ROH**-sis) Thickening or hardening of a tissue; in the nervous system, hardening of nervous tissue by fibrous and glial connective tissue.

sclerotherapy (**SKLAIR**-oh-**THAIR**-ah-pee) Injection of a solution into a vein to thrombose it.

scoliosis (skoh-lee-**OH**-sis) An abnormal lateral curvature of the vertebral column.

scoliotic (**SKOH**-lee-**OT**-ik) Pertaining to or suffering from scoliosis.

scrotal (**SKRO**-tal) Pertaining to the scrotum.

scrotum (**SKRO**-tum) Sac containing testes.

seasonal affective disorder (see-**ZON**-al af-**FEK**-tiv dis-**OR**-der) Depression that occurs at the same time every year, often in winter.

sebaceous glands (seh-**BAY**-shus GLANZ) Glands in the dermis that open into hair follicles and secrete an oily fluid called *sebum*.

seborrhea (seb-oh-**REE**-ah) Excessive amount of sebum.

seborrheic (seb-oh-**REE**-ik) Pertaining to seborrhea.

sebum (**SEE**-bum) Waxy secretion of the sebaceous glands.

secondary (**SEK**-ond-ah-ree) Diseases or symptoms following a primary disease or symptom.

secrete (seh-**KREET**) To produce a chemical substance in a cell and release it from the cell.

secretion (seh-**KREE**-shun) The production of a chemical substance in a cell and its release from the cell.

sedation (seh-**DAY**-shun) State of being calmed.

sedative (**SED**-ah-tiv) Agent that calms nervous excitement.

segment (**SEG**-ment) A section of an organ or structure.

segmentectomy (seg-men-**TEK**-toe-me) Surgical excision of a segment of a tissue or organ.

seizure (**SEE**-zhur) Event due to excessive electrical activity in the brain.

self-examination (**SELF**-ek-zam-ih-**NAY**-shun) Conduct an examination of one's own body.

self-mutilation (self-myu-tih-**LAY**-shun) Injury or disfigurement made to one's own body.

semen (**SEE**-men) Penile ejaculate containing sperm and seminal fluid.

semilunar (sem-ee-**LOO**-nar) Appears like a half moon.

seminal vesicle (**SEM**-in-al **VES**-ih-kull) Sac of the ductus deferens that produces seminal fluid.

seminiferous (sem-ih-**NIF**-er-us) Pertaining to carrying semen.

seminiferous tubule (sem-ih-**NIF**-er-us **TU**-byul) Coiled tubes in the testes that produce sperm.

seminoma (sem-ih-**NO**-mah) Neoplasm of germ cells of a testis.

senescence (seh-**NES**-ens) The state of being old.

senescent (seh-**NES**-ent) Growing old.

senile (**SEE**-nile) Characteristic of old age.

senility (seh-**NIL**-ih-tee) Mental disorders occurring in old age.

sensation (sen-**SAY**-shun) The conscious feeling of the effects of a stimulation.

sensorineural hearing loss (**SEN**-sor-ih-**NYUR**-al) Hearing loss caused by lesions of the inner ear or the auditory nerve.

sensory (**SEN**-soh-ree) Having the function of sensation; structures of the nervous system that carry impulses to the brain.

sepsis (**SEP**-sis) Presence of pathogenic organisms or their toxins in blood or tissues.

septicemia (sep-tih-**SEE**-mee-ah) Microorganisms circulating in, and infecting, the blood (blood poisoning).

septum (**SEP**-tum) A thin wall separating two cavities or tissue masses. Plural *septa*.

serotonin (ser-oh-**TOE**-nin) A neurotransmitter in the central and peripheral nervous systems.

serum (**SEER**-um) Fluid remaining after removal of cells and fibrin clot from blood.

shock (SHOCK) Sudden physical or mental collapse or circulatory collapse.

shunt (SHUNT) A bypass or diversion of fluid; for example, blood.

sigmoid (**SIG**-moyd) Sigmoid colon is shaped like an "S."

sigmoidoscopy (sig-moi-**DOS**-koh-pee) Endoscopic examination of the sigmoid colon.

sign (SINE) Physical evidence of a disease process.

silicosis (sil-ih-**KOH**-sis) Fibrotic lung disease from inhaling silica particles.

sinoatrial (SA) node (sigh-noh-**AY**-tree-al NODE) The center of modified cardiac muscle fibers in the wall of the right atrium that acts as the pacemaker for the heart rhythm.

sinus (**SIGH**-nus) Cavity or hollow space in a bone or other tissue.

sinus rhythm (**SIGH**-nus **RITH**-um) The normal (optimal) heart rhythm arising from the sinoatrial node.

sinusitis (sigh-nyu-**SIGH**-tis) Inflammation of the lining of a sinus.

Sjogren syndrome (**SHER**-gren **SIN**-drome) Dryness of the mucous membranes of the eye and mouth.

skeletal (**SKEL**-eh-tal) Pertaining to the skeleton.

skeleton (**SKEL**-eh-ton) The bony framework of the body.

Skene glands (SKEEN GLANZ) Paraurethral glands in the anterior wall of the vagina. Also called *paraurethral glands*.

smegma (**SMEG**-mah) Oily material produced by the glans and prepuce.

Snellen letter chart (**SNEL**-en) Test for acuity of distance vision.

snore (SNOR) Noise produced by vibrations in the structures of the nasopharynx.

sociopath (**SOH**-see-oh-path) Person with antisocial personality disorder.

somatic (soh-**MAT**-ik) Relating to the body in general; *or* a division of the peripheral nervous system serving the skeletal muscles.

somatostatin (**SOH**-mah-toh-**STAT**-in) Hormone that inhibits release of growth hormone and insulin.

somatotrophin (**SOH**-mah-toh-**TROH**-phin) Hormone of the anterior pituitary that stimulates the growth of body tissues. Also called *growth hormone*.

spasm (SPASM) Sudden involuntary contraction of a muscle group.

spasmodic (spaz-**MOD**-ik) Intermittent contractions.

spastic (**SPAS**-tik) Increased muscle tone on movement.

specific (speh-**SIF**-ik) Relating to a particular entity.

specificity (spes-ih-**FIS**-ih-tee) State of having a fixed relation to a particular entity.

sperm (SPERM) Mature male sex cell. Also called *spermatozoon*.

spermatic (**SPER**-mat-ik) Pertaining to sperm.

spermatid (**SPER**-mat-id) A cell late in the development process of sperm.

spermatocele (**SPER**-mat-oh-seal) Cyst of the epididymis that contains sperm.

spermatogenesis (**SPER**-mat-oh-**JEN**-eh-sis) The process by which male germ cells differentiate into sperm.

spermatozoa (**SPER**-mat-oh-**ZOH**-ah) Sperm (plural of *spermatozoon*).

spermicidal (sper-mih-**SIGH**-dal) Pertaining to the killing of sperm; *or* destructive to sperm.

spermicide (**SPER**-mih-side) Agent that destroys sperm.

sphenoid (**SFEE**-noyd) Wedge-shaped bone at the base of the skull.

sphincter (**SFINK**-ter) Band of muscle that encircles an opening; when it contracts, the opening squeezes closed.

sphygmomanometer (**SFIG**-moh-mah-**NOM**-ih-ter) Instrument for measuring arterial blood pressure.

spina bifida (**SPY**-nah **BIH**-fih-dah) Failure of one or more vertebral arches to close during fetal development.

spina bifida cystica (**SIS**-tik-ah) Meninges and spinal cord protruding through the absent vertebral arch and having the appearance of a cyst.

spina bifida occulta (**OH**-kul-tah) The deformity of the vertebral arch is not apparent from the surface.

spinal (**SPY**-nal) Pertaining to the spine.

spinal tap (**SPY**-nal TAP) Placement of a needle through an intervertebral space into the subarachnoid space to withdraw CSF.

spine (SPINE) The vertebral column; *or* a short bony projection.

spiral fracture (**SPY**-ral **FRAK**-chur) A fracture in the shape of a coil.

spirochete (**SPY**-roh-keet) Spiral-shaped bacterium causing a sexually transmitted disease (syphilis).

spirometer (spy-**ROM**-eh-ter) An instrument used to measure respiratory volumes.

spirometry (spy-**ROM**-eh-tree) Use of a spirometer.

spleen (SPLEEN) Vascular, lymphatic organ in the left upper quadrant of the abdomen.

splenectomy (sple-**NECK**-toe-me) Surgical removal of the spleen.

splenomegaly (sple-noh-**MEG**-ah-lee) Enlarged spleen.

spondylosis (spon-dih-**LOH**-sis) Degenerative osteoarthritis of the spine.

spongiosum (spun-jee-**OH**-sum) Spongelike tissue.

sprain (SPRAIN) A wrench or tear in a ligament.

sputum (**SPYU**-tum) Matter coughed up and spat out by individuals with respiratory disorders.

squamous cell (**SKWAY**-mus SELL) Flat, scalelike epithelial cell.

stabilize (**STAY**-bill-ize) To make or hold firm or steady.

stable (**STAY**-bel) Steady, not varying.

stage (STAYJ) Definition of the extent and dissemination of a malignant neoplasm.

staging (**STAY**-jing) Process of determination of the extent of the distribution of a neoplasm.

stapes (**STAY**-peez) Inner (medial) one of the three ossicles of the middle ear; shaped like a stirrup.

Staphylococcus (**STAF**-ih-loh-**KOK**-us) Genus of gram-positive bacteria that divide in more than one plane to form clusters. Plural *staphylococci.*

starch (STARCH) Complex carbohydrate made of multiple units of glucose attached together.

stasis (**STAY**-sis) Stagnation in the flow of any body fluid.

status (**STAT**-us) A state or condition.

status epilepticus (**STAT**-us ep-ih-**LEP**-tik-us) Latin phrase for being in a prolonged or recurrent seizure for longer than a specific time frame.

stem cell (STEM SELL) Undifferentiated cell found in a differentiated tissue that can divide to yield the specialized cells in that tissue.

stenosis (steh-**NOH**-sis) Narrowing of a canal or passage.

stent (STENT) Wire-mesh tube used to keep arteries open.

stereopsis (ster-ee-**OP**-sis) Three-dimensional vision.

stereotactic (**STER**-ee-oh-**TAK**-tic) A precise three-dimensional method to locate a lesion.

stereotype (**STER**-ee-oh-tipe) An image held in common by members of a group.

sterile (**STER**-il) Free from all living organisms and their spores; *or* unable to fertilize or reproduce.

sterility (ster-**RIL**-ih-tee) Inability to reproduce.

sterilization (**STER**-ih-lih-**ZAY**-shun) Process of making sterile.

sterilize (**STER**-ih-lize) To make sterile.

sternum (**STIR**-num) Long, flat bone forming the center of the anterior wall of the chest.

steroid (**STAIR**-oyd) Large family of chemical substances found in many drugs, hormones, and body components.

stethoscope (**STETH**-oh-skope) Instrument for listening to cardiac and respiratory sounds.

stimulant (**STIM**-you-lant) Agent that excites or strengthens.

stimulation (stim-you-**LAY**-shun) Arousal to increased functional activity.

stimulus (**STIM**-you-lus) Something that excites or strengthens the functional activity of an organ or part. Plural *stimuli.*

stoma (**STOW**-mah) Artificial opening.

strabismus (strah-**BIZ**-mus) Turning of an eye away from its normal position.

strain (STRAIN) Overstretch or tear in a muscle or tendon.

stratum basale (**STRAH**-tum bay-**SAL**-eh) Deepest layer of the epidermis, from which the other cells originate and migrate.

Streptococcus (strep-toe-**KOK**-us) Genus of gram-positive bacteria that grow in chains. Plural *streptococci.*

striated muscle (**STRI**-ay-ted **MUSS**-el) Another term for *skeletal muscle.*

stricture (**STRICK**-shur) Narrowing of a tube.

stridor (**STRY**-door) High-pitched noise made when there is a respiratory obstruction in the larynx or trachea.

stroke (STROHK) Acute clinical event caused by impaired cerebral circulation.

STYE (STEYE) Infection of an eyelash follicle.

subarachnoid space (sub-ah-**RACK**-noyd SPACE) Space between the pia mater and the arachnoid membrane.

subclavian (sub-**CLAY**-vee-an) Underneath the clavicle.

subcutaneous (sub-kew-**TAY**-nee-us) Below the skin. Also called *hypodermic.*

subdural space (sub-**DYU**-ral SPASE) Space between the arachnoid and dura mater layers of the meninges.

sublingual (sub-**LING**-wal) Underneath the tongue.

subluxation (sub-luck-**SAY**-shun) An incomplete dislocation when some contact between the joint surfaces remains.

submandibular (sub-man-**DIB**-you-lar) Underneath the mandible.

submucosa (sub-mew-**KOH**-sa) Tissue layer underneath the mucosa.

substernal (sub-**STER**-nal) Under (behind) the sternum or breastbone.

suction (**SUK**-shun) Use of a catheter to clear the upper airway or other tubes.

sulcus (**SUL**-cuss) Groove on the surface of the cerebral hemispheres that separates gyri. Plural *sulci.*

superficial (soo-per-**FISH**-al) Situated near the surface.

superior (soo-**PEER**-ee-or) Situated above.

supinate (**SOO**-pih-nate) Rotate the forearm so that the surface of the palm faces anteriorly in the anatomical position.

supination (soo-pih-**NAY**-shun) Process of lying face upward or of turning a hand or foot so that the palm or sole is facing up.

supine (soo-**PINE**) Lying face up, flat on your spine.

suprapubic (**SOO**-prah-pyu-bik) Above the symphysis pubis.

surfactant (sir-**FAK**-tant) A protein and fat compound that creates surface tension to hold the lung alveolar walls apart.

suture (**SOO**-chur) Two bones are joined together by a fibrous band continuous with their periosteum, as in the skull; *or* a stitch to hold the edges of a wound together; *or* to stitch the edges of a wound together. Plural *sutures.*

sympathetic (sim-pah-**THET**-ik) Division of the autonomic nervous system operating at an unconscious level.

sympathy (**SIM**-pah-thee) Appreciation and concern for another person's mental and emotional state.

symphysis (**SIM**-feh-sis) Two bones joined by fibrocartilage. Plural *symphyses*.

symptom (**SIMP**-tum) Departure from the normal experienced by a patient.

symptomatic (simp-toe-**MAT**-ik) Pertaining to the symptoms of a disease.

synapse (**SIN**-aps) Junction between two nerve cells or a nerve fiber and its target cell, where electrical impulses are transmitted between the cells.

syncope (**SIN**-koh-pee) Temporary loss of consciousness and posture due to diminished cerebral blood flow.

syndesmosis (sin-dez-**MOH**-sis) Binding together of two bones with ligaments. Plural *syndesmoses*.

syndrome (**SIN**-drohm) Combination of signs and symptoms associated with a particular disease process.

synovial (si-**NOH**-vee-al) Pertaining to synovial fluid and the synovial membrane.

synthesis (**SIN**-the-sis) The process of building a compound from different elements.

synthetic (sin-**THET**-ik) Built up or put together from simpler compounds.

syphilis (**SIF**-ih-lis) Sexually transmitted disease caused by a spirochete.

syringomyelia (sih-**RING**-oh-my-**EE**-lee-ah) Abnormal longitudinal cavities in the spinal cord that cause paresthesias and muscle weakness.

systemic (sis-**TEM**-ik) Relating to the entire organism.

systemic lupus erythematosus (sis-**TEM**-ik **LOO**-pus er-ih-**THEE**-mah-toe-sus) Inflammatory connective tissue disease affecting the whole body.

systole (**SIS**-toe-lee) Contraction of the heart muscle.

systolic (sis-**TOL**-ik) Pertaining to systole.

T

tachycardia (tack-ih-**KAR**-dee-ah) Rapid heart rate (above 100 beats per minute).

tachypnea (tack-ip-**NEE**-ah) Rapid breathing.

talipes (**TAL**-ip-eze) Deformity of the foot involving the talus.

talus (**TAY**-luss) The tarsal bone that articulates with the tibia to form the ankle joint.

tampon (**TAM**-pon) Plug or pack in a cavity to absorb or stop bleeding.

tamponade (tam-poh-**NAID**) Pathologic compression of an organ, such as the heart.

tapeworm (**TAPE**-worm) Intestinal parasitic worm.

tarsal (**TAR**-sal) Pertaining to the tarsus.

tarsus (**TAR**-sus) The collection of seven bones in the foot that form the ankle and instep; *or* the flat fibrous plate that gives shape to the outer edges of the eyelids.

tartar (**TAR**-tar) Calcified deposit at the gingival margin of the teeth.

Tay-Sachs disease (TAY SAKS diz-**EEZ**) Congenital fatal disorder of fat metabolism.

temperament (**TEM**-per-ah-ment) Predisposition to character or personality.

temporal (**TEM**-pore-al) Bone that forms part of the base and sides of the skull.

temporal lobe (**TEM**-pore-al LOBE) Posterior two-thirds of the cerebral hemispheres.

temporomandibular joint (TMJ) (**TEM**-pore-oh-man-**DIB**-you-lar JOYNT) The joint between the temporal bone and the mandible.

tendinitis (ten-dih-**NYE**-tis) Inflammation of a tendon. Also spelled *tendonitis*.

tendon (**TEN**-dun) Fibrous band that connects muscle to bone.

tenosynovitis (**TEN**-oh-sin-oh-**VIE**-tis) Inflammation of a tendon and its surrounding synovial sheath.

teratogen (**TER**-ah-toe-jen) Agent that produces fetal deformities.

teratogenesis (**TER**-ah-toe-**JEN**-eh-sis) Process involved in producing fetal deformities.

teratogenic (**TER**-ah-toe-**JEN**-ik) Pertaining to or capable of producing fetal deformities.

teratoma (ter-ah-**TOE**-mah) Neoplasm of a testis or ovary containing multiple tissues from other sites in the body.

testicle (**TES**-tih-kul) One of the male reproductive glands. Also called *testis*.

testicular (tes-**TICK**-you-lar) Pertaining to the testicle.

testis (**TES**-tis) A synonym for *testicle*. Plural *testes*.

testosterone (tes-**TOSS**-ter-own) Powerful androgen produced by the testes.

tetany (**TET**-ah-nee) Severe muscle twitches, cramps, and spasms.

tetralogy of Fallot (TOF) (te-**TRA**-loh-jee ov fah-**LOW**) Set of four congenital heart defects occurring together.

thalamus (**THAL**-ah-mus) Mass of gray matter underneath the ventricle in each cerebral hemisphere.

thalassemia (thal-ah-**SEE**-mee-ah) Group of inherited blood disorders that produce a hemolytic anemia.

thelarche (thee-**LAR**-key) Onset of breast development.

thenar (**THAY**-nar) The thenar eminence is the fleshy mass at the base of the thumb.

therapeutic (**THAIR**-ah-**PYU**-tik) Pertaining to the treatment of a disease or disorder.

therapy (**THAIR**-ah-pee) Systematic treatment of a disease, dysfunction, or disorder.

thoracentesis (**THOR**-ah-sen-**TEE**-sis) Insertion of a needle into the pleural cavity to withdraw fluid or air. Also called *pleural tap*.

thoracic (**THOR**-ass-ik) Pertaining to the chest (thorax).

thoracic cavity (**THOR**-ass-ik **KAV**-ih-tee) Space within the chest containing the lungs, heart, aorta, venae cavae, esophagus, trachea, and pulmonary vessels.

thoracoscopy (thor-ah-**KOS**-koh-pee) Examination of the pleural cavity with an endoscope.

thoracotomy (thor-ah-**KOT**-oh-me) Incision through the chest wall.

thorax (**THOR**-acks) The part of the trunk between the abdomen and the neck.

thrombin (**THROM**-bin) Enzyme that forms fibrin.

thrombocyte (**THROM**-boh-site) Another name for *platelet*.

thrombocytic (**THROM**-bo-**SIT**-ik) Pertaining to a thrombocyte (platelet).

thrombocytopenia (**THROM**-boh-site-oh-**PEE**-nee-uh) Deficiency of platelets in circulating blood.

thromboembolism (THROM-boh-EM-boh-lizm) A piece of detached blood clot (embolus) blocking a distant blood vessel.

thrombolysis (throm-BOH-lih-sis) Dissolving of a thrombus (clot).

thrombolytic (throm-boh-LIT-ik) Able to dissolve a thrombus.

thrombophlebitis (THROM-boh-fleh-BY-tis) Inflammation of a vein with clot formation.

thrombosis (throm-BOH-sis) Formation of a thrombus.

thrombus (THROM-bus) A clot attached to a diseased blood vessel or heart lining. Plural *thrombi*.

thrush (THRUSH) Infection with *Candida albicans.*

thymectomy (thigh-MEK-toe-me) Surgical removal of the thymus gland.

thymoma (thigh-MOH-mah) Benign tumor of the thymus.

thymus (THIGH-mus) Lymphoid and endocrine gland located in the mediastinum.

thyroid (THIGH-royd) Endocrine gland in the neck; *or* a cartilage of the larynx.

thyroid hormone (THIGH-royd HOR-mohn) Collective term for the two thyroid hormones, T3 and T4.

thyroid storm (THIGH-royd STORM) Medical crisis and emergency due to excess thyroid hormones.

thyroidectomy (thigh-royd-ECK-toe-me) Surgical removal of the thyroid gland.

thyroiditis (thigh-royd-EYE-tis) Inflammation of the thyroid gland.

thyrotoxicosis (THIGH-roe-toks-ih-KOH-sis) Disorder produced by excessive thyroid hormone production.

thyrotropin (thigh-roe-TROH-pin) Hormone from the anterior pituitary gland that stimulates function of the thyroid gland.

thyroxine (thigh-ROCK-sin) Thyroid hormone T4, tetraiodothyronine.

tibia (TIB-ee-ah) The larger bone of the lower leg.

tibial (TIB-ee-al) Pertaining to the tibia.

tic (TIK) Sudden, involuntary, repeated contraction of muscles.

tic douloureux (tik duh-luh-RUE) Painful, sudden, spasmodic involuntary contractions of the facial muscles supplied by the trigeminal nerve. Also called *trigeminal neuralgia.*

tinea (TIN-ee-ah) General term for a group of related skin infections caused by different species of fungi.

tinnitus (TIN-ih-tus) Persistent ringing, whistling, clicking, or booming noise in the ears.

tissue (TISH-you) Collection of similar cells.

tolerance (TOL-er-ans) The capacity to become accustomed to a stimulus or drug.

tomography (toe-MOG-rah-fee) Radiographic image of a selected slice of tissue.

tone (TONE) Tension present in resting muscles.

tongue (TUNG) Mobile muscle mass in the mouth; bears the taste buds.

tonic (TON-ik) State of muscular contraction.

tonic-clonic (TON-ik-KLON-ik) The body alternates between excessive muscular rigidity (tonic) and jerking muscular contractions (clonic).

tonic-clonic seizure (TON-ik-KLON-ik SEE-zhur) Generalized seizure due to epileptic activity in all or most of the brain.

tonometer (toe-NOM-eh-ter) Instrument for determining intraocular pressure.

tonometry (toe-NOM-eh-tree) The measurement of intraocular pressure.

tonsil (TON-sill) Mass of lymphoid tissue on either side of the throat at the back of the tongue.

tonsillectomy (ton-sih-LEK-toh-me) Surgical removal of the tonsils.

tonsillitis (ton-sih-LIE-tis) Inflammation of the tonsils.

topical (TOP-ih-kal) Medication applied to the skin to obtain a local effect.

torsion (TOR-shun) The act or result of twisting.

Tourette syndrome (tur-ET SIN-drome) Disorder of multiple motor and vocal tics.

toxic (TOK-sick) Pertaining to a toxin.

toxicity (tok-SIS-ih-tee) The state of being poisonous.

toxin (TOK-sin) Poisonous substance formed by a cell or organism.

trachea (TRAY-kee-ah) Air tube from the larynx to the bronchi.

tracheal (TRAY-kee-al) Pertaining to the trachea.

tracheostomy (tray-kee-OST-oh-me) Incision into the windpipe into which a tube can be inserted to assist breathing.

tracheotomy (tray-kee-OT-oh-me) Incision made into the trachea to create a tracheostomy.

tract (TRACKT) Bundle of nerve fibers with a common origin and destination.

traction (TRAK-shun) Pulling or dragging force.

trait (TRAYT) A discrete characteristic that has a known quality.

tranquilizer (TRANG-kwih-lie-zer) Agent that calms without sedating or depressing.

transdermal (tranz-DER-mal) Going across or through the skin.

transfusion (tranz-FYU-zhun) Transfer of blood or a blood component from donor to recipient.

transplant (TRANZ-plant) The tissue or organ used; *or* the act of transferring tissue from one person to another.

transplantation (TRANZ-plan-TAY-shun) The moving of tissue or an organ from one person or place to another.

transthoracic (tranz-thor-ASS-ik) Going through the chest wall.

transurethral (TRANZ-you-REE-thral) Procedure performed through the urethra.

transverse (tranz-VERS) Horizontal plane dividing the body into upper and lower portions.

transverse fracture (tranz-VERS FRAK-chur) A fracture perpendicular to the long axis of the bone.

tremor (TREM-or) Small, shaking, involuntary, repetitive movements of hands, extremities, neck, or jaw.

triceps brachii (TRY-sepz BRAY-key-eye) Muscle of the arm that has three heads or points of origin.

Trichomonas (trik-oh-MOH-nas) A parasite causing an STD.

trichomoniasis (TRIK-oh-moh-NIE-ah-sis) Infection with *Trichomonas vaginalis.*

tricuspid (try-KUSS-pid) Having three points; a tricuspid heart valve has three flaps.

trigeminal (try-GEM-in-al) The fifth (V) cranial nerve, which has three branches supplying the face.

triglyceride (try-GLISS-eh-ride) Lipid containing three fatty acids.

trimester (TRY-mes-ter) One-third of the length of a full-term pregnancy.

triplegia (try-**PLEE**-jee-ah) Paralysis of three limbs.

triplegic (try-**PLEE**-jik) Pertaining to or suffering from triplegia.

trochanter (troh-**KAN**-ter) One of two bony prominences near the head of the femur.

tropic (**TROH**-pik) Tropic hormones stimulate other endocrine glands to produce hormones.

tuberculosis (too-**BER**-kyu-**LOW**-sis) Infectious disease that can infect any organ or tissue.

tumor (**TOO**-mor) Any abnormal swelling.

tunica (**TYU**-nih-kah) A covering layer in the wall of a blood vessel or other tubular structure.

tunica vaginalis (**TYU**-nih-kah vaj-ih-**NAHL**-iss) The sheath of the testis and epididymis.

tympanic (tim-**PAN**-ik) Pertaining to the tympanic membrane (eardrum) or tympanic cavity.

tympanostomy (tim-pan-**OS**-toe-me) Surgically created new opening in the tympanic membrane to allow fluid to drain from the middle ear.

U

ulna (**UL**-nah) The medial and larger of the bones of the forearm.

ulnar (**UL**-nar) Pertaining to the ulna or to any of the structures (artery, vein, nerve) named after it.

ultrasonography (**UL**-trah-soh-**NOG**-rah-fee) Delineation of deep structures using sound waves.

ultraviolet (ul-trah-**VIE**-oh-let) Light rays at a higher frequency than the violet end of the spectrum.

umbilical (um-**BILL**-ih-kal) Pertaining to the umbilicus or the center of the abdomen.

umbilicus (um-**BILL**-ih-kuss) Pit in the abdomen where the umbilical cord entered the fetus.

unilateral (you-nih-**LAT**-er-al) Pertaining to one side.

urea (you-**REE**-ah) End product of nitrogen metabolism.

uremia (you-**REE**-me-ah) The complex of symptoms arising from renal failure.

ureter (you-**REE**-ter) Tube that connects a kidney to the urinary bladder.

ureteral (you-**REE**-ter-al) Pertaining to the ureter.

ureteroscope (you-**REE**-ter-oh-scope) Endoscope to view the inside of the ureter.

ureteroscopy (you-**REE**-ter-**OS**-koh-pee) To examine the ureter.

urethra (you-**REE**-thra) Canal leading from the bladder to the outside.

urethritis (you-ree-**THRI**-tis) Inflammation of the urethra.

urinalysis (yur-ih-**NAL**-ih-sis) Examination of urine to separate it into its elements and define their kind and/or quantity.

urinary (**YUR**-in-ary) Pertaining to urine.

urinate (**YUR**-in-ate) To pass urine.

urination (yur-ih-**NAY**-shun) The act of passing urine.

urine (**YUR**-in) Fluid and dissolved substances excreted by the kidney.

urological (yur-oh-**LOJ**-ih-kal) Pertaining to urology.

urologist (you-**ROL**-oh-jist) Medical specialist in disorders of the urinary system.

urology (you-**ROL**-oh-jee) Medical specialty of disorders of the urinary system.

urticaria (ur-tee-**KARE**-ee-ah) Rash of itchy wheals (hives).

uterine (**YOU**-ter-in) Pertaining to the uterus.

uterus (**YOU**-ter-us) Organ in which a fertilized egg develops into a fetus.

uvea (**YOU**-vee-ah) Middle coat of the eyeball—includes the iris, ciliary body, and choroid.

uveitis (you-vee-**EYE**-tis) Inflammation of the uvea.

uvula (**YOU**-vyu-lah) Fleshy projection of the soft palate.

V

vaccinate (**VAK**-sin-ate) To administer a vaccine.

vaccination (vak-sih-**NAY**-shun) Administration of a vaccine.

vaccine (**VAK**-seen) Preparation to generate active immunity.

vagina (vah-**JIE**-nah) Female genital canal extending from the uterus to the vulva.

vaginal (**VAJ**-ih-nal) Pertaining to the vagina.

vaginitis (vah-jih-**NIE**-tis) Inflammation of the vagina.

vaginosis (vah-jih-**NOH**-sis) A disease of the vagina.

vagus (**VAY**-gus) Tenth (X) cranial nerve; supplies many different organs throughout the body.

varicocele (**VAIR**-ih-koh-seal) Varicose veins of the spermatic cord.

varicose (**VAIR**-ih-kos) Characterized by or affected with varices.

varicosities (vair-ih-**KOS**-ih-teez) Collection of varicose veins.

varix (**VAIR**-iks) Dilated, tortuous vein. Plural *varices.*

vasectomy (vah-**SEK**-toe-me) Excision of a segment of the ductus deferens.

vasoconstriction (**VAY**-soh-con-**STRIK**-shun) Reduction in the diameter of a blood vessel.

vasodilation (**VAY**-soh-die-**LAY**-shun) Increase in the diameter of a blood vessel.

vasovasostomy (**VAY**-soh-vay-**SOS**-toe-me) Reanastomosis of the ductus deferens to restore the flow of sperm. Also called *vasectomy reversal.*

vegetative (**VEJ**-eh-tay-tiv) Functioning unconsciously, as plant life is assumed to do.

vein (VANE) Blood vessel carrying blood toward the heart.

vena cava (**VEE**-nah **KAY**-vah) One of the two largest veins in the body. Plural *venae cavae.*

venogram (**VEE**-noh-gram) Radiograph of veins after injection of radiopaque contrast material.

venous (**VEE**-nuss) Pertaining to a vein.

ventilation (ven-tih-**LAY**-shun) Movement of gases into and out of the lungs.

ventilator (**VEN**-tih-lay-tor) Device that breathes for the patient.

ventral (**VEN**-tral) Pertaining to the belly or situated nearer to the surface of the belly.

ventricle (**VEN**-trih-kel) Chamber of the heart (pumps blood) or brain (produces cerebrospinal fluid).

venule (**VEN**-yule or **VEEN**-yule) Small vein leading from the capillary network.

vernix caseosa (**VER**-nicks kay-see-**OH**-sah) Cheesy substance covering the skin of the fetus.

verruca (ver-**ROO**-cah) Wart caused by a virus.

vertebra (**VER**-teh-brah) One of the bones of the spinal column. Plural *vertebrae*.

vertebral (**VER**-teh-bral) Pertaining to a vertebra.

vertex (**VER**-teks) Topmost point of the vault of the skull.

vertigo (**VER**-tih-go) Sensation of spinning or whirling.

vesicle (**VES**-ih-kull) Small sac containing liquid; for example, a blister.

vestibular (ves-**TIB**-you-lar) Pertaining to the vestibule.

vestibule (**VES**-tih-byul) Space at the entrance to a canal.

vestibulectomy (ves-tib-you-**LEK**-toe-me) Surgical excision of the vulva.

villus (**VILL**-us) Thin, hairlike projection, particularly of a mucous membrane lining a cavity. Plural *villi.*

virus (**VIE**-rus) Group of infectious agents that require living cells for growth and reproduction.

viscera (**VISS**-er-ah) Internal organs, particularly in the abdomen.

visceral (**VISS**-er-al) Pertaining to the internal organs.

viscosity (viss-**KOS**-ih-tee) The resistance of a fluid to flow.

viscous (**VISS**-kus) Sticky fluid that is resistant to flow.

viscus (**VISS**-kus) Any single internal organ.

visual acuity (**VIH**-zhoo-al ah-**KYU**-ih-tee) Sharpness and clearness of vision.

vitamin (**VYE**-tah-min) Essential organic substance necessary in small amounts for normal cell function.

vitreous (**VIT**-ree-us) Vitreous humor is a gelatinous liquid in the posterior cavity of the eyeball with the appearance of glass.

vocal (**VOH**-kal) Pertaining to the voice.

void (**VOYD**) To evacuate urine or feces.

voluntary muscle (**VOL**-un-tare-ee **MUSS**-el) Muscle that is under the control of the will.

vomer (**VOH**-mer) Lower nasal septum.

vulva (**VUL**-vah) Female external genitalia.

vulvar (**VUL**-var) Pertaining to the vulva.

vulvodynia (vul-voh-**DIN**-ee-uh) Chronic vulvar pain.

vulvovaginal (**VUL**-voh-**VAJ**-ih-nal) Pertaining to the vulva and vagina.

vulvovaginitis (**VUL**-voh-vaj-ih-**NIE**-tis) Inflammation of the vulva and vagina.

W

warfarin (**WAR**-fuh-rin) Anticoagulant; also used as rat poison; trade name *Coumadin.*

Weber test (**VA**-ber) Test for sensorineural hearing loss.

wheal (**WHEEL**) Small, itchy swelling of the skin. Wheals raised by an injection do not itch. Also called *hives.*

whiplash (**WHIP**-lash) Symptoms caused by sudden, uncontrolled extension and flexion of the neck, often in an automobile accident.

white matter (**WITE MATT**-er) Regions of the brain and spinal cord occupied by bundles of axons.

whooping cough (**WHO**-ping KAWF) Infectious disease with spasmodic, intense cough ending on a whoop (stridor). Also called *pertussis.*

Wilms tumor (**WILMZ TOO**-mor) Cancerous kidney tumor of childhood. Also known as *nephroblastoma.*

wound (**WOOND**) Any injury that interrupts the continuity of skin or a mucous membrane.

X

xenograft (**ZEN**-oh-graft) A graft from another species. Also called *heterograft.*

Y

yeast (**YEEST**) Microscopic fungus.

Z

zygoma (zye-**GO**-mah) Bone that forms the prominence of the cheek.

zygomatic (zye-go-**MAT**-ik) Pertaining to the zygoma.

zygote (**ZYE**-goat) Cell resulting from the union of the sperm and egg.

Photo Credits

Front Matter

Page i: © Rick Brady/The McGraw-Hill Companies, Inc.; p. iv (top right): © Rick Brady/The McGraw-Hill Companies, Inc.; (center left): © Classic Collection/Shotshop GmbH/Alamy RF; p. v (top right): © Rick Brady/The McGraw-Hill Companies, Inc.; (bottom left): © Rick Brady/The McGraw-Hill Companies, Inc.; p. vi (top right): © Rick Brady/The McGraw-Hill Companies, Inc.; (bottom left): © Rick Brady/The McGraw-Hill Companies, Inc.; p. vii (top right): © ninsiri/Getty Images RF; (bottom left): © Rick Brady/The McGraw-Hill Companies, Inc.; p. viii (top right): © Rick Brady/The McGraw-Hill Companies, Inc.; (bottom left): © Rick Brady/The McGraw-Hill Companies, Inc.; p. ix (top right): © Rick Brady/The McGraw-Hill Companies, Inc.; (center left): © Rick Brady/The McGraw-Hill Companies, Inc.; (bottom right): © Rick Brady/The McGraw-Hill Companies, Inc.; p. x (top right): © Rick Brady/The McGraw-Hill Companies, Inc.; (center left): © Rick Brady/The McGraw-Hill Companies, Inc.; p. xiii: © Squared Studios/Getty Images RF.

Welcome

Page W-1: © Rick Brady/The McGraw-Hill Companies, Inc.; p. W-2 (top left): © Rick Brady/The McGraw-Hill Companies, Inc.; (bottom left): © Rick Brady/The McGraw-Hill Companies, Inc.; p. W-3 (top right): © Tony Freeman/PhotoEdit; (bottom right): © Rick Brady/The McGraw-Hill Companies, Inc.; p. W-6 (top left): © Rick Brady/The McGraw-Hill Companies, Inc.; (bottom left): © Rick Brady/The McGraw-Hill Companies, Inc.; p. W-7: © Vol. 66 PhotoDisc/Getty images RF; p. W-8: © Rob Melnychuk/Photodisc/Getty Images RF.

Chapter 1

Page 1: © Rick Brady/The McGraw-Hill Companies, Inc.

Chapter 2

Page 15: © Classic Collection/Shotshop GmbH/Alamy RF; p. 16: © Francis Leroy/Biocosmos/Science Source; p. 26 (top right): © Joe DeGrandis/The McGraw-Hill Companies, Inc.; (bottom left): © Eric Wise/The McGraw-Hill Companies, Inc.; (bottom right): © Joe DeGrandis/The McGraw-Hill Companies, Inc.; p. 28 (center left): The McGraw-Hill Companies, Inc.; (center right): The McGraw-Hill Companies, Inc.

Chapter 3

Page 31: © Rick Brady/The McGraw-Hill Companies, Inc.; p. 36: © Dr. P. Marazzi/SPL/Science Source; p. 38 (top left): © Biophoto Associates/Science Source; (center left): © James Stevenson/Science Source; (bottom left): © Mediscan/Alamy; (center right): © CMSP/Getty Images; (bottom right): © Logical Images; p. 40 (bottom right): © SPL/Science Source; (top left): © SPL/Science Source; (center left): © Dr. P. Marazzi/Science Source; (bottom left): © STEVE GSCHMEISSNER/Science Photo Library/Getty Images RF; (center right): © Eye of Science/Science source; p. 42 (top left): © Dr. P. Marazzi/Science Source; (center left): © Courtesy Dr. Maureen Mayes; (center right): © DaveBolton/E+/Getty Images RF; (bottom right): © Medical-on-line/Alamy; p. 44: © Dr. Harout Tanielian/Science Source; p. 46 (center right): © Dr. Harout Tanielian/Science Source; (bottom right): © Logical Images; p. 50 (bottom left): © Sheila Terry/

Science Source; (bottom center): © Dr. P. Marazzi/Science Source; (bottom right): © John Radcliffe Hospital/Science Source; p. 54: © BSIP/Getty Images.

Chapter 4

Page 57: © Rick Brady/The McGraw-Hill Companies, Inc.; p. 60: © Christine Ecke/The McGraw-Hill Companies, Inc.; p. 62 (bottom left): © Michael Klein/Photolibrary/Getty Images; (bottom right): © Joe DeGrandis/The McGraw-Hill Companies, Inc.; p. 74 (bottom left): © Zephyr/Science Source; (bottom center): © Dr. P. Marazzi/Science Source; (bottom right): © Aaron Roeth Photography RF; p. 78: © Andre Thijssen/Getty Images RF; p. 80: © AJPhoto/Science Source; p. 84: © Science Photo Library - DR. P. MARAZZI/Getty Images RF.

Chapter 5

Page 91: © Rick Brady/The McGraw-Hill Companies, Inc.; p. 94: © Rick Brady/The McGraw-Hill Companies, Inc.; p. 100: © Eric Wise/The McGraw-Hill Companies, Inc.; p. 106 (center left): © North Coast Medical; (bottom right): © Roger Ressmeyer/Eureka/Corbis.

Chapter 6

Page 109: © Rick Brady/The McGraw-Hill Companies, Inc.; p. 118: © Rick Brady/The McGraw-Hill Companies, Inc.; p. 122 (center left): © Ed Reschke; © Ed Reschke; (bottom right): © Alfred Pasieka/Science Source; p. 126: © Shelly Katz/The LIFE Images Collection/Getty Images; p. 134 (center left): © Dr. P. Marazzi/Science Source; (bottom left): © Nucleus Medical Art, Inc./Getty Images.

Chapter 7

Page 137: © ninsiri/Getty Images RF; p. 138: © Eric Wise/The McGraw-Hill Companies, Inc.; p. 140 (center left): © Bill Longcore/Science Source; (bottom center): © Meckes/Ottawa/Science source; p. 142 (top left): © Ed Reschke; © Ed Reschke; (bottom left): © Ed Reschke; (bottom center): © Ed Reschke; (bottom right): © Ed Reschke; p. 146 (center left): © Mediscan/Alamy; (center left): © Dr. P. Marazzi/Science Source; p. 156 (top left): © Dennis Strete/The McGraw-Hill Companies, Inc.; p. 158 (center left): © James Cavallini/Science Source; p. 162 (center right): © Eye of Science/Science Source; (center left): © ERproductions Ltd/Blend Images LLC RF; p. 164 (bottom right): © SPL/Science Source.

Chapter 8

Page 169: © Rick Brady/The McGraw-Hill Companies, Inc.; p. 176: © Gastrolab/Science Source; p. 178: © Electronic Publishing Services, Inc., NY/The McGraw-Hill Companies, Inc.; p. 182 (center right): © SCIEPRO/Getty Images RF; (bottom right): © SCIEPRO/Getty Images RF; p. 184 (bottom left): © Du Cane Medical Imaging Ltd./Science Source; (bottom right): © Wellcome Photo Library/Wellcome Images.

Chapter 9

Page 191: © Rick Brady/The McGraw-Hill Companies, Inc.; p. 198 (top right): © watanyou/Getty Images RF; (center right): © Scimat/

Science Source; (center right): © Mediscan/Alamy; (bottom right): © John Radcliffe Hospital/Science Source; p. 204: © CNRI/Science Source; p. 206 (center left): © Biophoto Associates/Science Source; (center right): © Educational Images LTD/Custom Medical Stock Photo/Newscom; p. 210: © Southern Illinois University/Science Source; p. 216: © CNRI/Science Source; p. 218 (bottom left): © Susan Leavines/Science Source; (bottom right): © Dr. P. Marazzi/SPL/Science Source; p. 220: © Phototake Inc./Alamy.

Chapter 10

Page 223: © Rick Brady/The McGraw-Hill Companies, Inc.; p. 232 (bottom left): © Phototake Inc./Alamy; (bottom center): © Phototake Inc./Alamy; p. 236: © Wellcome Photo Library/Wellcome Images; p. 238: © Dr. P. Marazzi/Science Source; p. 240: © James Cavallini/Science Source; p. 242 (center left): © Wellcome Images; (bottom left): © Simon Fraser/Newcastle Hospitals NHS/Science Photo Library/Science Source; p. 244 (center left): © ROBERTO SCHMIDT/Getty Images; (bottom right): © BSIP/Universal Images Group/Getty Images; p. 246: © Marcus E. Raichle; (top center): © Peyroux/AGE Fotostock RF; (top right): © CAVALLINI JAMES/BSIP SA/Alamy; p. 248 (bottom left): © George Rose/Getty Images News/Getty Images; p. 250 (top left): © Bojan Kontrec/Getty Images RF; (center left): © Benjamin Lowy/Getty Images News/Getty Images; (bottom right): © Will & Deni McIntyre/Science Source; p. 252 (top left): © Dr. P. Marazzi/Science Source; (center left): © Victor de Schwanberg/Science Source.

Chapter 11

Page 257: © Rick Brady/The McGraw-Hill Companies, Inc.; p. 258: © Joe DeGrandis/The McGraw-Hill Companies, Inc.; p. 260 (top left): © Phototake, Inc./Alamy; (center left): © Western Ophthalmic Hospital/Science Source; (bottom center): © KOKEL/BSIP SA/Alamy; (bottom right): © Dr. P. Marazzi/Science Source; p. 262 (center left): © Biophoto Associates/Science Source; (bottom left): © Matt Harris Photography/Alamy; p. 270 (bottom left): © Phototake Inc./Alamy; (bottom left): © National Eye Institute, National Institutes of Health; (bottom right): © Dr. P. Marazzi/Science Source; (bottom right): © National Eye Institute, National Institutes of Health; p. 272 (top left): © Steve Mason/Getty Images; (center left): © Paul Parker/Science Source; (bottom left): © KOKEL/BSIP SA/Alamy; (bottom right): © National Eye Institute, National Institutes of Health; p. 274: © Rick Brady/The McGraw-Hill Companies, Inc.; p. 279: © Rick Brady/The McGraw-Hill Companies, Inc.; p. 282: © Wellcome Images; p. 284: © Dr. G. Lacher/Science Source; p. 286 (center left): © Lester V. Bergman/Corbis; (bottom left): © SPL/Science Source; (bottom right): © Bo Veisland/Science Source.

Chapter 12

Page 293: © Rick Brady/The McGraw-Hill Companies, Inc.; p. 300 (top left): © Dr. M.A. Ansary/Science Source; (bottom left): © Dr. P. Marazzi/SPL/Science Source; (bottom right): © Mediscan/Alamy; p. 302: © Bachrach/Bettmann/Corbis; p. 308: © Oscar Gimeno Baldo/Alamy RF.

Chapter 13

Page 311: © Rick Brady/The McGraw-Hill Companies, Inc.; p. 314: © CNRI/Science Source; p. 316: © Mediscan/Alamy; p. 318: © Saturn Stills/Science Source; p. 324: © Saturn Stills/Science Source.

Chapter 14

Page 329: © Rick Brady/The McGraw-Hill Companies, Inc.; p. 334: © Brian Evans/Science Source; p. 338: © SPL/Science Source; p. 342 (bottom left): © Biophoto Associates/Science Source; (bottom center): © Centers for Disease Control and Prevention.

Chapter 15

Page 345: © Rick Brady/The McGraw-Hill Companies, Inc.; p. 348: © Dr. P. Marazzi/Science source; p. 354: © Alila Medical Images/Alamy RF; p. 356 (center left): © Wellcome Images; (bottom left): © Biophoto Associates/Science Source; p. 358: © Parviz M. Pour/Science Source; p. 360: © Jill Braaten/The McGraw-Hill Companies Inc.; p. 366: © Brand X Pictures/PunchStock; p. 368: © Science Source; p. 370: © Picture Partners/Science Source; p. 374 (center left): © Wellcome Images; (bottom left): © ALIX/Phanie/Science Source.

A

a/ae, 10
Ab, 146, 148, 152
Abbreviations box, 9
Abdomen, 29
Abdominal, 29
Abdominal cavity, 28
Abdominal quadrants, 28–29
Abdominal regions, 28
Abdominopelvic, 29
Abdominopelvic cavity, 28
Abdominoplasty, 54, 55
Abduction, 102, 103
ABG, 170, 186
Ablation, 127, 358, 359
ABO blood group, 148
Abortion, 370, 371
Abrasion, 48, 49, 54, 55
Absence seizures, 234
Absorption, 152, 153, 194, 204, 205, 216
   impairment of, 206
   process of, 212–215
Abstinence, 360
Abused substances, 252
AC, 70, 71
Accessory glands
   of eye, 260–261
   of male reproductive system, 330, 336, 337
Accessory organs, 192
   of digestive system, 192, 193
   of skin, 44–47
Accessory structures of eye, 258–263
Accommodate/accommodation/
      accommodative, 263
Accomodative esotropia, 262
ACE, 128
Acetabulum, 76, 77
Acetaminophen, 281
Acetone, 308, 309
Achilles tendon, 102, 103
Achondroplasia, 62, 63
ACL, 20, 22, 82, 84
Acne, 44, 45
Acoustic, 238, 239
Acquired immunodeficiency syndrome
      (AIDS), 164, 165, 342, 343
Acromegaly, 296, 297
Acromioclavicular (AC) joint, 70, 71
Acromion, 70, 71, 98
Acrophobia, 250, 251
ACTH, 296, 302
Active movement, 91, 93
Activities of daily living (ADL), 92, 106, 238
Acute, 281
Acute bronchitis, 182
Acute epiglottitis, 176
Acute glomerulonephritis, 314

Acute labyrinthitis, 290
Acute myocardial infarction (AMI), 8
Acute otitis media (AOM), 286
Acute renal failure (ARF), 316
Acute retention, 322
Acute rhinitis. *See* Rhinitis
Acute transverse myelitis, 242
Acyclovir, 276
AD, 288
Adaptive equipment, 104
Addiction, 252, 253
Addison disease, 302, 303
Adduction, 103
Adductor muscles, 102, 103
Adenocarcinoma, 184, 185, 206
Adenoidectomy, 157
Adenoids, 156, 157, 174, 175, 284, 285
ADH, 294, 296
Adipose tissue, 34, 35
ADL, 92, 106, 238
Adrenal, 302, 303
Adrenal glands, 294
Adrenaline, 302, 303
Adrenocortical, 302, 303
Adrenocortical hyperfunction, 302
Adrenocortical hypofunction, 302
Adrenocorticotropic, 297
Adrenocorticotropic hormone (ACTH), 296
Adult respiratory distress syndrome (ARDS),
      184, 188
AEDs, 118, 254
Affect, 249
Afferent, 155, 224, 225
Afferent lymphatic vessel, 154
Afferent nerves, 224
A-fib, 118
Agglutinate, 140, 141
Agglutination, 146, 147
Aging, in skin, 52
Agoraphobia, 250, 251
Agranulocyte, 142, 143
AIDS, 164, 165, 342, 343
Air cleanser, 172
Air moisturizer, 172
Air warmer, 172
Aldosterone, 302, 303
Alignment, of bones, 64, 65
Alimentary, 193
Alimentary canal, 192, 193
Allergen, 37, 152, 153
Allergenic, 37
Allergic, 37, 153
Allergic conjunctivitis, 270
Allergic dermatitis, 36
Allergic rhinitis, 172
Allergies, 37, 153, 164
Allergist, 139
Allograft, 52, 53

Alloimmune disorders, 164, 165
Alopecia, 46, 47
Alpha cells, 304
Alpha-glucosidase inhibitors, 308
ALS, 242
Altered mental state (AMS), 232, 234
Alveolar, 171
Alveolus/alveoli
   lung, 170, 171, 178
   mammary, 372
Alzheimer disease, 232, 233
Amblyopia, 262, 263
Ambulatory, 99
Ambulatory blood pressure monitor, 126
Amenorrhea, 354, 355
AMI, 8
Amino acids, 214, 215
Ammonia, 312, 313
Amniocentesis, 364, 365
Amnion, 366, 367
Amniotic, 367
Amniotic fluid abnormalities, 366, 367
Ampulla, 290, 291
Amputation, 88, 89, 106, 107, 306, 307
AMS, 232
Amylase, 194, 195
Amyotrophic, 243
Amyotrophic lateral sclerosis (ALS), 242
Anabolic steroids, 94
Anabolism, 18, 19
Anal, 193, 217
Anal canal, 216–218
Anal fissures, 218
Anal fistulas, 218
Analgesia, 35, 230, 231, 239
Analgesics, 34, 35, 238, 239
Anaphylactic, 165
Anaphylactic shock, 122, 164
Anaphylaxis, 164, 165
Anastomosis/anastomoses, 220, 221
Anatomical directional terms, 26–27
Anatomical planes, 26–27
Anatomical position, fundamental, 26
Anatomy, 27
Androgen, 44, 45, 332, 333
Anemia, 139, 140, 141
Anemic, 139
Anencephaly, 244, 245
Anesthesia, 230, 231
Aneurysm, 134, 135, 236, 237
Angina pectoris, 122
Angiogram, 126, 127, 273
Angiography, 127, 220, 247, 272, 273
Angioplasty, 127
Angiotensin-converting enzyme (ACE), 128
Ankle
   joint, 86, 87
   muscles, 102

W

X

Y

Z